Maternal and Child H

John Ehiri

Editor

Maternal and Child Health

Global Challenges, Programs, and Policies

Foreword by Paul Garner

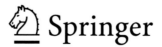 Springer

Editor
John Ehiri, PhD, MPH, MSc (Econ.)
Director, Professor
Division of Health Promotion Sciences
Mel and Enid Zuckerman College
  of Public Health
University of Arizona
1295 N. Martin Avenue
Tucson, AZ 85724
USA
jehiri@email.arizona.edu

ISBN 978-1-4614-9901-5   ISBN 978-0-387-89245-0 (eBook)
DOI 10.1007/b106524
Springer New York Dordrecht Heidelberg London

Printed on acid-free paper

Springer is part of Springer Science+Business Media (www.springer.com)

Foreword

There has been a crying need for a compendium of teaching and learning resources dedicated to critical global health issues confronting the most vulnerable members of our communities, women, infants, children, and adolescents. This book bridges this gap in literature by taking a global perspective, but weighting more of the content on the most pressing problems and possible solutions in middle- and low-income countries. From the outset, the book lays out the scene, first by respecting history and exploring the foundations of much of what we see today in the global health arena and then moving on to provide carefully researched appraisals of some of the most critical issues that the underpin achievement of maternal and child health-related Millennium Development Goals (MDGs) in middle- and low-income countries, including politics and power, specific disease conditions, programs, policies, and emerging concerns. Thus, it is right on target as a valuable educational resource for global health scholars, agencies, and frontline operatives who are striving to reduce global health inequities. A central theme of the book, among others, is that a systematic return to basic, evidence-based, cost-effective, and time-proven technologies will be an integral part of a sustainable response to global maternal and child health challenges. Revitalizing health systems in less-developed countries based on the tenets of the Alma Ata Declaration of Primary Healthcare, presented by the World Health Organization and United Nations Children's Fund over 30 years ago as the key to global health improvement, remains essential for attaining the maternal and child health-related MDGs.

Those who work in health care in developing countries are familiar with poorly equipped and scantly staffed health facilities that see hundreds of patients each day. Daily, they see the huge and often fluctuating burden of disease, the tragedy of infant deaths from infectious diseases, and the gross injustice of young women dying in childbirth. The result is that each year globally, more than 500,000 women, 99% in less-developed countries, die from pregnancy and childbirth-related complications. An additional 15–20 million suffer various debilitating consequences of pregnancy. Also globally, about 10 million children under the age of 5 die annually, mostly from lower respiratory infections, diarrheal diseases, malaria, measles, and undernutrition. The irony of this deplorable state of global maternal and child health is that simple, cost-effective interventions that can significantly improve survival and quality of life of women, infants, and children exist. Such interventions include access to clean water and basic sanitation, immunization, improved nutrition, and access to basic health-care services. Thus, for the most part, the underlying causes of morbidity and mortality among the maternal and child health population are inequity, poverty, shortage of health professionals, and dysfunctional health systems that are ill-equipped to effectively implement and maintain basic health-care services.

The concept of a global community is perhaps idealistic, but it helps international health and development agencies, health professionals, and policy planners to consider commonalities, rather than differences, between nations. Globalization is a term that is loosely used, but one of the important outcomes of the discourse is that it has facilitated a convergence of thoughts in that rather than dichotomizing the world into developing and developed, it fosters the understanding that we all have problems and solutions – whether in the realms of policy, public health, or clinical care – that are fundamentally common to all. Yet, variations exist between nations and even between regions in the same countries. The burden of ill health and premature death varies dramatically between countries and within social and economic strata in the same countries. Respecting these variations is essential to identifying the commonalities. It is thus noteworthy that the first part of this book is devoted to the issue of heterogeneity in the world's resources, systems of care, and health outcomes for women, infants, and children. Moving on to the second part, readers' attention is drawn to the fact that health is always within a context and that maternal and child health is critically influenced by power and politics within society. To provide specific examples, the book addresses the challenges posed by wars/ conflicts, globalization, gender equity, harmful traditional practices, and abortion. Adequate understanding of these contexts and their influences on maternal and child health is central to identifying and appraising priorities for action.

Equally, understanding the main disease burden among women and children and how interventions can influence health outcomes is core to global health practice. Selection of the eight diseases (malaria, HIV/AIDS, diarrheal diseases, malnutrition, tuberculosis, obstetric fistula, disabilities, and injuries) that are discussed in part three (specific disease concerns) is rational, given their contribution to the global burden of disease among women, infants, and children. The inclusion of tuberculosis and disabilities as they affect women and children globally is notable, given the limited focus on women and children in the current literature on these conditions.

How policies and programs are formulated and organized and who delivers them is central to the identification of appropriate and sustainable solutions. This is the focus of the fourth and final section of the book. Key challenges and emerging concerns in global maternal and child health programming are carefully chosen and substantively discussed in this part. Notable among the issues covered are such factors that have received minimal attention in existing global health textbooks, including the role of evidence-based policy and practice, challenges in making pregnancy safer, adolescent health, child maltreatment, children in difficult circumstances, and workforce training, deployment, and maintenance in the face of massive brain drain and health worker migration from developing countries to the developed world.

What is most exciting about this book is that it represents a global community of the best people in the field, individuals who understand the issues, have technical expertise, and can provide the reader with a clear, authoritative steer.

With all credit to the editor who has the global vision to bring this impressive array of authors together under a common theme, this book is a real contribution to help those who want to learn and perhaps become a part of the global community effort to tackle some of the biggest and most important problems in global health that face us today.

Paul Garner
Liverpool School of Tropical Medicine, England

Acknowledgments

This book was inspired by Greg R. Alexander, RS, MPH, ScD, Maternal and Child Health Epidemiologist, and former professor and chair, Department of Maternal and Child Health, University of Alabama at Birmingham School of Public Health. Greg, one of the most prominent perinatal epidemiologists nationally and globally, led groundbreaking studies on gestational age measurement, prenatal care, and racial and ethnic disparities in birth outcomes for nearly three decades until he passed away in February 2007. He would have been proud to see a profoundly researched, and well-documented textbook that is truly global in its authorship and content and, most importantly, that is devoted to issues of concern to the health of women, children, and adolescents.

This book is a collaborative enterprise. I would like to thank the contributors and colleagues who have made the completion of this work possible. My special thanks go to Sarah Windle, MPH, John Ilonze, MD, MPH, Katie Brigham, MPH, Rebecca Pass, MPA, and Catherine Lem, MPH, for their editorial assistance and for keeping tabs on references in the ever-changing drafts.

Finally, I am deeply indebted to my wife, Bridget, and to our children, Jenifer, Laurence, Amanda, and Paula, for their love, patience, understanding, and unflinching support.

Contents

Contributors

Rebecca Affolder The GAVI Alliance, Geneva, Switzerland

Ebere Anyanwu Medical Center for Immune and Toxic Disorders, Montgomery Colleges in Houston Texas, USA

Andrea Gottsegen Asnes Yale University School of Medicine, New Haven, Connecticut, USA

Robert E. Black Bloomberg School of Public Health, Johns Hopkins University, Baltimore, Maryland

Cynthia Boschi-Pinto World Health Organization, Geneva, Switzerland

Lisa Byers School of Social Work, University of Oklahoma, Tulsa, OK, USA

Andrew Cherry School of Social Work, University of Oklahoma, Tulsa, OK, USA

Ian G. Child University of Alabama at Birmingham, USA

Hoosen M. Coovadia Nelson R. Mandela School of Medicine, University of Natal, South Africa

Elke de Buhr Tulane University, New Orleans, USA

Emmanuel d'Harcourt International Rescue Committee, New York, USA

Mary Dillon School of Social Work, University of Oklahoma, OK, USA

John E. Ehiri Mel and Enid Zuckerman College of Public Health, University of Arizona, Tucson, Arizona, USA

Emmanuel Ezedinachi University of Calabar Teaching Hospital, Calabar, Nigeria

Nancy Gerein Nuffield Centre for International Health and Development, University of Leeds, England

Robert Gilman Bloomberg School of Public Health, Johns Hopkins University, Baltimore, Maryland, USA

Andrew Green Nuffield Centre for International Health and Development, University of Leeds, England, UK

Anne Hyre Jhpiego, Johns Hopkins University, Baltimore, Maryland, USA

Monir Islam World Health Organization, Geneva, Switzerland

Albrecht Jahn European Commission, Brussels, Belgium

Chuks Kamanu Abia State University Teaching Hospital Aba, Nigeria

Andrzej Kulczycki University of Alabama at Birmingham, USA

Claudio F. Lanata Nutritional Research Institute, Lima, Peru

John M. Leventhal Yale University School of Medicine, Yale University, New Haven, CT, USA

Julian Lob-Levyt GAVI Alliance, Geneva, Switzerland

Elizabeth Lule World Bank, Washington, DC, USA

Colin Mathers World Health Organization, Geneva, Switzerland

Martin Meremikwu University of Calabar Teaching Hospital (UCTH), Calabar, Cross River State, Nigeria

Caroline J. Min Mailman School of Public Health, Columbia University, New York

Tolib Mirzoev Nuffield Centre for International Health and Development, University of Leeds, England

Nancy Mock Tulane University, New Orleans, LA, USA

David Moore Imperial College London, England

Olaf Müller Ruprecht-Karls-University of Heidelberg, Germany

Marianne Nichol Queens University, Kingston, Canada

Mary Ann Pass University of Alabama at Birmingham, USA

Rebecca Pass United Nations World Food Programme, Dakar, Senegal

Stephen Pearson Nuffield Centre for International Health and Development, University of Leeds, England

William Pickett Queens University, Kingston, Canada

Susan Purdin International Rescue Committee, New York, USA

Joanna Raven Liverpool School of Tropical Medicine, England

Krishna Reddy Internal Medicine, Massachusetts General Hospital, Boston, MA, USA

Nigel C. Rollins University of KwaZulu-Natal, South Africa

James Rosen Independent Consultant and Economist, Washington DC, USA

Allan Rosenfield Mailman School of Public Health, Columbia University, New York, USA

Jeffrey M. Smith Jhpiego/Johns Hopkins University, Baltimore, Maryland, USA

Sally Theobald Liverpool School of Tropical Medicine, Liverpool, England

Alan Tita Obstetrics and Gynecology, University of Alabama, Birmingham, USA

Rachel Tolhurst Liverpool School of Tropical Medicine, Liverpool, England

L. Lewis Wall Washington University Medical School, St. Louis, Missouri, USA

Sarah Wamala Swedish National Institute of Public Health, Forskarens väg 3. SE-831 40 Östersund, Sweden

Amy T. Wilson Gallaudet University, Washington, DC, USA

Sarah Windle University of Alabama at Birmingham, USA

Victor Y.H. Yu Monash University, Australia

Michel Zaffran GAVI Alliance, Geneva, Switzerland

Introduction

Context

With increasing globalization, inequity, and escalating poverty, application of public health principles to the solution of maternal and child health problems that transcend national boundaries has become an issue of heightened interest among scholars and practitioners of public health. The fact that this interest is shared equally among scholars and practitioners in affluent and poor countries is noteworthy and well founded. For example, in affluent nations, there are regions, states, or counties with health outcomes (e.g., infant mortality rates and child undernutrition) that are comparable to those of for low-income countries. In addition, globalization, climate change, and the re-emergence of diseases previously thought to have been conquered in affluent nations mean that our understanding of the strategies for managing health conditions in resource-poor settings may have ready application in counties and neighborhoods in rich countries where poverty and inequity also abound. Thus, there is acceptance that acquisition of knowledge, skills, and competencies in addressing issues of global concern to maternal and child health populations is important for health professionals – whether they are working or intend to work domestically in rich nations or at foreign sites in resource-poor countries.

The phrase "global health" has gradually come to replace "*international health.*" Global health signifies the commonality of health challenges in both developed and less-developed countries, while international health often refers to health issues in other countries, especially in less-developed countries. In its 1997 report, *America's Vital Interest in Global Health*, the Institute of Medicine defined global health as health problems, issues, and concerns that transcend national boundaries and may be best addressed by cooperative actions (IOM 1997). Similarly, as the Global Burden of Disease Report (Murray and Lopez 1996) noted, health impacts across boundaries of geography, finance, and culture include impacts on the global ecosystem and other health determinants, such as poverty and genetics, a context that includes the whole world and produces its own institutional complexities. Global health has become a rallying point for organizations, professionals, and individuals with a passion for social justice and for alleviating pain and suffering among human populations, especially the poor and the most vulnerable members of our communities.

Maternal and Child Health has been the epicenter of international cooperation in health since the early eighteenth century. As Petersen and Alexander (2004) assert, much about public health in general is arguably about maternal and child health, and truly, much about global health is about maternal and child health. Maternal and child health represents the point at which all the disciplines of public health converge and operate synergistically in order to achieve public health goals (Alexander 2004). It has been defined as the professional and academic field that focuses on the determinants, mechanisms, and systems that operate and maintain the health, safety, well-being, and appropriate development of children and their families in countries and societies in order to enhance the future health and welfare of society and subsequent generations (Alexander et al. 2004). In as much as global health policies and programs are rooted in a social justice philosophy and the protection of vulnerable populations, maternal and child health embodies the concept of global advocacy for the largest vulnerable populations in both developed and less-developed countries, notably women, children, and adolescents.

At the biological level, mothers everywhere conceive, progress through pregnancy, and typically deliver a single infant in fundamentally the same way. Yet unacceptable disparities exist in birth outcomes between women in rich and poor countries and even between women from rich and poor households in the same country or region. Each year globally, there are at least 3.2 million stillborn babies, more than 4 million neonatal deaths, and more than half a million maternal deaths. The vast majority of these deaths are preventable, and the countries with the highest burdens of maternal and child morbidity and mortality are those who currently appear to be making the least progress in reducing these rates.

Concern for the health of every child is paramount for the mother and her nation because the country's future ultimately depends upon the achievements of her child. A healthy child needs a healthy mother, and an environment free from harmful traditional practices and violence, which provides adequate shelter, nutrition, clean water, basic school education, preventive, and therapeutic health services. For maintenance of maternal health, the mother also needs a satisfying job with adequate pay and a community that acknowledges her rights and provides equal opportunities for all.

The reality, however, is that our globe is a fundamentally complex and heterogeneous place with extreme disparities in physical geography, exploitable resources, honest and skillful governance, education, and promises of income opportunities that do more than just sustain life. These inequities lead to a wide range of outcomes and to the tragic fact that in less-developed countries, a child under 5 years of age died every 3 seconds yesterday, will do so today, and will die tomorrow and as far as the eyes can see into the future unless pragmatic preventive actions are taken now, including among other things, the elimination of global poverty. To paraphrase Wennberg (1998), "...for medical care, geography is our destiny," and so is poverty. Causes of mortality that have largely disappeared in the developed world today, or that are readily and inexpensively immunizable or treatable, continue to kill millions of women and children for lack of resources and for simple operational reasons. In many less-developed countries, if the cure for any major contributor to the burden of disease were an aspirin and a glass of water given to everyone four times a year by a roving caregiver with minimal medical training, we could not consistently deliver it.

A significant proportion of the United Nation's Millennium Development Goals and Targets have major bearing on the health of women and children. Although we are halfway to the 2015 target, we already know that in some parts of Asia and almost all of sub-Saharan Africa, we will likely fail to meet our goals, given a context in which nearly half of the population is malnourished; millions have limited access to portable water, and live on less than US $1 a day (World Bank 2004).

In the richest countries, life expectancy is almost double that of the poorest: infant mortality rates and mortality for children under 5 years of age are over a hundred times less than the rates in the poorest countries. Maternal mortality is very rare in the richest nations. Yet, several puzzling situations also persist in these affluent nations, notably the following: (i) there is a twofold difference in infant mortality rates between Far Eastern and Scandinavian countries and the United States; (ii) there is a twofold difference between infant mortality and low-birth-weight rates of white and black births in the United States, but rates of white and Hispanic births are almost equal; and (iii) despite all the medical and technological innovations and the huge resources expended on clinical interventions in the richest nations, none has shown any significant reduction in low-birth-weight rates over the past 30 years. Thus, these phenomena lend credence to the widely acknowledged axiom that the causes of health and illness in human populations do not just lie in biological and genetic factors but also in (i) the environment (physical, chemical, biological); (ii) personal choices, lifestyles, and behaviors; (iii) family and community support; (iv) the psychology of inequality; (v) the social philosophy of government; and (vi) each nation's health-care system. This therefore calls for greater policy and programmatic attention to economic and social determinants of health among the maternal and child health populations. The challenge ahead is to refocus program content and to balance the drive for the development of new technologies with establishment of viable organizational strategies that build health systems and ensure effective and efficient continuum of services. Strategies for improvement should include revising the structure, content, and most importantly, implementation of current maternal and newborn health programs, developing funded national implementation plans to achieve universal coverage for maternal and newborn health-care services, and initiating action to muster the political commitment needed to achieve and sustain these systems and programs. Much of the challenge, in fact, is to accommodate both programmatic and systemic concerns which are organizational rather than technical problems.

Rationale and Target Audience for the Book

Although there are many textbooks on the general topic of global health, there has been a paucity of textbooks or other compendium of training resources that are specifically dedicated to the field of global maternal and child health, apart from scattered reports of agencies and professionals working in the field. This book has been purposefully conceptualized to address this apparent deficit in the global health literature. It is intended as a reference textbook for graduate and advanced undergraduate public health students; instructors designing courses on critical issues in global maternal and child health; frontline professionals seeking information on evidence-based maternal and child programs and policies; and policy makers sifting through priorities for research and development in this field. Unlike many textbooks that would require significant additional support materials to carry students through a full semester course, this book has been structured to sustain up to two semester courses in global health without the usual dire need for significant additional reading resources. Nevertheless, all chapters are adequately referenced, thus providing the opportunity for follow-up research, analysis, and synthesis. To help guide course instructors, each chapter has learning objectives, key terms, and discussion questions. Contributors are some of the world's most respected experts, carefully selected to represent different global geographic regions and to ensure complementarity not only of professional disciplines but most importantly, academic and field practice perspectives. Authors are individuals who have won teaching, research, and public health service awards and are internationally recognized as authorities in global health research, practice, policy, and leadership. They have diverse qualifications and skills in maternal and child health in addition to prior or current leadership positions in maternal and child health-related organizations and programs globally.

Content and Layout

The chapters are grouped into four parts that represent interrelated thematic areas viz. (i) the world's heterogeneity; (ii) politics, power, and maternal and children health; (iii) specific disease concerns; and (iv) programs, policies, and emerging concerns.

Part I: The World's Heterogeneity

This part contains six chapters that present an overview of the world's complexity and macrolevel factors that impact maternal and child health. It deals with the heterogeneity of the world's geography and its resources, health systems, living and working environments, economic strengths, and their impacts on maternal and child health outcomes.

In Chapter 1, Allan Rosenfield and Caroline Min of Columbia University present an account of the history of international cooperation in maternal and child health. They provide an overview of how maternal and child health gained recognition in industrialized countries and later became a focal point of development assistance to low-income countries. They discuss cooperation in maternal and child health within the context of shifting ideologies in global public health and present a chronology of significant events, policies, and programmatic initiatives that demonstrate how the maternal and child health agenda has evolved over the past 60 years.

The global burden of disease among women, children, and adolescents is presented in Chapter 2. Colin Mathers, Coordinator for Epidemiology and Burden of Disease in the Information, Evidence and Research Cluster at the World Health Organization office in Geneva, presents an analysis of major diseases and injuries that contribute to morbidity and mortality among children (ages 0–9 years), adolescents (ages 10–19 years), and women (ages 20 and over) for different World Bank geographic regions (Africa, East Asia and the Pacific, Europe and Central Asia, Latin America and the Caribbean, Middle East and North Africa, and South Asia). The chapter highlights how much of the global mortality among the maternal and child health population is concentrated within middle- and low-income countries, particularly in South Asia and sub-Saharan Africa. As he demonstrates, infectious diseases continue to be the major causes of mortality among children under the age of 5, with five largely preventable conditions (lower respiratory infections, diarrheal diseases, malaria, HIV/AIDS, and measles) accounting for 70% of all child deaths in sub-Saharan Africa. As the chapter shows, morbidity and mortality among the different maternal and child health subpopulation groups are influenced by different sets of factors. For children under the age of 10 years, the most important factors are undernutrition, unsafe water, and sanitation-related conditions. For adolescents aged 10–19 years, mental disorders (particularly depression, schizophrenia, and bipolar disorders), injuries (especially road traffic accidents), violence, suicide, and alcohol use disorders are the most important factors. Among women aged 20–59 years, HIV/AIDS is the leading cause of burden of disease, particularly in sub-Saharan Africa.

In recognition of the importance of the perinatal period in the field of maternal and child health, Chapter 3 is devoted to an overview of perinatal mortality, stillbirths, and neonatal mortality. Causes of perinatal mortality as well as low cost, evidence-based interventions for promoting neonatal survival across the prenatal, antenatal, intrapartum, and postpartum stages are examined. It is concluded that strategies which address inequalities both within a country and between countries are necessary for achievement of improvement in global perinatal health.

To review progress, challenges, and priorities for future investments in rich countries, Ian Child and John Ehiri focus on the different ways that maternal and child health services operate in member states of the Organization for Economic Cooperation and Development (OECD) in Chapter 4. They present a brief overview of health and income inequity among the different member nations of OECD and between OECD and the rest of the world. The chapter includes in-depth analysis of the structure and financing of health care in OECD countries, health status indicators, models for delivery of maternal and child health services, and the role of social determinants on maternal and child health outcomes. The chapter highlights the puzzling fact that despite the multiplicity of pre- and postnatal care approaches, technological improvements, increased expenditure, and intensity of care over the last 30 years, no significant improvement in the proportion of infants born with low birth weight has been observed in any high-income OECD country. The chapter concludes with a call for greater policy and programmatic attention to economic and social determinants of maternal and child health.

Nancy Gerein and her colleagues from the Nuffield Centre for International Health and Development at the University of Leeds, England, analyze the impact of health systems on maternal and child health in Chapter 5. They begin with a discussion of the main elements of a health-care system versus a health system, examining the key differences between the two. They use a conceptual model to characterize the different elements of the health system from both the biomedical and the holistic perspectives. The mechanisms by which the elements interact to influence access, quality, use of health services, and ultimately the health of mothers and children are analyzed. They discuss major challenges for health-care systems in improving the health of mothers and children and conclude with an analysis of the role of the health system in achieving Millennium Development Goals (MDGs) related to maternal and child health.

Mary Ann Pass, Professor of Maternal and Child Health at the University of Alabama at Birmingham, and her colleague Rebecca Pass conclude Part I with their review of the impact of the environment on maternal and child health in Chapter 6. They highlight disparities in environmental health risks for maternal and child health populations in different geographic and economic regions of the world. The chapter analyzes the contributions of unclean water, poor sanitation, poor hygiene practices, water-, soil-, and air-borne diseases, overcrowding and pollution to poor maternal and child health outcomes and examines how women and children in developed and less-developed nations are exposed to ambient atmospheric pollution from industry and power plants, accidental and deliberate chemical and petroleum pollution of water tables, asbestos and lead contamina-tion in older houses, tobacco smoke, radiation, and high risk of traffic accidents.

Part II: Politics, Power, and Maternal and Child Health

While it could be argued that virtually all of the themes covered in this book are influenced by politics and power at the global, national, and local levels, this part of the book is devoted to the specific impacts of globalization, wars and conflicts, gender inequity, harmful traditional practices, and abortion politics on the health of women and children.

In Chapter 7, Emmanuel D'Harcourt and Susan Purdin of International Rescue Committee present an analysis of the nature and emerging trends in modern conflicts, drawing on their vast experiences in frontline emergency rescue missions in recent and current conflict and emergency situations around the world. The impact of conflicts is delineated from the perspective of direct trauma and the indirect effects of malnutrition, displacement, rape, increased vulner-ability to infectious diseases, and adverse obstetric conditions. They also discuss the relationship between war and poverty. They present a causal model with which they analyze the pathways by which conflict affects the health and well-being of women, children, and adolescents through food insecurity, economic collapse, decline in habitat, diversion of public spending, destruction of infra-structure, and loss of qualified personnel. They conclude with an analysis of strategies for mitigating the impact of conflict on maternal and child health, including how to respond to immediate needs in acute complex emergencies, provision of routine care in nonroutine conditions, primary health care, and postconflict healing and rebuilding.

The impact of globalization on maternal and child health is presented in Chapter 8. Here, Dr. Sarah Wamala examines how globalization directly affects the health and well-being of women through changing occupational roles, evolu-tions in food production, preparation and consumption patterns, and migration. The indirect effects of privatization and such international policy mechanisms as the Structural Adjustment Programs (SAPs) on availability of services and provision of care are also analyzed. The chapter reviews potential public health practice and policy responses and examines the extent to which the Millennium Development Goals contribute toward alleviation of the adverse impact of globalization on the health of women and children.

Sally Theobald and her colleagues in the Gender and Health Research Group at the Liverpool School of Tropical Medicine, England, introduce the concept of gender equity and gender power relations in Chapter 9. They begin with definitions of such key concepts as sex, gender, gender roles and relations, women's health and gender analysis, gender equity, gender mainstreaming, gender divisions of labor, gender norms and identities, bargaining positions, and access to, and control over, resources. With specific examples, they illustrate how these concepts interact to influence and shape maternal, infant, and child health status and access to health care. They discuss the importance of understanding and mainstreaming gender into global health at the policy, health provider, and community levels, using cross-cutting approaches.

Chapter 10 examines the impact of harmful traditional practices on maternal and child health, using female genital mutilation (FGM) as an example. Beginning with a brief overview of harmful traditional practices, Sarah Windle and her colleagues at the University of Alabama at Birmingham (UAB) discuss relevant terms, definitions, and types of FGM. First, the origin and prevalence of FGM are explored. Second, the health consequences and issues related to care of victims are discussed, and finally, factors contributing to FGM are critically analyzed. They examine the policy and practice options for eliminating FGM and review examples of interventions in order to identify best practices for prevention. Recognizing that there is no simple solution to the problem, they argue that interventions for preventing FGM should be nondirective, culturally sensitive, and multifaceted to be of practical relevance. The authors assert that such interventions should not only motivate change but should also provide alternative options and help communities to establish the practical means by which change can occur. Potentially effective prevention interventions targeted at local practitioners of FGM, parents, at-risk adolescents, health and social workers, governments, religious authorities, the civil society, and communities are presented.

In Chapter 11, Andrzej Kulczycki concludes Part II with a global overview of abortion, examining its history and incidence, why women have abortions, and who has abortions. He discusses abortion laws and policies, their implementation and public health implications, safe and unsafe abortion, abortion-related mortality and morbidity, conditions under which abortions occur around the world, and the implications for maternal health. He then examines abortion techniques, safety, and trends toward earlier abortion in countries where abortion is safe and available. He concludes with a discussion of post-abortion care – its evolution, current best practices, and examples.

Part III: Specific Disease Concerns

This part contains eight chapters that focus on some of the major diseases that make the most significant contribution to the global burden of disease among MCH populations, notably malaria, diarrheal diseases, HIV/AIDS, tuberculosis, malnutrition, and injuries. It also includes chapters on obstetric fistula and disabilities, which are less emphasized in global maternal and child health but nonetheless, are major causes of pain and suffering among women, children, and adolescents.

In Chapter 12, Martin Meremikwu and his colleagues discuss the global burden of malaria, its clinical manifestations, and health consequences, including anemia, splenomegaly, and adverse pregnancy and birth outcomes. They analyze mechanisms and consequences of HIV and malaria coinfection as well as malaria treatment and control options. They also discuss the challenges posed by vector resistance to insecticides, parasite resistance to antimalarials, climate change, wars/conflicts, and HIV/AIDS which increase susceptibility to malaria and consume resources available for control and prevention efforts. Also discussed are social, cultural, and economic limitations associated with community delivery of malaria treatment through existing primary health-care systems, the prospect of scaling up control and prevention efforts through vaccine development, and the use of artemisinin-based combination treatments (ACTs). The chapter concludes with a call for wider use of insecticide-treated bednets and for donors and governments to develop effective mechanisms to monitor and ensure access to effective treatment and prevention for children, adolescents, pregnant women, and children in difficult circumstances. The need to strengthen health systems to ensure optimization of prevention and treatment efforts for these vulnerable populations is also emphasized.

While the introduction of oral rehydration solution (ORS) has helped to significantly reduce global child mortality from diarrhea, morbidity from diarrhea has not declined markedly over the past two decades. In Chapter 13, three of the world's leading experts on this subject, Cynthia Boschi-Pinto, Claudio Lanata, and Robert Black provide a comprehensive overview of the current status of the global burden of childhood diarrhea, highlighting evidence of the relationship between diarrheal diseases and child health. They begin with definitions and descriptions of clinical manifestations of childhood diarrhea and provide an exposition on the global burden of childhood diarrheal morbidity and mortality in different world regions and by age groups. They highlight the unequal distribution of diarrhea between resource-rich and resource-poor countries and examine the relative contributions of different diarrheal disease pathogens and various hypothesized risk factors. They conclude with an appraisal of the evidence base of various treatment and prevention options, including promotion of exclusive breastfeeding, hand washing, vaccines, oral rehydration therapy (ORT), zinc supplementation, and improved access to basic care.

Krishna Reddy (Harvard Medical School), David Moore (Imperial College London), and Robert Gilman (Hopkins) discuss tuberculosis (TB) in women and children in Chapter 14. They present a global overview of the prevalence and trends in tuberculosis among children and the challenges of tracking TB among children due to the difficulty of diagnosis, lack of commonly used standard case definitions, inadequate surveillance in less-developed countries, and neglect of childhood TB control programs. They review risk factors for TB among children, pathogenesis of the condition, the relationship between HIV and TB as well as problems posed by multidrug-resistant TB. They examine options for treatment and prevention of childhood TB and related challenges. Also discussed are the effects of pregnancy on TB. Here, they examine the historical perspectives of research on the topic as well as clinical features and diagnosis of TB among pregnant and nonpregnant women. They present evidence from research on perinatal and maternal outcomes of TB in pregnancy and factors that influence such outcomes. They conclude with an examination of issues around treatment of both latent and active TB in pregnancy.

In Chapter 15, Hoosen M. (Jerry) Coovadia and Nigel Rollins of the Nelson R. Mandela School of Medicine, University of KwaZulu Natal, Durban, South Africa, review the global burden of HIV/AIDS with a focus on women, children, and adolescents. They begin with a discussion of the prevalence of HIV/AIDS among women, highlighting the factors that increase women's vulnerability to the disease. They discuss strategies for prevention of HIV among women, emphasizing the need for improved antenatal care services with effective counseling on options for prevention of mother-to-child transmission and cervical barrier methods of prevention (e.g., diaphragms, microbicides, and HIV vaccine), detection and treatment of sexually transmitted infections, especially those due to herpes virus 2, and use of female condoms. Also presented is an overview of the global burden of HIV/AIDS and its impact on children and adolescents. They discuss strategies for comprehensive management of children at risk for HIV/AIDS and conclude with an examination of the impact of HIV/AIDS on the family and community, highlighting the challenge posed by the increasing scale of AIDS orphans globally. They recommend that prevention programs targeting women and children be focused on creating social, political, economic, and cultural environments that empower women, challenge stigma and discrimination among women, and aggressively combat poverty, gender, and racial inequalities.

Chapter 16 by Olaf Müller and his colleague Albrecht Jahn presents a global overview of malnutrition (undernutrition and obesity), its multiple direct and indirect causes, manifestations, management, and prevention. They examine the relationship between malnutrition and Millennium Development Goal targets related to maternal and child health. The chapter concludes with a synthesis of intervention strategies that could significantly contribute to achievement of the Millennium Development Goal target of reducing by half of 1990 figures, the proportion of people who suffer from hunger.

L. Lewis Wall presents an overview of the global burden of obstetric fistula in Chapter 17. Using the Worldwide Fistula Fund's pathways to the development of obstetric fistula, he analyzed the biomedical and sociocultural causes of obstetric fistula, including the role of obstructed labor, women's low status in society, malnutrition, illiteracy, limited access to emergency obstetric services, early marriage, and traditional harmful practices. He discusses the consequences (medical and social) of obstetric fistula as well as treatment options and challenges. He concludes with an appraisal of short- and long-term prevention strategies as they relate to the provision of appropriate and timely obstetric services, health systems development, and cultural changes that institutionalize gender equity from birth through the life course.

The much neglected problem of disabilities among women and children is presented in Chapter 18. Here, Amy Wilson of Gallaudet University, a world leader in liberal arts education and career development for deaf and hard-of-hearing students, discusses the definition and causes of disability, global prevalence of disabilities, and the relationship between poverty and disability. She examines how local concepts and beliefs frame a society's perspective of disability and how this perspective affects the status of women and children with disabilities. She reviews the barriers posed by lack of national disability policies or laws, and the nonenforcement of such policies and laws where they exist. International and national efforts and strategies to improve inclusion and access to health and social care for women and children with disabilities are discussed.

Injuries, a major contributor to the burden of disease among children and adolescents, are presented in Chapter 19 by Wilson Pickett and Marianne Nichol. They provide a profile of the occurrence of unintentional injuries in populations of children and analyze their underlying determinants as well as possible approaches to prevention. They present rates of fatal and traumatic injury across countries and discuss leading external causes and consequences of traumatic injuries by age, sex, and other known disparities. Current evidence surrounding the relative effects of different preventive approaches is reviewed and a summary of suggested implications for practice, policy, and research is presented. They conclude with a call for effective prevention strategies to consider engineered changes to the physical environment and legislation, nested within the framework of education and sustainable behavior change.

Part IV: Programs, Policies, and Emerging Concerns

The fourth and final part of the book contains 10 chapters that address a range of maternal and child health programmatic and policy issues, including implementation of evidence-based interventions, teenage pregnancy prevention, the challenge of making pregnancies safer, progress and challenges related to effective and efficient application of currently available vaccines, issues related to integrated management of childhood illnesses, and adolescent health. This part also addresses the problems of child maltreatment, children in difficult circumstances, the challenges of training and deploying the maternal and child health workforce in the face of increasing brain drain and health worker migration, and the need for global maternal and child health policy that is underpinned by the tenets of Alma Ata's Declaration of primary health care.

Maternal and child health programs in many less-developed countries provide largely curative and preventive interventions that are already known to be effective. This means that achievement of quality in maternal and child health services requires identification of these evidence-based practices and implementing them according to established standards. In Chapter 20, Alan Tita and John Ehiri provide a synthesis of the status of evidence-based global maternal and child health practice and policy, with particular reference to less-developed countries. They approach the discussion from the perspectives of two main maternal and child health practice domains (maternal and perinatal health, and infant and child health) that chronologically relate to the continuum of pregnancy, delivery and birth, and child development. They examine the meaning of evidence-based care and discuss its advantages, methods, and limitations. They trace some of the key historical milestones in the development of evidence-based maternal and child health and provide an outline of some specific maternal and child health interventions that are currently considered evidence based.

In Chapter 21, Andrew Cherry his colleagues explore issues related to the problem of teen pregnancy from a global perspective, examining regional and cross-national themes, trends, progress, and challenges. They highlight the social, economic, and cultural determinants of teen pregnancy and analyze programs and policies designed to reduce the health, economic, and social risks among pregnant teens. Teen pregnancy situation in different regions of the world is presented, using the United States (North America), United Kingdom and Russia (Europe and Central Asia), Vietnam and Japan (East Asia and the Pacific), India (South Asia), Mexico (Central and South America), Nigeria (Africa), and Egypt (Middle East and North Africa) as examples.

Progress and challenges in making pregnancies safer are discussed in Chapter 22. Here, Monir Islam of the World Health Organization discusses the global problem of maternal mortality, highlighting inequities that exist between and within regions, countries, and populations. Using McCarthy and Maine's (1992) framework for analyzing determinants of maternal mortality, he examines the role of distant factors (e.g., socioeconomic status) and how they interact with intermediate factors (e.g., access to care and health behavior) as well as indeterminate factors to influence maternal and child health outcomes. He reviews progress made globally in averting maternal mortality and the threats to this progress, including wars and conflicts, emerging and re-emerging diseases (e.g., malaria and HIV/AIDS). He concludes with a synthesis of gaps in programs and policies and recommends measures for achieving Millennium Development Goals related to reduction of maternal mortality.

Although significant progress has been made in global immunization coverage, immunizable diseases remain the leading causes of maternal and child mortality in less-developed countries. In Chapter 23, Rebecca Affolder, executive secretary of GAVI Alliance in Geneva, and her colleagues present a historical perspective on the emergence of vaccines as a means of disease control and prevention over the past two centuries. Beginning with the discovery of smallpox vaccine by Edward Jenner in 1796, they identify and discuss important milestones in widespread use of vaccines in global health. Inequity in access to vaccines between rich and poor countries and the underpinning factors are discussed, including lack of safety and quality assurance systems in poor countries, focus of research and development on rich nations' priorities, and the diversion of scarce resources to other emerging global health priorities. They discuss various innovative options for financing wider access to new and underused vaccines in poor countries and conclude with an examination of issues of sustainability in vaccine development, procurement, management, and integration into routine care in resource-poor settings.

In Chapter 24, Elizabeth Lule of the World Bank and her colleague James Rosen present a global demographic profile of adolescents and examine the rationale for attention to promotion of adolescent health by national governments and international health agencies. Major health problems confronting adolescents are analyzed as they vary by region and between developed and less-developed countries. Specific conditions contributing to the global burden of disease among adolescents (mental disorders, intentional and unintentional injuries, malnutrition, tobacco, alcohol and drug use, sexual and reproductive health concerns) are discussed, and the effectiveness of programs to address these conditions as well as policy and program gaps are appraised.

Physical and emotional maltreatment, sexual abuse, and negligent treatment of children, as well as their commercial and other exploitation, constitute a health challenge that prevalent in all parts of the world. While deaths associated with child maltreatment represent only the tip of iceberg, millions of children are victims of nonfatal abuse and neglect. Ill-health associated with child abuse contributes significantly to the global burden of disease among children and increases their predisposition to serious illnesses in adulthood. An overview of the global problem of child maltreatment is presented in Chapter 25 by Andrea Asnes and John Leventhal of Yale University School of Medicine. They begin with an examination of the challenges in building consensus on a universal operational definition of child maltreatment. Types of childhood maltreatment and the scope of the problem are analyzed from a global perspective. The health and economic consequences of the problem are reviewed as are the concomitant risk factors, including those related to children, their parents, families, and the society. They conclude with an appraisal of strategies for prevention, highlighting actions at (i) the societal and community level (e.g., promotion of social, economic, and cultural rights, reducing income and gender inequalities, and eradicating cultural acceptance of violent or exploitative behavior toward children); (ii) the relationship level (e.g., early and frequent home visiting by trained providers who are able to establish a relationship with the parent(s) and teach effective parenting); and (iii) the individual level (e.g., education of children about how to avoid unsafe situations and protect themselves when confronted with threatening situations).

In Chapter 26, Nancy Mock and Elke de Buhr of Tulane University present a review of definitional and methodological difficulties associated with identifying and enumerating children in difficult circumstances. They examine trends in the evolution of the problem and its public health impact, and analyze the status of policies and strategies to protect and promote the health of children in difficult circumstances.

The integrated management of childhood illnesses (IMCI) initiative was introduced by the World Health Organization (WHO) and the United Nations Children's Fund (UNICEF) in the 1990s in response to the limitations of the child survival revolution of the 1980s that was based on disparate vertical programs. Thus, it represents a major policy shift in international approach to child health management and now represents the guiding principle of many technical assistance projects in support of child health in less-developed countries. In Chapter 27, Martin Meremikwu and John Ehiri present a historical perspective on this initiative and examine its evidence base. They describe field implementation case studies and conclude with an appraisal of the current status of the initiative. Prospects for scaling it up to improve child health globally are also discussed.

The performance of health-care systems depends ultimately on the knowledge, skills, and motivation of the people responsible for delivering services: health and social care personnel. In Chapter 28, Jeff Smith and Anne Hyre of Jhpiego, Johns Hopkins University, provide a review of some of the critical issues in health sector human resource planning, development, and maintenance that underpin the provision of high-quality maternal and child health services in less-developed countries. They explore elements of successful training programs as well as issues around the deployment, integration, supervision, support, and retention of maternal and child health workers. They examine factors that influence the performance of maternal and child health workers and discuss gender in relation to maternal and child health workforce capacity building. They conclude with a review of the relationship between maternal and child health human resource development and service provision at the local community level.

In the concluding portion of this book (Chapter 29), John Ehiri determinants presents a critical review of current strategies for promoting child health in developing countries and examines the environmental, social, and political factors that influence child health. The demise of Primary Healthcare, a strategy that over 20 years, ago was declared the model for achieving the goals of health for all, is reviewed. He asserts that after several years of investment in disease-focused vertical interventions, preventable diseases still remain a major challenge for women, infants, and children. He concludes with a call for return to the tenets of the Alma Ata Declaration of Primary Health, which emphasizes action on social, environmental, and economic determinants of health (including poverty alleviation), a focus on health systems development, and access to basic health care.

References

Alexander GR (2004) Maternal and child health (MCH). Encyclopedia of health care management. Thousand Oaks, CA: Sage Publications.

Institute of Medicine (1997) America's vital interest in global health: protecting our people, enhancing our economy, and advancing our international interests. Washington, DC: National Academy Press

McCarthy J, Maine D (1992) A framework for analyzing the determinants of maternal mortality. Studies in Family Planning, 23(1), 23–33

Murray CJL, Lopez AD (Eds.) (1996) The global burden of disease. Vol. 1. Cambridge, MA: Harvard University Press

Petersen DJ, Alexander GR (2004) Editorial – Charting a future course for the MCH journal. Maternal and Child Health Journal 8:1; 1–3

Wennberg DE (1998) Variation in the delivery of health care: the stakes are high (editorial). Annals of Internal Medicine 128:866–868

World Bank (2004) World Development Report 2004: making services work for poor people. Washington DC: The World Bank

Part I
The World's Heterogeneity

Chapter 1
A History of International Cooperation in Maternal and Child Health

Allan Rosenfield and Caroline J. Min

Learning Objectives After reading this chapter and answering the discussion questions that follow, you should be able to

- Discuss how maternal and child health gained recognition in industrialized countries and subsequently became a focal point of development assistance to less developed countries.
- Identify significant milestones in international cooperation in maternal and child health (including specific programs and initiatives) to illustrate how maternal and child health agenda has evolved over the past 60 years.
- Evaluate current international cooperation in maternal and child health within the context of shifting ideologies in global health.

Introduction

Prior to the twentieth century, the health of mothers and children was generally considered a domestic concern. Childbirth was supervised by midwives, traditional birth attendants (TBAs), or relatives, with physicians gradually attending a greater share of deliveries in industrialized countries. Before the introduction of scientific medicine, care for sick children was rudimentary and it was commonly accepted that a significant number of children would not survive childhood. The nineteenth century brought discoveries in bacteriology and other medical developments, as well as sanitary reforms, yet infant mortality rates remained high. Pediatric

C.J. Min (✉)
Columbia University, New York, USA

hospitals were established in growing numbers, but by themselves they did not have much influence on child mortality rates (Williams et al. 1994).

Toward the late 1800s (Box 1.1), leaders across Europe began to take a keen interest in the health of children. High rates of infant mortality combined with declining rates of birth aroused fears among politicians that their nations would fall behind in the race for economic and military supremacy, which required a robust adult population and, thus healthy children and healthy mothers to bear them. Fears of national deterioration were especially strong among the French in the wake of their defeat in the Franco-Prussian War (1870–1871), and later among the British after their poor showing in the Boer War (1899–1902) and their difficulties in recruiting able-bodied soldiers (Dwork 1987).

Newly established infant welfare programs quickly attracted the attention of physicians, philanthropists, and reformers, as well as government officials. In 1892, Pierre Budin at the Charité Hospital in Paris organized the first *consultation de nourrissons* or infant health consultation (Dwork 1987). Mothers who gave birth at the hospital were asked to return each week to have their babies weighed and examined. Budin educated mothers on the importance of breastfeeding or providing infants with sterilized milk, and the basics of infant care. In 1894, Léon Dufour in Fécamp, Normandy, opened a milk station, or *goutte de lait*, where he distributed sterilized milk and provided weekly medical care for infants. *Consultations de nourrissons* and *goutte de lait* clinics were highly successful in reducing morbidity and mortality rates for enrolled infants compared to rates for the general infant population, and they quickly proliferated throughout the country with

J.E. Ehiri (ed.), *Maternal and Child Health*, DOI 10.1007/b106524_1,
© Springer Science+Business Media, LLC 2009

Box 1.1 Milestones in Global Cooperation in MCH

- 1892 – Pierre Budine organized the first *consultation de nourrisons*, or infant health consultation.
- 1894 – Leon Dufour opened the first milk station.
- 1946 – The United Nations International Children's Emergency Fund was founded to provide relief to children and orphans of the world wars.
- 1948 – The Universal Declaration of Human Rights was adopted by the UN General Assembly.
- 1948 – The World Health Organization was founded.
- 1955 – The WHO and UNICEF launch an unsuccessful campaign to eradicate malaria.
- 1961 – The US Agency for International Development (USAID) was established.
- 1965 – China develops the "barefoot doctors".
- 1967 – The World Health Organization launched the smallpox eradication program (January 1)
- 1974 – The WHO launched Expanded Programme on Immunization (EPI).
- 1977 – Smallpox certified globally eradicated – marking one of the most successful public health programs in history.
- 1978 – The WHO and UNICEF co-sponsor the International Conference on Primary Health Care in Alma-Ata, Kazakhstan, which leads to the Declaration of Alma-Ata (see Box 1.2).
- 1982 – The child survival revolution, GOBI-FFF, launched by James P. Grant, then Executive Director of UNICEF.
- 1984 – A Task Force on Child Survival and Development established to coordinate immunization activities of major international agencies.
- 1987 – The World Bank, the WHO, and the United Nations Population Fund (UNFPA) sponsored an international conference in Nairobi that became the launching point of the Safe Motherhood Initiative.
- 1990 – The World Summit for Children in New York set forth goals to be achieved by 2000, including a goal to reduce the under-5 mortality rate by one-third or to 70 deaths per 1,000 live births, whichever is less.
- 1989 – The UN General Assembly adopted the Convention on the Rights of the Child.
- 1994 – The International Conference on Population and Development (ICPD) in Cairo led to the current definition of reproductive health and reproductive rights (see Box 1.4), reaffirmed at the 1995 Fourth World Conference for Women in Beijing.
- 1996 – The WHO and UNICEF introduced the Integrated Management of Childhood Illness initiative (IMCI), one of the predominant strategies for addressing child health today.
- 1997 – A Safe Motherhood Technical Consultation was convened in Colombo, Sri Lanka, and new strategic priorities were set, including the acknowledgment of maternal mortality as a social injustice.
- 1999 – The Bill and Melinda Gates Foundation launched the Global Alliance for Vaccines and Immunization (GAVI) now known as the GAVI Alliance.
- 1999 – The Bill and Melinda Gates Foundation funded Columbia's Mailman School of Public Health to launch Averting Maternal Death & Disability (AMDD).
- 2000 – World leaders at the UN Millennium Summit developed the Millennium Development Goals (MDGs).
- 2002 – The UNV Secretary-General commissioned the UN Millennium Project to develop a concrete action plan to achieve the MDGs (see Box 1.5).
- 2005 – The Partnership for Maternal, Newborn and Child Health was launched to harmonize and accelerate efforts toward achieving MDG-4 and MDG-5.

both private and public funding (Dwork 1987). Milk depots were opened in England and the United States, which soon began using health visitors or visiting nurses to provide home-based consultations on infant care. By the early twentieth century, local authorities were providing infant health services in one form or another in the industrialized countries of Europe and in the United States. The loss of lives during the First World War hastened the development of more comprehensive infant and child welfare programs (Dwork 1987).

Public interest in maternal and child health was also motivated by other humanitarian concerns. New and more comprehensive reports on the high levels of infant and maternal mortality in England, the United States, and other countries stimulated action at the local and national levels. Medical associations, charities, women's groups, and other segments of civil society took an active interest, often as part of social reform movements of that era. For example, a number of committees and associations, both medical and lay, were formed in various European countries expressly to improve maternal health. Advocacy was often instrumental in introducing legislation and securing funds to address the issue (Van Lerberghe and De Brouwere 2001). MCH was given formal recognition in the United States following the emergence of child labor abolition and the pressure exerted by progressive reform movements, leading to the establishment of the Federal Children's Bureau in 1912 (Lindenmeyer 1997). During this time, cooperation between nations on matters of health focused on the control of communicable diseases to facilitate trade and commerce. International Sanitary Conferences, beginning in 1851, were convened periodically to discuss quarantine and other measures to control cholera, plague, and yellow fever (Howard-Jones 1975). International health bodies, such as the Pan American Sanitary Bureau (1902) and the Office International d'Hygiène Publique (1907), were created mainly to collect and disseminate new knowledge on infectious diseases. After the First World War, the League of Nations was created along with a subdivision, the Health Organization, whose chief activities included the formation of expert committees to study selected diseases and topics. The League of Nations collapsed after failing to prevent the outbreak of another world war (Simonds 1934).

The end of the Second World War ushered in a new era of international cooperation in health, within which assistance to mothers and children, as a moral obligation, would figure prominently. The United Nations (UN) was established in 1945 and the United Nations International Children's Emergency Fund (UNICEF) was founded a year later to provide relief to the thousands of children and orphans left vulnerable by the war. Its earliest programs involved providing aid, in the form of dried milk, to both Western and Eastern European countries. UNICEF endured to take on a broader role in protecting children all around the world, later changing its name to the United Nations Children's Fund (while retaining its original acronym). The World Health Organization (WHO), a specialized UN agency, came into being in 1948 to help all people attain "the highest possible level of health", including a function "to promote maternal and child health and welfare" (World Health Organization 1948). The Universal Declaration of Human Rights, adopted by the United Nations General Assembly in 1948, included the acknowledgment that "motherhood and childhood are entitled to special care and assistance" (United Nations 1948).

Maternal and child health had evolved into an international priority, but the exact strategies for promoting MCH would be debated and transformed repeatedly in the coming decades. Cooperation in MCH has not been limited to the work of the UN or other multilateral organizations. During the first half of the twentieth century, many of the nations now categorized as developing countries were colonies or protectorates. After the independence movements of the late 1940s to the early 1960s, industrialized nations began to provide aid directly to developing countries on a one-to-one basis, a form of assistance known as bilateral aid. The US Agency for International Development (USAID), for example, was established in 1961 to provide economic and social development assistance to other nations and has funded a number of MCH programs in developing countries (USAID 2008). Non-governmental organizations (NGOs), or civil society organizations (CSOs), have also been influential in shaping the global MCH agenda.

From Vertical, Disease Control Programs to Primary Health Care

The first international programs that were implemented, beyond war relief efforts, focused on the control or eradication of specific diseases not only in Europe but also in Asia, Africa, and Latin America. Technological breakthroughs, including new and cheaper drugs and vaccines, offered a way to address epidemic diseases on a grand scale. Mass disease campaigns were often "vertical" programs, i.e., they utilized financial and logistical resources separate from those of other programs or regular health services. This was often at the insistence of donors who preferred having specific objectives and who believed that most countries lacked infrastructures capable of reaching large segments of the population. Tuberculosis, yaws, and other diseases came under attack, with generally successful results. Even child malnutrition was addressed as a disease with protein as its technical solution. During its first two decades, UNICEF's efforts to improve child nutrition consisted of providing milk to children and pregnant and nursing women (UNICEF 2008a).

However, vertical programs often did little to develop existing health systems. The campaign to eradicate malaria, launched in 1955 by the WHO and UNICEF, was a noteworthy failure (Brown 2002). It demonstrated that not all diseases could be tamed by the transfer of technology, in this case DDT spraying in the absence of well-functioning healthcare infrastructures to support and sustain efforts. The campaign, as well as others like it, ignored the social, economic, and cultural dimensions of disease. Nonetheless, disease-specific campaigns continued to be implemented. The smallpox eradication program, concluded in the late 1970s, was one of the most successful public health programs in history. A global initiative is currently underway to eradicate poliomyelitis which is now endemic in only a handful of countries. However, the need for a more integrated and long-term approach to delivering healthcare services has been increasingly acknowledged by international policymakers and health planners.

Like their older counterparts, newly independent nations sought a different model of health care, part of a broader push for "development" aimed at improving the economic and social conditions of even the poorest citizens. Under colonial rule, health services were largely intended for European military and civilian populations. They emphasized high technology and curative care in large, urban hospitals. Developing countries planned to expand basic curative and preventive health services in rural areas, where most of the population lived, through a network of health posts or health centers staffed by auxiliary health workers (known as medical assistants or health assistants). They invested in the development of community health workers, who were volunteers, selected by their own communities and trained to provide health education and basic services to their neighbors. The most successful and inspiring community-based health initiative was the "barefoot doctors" program in China which stressed meeting the basic health needs of all people. Thousands of peasants were trained in basic medical practices and preventive medicine including proper hygiene, diagnosing infectious disease, family planning, and maternal and child care. They continued their work alongside other farmers in the fields, providing readily accessible health care for most peasants, including mothers and children. In reality, however, most developing countries continued to spend a large share of health budgets on urban, tertiary hospitals while neglecting care for poor and rural populations.

The call for an integrated, more equitable approach to health care reached a climax in 1978 at the International Conference on Primary Health Care in Alma-Ata, Kazakhstan, co-sponsored by the WHO and UNICEF and attended by representatives of over 130 countries and 60 organizations (WHO/UNICEF 1978). The Declaration of Alma-Ata affirmed the goal of health for all by 2000 and outlined a strategy for meeting this ambitious goal – primary health care (PHC) (Box 1.2). More than just an organizational strategy, PHC envisioned a process of decision making that valued the community as a key actor. It recognized the underlying social, economic, and political dimensions of health and, therefore, the need for a multi-sectoral approach. While PHC has often been interpreted as merely community-based, preventive health care, the declaration recognized the provision of curative and rehabilitative services to address health problems in the community. It stated that PHC should

Box 1.2 Declaration of Alma-Ata

"Primary healthcare is essential healthcare based on practical, scientifically sound and socially acceptable methods and technology made universally accessible to individuals and families in the community through their full participation and at a cost that the community and country can afford to maintain at every stage of their development in the spirit of self-reliance and self-determination. It forms an integral part both of the country's health system, of which it is the central function and main focus, and of the overall social and economic development of the community. It is the first level of contact of individuals, the family and community with the national health system bringing healthcare as close as possible to where people live and work, and constitutes the first element of a continuing healthcare process." (Article VI)

"[Primary healthcare] includes at least: education concerning prevailing health problems and the methods of preventing and controlling them; promotion of food supply and proper nutrition; an adequate supply of safe water and basic sanitation; maternal and child healthcare, including family planning [emphasis added]; immunization against the major infectious diseases; prevention and control of locally endemic diseases; appropriate treatment of common diseases and injuries; and provision of essential drugs." (Article VII, 3).

Source: WHO/UNICEF (1978)

be sustained by "functional and mutually supportive referral systems, leading to the progressive improvement of comprehensive healthcare for all" (WHO/UNICEF 1978).

Almost immediately, the concept of primary health care was challenged. It was argued by some that PHC was too ambitious to be attainable in the near future. Instead, as an interim measure, a few conditions responsible for the greatest mortality and morbidity and for which efficacious and relatively inexpensive interventions exist should be prioritized, an idea referred to as selective primary health care (Walsh and Warren 1979). A debate on comprehensive versus selective primary health care followed. However, UNICEF soon adopted the selective approach as the foundation of its child survival revolution. In the 1980s, developing countries were suffering from global recession and were immersed in foreign debt. In order to receive bailout loans, countries were forced to adopt highly controversial stabilization and structural adjustment programs promoted by the World Bank and the International Monetary Fund (IMF). Among other conditions, these programs required sharp cuts in public spending on health, education, and other social sectors. Issues and concerns surrounding structural adjustment programs and MCH are

dealt with in more detail in Chapter 8 (Globalization). PHC helped to bring attention to issues of community participation, equity, and universal access. But PHC was not widely or consistently implemented and soon lost ground.

The Child Survival Revolution

In 1982, James P. Grant, then Executive Director of UNICEF, launched an initiative known as the child survival revolution (UNICEF 1983). Although child mortality rates in low-income countries were reduced by half between the end of Second World War and the early 1970s, progress was not maintained and almost 15 million children still died each year from malnutrition and infection. UNICEF called for massive coverage of four interventions that could significantly reaccelerate progress in child health and nutrition, collectively known by the acronym GOBI:

Growth monitoring
Oral rehydration therapy (ORT) (Box 1.3)
Breastfeeding
Immunization

Box 1.3 Oral Rehydration Therapy

Oral rehydration therapy (ORT) is a combination of salt water and glucose in the right proportions that enables the liquid to be absorbed through the intestinal wall. It is used to treat dehydration caused by diarrheal infections. ORT was discovered in the late 1960s by researchers at the Cholera Research Laboratory in Dhaka, Bangladesh (later renamed the International Centre for Diarrheal Disease Research, Bangladesh) and the Infectious Diseases Hospital in Calcutta. During the Bangladesh war of independence in 1971, ORT was applied in refugee camps to combat outbreaks of cholera and was found to be extremely effective. ORT is considered to be one of the most important medical breakthroughs of the twentieth century.

These interventions were chosen because they were low cost, low risk, effective, and feasible to implement (UNICEF 2008b). Food supplementation, family planning, and female education (GOBI-FFF) were subsequently added to the package in response to concerns that GOBI was too narrow in its focus. However, international agencies, donors, and ministries of health focused primarily on two components, ORT and immunization, referred to as the "twin engines" of the revolution (UNICEF 2008b). Some health professionals and policymakers criticized child survival programs for being top-down, vertical programs, a reversion to the mass disease campaigns of the 1950s. Nonetheless, the child survival campaign generated a great degree of political and popular support worldwide, and Jim Grant's energetic leadership and personal commitment to the cause was credited with much of its success.

The WHO's Programme for the Control of Diarrheal Diseases helped countries to develop training courses for health workers on how to administer ORT, while UNICEF supported the production of packets of oral rehydration salts. Between 1979 and 1992, the supply of packets increased from 51 to 800 million. The number of worldwide deaths due to diarrhea among children under 5 years of age fell from 4.6 million in 1980 to 3.3 million in 1990, a result of the widespread introduction of ORT and other complementary activities (Victora et al. 2000). Local NGOs were involved in spreading knowledge about ORT directly to the village level. Most notably, BRAC (formerly the Bangladesh Rural Advancement Committee) carried out a nationwide campaign in Bangladesh in the 1980s to educate women in rural areas on how to mix and administer

oral rehydration solution using commonly available ingredients and simple measurements. Between 1980 and 1990, BRAC brought the message of ORT to over 12 million mothers (Chowdhury and Cash 1996).

Before the WHO launched its Expanded Programme on Immunization (EPI) in 1974, only a small proportion of children in developing countries were being immunized (UNICEF 2008c). EPI set out to achieve universal immunization coverage against six major diseases: tuberculosis, diphtheria, pertussis, tetanus, polio, and measles. In 1984, a Task Force on Child Survival and Development was established to help develop and coordinate the immunization activities of the major international agencies, including WHO, UNICEF, the Rockefeller Foundation, the United Nations Development Programme (UNDP), and the World Bank. The scope of the Task Force's work eventually expanded to address other aspects of global health. Global immunization coverage increased dramatically to almost 75% by 1990, helping to avert millions of child deaths, but remained level at 70–75% during the 1990s with wide variations in coverage between regions (UNICEF 2001). The GAVI Fund (formerly known as the Global Alliance for Vaccines and Immunization) was established in 1999 by the Bill & Melinda Gates Foundation to help break the stagnation and widen children's access to vaccines in poor countries. The GAVI Fund is now a public–private partnership made up of national governments, UNICEF, WHO, the World Bank, the Bill & Melinda Gates Foundation, the vaccine industry, public health institutions, and NGOs (see Chapter 23 – Immunization).

One of the predominant strategies for addressing child health today is the Integrated Management of Childhood Illness (IMCI) initiative (Chapter 27). The introduction of IMCI by the WHO and UNICEF in the mid-1990s was a change of course from other major child health initiatives (Tulloch 1999). IMCI integrates disease control programs into a package of basic services and now includes household- and community-level components. Health workers are trained in comprehensive case management skills to accurately diagnose and treat a range of problems as well as promote preventive measures. IMCI originally focused on facility-based interventions for pneumonia, diarrhea, malaria, and measles, as well as malnutrition. Newer options, such as early childhood development and the treatment of HIV/AIDS, can be included in a country's IMCI package. In addition to training health workers, IMCI aims to strengthen health systems by developing referral mechanisms for severely ill children, ensuring the widespread availability of drugs and supplies, improving supervision of staff, and emphasizing monitoring and evaluation. Community-based interventions promote key household and community practices linked to the prevention and treatment of common childhood illnesses. The IMCI strategy has been adopted in more than 100 countries (PAHO 2008).

The campaign for child survival reached its political peak in 1990 when 71 heads of state and government pledged their support at the World Summit for Children in New York, one of the largest gatherings of world leaders ever assembled at the UN. The summit set forth goals to be achieved by 2000, including a goal to reduce the under-5 mortality rate by one-third or to 70 deaths per 1,000 live births, whichever is less. A year earlier, in 1989, the UN General Assembly adopted the Convention on the Rights of the Child which came into force as international law in 1990 and was eventually ratified by almost all nations – a remarkable achievement (the United States has yet to ratify the convention). The convention outlines the basic human rights of children everywhere and protects these rights by setting standards in health care, education, and legal, civil, and social services.

Substantial progress was made in the decade following the launch of the child survival revolution. However, since the mid-1990s, progress in reducing child mortality has slowed in many countries and reversed in some, and the World Summit goal for reducing child mortality was not achieved. The under-5 mortality rate fell from 117 deaths per 1,000 live births in 1980 to 93 per 1,000 in 1990. However, instead of a one-third reduction, under-5 mortality declined by only 11% between 1990 and 2000 to 83 deaths per 1,000 births (UNICEF 2001). More than 10 million children under 5 years of age still die each year worldwide, and significant challenges remain in particular regions and countries. Members of the international health community have called for a renewed commitment to child survival – a second revolution – including increased efforts to reduce inequities in child health status and strengthen health systems to deliver more coordinated services for children.

Where Is the "M" in MCH?

Over 500,000 women die each year from pregnancy-related causes; almost all maternal deaths occur in developing regions (World Health Organization 2004). For every woman who dies, many others suffer from debilitating complications, including vesico-vaginal fistula and recto-vaginal fistula. While international agencies and donors were mounting enormous efforts to reduce child mortality, the problem of maternal mortality and morbidity barely registered on the public health agenda. In 1985, an influential article was published in *The Lancet* that highlighted the tragedy of maternal mortality and called on the World Bank to make maternity care one of its priorities (Rosenfield and Maine 1985). The same year, women's health and advocacy groups from around the world gathered together at a conference in Nairobi to mark the end of the UN Decade for Women, an initiative to help focus more attention on women's health and rights. The announcement there of the estimated number of maternal deaths occurring in developing countries gave rise to calls for more action to prevent this tragedy.

There are a number of reasons why maternal mortality received little attention among politicians and policymakers. First, the scale of the problem was unclear in most developing countries until the 1980s because of poor or non-existent vital registration systems. In the mid-1980s, the WHO supported the first community studies on levels of maternal mortality in developing countries and, with the limited information available from vital registration systems and hospital-based studies, was able to generate global and regional estimates of maternal mortality (World Health Organization 1986). In 1996, the WHO and UNICEF published revised global and regional totals of maternal mortality and included, for the first time, individual country estimates (World Health Organization 1996). The availability of data, particularly at the country level, was critical in drawing more attention to the issue. While techniques for measuring maternal mortality have improved somewhat, information is still extremely difficult to collect and available data continue to be rough estimates.

Second, while relatively simple preventive measures can substantially reduce mortality among infants and young children, this is not the case with maternal mortality. The major direct causes of maternal death are hemorrhage, infection, eclampsia, obstructed labor, and complications of unsafe abortion (Khan and Wojdyla 2006). Women who develop life-threatening complications during pregnancy or childbirth need access to the appropriate medical interventions, later referred to as emergency obstetric care (EmOC). International agencies, donors, and health professionals believed it was more feasible to address the problem of child mortality, which responded relatively quickly and successfully to preventive measures delivered by vertical programs. Also, while interpretations of PHC varied, the idea of promoting medical treatment found little support at the time. The few measures targeted to mothers, antenatal consultations and education, had little impact on maternal mortality and were largely aimed at improving infant health (Van Lerberghe and De Brouwere 2001). Family planning programs (MCH/FP) were also heavily emphasized in developing countries beginning in the 1960s. Family planning reduces the number of unwanted and unplanned pregnancies and, consequently, the number of maternal deaths, women who are pregnant and develop life-threatening complications and need access to the appropriate care.

Third, discrimination against women is embedded in the social, economic, and cultural fabric of most societies, and women's contributions to society are often unrecognized or undervalued. As Halfdan Mahler, former Director-General of WHO, put it, maternal mortality "has been neglected because those who suffer it are neglected people, with the least power and influence over how national resources shall be spent; they are the poor, the rural peasants, and, above all, women" (Mahler 1987). Allan Rosenfield, former Dean of Columbia's Mailman School of Public Health, stated on several occasions that poor rural women have been ignored and that they have a basic human right to access to effective maternal health care.

The Safe Motherhood Initiative

The "Where is the M in MCH" paper, mentioned above, strongly recommended that the World Bank play a major role in this area. A meeting was held at the World Bank which led to consideration of an international conference. In response to mounting concerns, the World Bank, the WHO, and the United Nations Population Fund (UNFPA) in 1987 sponsored an international conference in Nairobi to raise global awareness of the state of maternal health in developing countries and to mobilize support. The conference issued a call to action and became the launching point of the Safe Motherhood Initiative (Chapter 22 – Making Pregnancy Safer), which set a goal to reduce maternal mortality by 50% by the year 2000. UNDP, UNICEF, International Planned Parenthood Federation, and the Population Council joined the three original co-sponsors in the formation of a Safe Motherhood Inter-Agency Group. A series of national and regional safe motherhood meetings followed that helped to increase global recognition of the problem.

In the early years of the Safe Motherhood Initiative, UN bodies, donors, and ministries of health continued to support two strategies already being implemented: antenatal care with a focus on screening and the training of traditional birth attendants (TBAs) in safe and hygienic practices. Both interventions fit within the perceived ideal of primary health care and were also thought to be cost-effective. Antenatal screening, an approach supported by the first WHO expert committee on motherhood in the early 1950s (WHO 1952), became accepted wisdom despite some evidence of its ineffectiveness. The idea was to persuade all women to attend at least one antenatal visit during their pregnancy. A screening test would be conducted and those women identified as high risk could then be monitored and treated or advised to give birth at a health facility. However, many direct obstetric complications can be neither predicted nor prevented. Many women who develop complications have few or no risk factors, and most women with risk factors have uneventful pregnancies.

The training of TBAs, which became common in the 1970s, was considered a rational approach to reducing maternal mortality in countries where there is a shortage of professional health workers and where the majority of women deliver at home. TBAs live and provide services in rural areas where women have the least access to medical care; they are accepted members of the community and they are reimbursed by women and their families and do not need government salaries. It was thought that TBAs could be used to refer women with complications to a facility for treatment and that they could also be trained to use hygienic practices and avoid harmful ones, such as pushing on the abdomen to hasten delivery. However, most TBA training programs neither ensured effective supervision nor provided the appropriate linkages to referral services. For most of the complications of pregnancy and childbirth, there is little that TBAs can do to save women's lives.

A Safe Motherhood Technical Consultation was convened in Colombo, Sri Lanka, in 1997 to review key lessons learned from the Initiative's first 10 years and to develop a consensus on the most effective strategies. By this time, it was apparent that little progress was being made (Maine and Rosenfield 1999). Strategic priorities were not clearly defined at the outset and some broadened the safe motherhood agenda to include a range of activities aimed at improving women's health and social status, including nutrition and education for young girls. Though commendable, these activities cannot substantially reduce levels of maternal mortality. This lack of focus was, in part, fueled by the mistaken idea that maternal mortality can be reduced by general socioeconomic development. However, the experience of countries in Europe and North America has shown that levels of maternal mortality are primarily affected by access to medical interventions, not

improvements in living standards. Such a broad agenda led some policymakers and program managers to believe that safe motherhood was already a part of their programs (e.g., family planning, antenatal care, and nutrition), while others considered the agenda too complex and too costly to implement. In contrast, UNICEF provided donors and ministries of health with a priority list of interventions – GOBI – that could prevent childhood deaths from the most common causes.

Furthermore, fears that targeting maternal mortality would force developing countries to revert to an emphasis on large, curative hospitals persist. While emergency obstetrical care, such as a cesarean delivery for obstructed labor, must take place in a properly equipped facility, many life-saving procedures can be implemented in health centers or the most peripheral levels of the healthcare system, supported by strong referral mechanisms. In most rural areas in developing countries, there are almost no obstetricians and very few physicians. To make emergency obstetrical care available, including cesarean sections, Mozambique (and later Tanzania and Malawi) trained community health workers to be able to provide such care (Pereira et al. 2007). This program, which was started about 15 years ago, has been highly successful as communities can also play an important role in helping to ensure that pregnant women who develop complications receive timely care, although distance from adequate facilities can still be a barrier in rural areas. It should also be noted that many safe motherhood programs gave little attention to the management of complications from unsafe abortion because of the political sensitivities that surround this issue.

The Sri Lanka meeting focused on a number of key action messages (Starrs 1998). Specific messages recognized that every pregnancy faces risks and, therefore, programs should stop using risk screening tools as a means to reduce maternal mortality. Ensuring skilled attendance at delivery was emphasized. The definition of a skilled attendant, a health worker with midwifery skills, excludes TBAs and, accordingly, donors and governments have abandoned large-scale TBA training programs. Furthermore, maternal mortality was framed as a social injustice. A human rights approach obligates governments to use all political and legal means available to provide appropriate health services to all women. Today, international efforts to reduce maternal mortality focus on ensuring a skilled attendant at all deliveries and increasing access to emergency obstetric care.

A number of organizations have been involved in maternal health programs over the past 20 years, including broad-based coalitions and partnerships. For example, local NGOs have been involved in public education campaigns and other activities. The White Ribbon Alliance for Safe Motherhood promotes awareness about maternal mortality and includes international and local NGOs, UN agencies, bilateral agencies, and other organizations and individuals. Major donors such as the World Bank, USAID, and the Department for International Development (United Kingdom) have supported intensive maternal health projects in a number of countries.

The International Conference on Population and Development (ICPD)

In the 1960s, fearing the economic and social consequences of rapid population growth, many countries declared national population policies and established family planning programs with the support of a variety of donors, particularly USAID. Dismayed by the focus on meeting demographic targets, an international women's health movement emerged that sought to shift the rationale for family planning programs from population control to women's health and rights. The 1994 International Conference on Population and Development (ICPD) in Cairo marked the culmination of advocacy efforts and a significant shift in ideology. The conference was attended by delegates of over 180 countries as well as representatives of approximately 1,200 NGOs. Both family planning and safe motherhood, along with sexual health, were incorporated under the concept of reproductive health (Box 1.4). ICPD was also the first major international conference to formally articulate a human rights approach to the provision of reproductive health services. These concepts were reaffirmed at the 1995 Fourth World Conference for Women in Beijing.

The ICPD Programme of Action called on countries to reduce maternal mortality by one-half of their 1990 levels by the year 2000 and a further one-half by 2015. Operationally, ICPD did not result in any real integration of family planning and maternal health programs. Reproductive health programs have focused on family planning and the prevention and management of sexually transmitted diseases. Legal safe abortion services, post-abortion care, and, to a lesser extent, issues such as female genital mutilation and violence have also been part of the agenda.

The Millennium Development Goals (MDGs)

In 2000, world leaders gathered at the UN Millennium Summit to discuss the major development challenges heading into the twenty-first century. Representatives of 189 countries adopted the Millennium Declaration as a blueprint for action, from which eight Millennium Development Goals (MDGs) were established (Box 1.5). The MDGs have a target date of 2015 and synthesize many of the commitments made at the international conferences and summits of the 1990s. Both maternal and child health are emphasized, while reproductive health is conspicuously absent from the list. Reproductive health advocates have argued, however, that achievement of the MDGs requires full implementation of the ICPD Programme of Action. Nevertheless, the MDGs are currently at the center of the global health and development agenda and have galvanized an unprecedented level of support. They are being used to reframe the work of UN agencies, governments, and organizations, and tracking progress in all parts of the world is a priority. MDGs 4 and 5 relate directly to MCH, while many of the other MDGs, including MDG 1, are significant. The inclusion of maternal health within the MDG framework was a highly significant development, although progress toward meeting MDG-5 has been slow, particularly in sub-Saharan Africa and parts of Asia.

In 2002, the United Nations Secretary-General commissioned the UN Millennium Project to develop a concrete action plan to achieve the MDGs. The project established 10 thematic taskforces to conduct extensive research on their respective topics and produce recommendations. The Task Force on Child Health and Maternal Health

Box 1.4 Definition of Reproductive Health and Reproductive Rights

The ICPD Programme of Action defined reproductive health and reproductive rights as follows:
"Reproductive health is a state of complete physical, mental and social well-being and not merely the absence of disease or infirmity, in all matters relating to the reproductive system and to its functions and processes. Reproductive health therefore implies that people are able to have a satisfying and safe sex life and that they have the capability to reproduce and the freedom to decide if, when and how often to do so. Implicit in this last condition are the right of men and women to be informed and to have access to safe, effective, affordable and acceptable methods of family planning of their choice, as well as other methods of their choice for regulation of fertility which are not against the law, and the right of access to appropriate health-care services that will enable women to go safely through pregnancy and childbirth and provide couples with the best chance of having a healthy infant [emphasis added]. In line with the above definition of reproductive health, reproductive healthcare is defined as the constellation of methods, techniques and services that contribute to reproductive health and well-being by preventing and solving reproductive health problems. It also includes sexual health, the purpose of which is the enhancement of life and personal relations, and not merely counseling and care related to reproduction and sexually transmitted diseases." (paragraph 7.2)
"Bearing in mind the above definition, reproductive rights encompass certain human rights that are already recognized in national laws, international human rights documents and other consensus documents. These rights rest on the recognition of the basic right of all couples and individuals to decide freely and responsibly the number, spacing and timing of their children and to have the information and means to do so, and the right to attain the highest standard of sexual and reproductive health. It also includes their right to make decisions concerning reproduction free of discrimination, coercion and violence, as expressed in human rights documents. In the exercise of this right, they should take into account the needs of their living and future children and their responsibilities towards the community. The promotion of the responsible exercise of these rights for all people should be the fundamental basis for government- and community-supported policies and programs in the area of reproductive health, including family planning." (paragraph 7.3)
   Source: United Nations (1944)

emphasized the importance of strengthening health systems in developing countries in order to achieve meaningful and sustainable progress toward reducing child and maternal mortality (Freedman and Waldman 2005). The task force recommended the rapid scale-up of interventions such as IMCI and the universal provision of emergency obstetric care.

Newborn Survival and the Continuum of Care

Until recently, the health of newborns was virtually neglected by policymakers and program managers. Of the more than 10 million children who die each year before the age of 5 years, 4 million (38%) die

within the first month of life or the neonatal period. Approximately three quarters of neonatal deaths occur in the first week after birth. Four million babies are stillborn (Lawn et al. 2005). Effective, low-cost, feasible interventions do exist and can significantly reduce neonatal mortality if universally implemented. They include tetanus toxoid vaccination, antibiotics for infections, exclusive breastfeeding, and kangaroo mother care for low birth weight babies (a method that encourages skin-to-skin contact between mothers and their newborns to reduce hypothermia, encourage breast feeding, and prevent infection). Skilled attendants at childbirth are critical for both mothers and newborns, but maternal health programs have focused on bringing mothers safely through pregnancy and childbirth. At the same time, newborn health has not been

Box 1.5 United Nations Millennium Development Goals

Goal 1: Eradicate extreme poverty and hunger.
Goal 2: Achieve universal primary education.
Goal 3: Promote gender equality and empower women.
Goal 4: Reduce child mortality.
Target:
Reduce by two thirds the under-five mortality rate

Indicators:
Under-five mortality rate; Infant mortality rate.
Proportion of 1-year olds immunized against measles.

Goal 5: Improve maternal health
Targets:
Reduce by three quarters the maternal mortality ratio.

Indicators:
Maternal mortality ratio.
Proportion of births attended by skilled health personnel.

Goal 6: Combat HIV/AIDS, malaria and other diseases.
Goal 7: Ensure environmental sustainability.
Goal 8: Develop a Global Partnership for Development.

Source: The United Nations Development Programme (2003)

integrated into conventional child health programs, which focus on vaccine-preventable diseases, diarrhea, and acute respiratory tract infections. In order to achieve MDG-4 which aims to reduce child mortality by two-thirds by 2015, significant reductions in neonatal mortality must be achieved.

More efforts have been made to incorporate newborn health into MCH programs. For example, IMCI (Chapter 27) is developing new guidelines that address the care of sick newborns. In 2005, the Partnership for Maternal, Newborn and Child Health was launched to harmonize and accelerate efforts toward achieving MDG-4 and MDG-5. The partnership is the result of a merger between three existing consortiums on safe motherhood, child survival, and newborn health and consists of more than 80 members, including governments, UN agencies, NGOs, professional associations, bilateral agencies, foundations, and academic and research institutions. The WHO has recently advocated for a repositioning of MCH to MNCH (maternal, newborn, and child health) to reflect a more seamless

continuum of care for mothers and children from pregnancy to childbirth and the immediate postnatal period to childhood (World Health Organization 2005). The turnover between maternal and child health services is critical, but there is still no clear consensus on who should provide care and where, to newborns, especially during the first week after birth.

Conclusion – Moving Forward in International MCH

A review of international policies and programs in MCH reveals a number of significant developments. Cooperation has grown to include many different agents, from UN agencies and governments to local NGOs. A number of partnerships have emerged that include a broad range of organizations and interests. Maternal health issues have become prominent on the global health agenda, and the approaches needed to prevent maternal deaths are better understood. Neonatal mortality is receiving due attention as a public health problem. Reducing maternal and child mortality is no longer merely a technical issue but a human rights imperative. The need to strengthen the capacity of health systems to deliver services is also widely acknowledged.

Nonetheless, many issues that have arisen in the past remain. The merits of disease-specific versus integrated approaches are still debated, although the reality is that both will continue to be used to formulate MCH programs and policies. And while competition for global attention and, more concretely, resources is not necessarily intentional, constrained budgets in developing countries and inadequate funding levels will continue to make priority setting in MCH difficult. Cooperation in MCH will, therefore, require more intense advocacy efforts to increase the pool of funding available to address the broad range of problems. All the various actors will need to address other strategic issues as well, such as how to develop an adequate health-care workforce to handle the myriad of demands and how to scale up and more equitably deliver effective interventions.

Key Terms

Alma-Ata Declaration	International Monetary Fund	Integrated Management of
Averting Maternal Death and	League of Nations	Childhood Illnesses
Disability (AMDD)	Midwives	(IMCHI)
Barefoot doctor	Newborn survival	United Nations Children's
Child survival revolution	Pan American Sanitary Bureau	Fund (UNICEF)
Emergency Obstetric Care	Primary health care	United States Agency for
(EmOC)	Reproductive rights	International Development
Expanded Programme on	Safe motherhood	(USAID)
Immunization (EPI)	Sanitary reforms	Universal Declaration of
Global Alliance for Vaccines	Traditional birth attendants	Human Rights
and Immunization (GAVI)	(TBAs)	World Bank
GOBI-FFF	United Nations Decade for	World Health Organization
Infant mortality rate	Women	

Questions for Discussion

- The end of the Second World War ushered in a new era of international cooperation in health within which assistance to mothers and children featured prominently as a moral obligation. Discuss.
- Identify and discuss the intervention programs of the child survival revolution. What were the major criticisms of these intervention approaches?
- Why were many vertical, disease control programs supported by international donor agencies regarded as largely ineffective in sustainably reducing the burden of disease and mortality among women and children in less developed countries?

- What were the major reasons why maternal mortality received little attention among politicians and policy makers until the 1980s?
- Reducing maternal and child mortality is no longer merely a technical issue but a human rights imperative. Discuss.

References

Brown A (2002) Personal experiences in the malaria eradication campaign 1955–1962. Journal of the Royal Society of Medicine, 95:3; 154–156

Chowdhury AMR, Cash RA (1996) A simple solution: Teaching millions to treat diarrhea at home. Bangladesh: University Press Ltd., Dhaka

Dwork D (1987) War is good for babies and other young children: A history of the infant and child welfare movement in England 1898–1918. London: Tavistock Publications

Freedman L, Waldman R (2005) Who's got the power? Transforming health systems for women and children. UN Millennium Project Task Force on Child Health and Maternal Health, New York http://www.unmillenniumproject.org/documents/maternalchild-frontmatter.pdf, cited 9 July 2008

Howard-Jones N (1975) The scientific background of the International Sanitary Conferences, 1851–1938. Geneva: World Health Organization

Khan PS, Wojdyla D (2006) WHO analysis of causes of maternal death: A systematic review. The Lancet, 367:9516; 1066–1074

Lawn JE, Cousens, S, Zupan J (2005) for the Lancet Neonatal Survival Steering Team 1.4 million neonatal deaths: When? Where? Why? Lancet, 365; 891–900

Lindenmeyer L (1997) A Right to Childhood: The U.S. Children's Bureau and Child Welfare, 1912–1946. Urbana, IL: University of Illinois Press

Mahler H (1987) The Safe Motherhood Initiative: a call to action. The Lancet, 1, 668–670

Maine D, Rosenfield A (1999) The Safe Motherhood Initiative: Why has it stalled? American Journal of Public Health, 89(4), 480–482

Pan American Health Organization (2008) About Integrated Management of Childhood Illness (IMCI). http://www.paho.org/English/ad/dpc/cd/imci-aiepi.htm, cited 9 July 2008

Pereira C, Cumbi A, Malalane R (2007) Meeting the need for emergency obstetric care in Mozambique: work performance and histories of medical doctors and assistant medical officers trained for surgery. British Journal of Obstetrics and Gynaecology, 114:12, 1530–1533

Rosenfield A, Maine, D (1985) Maternal mortality – a neglected tragedy. Where is the M in MCH? The Lancet, 2:83–85

Simonds F (1934) The Collapse of the Peace Movement. Annals of the American Academy of Political and Social Science, 174:116–120

Starrs A (ed.) (1998) The safe motherhood action agenda: priorities for the next decade. Report on the safe motherhood technical consultation, 18–23 October, 1997, Colombo, Sri Lanka. New York: Family Care International. http://www.popline.org/docs/1365/149862.html, cited 9 July 2008

Tulloch J (1999) Integrated approach to child health in developing countries. The Lancet 354(Suppl. 2), 16–20

United Nations Children's Fund (UNICEF) (1983) The state of the world's children, 1982-83. New York: Oxford University Press. http://www.popline.org/docs/013147, cited 9 July 2008

United Nations Children's Fund (UNICEF) (2001) Progress since the World Summit for Children: a statistical review. New York: UNICEF. http://www.unicef.org/specialsession/about/sgreport-pdf/sgreport_adapted_stats_eng.pdf, cited 9 July 2008

United Nations Children's Fund (UNICEF) (2008a) Our history. http://www.unicef.org/about/who/index_history.html, cited 9 July 2008

United Nations Children's Fund (UNICEF) (2008b) UNICEF'S GOBI-FFF programs. http://rehydrate.org/facts/gobi_fff.htm, cited 9 July 2008

United Nations Children's Fund (UNICEF) (2008c) Expanding immunization coverage. http://www.unicef.org/immunization/index_coverage.html, cited 9 July 2008

United Nations Development Programme (UNDP) (2003) Human Development Report: Millennium Development Goals: A Compact among Nations to End Human Poverty: Oxford University Press, New York

United Nations (1948) The Universal Declaration of Human Rights. Office of the High Commissioner for Human Rights. New York: United Nations. http://www.unhchr.ch/udhr/index.htm, cited 17 November 2008

United Nations (1994) Report of the International Conference on Population and Development (Document A/CONF.171/13): United Nations, New York

USAID (2008) About USAID this is USAID. Washington, D.C.: United States Agency for International Development (USAID) http://www.usaid.gov/about_usaid/, cited 9 July 2008

Van Lerberghe W, De Brouwere V (2001) Of blind alleys and things that have worked: history's lessons on reducing maternal mortality. In: De Brouwere V, Van Lerberghe W, eds. Safe Motherhood Strategies: A Review of the Evidence. ITG Press, Antwerp

Victora CG, Bryce J, Fontaine O et al. (2000) Reducing deaths from diarrhoea through oral rehydration therapy. Bulletin of the World Health Organization, 78:10; 1246–1255

Walsh JA, Warren KS (1979) Selective primary healthcare: an interim strategy for disease control in developing countries. New England Journal of Medicine, 301:18; 967–974

WHO/UNICEF (1978) Declaration of Alma-Ata. International Conference on Primary Healthcare, Alma-Ata, USSR, 6-12 September 1978. http://www.who.int/hpr/NPH/docs/declaration_almaata.pdf, cited 9 July 2008

WHO/UNICEF (1996) Revised 1990 estimates of maternal mortality: a new approach by WHO and UNICEF. Geneva: World Health Organization. http://whqlibdoc.who.int/hq/1996/WHO_FRH_MSM_96.11.pdf, cited 9 July 2008

Williams CD, Baumslag N, Jelliffe DB (1994) Mother and Child Health: Delivering the Services. New York: Oxford University Press

WHO General Assembly (1948) Universal Declaration of Human Rights, Article 25. New York: United Nations, 1948. http://www.un.org/Overview/rights.html, cited 9 July 2008

World Health Organization (1948) Constitution of the World Health Organization, Article 2(l). Geneva: World Health Organization, 1948 http://www.yale.edu/lawweb/avalon/decade/decad051.htm#art2, cited 9 July 2008

World Health Organization (1952) Expert Committee on Maternity Care: First Report. A Preliminary Survey. Geneva: World Health Organization (WHO Technical Report Series, No. 51)

World Health Organization (1986) Maternal Mortality Rates: A Tabulation of Available Information. Division of Family Health, World Health Organization WHO Document FHE/86.3. Geneva: World Health Organization. http://www.popline.org/docs/044860, cited 9 July 2008

World Health Organization (2004) Maternal Mortality in 2000: Estimates Developed by WHO, UNICEF and UNFPA. Geneva: World Health Organization, 2004. http://www.reliefweb.int/library/documents/2003/who-saf-22oct.pdf, cited 9 July 2008

World Health Organization (2005) The World Health Report 2005: Make Every Mother and Child Count. Geneva: World Health Organization. http://www.who.int/entity/whr/2005/whr2005_en.pdf, cited 9 July 2008

Chapter 2
Global Burden of Disease Among Women, Children, and Adolescents

Colin Mathers

Learning Objectives After reading this chapter and answering the discussion questions that follow, you should be able to

- Identify and discuss the conditions that contribute the most significantly to loss of health for children (ages 0–9 years), adolescents (ages 10–19 years), and women (ages 20 years and over) in different regions of the world.
- Appraise the burden of disease attributable to key risk factors for children, adolescents, and women in different regions of the world.
- Discuss the global distribution of mortality among children, women, and adolescents.
- Evaluate the importance of the global burden of disease studies and the implications for global health policy.

Introduction

Using the latest available estimates of mortality and disease burden from World Health Organization's (WHO) Global Burden of Disease (GBD) study for the year 2002, this chapter presents an analysis of major diseases and injuries that contribute most significantly to loss of health for children (ages 0–9 years), adolescents (ages 10–19 years), and women (ages 20 and over) for different regions of the world. The chapter draws heavily on an extensive WHO study of risk factors to provide further information

on attributable disease burden for selected key risk factors for children, adolescents, and women in different geographic regions of the world. As the analyses reveal, much of the global mortality among children is concentrated in middle- and low-income countries, particularly in south Asia and sub-Saharan Africa. Infectious diseases are the principal causes of mortality among children under 5, with five largely preventable conditions (lower respiratory infections, diarrheal diseases, malaria, HIV/AIDS, and measles) accounting for 70% of all child deaths in sub-Saharan Africa. A third of the mortality among children under the age of 10 was attributable to underweight, with unsafe water, sanitation, and hygiene accounting for another 13%. For adolescents aged 10–19, mental disorders (particularly depression, schizophrenia, and bipolar disorders), injuries (especially road traffic accidents), violence, and suicide were the leading causes of burden of disease. Alcohol use disorders were the second leading cause of burden of disease in adolescents in high-income countries. Globally among women aged 20–59, HIV/AIDS was the leading cause of burden of disease; it is responsible for one-half of deaths and disability-adjusted life years (DALYs) in this age group in sub-Saharan Africa.

Detailed description of the level and distribution of diseases, injuries, and their causes are important inputs to public health policies and programs. When we are interested in assessing all important causes of loss of health, the statistics that must be compared rapidly become large, and we face difficulties in comparing indicators relating to different health states, mortality risks, or disease events. Such statistics also suffer from several other limitations that reduce their practical value for policy making.

C. Mathers (✉)
Information, Evidence and Research Cluster, World Health Organization, Geneva, Switzerland

J.E. Ehiri (ed.), *Maternal and Child Health*, DOI 10.1007/b106524_2,

First, they are partial and fragmented. Basic information on causes of death are not available for all important causes in many countries, and mortality statistics fail to capture the impact of non-fatal conditions, such as mental disorders, musculoskeletal disorders, blindness, or deafness. Second, analyses of incidence, prevalence, or mortality for single causes often result in under- or over-estimates, when not constrained to fit within demographically plausible limits or to be internally consistent.

Diseases that cause a large number of deaths are clear public health priorities, but mortality statistics alone do not capture the burden of disease caused by chronic diseases, injuries, and mental health disorders. A substantial body of work in the last two decades has focused on the quantification of burden of disease using a summary measure that includes both disability (or loss of full health) and premature death and gives extra weight to diseases that primarily affect younger people, since mortality at younger ages results in a greater loss of years of life.

Global Burden of Disease (GBD) Studies

The initial Global Burden of Disease (GBD) Study was commissioned by the World Bank to provide a comprehensive assessment of disease burden in 1990 from more than 100 diseases and injuries, and from 10 selected risk factors (Murray and Lopez 1996a, b). As well as generating a comprehensive and consistent set of estimates of mortality and morbidity by age, sex, and region for the world, the GBD study introduced a new metric – the disability-adjusted life year (DALY) – to simultaneously quantify the burden of disease from premature mortality and the non-fatal consequences of over 100 diseases and injuries.

The WHO has undertaken a new assessment of the global burden of disease for the years 1999–2002, with annual assessments published in Annex Tables to the World Health Reports from 1998 to 2004 (World Health Organization 2004). Additionally, a major and expanded research program, the Comparative Risk Assessment (CRA) project, was undertaken to quantify the global and regional attributable mortality and burden for 26 major risk factors (Ezzati et al. 2004). These assessments were used as the framework for cost-effectiveness and priority setting analyses carried out for the Disease Control Priorities Project, a joint project of the World Bank, the World Health Organization, and the National Institutes of Health, funded by the Gates Foundation. The GBD results were documented in detail, with information on data sources and methods as well as uncertainty and sensitivity analyses, in a book published as part of the Disease Control Priorities Project (Lopez et al. 2006). The estimates for 2002 remain the latest available at the time of writing, although an incremental update which will include 2004 results will soon be available.

The Disability-Adjusted Life Year (DALY)

The disability-adjusted life year (DALY) extends the concept of potential years of life lost due to premature death (PYLL) to include equivalent years of "healthy" life lost from living in states of poor health or disability. One lost DALY can be thought of as one lost year of "healthy" life (either through death or illness/disability), and total DALYs (the burden of disease) as a measurement of the gap between the current health of a population and an ideal situation where everyone in the population lives into old age in full health. DALYs for a specific disease or injury cause are calculated as the sum of the years of life lost due to premature mortality (YLL) from that cause and the years lost due to disability (YLD) for incident cases of the disease or injury. The YLL are calculated from the number of deaths, d_x, at each age x multiplied by a global standard life expectancy, L_x, which is a function of age x:

$$YLL_x = \sum_x d_x \times L_x$$

The loss function L_x was specified in terms of the life expectancies at various ages in standard life tables with life expectancy at birth fixed at 82.5 years for females and 80.0 years for males, rather than using an arbitrary age cutoff such as 70 years. The loss function was specified to be the same for all deaths of a given age and sex, in all regions of the world (Murray and Lopez 1996b). Because YLL measure the incident stream of lost years of life due to deaths, an incidence perspective is taken for the calculation of YLD. The YLD for a particular cause in a particular time period are calculated by multiplying the number of incident cases i_x, at each age x in that period by the average duration of the disease for each age of incidence, l_x, and a weight factor dw_x that reflects the severity of the disease on a scale from 0 (full health) to 1 (dead):

$$YLD_x = \sum_x i_x \times l_x \times dw_x$$

YLD are calculated either for the average incident case of the disease or for one or more disabling sequelae of the disease. For example, YLD for diabetes are calculated by adding the YLD for uncomplicated cases and the YLD for sequelae such as diabetic neuropathy, retinopathy, and amputation. The "valuation" of time lived in non-fatal health states formalizes and quantifies social preferences for different states of health as *disability weights* (dw_x). These weights can also be described as health state valuations or health state preferences. In the formulation of the DALY, the disability weight is conceived of as quantifying the relative loss of health for different conditions or states and does not carry any implication about quality of life or the overall value of a life lived in particular health or disability states.

The disability weights used in the GBD for 2002, and the methods used to obtain them, are described elsewhere (Mathers et al. 2006). Murray and Lopez chose to apply a 3% time discount rate to the years of life lost in the future to estimate the net present value of years of life lost in calculating DALYs. Based on a number of studies that suggest the existence of a broad social preference to value a year lived by a young adult more highly than a year lived by a young child or an older person, Murray incorporated non-uniform age weights. When discounting and age weighting are both applied, a death in infancy corresponds to 33 DALYs, while deaths at ages 5–20 equate to around 36 DALYs. Discounting and age weighting essentially modify the loss function, L_x, in the calculation of YLL and the average duration, l_x, in the calculation of YLD. A more complete account of

the DALY, calculation formulae, and the philosophy underlying parameter choices is given by Murray (1996).

Data Sources and Methods

The GBD study developed methods and approaches to make estimates for causes of burden for which there was limited data and considerable uncertainty, to ensure that causes with limited information were not implicitly considered to have zero burden and hence ignored by health policy makers (Murray et al. 2003). The basic philosophy guiding the GBD approach is that there is likely to be useful information content in many sources of health data, provided they are carefully screened for plausibility and completeness and that internally consistent estimates of the global descriptive epidemiology of major conditions are possible with appropriate tools, investigator commitment, and expert opinion. Diseases and injuries are classified in the GBD using a tree structure based on the International Classification of Diseases. The highest level of aggregation consists of three broad cause groups: Group I (communicable, maternal, perinatal, and nutritional conditions), Group II (non-communicable diseases), and Group III (injuries). Group I causes are those conditions that typically decline at a faster pace than all-cause mortality during the epidemiological transition and occur largely in poor populations (see Table 2.1).

The GBD study produced comprehensive estimates for mortality and YLL by country, cause, and sex for 5-year age groups up to age 85 years and over. For incidence, prevalence, and YLD, estimates were made for 17 geographic regions and for 8 age groups: 0–4, 5–14, 15–29, 30–44, 45–59, 60–69, 70–79, and 80+. For the purposes of this chapter, the YLD estimates were imputed to the age groups 0–4, 5–9, 10–19, and 20–29 as follows: For cause–age–sex groups where the YLD/YLL ratio was less than 5, YLD were imputed to 5-year age groups using the YLL estimates for the 5-year age groups and the YLD/YLL ratio for the relevant broader age group. For other cause–age–sex groups where the DALY was dominated by non-fatal loss of health, the YLD rate per capita was assumed to be constant for the 5-year age groups within the

Table 2.1 Estimated global deaths and burden of disease by cause for children, adolescents, and women, 2002. Within each major group, disease and injury causes resulting in greater than 1% of total deaths or DALYs for all ages combined are shown, ranked within each group by global DALYs

	Children aged 0–9		Adolescents aged 10–19		Women aged 20 and over		All ages, both sexes	
	Deaths ('000)	DALYs ('000)	Deaths ('000)	DALYs ('000)	Deaths ('000)	DALYs ('000)	Deaths ('000)	DALYs ('000)
All causes				– Number (thousands) –				
Total number (thousands)	11,401	501,067	1,380	116,331	21,035	413,737	57,243	1,490,168
Rate per 1,000 population	9.3	409.9	1.2	98.1	10.9	215.2	9.2	239.4
Selected cause groups								
I. Communicable, maternal, perinatal, and nutritional conditions								
Group I total	9,905	388,643	533	31,656	3,920	104,146	18,538	612,185
Perinatal conditions*	2,462	97,300	0	2	0	1	2,462	97,303
Lower respiratory infections	1,986	71,410	155	6,315	918	7,847	3,947	93,617
HIV/AIDS	434	15,244	54	2,171	1,127	33,036	2,919	85,581
Diarrheal diseases	1,686	59,378	4	1,137	87	1,781	1,869	64,368
Malaria	827	31,634	11	991	36	1,037	908	34,604
Tuberculosis	62	2,460	55	2,447	479	10,405	1,566	34,726
Maternal conditions	0	113	66	7,787	444	25,698	510	33,599
Measles	599	21,004	9	346	0	1	607	21,352
Protein-energy malnutrition	166	15,537	18	661	39	335	260	16,883
II. Non-communicable diseases								
Group II total	961	76,144	300	56,402	15,848	273,930	33,537	696,298
Unipolar depressive disorders	0	3,003	0	11,775	7	32,347	13	67,052
Ischemic heart disease	8	420	14	863	3,395	23,691	7,208	58,632
Cerebrovascular disease	17	582	14	502	2,946	23,298	5,509	49,169
Chronic obstructive pulmonary disease	4	154	1	149	1,333	12,268	2,748	27,721
Hearing loss, adult onset	–	–	–	447	–	12,465	–	25,948
Cataracts	–	152	–	721	–	13,751	–	25,152
Alcohol use disorders	0	126	0	3,424	13	2,493	91	20,258
Diabetes mellitus	4	199	5	423	542	8,244	988	16,161

Table 2.1 (continued)

	Children aged 0–9		Adolescents aged 10–19		Women aged 20 and over		All ages, both sexes	
	Deaths ('000)	DALYs ('000)	Deaths ('000)	DALYs ('000)	Deaths ('000)	DALYs ('000)	Deaths ('000)	DALYs ('000)
Schizophrenia	0	803	0	5,241	12	5,298	23	16,090
Asthma	6	4,049	12	4,108	110	3,086	240	15,285
Osteoarthritis	0	5	0	485	3	8,730	5	14,809
Congenital heart anomalies	230	14,401	11	408	11	256	262	15,309
Vision disorders, age related	–	54	–	296	–	7,686	–	14,102
Bipolar disorder	0	356	0	4,613	1	4,450	1	13,903
Cirrhosis of the liver	30	1,206	14	669	256	4,158	786	13,973
Lung cancer	1	34	1	35	353	3,226	1,243	11,228
Nephritis and nephrosis	22	997	15	745	315	3,133	677	8,393
Stomach cancer	0	14	2	57	326	3,016	850	8,094
Hypertensive heart disease	2	84	2	72	490	3,714	911	7,643
Liver cancer	2	83	4	139	188	1,981	618	7,135
Colon and rectum cancer	0	3	1	37	299	2,684	622	5,817
III. Injuries								
Group III total	535	34,507	547	33,890	1,268	33,267	5,168	181,685
Road traffic accidents	136	7,207	138	7,066	229	5,915	1,192	38,630
Violence	20	1,074	66	3,981	90	2,636	559	21,372
Self-inflicted injuries	2	149	83	3,700	286	6,373	873	20,765
Falls	30	4,342	19	3,376	137	2,834	392	16,158
All causes								

* Includes "causes arising in the perinatal period" as defined in the International Classification of Diseases and does not include all causes of deaths occurring in the perinatal period.

Source: World Health Organization (2004)

broader YLD age range. Results are presented using World Bank geographic regions to group low- and middle-income countries. High-income countries in all regions are separately grouped as a single "high-income" group. Definitions of these regions are given by Lopez et al. (2006).

Estimation of Mortality Levels and Causes of Death

For the most recent GBD estimates at the WHO, life tables specifying mortality rates by age and sex for 192 WHO Member States were developed for 2002 from available death registration data (112 member states), sample registration systems (India, China), and data on child and adult mortality from censuses and surveys such as the Demography and Health Surveys (DHS) and UNICEF's Multiple Indicator Cluster Surveys (MICS). Death registration data containing usable information on cause of death distributions were available for 107 countries, the majority of these in the high-income group, Latin America and the Caribbean, and Europe and central Asia. Population-based epidemiological studies, disease registers, and notification systems (in excess of 2,700 data sets) contributed to the estimation of mortality due to 21 specific communicable causes of death, including HIV/ AIDS, malaria, tuberculosis, childhood immunizable diseases, schistosomiasis, trypanosomiasis, and Chagas disease. Almost one-third of these data sets related to sub-Saharan Africa. In order to address information gaps relating to other causes of death for populations without useable death registration data, models for estimating broad cause-of-death patterns based on GDP and overall mortality levels were used (Mathers et al. 2006).

Calculating Years Lived with Disability (YLD)

Estimating YLD requires systematic assessments of the available evidence on incidence, prevalence, duration, and severity of a wide range of conditions, often based on inconsistent, fragmented, and partial data available from different studies. Data sources included disease registers, epidemiological studies, health surveys, and health facility data (where relevant). Two key tools in dealing with limited or missing data were to carefully screen sources of health data for plausibility and completeness, drawing on expert opinion and on cross-population comparisons, and to explicitly ensure the internal consistency of estimates of incidence, prevalence, case fatality, and mortality for each specific disease cause. A software tool called DisMod was developed for the GBD study to help model the incidence and duration parameters needed for YLD calculations from available data, to incorporate expert knowledge, and to check the consistency of different epidemiological estimates and ensure that the estimates used were internally consistent (Barendregt et al. 2003).

Epidemiological estimates for incidence, prevalence, and YLD were first developed for 17 groupings of countries, and then imputed to country populations using available country-level information and methods to ensure consistency with the country-specific mortality estimates. The resulting country-level estimates were then used to prepare regional estimates for the World Bank country groups. Around 8,700 data sets were used to quantify the YLD estimates for GBD 2000–2002, of which more than 7,000 related to Group I causes. One-quarter of the data sets relate to populations in sub-Saharan Africa and around one-fifth to populations in high-income countries. Together with the more than 1,370 additional data sets used for the estimation of YLL, the 2000–2002 GBD Study incorporated information from over 10,000 data sets relating to population health and mortality. This almost certainly represents the largest synthesis of global information on population health ever carried out. Cause-specific data sources and methods are documented in more detail by Mathers et al. (2006).

Disease Burden from Risk Factors

There are many published analyses of disease and mortality attributable to individual risk factors such as tobacco smoking or unsafe water and sanitation, usually for specific populations. It is usually difficult to compare such estimates across risk factors due to different definitions and treatments of "hazardous exposure" and to differences in health outcome measures used. As part of the Global Burden of Disease project, a unified framework for Comparative Risk Assessment (CRA) was developed using a systematic and consistent approach to the assessment of the changes in population health (deaths or DALYs) which would result from modifying the population distribution of exposure to a risk factor or a group of risk factors (Ezzati et al. 2003). In the CRA framework, the burden of disease due to the observed exposure distribution in a population is compared with the burden from an alternative "theoretical minimum risk" distribution which is defined consistently for different risk factors.

The CRA project included 26 selected risk factors presented in Table 2.3. The criteria for selection of risk factors included that they were not too specific or broad, that the likelihood of causality was high based on scientific knowledge, that sufficient data on exposure levels and relative risks of health outcomes were available, and that they were potentially modifiable. For many of these risk factors, the counterfactual distribution is zero exposure (e.g., 100% of the population being never smokers). For some risk factors, where zero exposure is an inappropriate choice [e.g., body mass index (BMI), high blood pressure, or outdoor air pollution (where there is a physical lower limit to particulate matter concentration)], the lowest levels observed in specific low-risk populations and epidemiological studies were used to choose the theoretical minimum risk distribution. The counterfactual exposure distributions are specified elsewhere (Ezzati et al. 2002).

The proportional reduction in disease or death that would occur if exposure to a risk factor or group of risk factors were reduced to the counterfactual distribution is referred to as the population attributable fraction (PAF) and is given by the following relationship:

$$PAF = \frac{\int\limits_{x=0}^{m} RR(x)P(x)\,dx - \int\limits_{x=0}^{m} RR(x)P'(x)\,dx}{\int\limits_{x=0}^{m} RR(x)P(x)\,dx}$$

x: risk factor exposure level
$P(x)$: population distribution of exposure
$P'(x)$: counterfactual distribution of exposure
$RR(x)$: relative risk of mortality from site-specific cancer at exposure level x
m: maximum exposure level

For risk factors with discrete exposure levels, a similar equation can be written with summation over the discrete levels, rather than integration. Because most diseases are caused by multiple risk factors acting together, and because some risk factors act through others, PAFs for multiple risk factors for the same disease can add to more than 100% (Murray and Lopez 1999). In other words, the joint attributable burden of several risk factors combined may be less than the sum of the individual attributable burdens. For this reason, attributable burden estimates for individual risk factors presented below should not be added across risk factors. For each risk factor, between 1999 and 2002, an expert group conducted a comprehensive review of published literature as well as sources such as government reports, international databases to obtain data on risk factor exposure and the magnitude of hazardous effects (relative risk, RR, or absolute hazard size when appropriate) (Ezzati et al. 2004). This chapter presents some summary results for the mortality and burden of disease in the year 2002 attributable to the 26 selected risk factors. This measures the reduction in the current (2002) disease or death if the current and *past* exposure to the risk factor had been equal to a counterfactual distribution. The results presented here are based on the analyses carried out for the year 2000 for the CRA project. Age–sex–cause-specific PAFs calculated for the year 2000 for 14 subregions of the 6 WHO regions were applied to country-specific estimates of mortality and burden of disease for the year 2002 for each country in each of the 14 subregions. The results were aggregated for high-, low-, and middle-income countries.

Global Burden of Disease – An Overview

Just over 57 million people died in 2002, 10.4 million (or nearly 20%) of whom were children less than 5 years of age. Of these child deaths, 99%

occurred in low- and middle-income countries. Child and adolescent deaths under age 20 comprise just 1.5% of deaths in high-income countries, but more than 25% in low- and middle-income countries (Fig. 2.1). About 70% of deaths in high-income countries occurred beyond 70 years of age, compared to 30% in other countries. A key point is the comparatively high number of deaths in low- and middle-income countries at young and middle adult ages. The causes of death at these ages, as well as in childhood, are thus important in assessing public health priorities. Measured in

DALYs, 21% of total disease and injury burden for the world in 2002 was in children aged less than 10 years, 7.5% in adolescents aged 10–19 years, and 34% in women aged 20 years and over. The global disease burden for children fell almost entirely in low- and middle-income countries (Fig. 2.2). Table 2.1 summarizes estimated numbers of deaths and DALYs in 2002 for diseases and injuries which caused more than 1% of global deaths or DALYs.

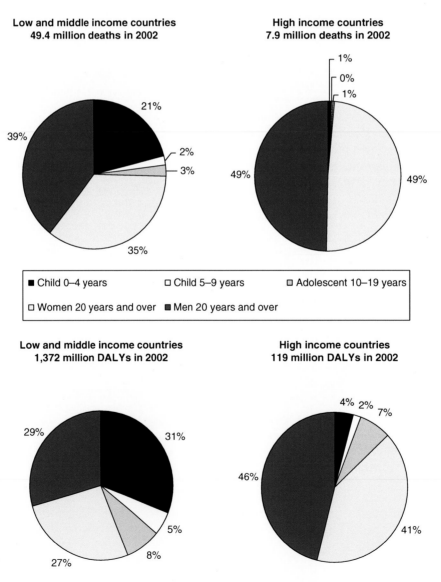

Fig. 2.1 Age–sex distribution of total deaths in low- and middle-income countries and in high-income countries, 2002

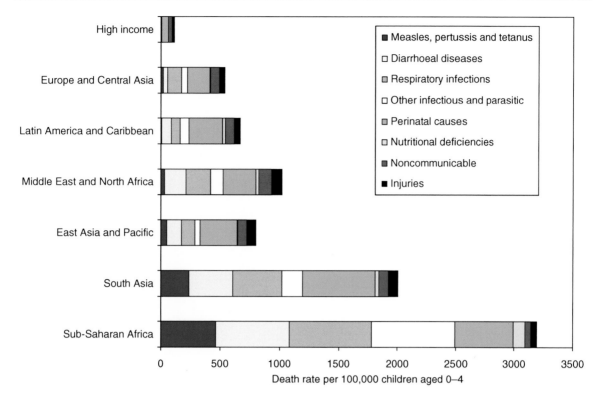

Fig. 2.2 Death rates by disease group and region for children aged 0–4 years, 2002. For all the World Bank geographical regions, high-income countries have been excluded and are shown as a single group at the top of the graph. Source: World Health Organization (2004)

The Burden of Disease in Children

Of the estimated 11.4 million deaths of children under age 10 in 2002, over 90% (or 10.4 million) were among children aged 0–4 years and 99% of these deaths occurred in low- and middle-income countries. The risk of a child dying before age 5 ranged from 17% in sub-Saharan Africa to 0.7% in high-income countries in 2002. Globally, conditions arising in the perinatal period such as prematurity, birth asphyxia, and severe neonatal infections were the leading cause of death under age 5, responsible for 2.5 million deaths (Table 2.1). Lower respiratory infections, principally pneumonia, diarrheal diseases, malaria, HIV/AIDS, and measles were the next leading causes. Collectively these five largely preventable causes were responsible for 70% of all child deaths.

Infectious and parasitic diseases remain the major killers of children in the developing world (Fig. 2.2 and Table 2.1). Although notable success has been achieved in certain areas (e.g., polio), communicable diseases still represent 7 out of the top 10 causes and cause about 60% of all child deaths. Overall, the 10 leading causes represent 83% of all child deaths under age 5. In contrast, in high-income countries perinatal conditions and congenital anomalies are the leading causes of child death (Table 2.2).

About 90% of all HIV/AIDS and malaria deaths in children in developing countries occurred in sub-Saharan Africa, where 23% of the world's births and 43% of the world's child deaths are found. The immense surge of HIV/AIDS mortality in children in recent years means that HIV/AIDS is now responsible for around 300,000 child deaths annually in sub-Saharan Africa and nearly 7% of all child deaths in the region. Some progress has been observed against diarrheal diseases and measles. While incidence is thought to have remained stable, mortality from diarrheal diseases has fallen from 2.5 million deaths in 1990 to about 1.7 million deaths in 2002, accounting for 15% of all child deaths under age 10.

Table 2.2 Leading causes of mortality by income group among children aged 0–4 years, 2002

Low- and middle-income countries				High-income countries			
	Cause	Deaths (thousands)	Percent of total deaths		Cause	Deaths (thousands)	Percent of total deaths
1	Perinatal conditions[a]	2,431	23.4	1	Perinatal conditions[a]	30.7	43.9
2	Lower respiratory infections	1,803	17.3	2	Congenital anomalies	16.9	24.2
3	Diarrheal diseases	1,681	16.2	3	Road traffic accidents	1.7	2.4
4	Malaria	822	7.9	4	Lower respiratory infections	1.5	2.2
5	Measles	537	5.2	5	Endocrine disorders	1.5	2.2
6	Congenital anomalies	408	3.9	6	Drownings	1.2	1.7
7	HIV/AIDS	340	3.3	7	Violence	1.0	1.5
8	Whooping cough	294	2.8	8	Meningitis	0.8	1.1
9	Tetanus	198	1.9	9	Leukemia	0.6	0.8
10	Protein-energy malnutrition	148	1.4	10	Inflammatory heart diseases	0.6	0.8

[a]Includes "causes arising in the perinatal period" as defined in the International Classification of Diseases and does not include all causes of deaths occurring in the perinatal period.
Source: World Health Organization (2004)

There has also been a significant decline in deaths from measles, although more than half a million children under 5 years were killed by measles in 2002. Malaria deaths are thought to have increased during the 1990 s to around 820,000 deaths among children under 5 years of age in 2002, nearly 8% of all under-5 deaths.

Many Latin American and some Asian and Middle-Eastern countries have partly shifted toward the cause-of-death pattern observed in high-income countries. Here, conditions arising in the perinatal period, including birth asphyxia, birth trauma, and low birth weight, have replaced infectious diseases as the leading causes of death and are now responsible for 21–36% of deaths. Such a shift in the cause-of-death pattern has not occurred in sub-Saharan Africa, where perinatal conditions rank in fourth place.

The Burden of Diseases and Injuries in Children

The leading causes of burden of disease in children aged 0–9 years, as measured in DALYs, are almost the same as for mortality, except that protein-energy malnutrition ranks somewhat higher as the seventh leading cause because of the considerable disability associated with lifelong stunting and, for many cases of severe stunting, associated cognitive impairment. Malnutrition (resulting in underweight) is also a risk factor for deaths from infectious causes as discussed in the following section. More than 85% of the burden of disease among children aged 0–9 is concentrated in children aged 0–4. Because DALYs are calculated using an incidence perspective, this means that 85% of lost years of healthy life are due to incident disease, injury, and mortality below age 5. However, there will be prevalent disability among children aged 5–9 years due to infectious diseases, nutritional deficiencies, congenital malformations, etc., present at birth or incident in the first 5 years. Almost 50% of the burden of disease in children aged 0–4 years is attributable to just seven infectious diseases: lower respiratory infections, diarrheal diseases, malaria, measles, whooping cough, HIV/ AIDS, and tetanus. Injuries become relatively more important for children aged 5–9 years. Among the top 10 causes of DALYs for this age group are road traffic accidents, falls, and fires. Although injuries become more important for boys beyond infancy, the causes of burden of disease are broadly similar for boys and girls.

Fig. 2.3 Mortality attributable to 10 leading global risk factors for children aged 0–9 years, as a percent of global deaths for children aged 0–9 years. The figure shows the estimated mortality and disease burden attributable to each risk factor considered individually. Source: World Health Organization (2004)

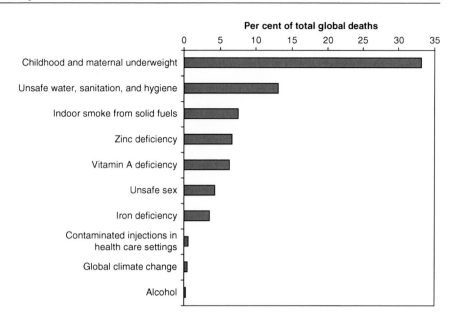

Leading Risk Factors for Mortality and Burden of Disease in Children

One-third of child deaths under age 10 in 2002 were attributable to underweight (primarily due to protein-energy malnutrition). Micronutrient deficiencies were also among the leading risk factors for child mortality (e.g., vitamin A deficiency [6.3%], zinc deficiency [6.7%], and iron deficiency [3.6%]) (Fig. 2.3 and Table 2.3). Unsafe water, sanitation, and hygiene was the second leading risk factor responsible for child deaths through diarrheal diseases primarily [13.0%] followed by indoor smoke from household use of solid fuels [7.5%] and unsafe sex [4.3%]. The mortality and burden of disease attributable to all these risks was primarily concentrated in south Asia and sub-Saharan Africa.

The Burden of Disease in Adolescents

While death rates and burden of disease rates are lower for adolescents than for children or adults aged 20 years and over, many of these deaths are preventable and strong regional differences remain (Fig. 2.4). The regional differentials are lower than for child deaths, and total death rates for

adolescents are very similar in all developing regions at just under 1 per 1,000 population except for south Asia, where the rate is twice as high, and sub-Saharan Africa, where it is almost three times as high. HIV/AIDS, tuberculosis, and maternal deaths explain much of the excess death rate in sub-Saharan Africa, along with higher rates from other infectious diseases and violence and war. For south Asia, the excess death rate is associated with high infectious disease death rates and with high injury death rates. Globally, lower respiratory infections and road traffic accidents were the leading causes of death in adolescents (Table 2.1). These were followed by suicide (6%), drownings (6%), and interpersonal violence (5%) (WHO 2004).

Road traffic accidents were the second leading cause of burden of disease in this age group, after unipolar major depression (Table 2.4). Injuries comprised four out of the ten leading causes of DALYs for adolescents as well. Several mental disorders also appear in the top 10 causes of burden including depression, schizophrenia, bipolar disorder, and alcohol use disorders (dependence and problem use of alcohol). Alcohol use disorders were the second leading cause of burden of disease in adolescents in high-income countries; in low- and middle-income countries they were only the 11th leading cause.

Table 2.3 Attributable global deaths (000) and DALYs (000) by risk factor – for children, adolescents, and women, 2002. The combined effects of any group of risk factors in this table will often be less than the sum of their separate effects

All causes	Children aged 0–9		Adolescents aged 10–19		Women aged 20 and over		All ages, both sexes	
	Deaths ('000)	DALYs ('000)	Deaths ('000)	DALYs ('000)	Deaths ('000)	DALYs ('000)	Deaths ('000)	DALYs ('000)
Childhood and maternal under-nutrition								
Childhood and maternal underweight	3,778	139,272	–	–	–	–	3,778	139,272
Iron deficiency	410	16,046	16	2,697	144	6,090	603	27,489
Vitamin A deficiency	718	25,018	15	551	90	2,599	823	28,177
Zinc deficiency	762	27,160	–	–	–	–	762	27,160
Other diet-related risks and physical inactivity								
High blood pressure	–	–	–	–	4,250	29,202	7,984	61,746
High cholesterol	–	–	–	–	2,077	16,200	4,018	36,495
Overweight and obesity	–	–	–	–	1,227	15,782	2,225	29,065
Low fruit and vegetable intake	–	–	5	241	1,165	10,434	2,526	24,855
Physical inactivity	–	–	3	188	980	8,942	1,981	19,560
Sexual and reproductive health risks								
Unsafe sex	492	18,217	55	4,014	1,380	39,367	3,162	95,005
Lack of contraception	–	–	13	1,551	149	7,501	162	9,052
Addictive substances								
Tobacco	–	–	–	–	1,029	11,545	5,039	61,284
Alcohol	25	1,338	85	7,600	379	8,410	2,199	61,557
Illicit drugs	0	87	6	1,740	50	2,410	247	12,336
Environmental risks								
Unsafe water, sanitation, and hygiene	1,483	52,213	4	992	76	1,547	1,643	56,554
Urban outdoor air pollution	22	735	–	–	359	2,339	769	6,079
Indoor smoke from solid fuels	851	29,948	–	–	549	4,522	1,592	36,430
Lead	2	9,793	2	85	80	1,058	246	13,172
Global climate change	62	2,494	1	105	3	111	70	2,808
Occupational risks								
Occupational airborne particulates	–	–	1	363	95	1,091	377	5,092
Occupational carcinogens	–	–	1	21	21	218	121	1,181
Occupational ergonomic stressors	–	–	0	96	0	312	1	854
Occupational noise	–	–	–	111	–	1,341	–	4,278
Occupational risk factors for injuries	–	–	27	1,518	17	636	315	10,767
Other selected risks to health								
Unsafe healthcare injections	66	2,356	12	506	153	2,789	543	10,908
Childhood sexual abuse	–	–	6	1,362	38	4,563	82	8,595

Source: World Health Organization (2004)

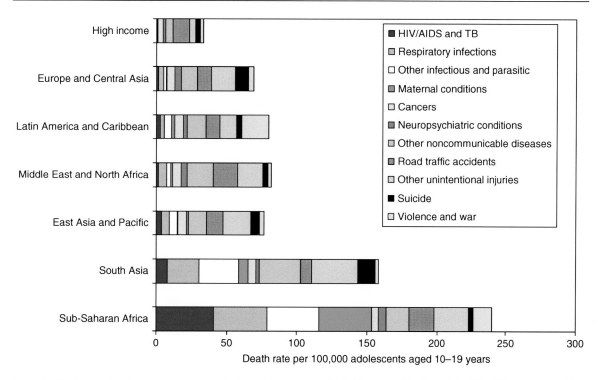

Fig. 2.4 Death rates by disease group and region for adolescents aged 10–19 years, 2002. For all the World Bank geographical regions, high-income countries have been excluded and are shown as a single group at the top of the graph. Source: World Health Organization (2004)

Table 2.4 Leading causes of disease burden by income group among adolescents aged 10–19 years, 2002

	Low- and middle-income countries				High-income countries		
	Cause	*DALYs (thousands)*	*Percent of total DALYs*			*Cause*	*DALYs (thousands)*	*Percent of total DALYs*
1	Unipolar depressive disorders	10,316	9.6	1	Unipolar depressive disorders	1,458	17.4
2	Road traffic accidents	6,443	6.0	2	Alcohol use disorders	820	9.8
3	Lower respiratory infections	6,294	5.8	3	Road traffic accidents	623	7.4
4	Schizophrenia	4,766	4.4	4	Asthma	521	6.2
5	Bipolar disorder	4,193	3.9	5	Schizophrenia	474	5.7
6	Violence	3,856	3.6	6	Migraine	468	5.6
7	Asthma	3,587	3.3	7	Bipolar disorder	420	5.0
8	Self-inflicted injuries	3,489	3.2	8	Drug use disorders	295	3.5
9	Falls	3,226	3.0	9	Panic disorder	228	2.7
10	Drownings	2,977	2.8	10	Self-inflicted injuries	211	2.5

Source: World Health Organization (2004)

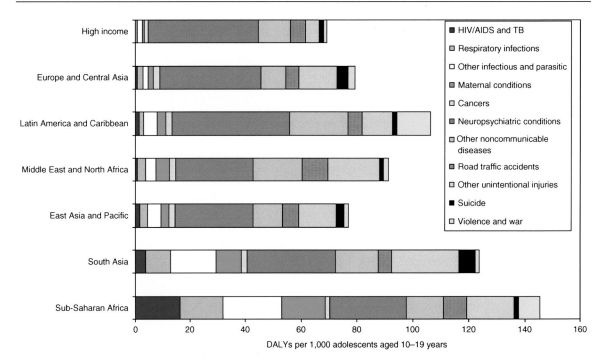

Fig. 2.5 DALYs per 1,000 population, by region and cause group, adolescents aged 10–19 years, 2002. For all the World Bank geographical regions, high-income countries have been excluded and are shown as a single group at the top of the graph. Source: World Health Organization (2004)

Interpersonal violence and war are disproportionately large contributors to adolescent burden of disease in Latin America and the Caribbean and in sub-Saharan Africa (Fig. 2.5). In sub-Saharan Africa, where there were significant conflict levels in a number of large countries, war and civil conflict were responsible for almost as much burden of disease as interpersonal violence. In Latin America, interpersonal violence is far more important, responsible for twice as many DALYs as road traffic accidents in the age group 10–19 years. Unintentional injuries other than road traffic accidents are also responsible for a much higher burden of disease in south Asia than in other regions.

Leading Risk Factors for Mortality and Burden of Disease in Adolescents

Among the selected 26 risk factors quantified in the CRA project, the leading attributable cause of mortality in adolescents was alcohol, responsible for around 6% of deaths in the age group 10–19 years.

This was followed by unsafe sex (4% of deaths) and selected occupational risks (totaling 2% of deaths). Alcohol was also the leading risk factor for burden of disease, responsible for an estimated 6.5% of DALYs in ages 10–19 (Fig. 2.6). These DALYs include the direct burden of alcohol dependence and problem use, as well as the attributable DALYs from causes such as road traffic accidents, which were estimated to already be responsible for increased burden of disease among this population group. Other important risk factors in this age range include unsafe sex, iron deficiency, occupational risks, illicit drugs, and lack of contraception.

The Burden of Disease in Women

Table 2.5 shows the 20 leading causes of deaths and DALYs among women aged 20–59 years worldwide for 2002. Despite a global trend of declining communicable disease burden in adults, HIV/AIDS has become the leading cause of mortality and the single most important contributor to the burden of disease

Fig. 2.6 DALYs attributable to 10 leading global risk factors for adolescents aged 10–19 years, as a percent of global DALYs for adolescents. The figure shows the estimated disease burden attributable to each risk factor considered individually. Source: World Health Organization (2004)

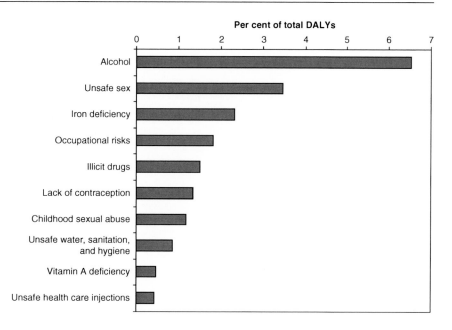

among women aged 20–59. Nearly 90% of the 1.1 million adult female deaths from HIV/AIDS globally in 2002 occurred in sub-Saharan Africa. In this region, HIV/AIDS accounted for almost half of deaths of adult women (aged 20–59). Owing to the impact of HIV/AIDS, there has been a reversal in mortality trends among women in this region and life expectancies for many countries have declined since 1990.

Injuries were also an important cause of death and burden of disease (Table 2.6). Road traffic accidents and self-inflicted injuries (suicide) were among the 10 leading causes of death, and fires and violence were also in the top 20 causes. Suicide was the fifth leading cause of death for women in this age group, after HIV/AIDS, ischemic heart disease, stroke, and tuberculosis. Other chronic diseases in the top 10 causes of death included breast cancer and chronic obstructive lung disease.

The overall death rate from all causes varied greatly across the regional groupings of low- and middle-income countries (Fig. 2.7) and between them and high-income countries. HIV/AIDS was largely responsible for the very high death rate in sub-Saharan Africa relative to other low-income countries, although other infectious diseases were

also a greater cause of death, as they were in south India. Maternal conditions, associated with pregnancy and childbirth, were also important in south Asia and Africa. Cardiovascular diseases were an important cause of death in all middle- and low-income regions of the world, but highest rates were in Europe and central Asia, reflecting the high rates of cardiovascular disease in former Soviet and Eastern European countries.

In developing countries, non-communicable diseases were responsible for more than 60% of deaths in women aged 20–59 in all regions except south Asia and sub-Saharan Africa, where Group I causes including HIV/AIDS remained responsible for two-fifths and three-quarters of deaths, respectively (Fig. 2.7). In other words, the epidemiologic transition is already well established in most developing countries. Maternal conditions were estimated to be responsible for 2.9% of deaths worldwide in females aged 20 and older in 2005 or 444,000 deaths. Among reproductive-age women aged 20–44, these conditions were responsible for 13.1% of deaths. The most common causes of maternal mortality include post-partum hemorrhage (25%), eclampsia (12%), unsafe abortions (13%), infections (15%), and obstructed labor (8%) (World Health Organization 2005).

Table 2.5 Twenty leading causes of mortality and disease burden in the world among women aged 20–59 years, 2002

	Mortality				Burden of disease		
	Cause	*Deaths (thousands)*	*Percent of total deaths*		*Cause*	*DALYs (thousands)*	*Percent of total DALYs*
1	HIV/AIDS	1,112	17.7	1	HIV/AIDS	32,871	10.8
2	Ischemic heart disease	416	6.6	2	Unipolar depressive disorders	30,086	9.9
3	Tuberculosis	325	5.2	3	Cataracts	9,295	3.1
4	Cerebrovascular disease	321	5.1	4	Tuberculosis	9,163	3.0
5	Self-inflicted injuries	214	3.4	5	Hearing loss, adult onset	9,028	3.0
6	Breast cancer	205	3.3	6	Ischemic heart disease	8,508	2.8
7	Lower respiratory infections	174	2.8	7	Cerebrovascular disease	7,812	2.6
8	Road traffic accidents	163	2.6	8	Osteoarthritis	6,189	2.0
9	COPD	145	2.3	9	Self-inflicted injuries	5,877	1.9
10	Maternal hemorrhage	130	2.1	10	COPD	5,631	1.9
11	Cirrhosis of the liver	112	1.8	11	Road traffic accidents	5,403	1.8
12	Diabetes mellitus[a]	107	1.7	12	Schizophrenia	5,238	1.7
13	Cervix uteri cancer	105	1.7	13	Maternal sepsis	5,120	1.7
14	Fires	104	1.7	14	Vision disorders, age related	4,851	1.6
15	Nephritis and nephrosis	90	1.4	15	Diabetes mellitus[a]	4,808	1.6
16	Lung cancer	87	1.4	16	Bipolar disorder	4,444	1.5
17	Stomach cancer	85	1.4	17	Lower respiratory infections	4,423	1.5
18	Hypertensive heart disease	72	1.1	18	Breast cancer	4,278	1.4
19	Violence	72	1.1	19	Maternal hemorrhage	3,907	1.3
20	Rheumatic heart disease	71	1.1	20	Anemia	3,659	1.2

[a]Does not include renal failure deaths attributable to diabetic nephropathy or cardiovascular disease deaths attributable to diabetes mellitus as a risk factor.
Source: World Health Organization (2004)

Diabetes caused around 550,000 deaths in women aged 20 years and over. Diabetes increases the risk of cardiovascular disease and the total attributable deaths are likely to be more than double the direct deaths. Together, cardiovascular disease and diabetes were responsible for more than two in five deaths among women aged 20 years and over. Just fewer than 1 million women aged 20–59 died of cancer in 2002. The most common cancers were breast cancer (22% of cancer deaths in women aged 20-59), cervical cancer (11%), lung cancers (9%), and stomach cancers (9%), but there are significant regional variations in the prevalence of cancer by site.

Disability and Burden of Disease

Among the 10 leading causes of burden of disease for adult women aged 20–59 are four non-fatal conditions: unipolar depressive disorders,

Table 2.6 Leading causes of disease burden among women aged 60+ years in the world, 2002

Low- and middle-income countries			High-income countries		
Cause	DALYs (thousands)	Percent of total DALYs	Cause	DALYs (thousands)	Percent of total DALYs
1 Ischemic heart disease	2,979	20.2	1 Cerebrovascular disease	15,486	14.0
2 Cerebrovascular disease	2,625	17.8	2 Ischemic heart disease	15,183	13.7
3 COPD	1,188	8.0	3 COPD	6,637	6.0
4 Lower respiratory infections	744	5.0	4 Alzheimer and other dementias	5,468	4.9
5 Diabetes mellitus[a]	436	3.0	5 Cataracts	4,456	4.0
6 Hypertensive heart disease	418	2.8	6 Hearing loss, adult onset	3,437	3.1
7 Breast cancer	270	1.8	7 Diabetes mellitus[a]	3,437	3.1
8 Lung cancer	265	1.8	8 Lower respiratory infections	3,424	3.1
9 Alzheimer and other dementias	244	1.7	9 Vision disorders, age related	2,835	2.6
10 Stomach cancer	240	1.6	10 Osteoarthritis	2,541	2.3

[a]Does not include renal failure deaths attributable to diabetic nephropathy or cardiovascular disease deaths attributable to diabetes mellitus as a risk factor.

Source: World Health Organization (2004)

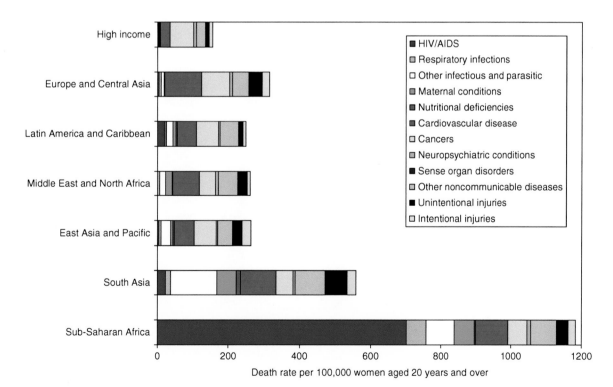

Fig. 2.7 Death rates by disease group and region for women aged 20–59 years, 2002. For all the World Bank geographical regions, high-income countries have been excluded and are shown as a single group at the top of the graph. Source: World Health Organization (2004)

Fig. 2.8 Global YLD, YLL, and DALYs for major disease groups, women aged 20–59 years, 2002. DALYs are the sum of years of life lost due to premature mortality (YLL) and years lived with disability (YLD). Source: World Health Organization (2004)

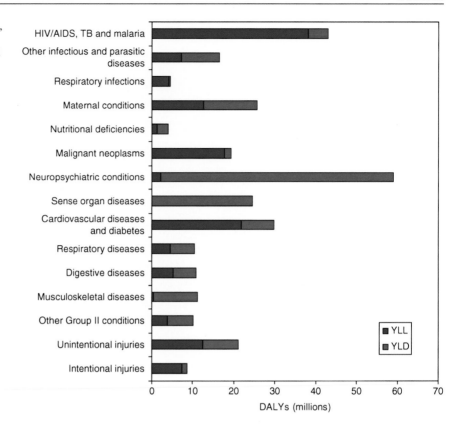

cataracts, adult-onset hearing loss, and osteoarthritis. Figure 2.8 summarizes the contributions of premature mortality (YLL) and disability (YLD) to the burden of disease for the various major cause groups. In all regions, neuropsychiatric conditions are the most important causes of disability, accounting for over 37% of YLDs among women aged 20–59 years. While depression is the leading cause of disability for both males and females, the burden of depression is 50% higher for females than males, and females also have higher burden from anxiety disorders, migraine, and senile dementias. In contrast, the male burden for alcohol and drug use disorders is nearly six times higher than that for females, and accounts for one-quarter of the male neuropsychiatric burden. Vision disorders, hearing loss, and musculoskeletal disorders are also important causes of YLD, particularly for women, in both developed and developing countries. The burden of non-communicable diseases accounted for just

over one-half of the global burden of disease for women aged 20–59 in 2002, and close to one-third of the non-communicable disease burden was due to neuropsychiatric conditions (Fig. 2.9).

Mortality and Burden of Disease for Adult Women Aged 60 Years and Over

The risk of death rises rapidly with age among women aged 60 and over in all regions. Globally, 60-year-old women have an 18% chance of dying before their 70th birthday. Regional variations in risk of death at older ages are smaller than at younger ages, although death rates at older ages are significantly lower in high-income countries where a 60-year-old woman has on average, a 9% chance of dying before age 70. Historical data from countries such as Australia and Sweden show that life expectancy at age 60 changed slowly

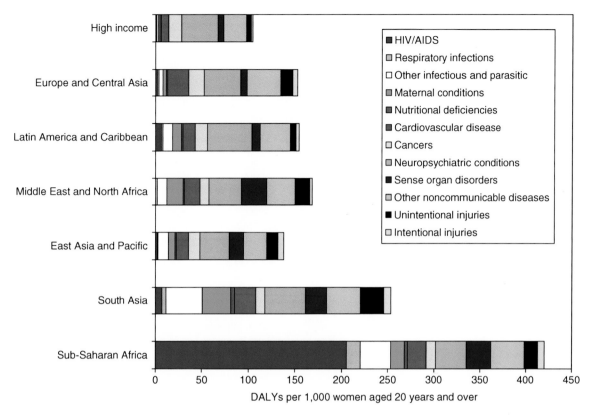

Fig. 2.9 DALYs per 1,000 population, by disease group and region for women aged 20–59 years, 2002. For all the World Bank geographical regions, high-income countries have been excluded and are shown as a single group at the top of the graph. Source: World Health Organization 2004

during the first six to seven decades of the 20th century but since around 1970 has started to increase substantially. Life expectancy at age 60 has now reached 27 years in Japan. In Eastern Europe from 1990 onward, Poland and Hungary have started to experience similar improvements in mortality for older women, but Russia has not.

Female deaths at ages 60 years and over are predominantly due to chronic (non-communicable diseases) and globally the leading causes of death in 2002 were ischemic heart disease, cerebrovascular disease, and chronic respiratory disease. Together with diabetes mellitus, these causes were responsible for just under one-half of all female deaths at ages 60 and greater. Other leading causes of death included acute lower respiratory infections (pneumonia and influenza), breast cancer, lung cancer, stomach cancer, and senile dementia. Chronic obstructive pulmonary disease (COPD) was responsible for about 1.3 million female deaths in 2002.

The primary risk factor for COPD is tobacco use, and as more females smoke, the prevalence of COPD will increase.

While Alzheimer disease and other dementias were the leading cause of YLD for older females, sight and hearing loss disorders accounted for four of the ten leading causes of disability. Other important causes included cerebrovascular disease, diabetes, and chronic lung disease. YLD rates were higher in low- and middle-income countries than in high-income countries in 2002 although their variation across regions was much lower than for YLL rates. The prevalence of disabling conditions such as dementia and musculoskeletal disease was higher in high-income countries due to the higher proportions of older women in their populations and, for dementia, to higher age-specific prevalence rates than in low- and middle-income countries. This was offset by lower contributions to disability in high-income countries from conditions such as cardiovascular and chronic respiratory diseases, and long-term sequelae of communicable diseases and nutritional deficiencies. In other words, women living in developing countries not only face shorter life expectancies than those in developed countries but also live a higher proportion of their lives in poor health.

In terms of overall DALYs for women aged 60 years and older, ischemic heart disease, cerebrovascular disease, and chronic obstructive pulmonary disease were the three leading causes (together responsible for one-third of all DALYs in this age group), followed by Alzheimer and other dementias, and cataracts. Vision disorders, including cataracts and age-related vision disorders, were responsible for 7% of the total DALYs, around double the burden of hearing loss.

Burden of Disease Attributable to Selected Risk Factors for Women Aged 20 Years and Over

The leading global causes of mortality and disease burden for women aged 20 years and over included risk factors for communicable, maternal, perinatal, and nutritional conditions (e.g., unsafe sex; indoor smoke from household use of solid fuels; and iron deficiency), whose burden is primarily concentrated in the low-income and high-mortality regions of sub-Saharan Africa and east Asia, as well as risk factors for non-communicable diseases (e.g., high blood pressure and cholesterol, tobacco and alcohol use, and overweight and obesity) which affect most regions. High blood pressure was the single leading global cause of mortality for adult women, responsible for 20% of all deaths, although most of these are at older ages. In terms of DALYs, which measure lost years of full health, high blood pressure is second behind unsafe sex (Fig. 2.10a, b)

Leading causes of burden of disease in low- and middle-income countries were unsafe sex (10%), high blood pressure (7%), high serum cholesterol (3.8%), and high body mass index – or overweight and obesity (3.2%). The relative contribution of unsafe sex was disproportionately larger (40%) in sub-Saharan Africa where HIV/AIDS prevalence is

the highest, making it the leading cause of burden of disease in these countries. In high-income countries, smoking (9%), high blood pressure (8%), high BMI (7%), high cholesterol (4.6%), and alcohol use (4.2%) were consistently the leading causes of loss of healthy life, contributing mainly to non-communicable diseases and, to a lesser extent, injuries.

Discussion and Conclusions

The analysis presented here has confirmed some of the conclusions of the original GBD study about the importance of including non-fatal outcomes in a comprehensive assessment of global population health and has confirmed the growing importance of non-communicable diseases for women in low- and middle-income countries, but has also documented some dramatic changes in women's health in some regions since 1990. Among the key findings are the following:

- The vast majority of child deaths are concentrated in middle- and low-income countries, particularly in south Asia and sub-Saharan Africa. Infectious diseases remain the principal killers of children under 5. Just five largely preventable conditions were responsible for 70% of all child deaths in 2002: lower respiratory infections, diarrheal diseases, malaria, HIV/AIDS, and measles.
- One-third of child deaths under age 10 in 2002 were attributable to underweight, and another 13% to unsafe water, sanitation, and hygiene.
- Mental disorders, particularly depression, schizophrenia, and bipolar disorders, and injuries, particularly road traffic accidents, violence, and suicide, were the leading causes of burden of disease in adolescents aged 10–19 in 2002. Alcohol use disorders were the second leading cause of burden of disease in adolescents in high-income countries.
- HIV/AIDS is now the leading cause of burden of disease among women aged 20–59 years globally, and responsible for one-half of deaths and DALYs in this group in sub-Saharan Africa.
- The epidemiological transition in low- and middle-income countries has resulted in a 20%

Fig. 2.10a, b Mortality attributable to 10 leading global risk factors for women aged 20 years and over, as a percent of global deaths for women aged 20 years and over. The figure shows the estimated mortality and disease burden attributable to each risk factor considered individually. Source: World Health Organization (2004)

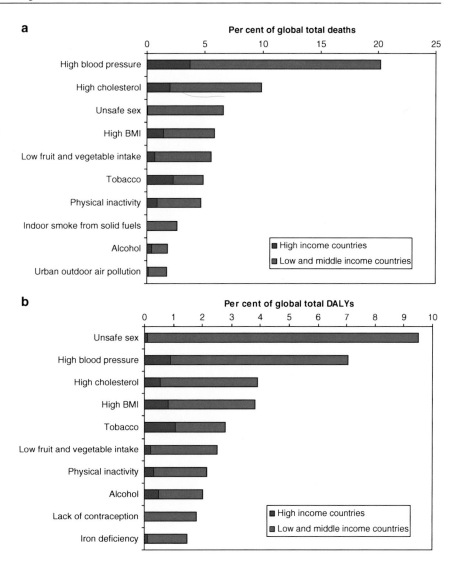

reduction since 1990 in the per capita disease burden due to Group I causes (communicable, maternal, perinatal, and nutritional conditions). Without the HIV/AIDS epidemic, this reduction would have been substantially greater, at 30% over the last 11 years. Several of the "traditional" infectious diseases such as tuberculosis and malaria have not declined, in part because of weak public health services and the increased numbers of women with immune systems weakened by HIV/AIDS.

- The per capita disease burden in Europe and central Asian countries has increased since

1990, so that women in this region now have similar levels of health to other low- and middle-income countries of the world apart from those in south Asia and sub-Saharan Africa.

- Women aged 20–59 in low- and middle-income countries have substantially greater mortality risks and disease burden from non-communicable diseases than those in high-income countries.

- Injury deaths are noticeably higher for women in some parts of Asia and the Middle East and North Africa, in part due to high levels of suicide and violence. This higher burden of injury deaths in combination with higher rates of infant and child mortality for girls result in the narrowest differential between male and female healthy life expectancy for any of the low- and middle-income regions.

- High blood pressure is the leading risk factor for attributable mortality for women aged 20 years and over, responsible for an estimated 20% of deaths in 2002. In terms of burden of disease, unsafe sex was the leading risk factor, responsible for 10% of DALYs.
- Sense organ disorders, principally hearing and sight loss, contribute significantly to disability among older women in all regions of the world. Levels of non-fatal health loss are proportionately greater in lower income countries than in high-income countries, contrary to the perception that disability is associated with older populations.

The GBD analyses have been criticised for making estimates of mortality and burden of disease for regions with limited, incomplete, and uncertain data (Cooper et al. 1998). Murray and colleagues have argued that health planning based on uncertain assessments of the available evidence, which attempt to synthesize it while ensuring consistency and adjustment for known biases, will almost always be more informed than planning based on ideology (Murray et al. 2003). The GBD analytic approach has been strongly influenced by demographic and economic traditions of making the best possible estimates of quantities of interest for populations from the available data, using a range of techniques depending on the type and quality of evidence.

While methodological and data developments over the past decade have improved the empirical base for disease burden assessment, there are still very substantial data gaps and uncertainties, particularly for causes of death and levels of adult mortality in Africa and parts of Asia. Improving the population-level information on causes of death and on the incidence, prevalence, and health states associated with major disease and injury causes remains a major priority for national and international health and statistical agencies. At the time of writing, the Gates Foundation has decided to provide substantial funding for an international collaborative effort, led by Chris Murray and with the WHO collaboration, to carry out a complete revision and update of the Global Burden of Disease over the next 3 years, taking advantage of recent developments in data collection and analysis methods. Despite the uncertainties in the 2002 estimates, the results summarized here suggest that further gains in health for children, adolescents, and women in developing countries could be achieved. Intervention choices and priorities can be better guided by information about potential costs and gains, including a comprehensive understanding of disease burden. More rational application of the available information and knowledge in this area would accelerate progress toward millennium development goals and reduce the persistent differentials in health that show little tendency to narrow under current health policies.

Key Terms

Age weighting	Global descriptive	Observed exposure distribution
Alcohol	epidemiology	Plausibility
Attributable mortality	Hazardous exposure	Population attributable
Bipolar disorders	High-income countries	fraction (PAF)
Body mass index (BMI)	HIV/AIDS	Population distribution of
Burden of disease	Hygiene	exposure
Causality	Incidence	Potential years of life lost to
Cause-of-death patterns	Individual attributable burden	premature death (PYLL)
Central America	Infectious diseases	Premature death
Chronic diseases	Injuries	Prevalence
Comparative Risk Assessment	Internally consistent estimates	Quality of life
(CRA)	International Classification of	Relative loss of health
Counterfactual distribution	Diseases (ICD)	Relative risk
Death registration	Latin America and the	Retinopathy
Demography and Health	Caribbean	Risk factor exposure level
Surveys	Life expectancy	Risk factors
Depression	Low-income countries	Sanitation
Diabetic neuropathy	Lower respiratory tract	Schizophrenia
Diarrheal diseases	infections	Sensitivity analysis
Disability	Malaria	Standard life table
Disability-adjusted life years	Maximum exposure level	Sub-Saharan Africa
(DALYs)	Measles	Suicide
Disability weights	Mental disorders	Theoretical minimum risk
Discounting	Middle-income countries	Theoretical minimum risk
Discrete exposure levels	Multiple Indicator Cluster	distribution
Disease control priority	Survey	Underweight
Disease notification systems	Musculoskeletal disorders	Unsafe water
DisMod	Non-fatal conditions	Valuation
Epidemiological transition	Non-uniform age weights	Violence
Global Burden of Disease	North Africa and the Middle	Years of life lost to premature
Study	East	mortality (YLL)

Questions for Discussion

1 Write short explanatory notes to summarize your understanding of the following terms:

   a. Disability-adjusted life years
   b. Epidemiological transition
   c. Population attributable fraction (PAF)
   d. Comparative Risk Assessment (CRA)

2 In what ways can information on global burden of disease aid global health policy? What are the limitations of global burden of disease estimates?

3 Identify the major causes of global burden of morbidity and mortality for the following age groups:

   a. Children aged 0–9 years
   b. Adolescents aged 10–19 years
   c. Women aged 20 years and older

4 Discuss the major features of disease burden and risk factors in low-income countries compared to high-income countries.

References

Barendregt J, van Oortmarssen GJ et al. (2003) A generic model for the assessment of disease epidemiology: the computational basis of DisMod II. Population Health Metrics, 1, 4

Cooper RS, Osotimehin B et al. (1998) Disease burden in sub-Saharan Africa: what should we conclude in the absence of data? The Lancet, 351(9097), 208–210

Ezzati M, Vander Hoom S, Rodgers A et al. (2002) Comparative Risk Assessment Collaborative Group. Selected major risk factors and global and regional burden of disease. Lancet, 360(9343), 1347–1360

Ezzati M, Vander Hoom S, Rodgers A et al. (2003) Comparative Risk Factors Collaborating Group. Estimates of global and regional potential health gains from reducing multiple major risk factors. The Lancet, 362, 271–280

Ezzati M, Lopez AD, Rodgers A, et al. (2004) Comparative Quantification of Health Risks: Global and Regional Burden of Disease Attributable to Selected Major Risk. World Health Organization, Geneva

Lopez AD, Mathers CD, Ezziati M et al. (2006) Global Burden of Disease and Risk Factors. Oxford University Press, New York

Mathers CD, Lopez AD, Murray CJL (2006) The burden of disease and mortality by condition: data, methods and results for 2001. In Global Burden of Disease and Risk Factors, Lopez AD et al. (eds.). Oxford University Press, New York, pp. 45–240

Murray CJL (1996) Rethinking DALYs. In The Global Burden of Disease, vol. 1 Murray CJL, Lopez AD (eds.). Harvard University Press, Cambridge, pp. 1–98

Murray CJL, Lopez AD (1996a) Global Health Statistics. Harvard University Press, Cambridge

Murray CJL, Lopez AD (1996b) The Global Burden of Disease: A Comprehensive Assessment of Mortality and Disability from Diseases, Injuries and Risk Factors in 1990 and projected to 2020. Harvard University Press, Cambridge

Murray CJL, Lopez AD (1999) On the comparable quantification of health risks: lessons from the global burden of disease study. Epidemiology 10(5), 594–605

Murray CJL, Mathers CD, Salomon JA (2003) Towards evidence-based public health. In Health Systems Performance Assessment: Debates, Methods and Empiricism. Murray CJL, Evans D (eds.). World Health Organization, Geneva

World Bank (1993) World Development Report 1993. Investing in Health. Oxford University Press for the World Bank, New York, http://files.dcp2.org/pdf/World-DevelopmentReport1993.pdf, cited 7 July 2008

World Health Organization (2004) World Health Report 2004: Changing History. World Health Organization, Geneva, http://www.who.int/whr/2004/en/, cited 7 July 2008

World Health Organization (2005) World Health Report 2005: Make Every Mother and Child Count. World Health Organization, Geneva, http://www.who.int/whr/2005/en/index.html, cited 7 July 2008

Chapter 3
Promotion of Global Perinatal Health

Victor Y.H. Yu

Learning Objectives After reading this chapter and answering the discussion questions that follow, you should be able to

- Present an overview of perinatal mortality rates, stillbirth rates, and neonatal mortality rates in different geographical and economic regions of the world.
- Identify and discuss factors that influence perinatal survival from a global perspective.
- Identify and evaluate the evidence base of specific low-cost interventions to improve perinatal health.

Introduction

Globally, there are 141 million annual live births; 127 million (90%) of which occur in developing countries. These regions also have a higher rate of contribution to the 7.5 million annual perinatal deaths and 5.1 million neonatal deaths. The perinatal mortality rate (PMR) and the neonatal mortality rate (NMR) have often been used as indicators of the standard of a country's social, educational, and health-care systems. Developing regions of the world, and particularly rural areas, where there are few skilled birth attendants experience disproportionately high perinatal mortality rates. This chapter presents an overview of perinatal health, providing data on perinatal mortality rates, stillbirth rates, and neonatal mortality rates across the globe. Underlying causes of stillbirths and neonatal deaths

are exacerbated by lack of health-care and poorly distributed health-care access and funding. Discrepancies in data collection and measurement in some regions and the resulting lack of comparable data pose challenges to assessment and response to perinatal mortality. Sixteen low-cost, community-based interventions with proven efficacy for neonatal survival have been identified across the prenatal, antenatal, intrapartum, and postpartum stages. Standardizing and improving available data and directing more funding to prevention of perinatal mortality are key factors in reducing mortality rates. Strategies that address inequalities both within a country, and between countries are necessary if there is going to be further improvement in global perinatal health.

Perinatal mortality refers to death in the perinatal period that includes late pregnancy, birth, and the neonatal period. By avoiding the difficult judgment of whether a fetus exhibits signs of life or not at birth, it is a useful measure for comparison of reproductive loss and perinatal health between countries. Although the global perinatal mortality rate (PMR) has fallen by about 10% in the last decade, the total number of perinatal deaths has remained unchanged because the number of births has increased in the same period. No systematic global estimates of stillbirths exist, and any statistical modeling used to predict stillbirth number and stillbirth rate (SBR) probably underestimates both figures. Epidemiological data on the estimated 450 neonatal deaths every hour around the world remain sparse, but most of these deaths are considered preventable and, halving of the global neonatal mortality rate (NMR) is an achievable goal. In this chapter, published data on perinatal outcomes (including available estimates of global and regional PMR, SBR, and NMR) are

Victor Y.H. Yu (✉)
Monash University, Australia

J.E. Ehiri (ed.), *Maternal and Child Health*, DOI 10.1007/b106524_3,
© Springer Science+Business Media, LLC 2009

reviewed, problems and obstacles associated with the promotion of perinatal health are described, and strategies that are potentially effective in improving perinatal health in the future are suggested. Box 3.1 presents definitions of common terminologies used in the field of perinatology.

Box 3.1 Definition of Terms

Live birth: Live birth is the complete expulsion or extraction from its mother, of a product of conception, irrespective of the duration of the pregnancy, which, after such separation, breathes or shows any other evidence of life, such as beating of the heart, pulsation of the umbilical cord, or definite movement of voluntary muscles, whether or not the umbilical cord has been cut or the placenta is attached; each product of such a birth is considered live-born.
   Fetal death: Fetal death is death prior to the complete expulsion or extraction from its mother of a product of conception, irrespective of the duration of pregnancy; the death is indicated by the fact that after such separation the fetus does not breathe or show any other evidence of life, such as beating of the heart, pulsation of the umbilical cord, or definite movement of voluntary muscles.
   Birth weight: The first weight of the fetus or newborn obtained immediately after birth.

Low birth weight: Less than 2500 g (up to, and including 2499 g).
   Very low birth weight: Less than 1500 g (up to, and including 1499 g).
   Extremely low birth weight: Less than 1000 g (up to, and including 999 g).

Gestational age: The duration of gestation is measured from the first day of the last normal menstrual period.

Pre-term: Less than 37 completed weeks (less than 259 days) of gestation.
   Term: From 37 completed weeks to less than 42 completed weeks (259–293 days) of gestation.
   Post-term: Forty-two completed weeks or more (294 days or more) of gestation.
   Perinatal period: The perinatal period commences at 22 completed weeks (154 days) of gestation (the time when birth weight is normally 500 g), and ends seven completed days after birth.
   Neonatal period: The neonatal period commences at birth and ends 28 completed days after birth.
   Neonatal deaths: Deaths among live-births during the first 28 completed days of life; may be subdivided into early neonatal deaths, occurring during the first seven days of life, and late neonatal deaths, occurring after the seventh day but before 28 completed days of life.

Fetal death ratio

$$\frac{\text{Fetal deaths}}{\text{Live-births}} \times 1000$$

Fetal death rate

$$\frac{\text{Fetal deaths}}{\text{Total births}} \times 1000$$

Fetal death rate, weight-specific

$$\frac{\text{Fetal deaths weighing 1000 g and over}}{\text{Total births weighing 1000 g and over}} \times 1000$$

Early neonatal mortality rate

$$\frac{\text{Early neonatal deaths}}{\text{Live-births}} \times 1000$$

Early neonatal mortality rate, weight-specific

$$\frac{\text{Early neonatal deaths of infants weighing 1000 g and over at birth}}{\text{Live-births weighing 1000 g and over}} \times 1000$$

Perinatal mortality ratio

$$\frac{\text{Fetal deaths and early neonatal deaths}}{\text{Live-births}} \times 1000$$

Perinatal mortality rate

$$\frac{\text{Fetal deaths and early neonatal deaths}}{\text{Total births}} \times 1000$$

Perinatal mortality rate, weight-specific

$$\frac{\text{Fetal deaths weighing 1000 g and over, plus early neonatal deaths of infants weighing 1000 g and over at birth}}{\text{Total births weighing 1000 g and over}} \times 1000$$

Neonatal mortality rate

$$\frac{\text{Neonatal deaths}}{\text{Live-births}} \times 1000$$

Neonatal mortality rate, weight-specific

$$\frac{\text{Neonatal deaths of infants weighing 1000 g and over at birth}}{\text{Live-births weighing 1000 g and over}} \times 1000$$

Infant mortality rate

$$\frac{\text{Deaths under one year of age}}{\text{Live-births}} \times 1000$$

Infant mortality rate, weight-specific

$$\frac{\text{Infant deaths among live-births weighing 1000 g and over at birth}}{\text{Live-births weighing 1,000 g and over}} \times 1000$$

Source: World Health Organization (2006)

Perinatal Outcome

Perinatal Deaths

The Maternal and Safe Motherhood Program of the World Health Organization (WHO) gave an estimate of 7.5 million annual perinatal deaths and a global PMR of 53 per 1,000 births (WHO 1996). Great disparities were reported to exist in PMR between the five world regions: Africa (75 per 1,000), Asia–Oceania (53 per 1,000), Central and South America (39 per 1,000), Europe (13 per 1,000), and North America (9 per 1,000). The differences in PMR could partly be explained by the proportion of developed and developing countries in these world regions. The PMR in developing countries was estimated to be 5.2 times higher than that, in developed countries. This discrepancy has progressively worsened in recent years, because over a period, when a 35% reduction in PMR was observed in developed countries, developing countries saw only an 11% reduction in PMR (Yu 2003).

The world region with the largest number of annual births is the Asia–Oceania region. Therefore, although its PMR is not the highest but second to that of Africa, it has the greatest number of perinatal deaths among the five regions. Further analysis of the five sub-regions within the Asia–Oceania region has shown that south Asia has the highest estimated PMR (66 per 1,000) followed by west Asia and Oceania (44 per 1,000), east Asia (41 per 1,000), and Southeast Asia (37 per 1,000). Within the Asia–Oceania region, there are only five places that have a PMR below 10 per 1,000: Australia, Hong Kong, Japan, New Zealand and Singapore. However, the number of births in these places with a more favorable PMR was relatively low: Australia (260,000), Hong Kong (300,000), Japan (1.3 million), New Zealand (60,000), and Singapore (40,000). In total, less than 1.7 million or just over 2% of the annual births in the Asia–Oceania region were from these five places. In contrast to these low PMR settings, countries in the sub-region of south Asia such as Bangladesh, Pakistan, Nepal, and India have an estimated PMR of 65–85 per 1,000. Sri Lanka was the one exception with a relatively low PMR of 25 per 1,000. Countries in the sub-region of west Asia could be divided into three groups. The first group with the highest PMRs included Yemen, Turkey, Syria, and Iraq (40–70 per 1,000). The second group with medium-high PMRs included Iran, Jordan, Oman, and Saudi Arabia (30 per 1,000). The third group with medium-low PMRs included Bahrain, Kuwait, and United Arab Emirates (20 per 1,000). The sub-region of east Asia has always been dominated by China with over twenty million annual births and an estimated PMR of 45 per 1,000. Excluding Hong Kong and Japan, South Korea has the best PMR in east Asia (15 per 1,000). Countries in the sub-region of Southeast Asia have a relatively wide range of estimated PMRs. The highest was found in Laos and Cambodia (65–90 per 1,000), medium high in Indonesia and Myanmar (45–55 per 1,000), and medium low in Vietnam, Philippines, and Thailand (20–25 per 1,000). Excluding Australia, New Zealand, and Singapore, Malaysia has the best PMR in Southeast Asia (20 per 1,000).

Stillbirths

The most recently published global estimate of 3.2 million stillbirths (uncertainty interval 2.5–4.1 million) is similar to the WHO estimate of 3.3 million in 2005, which is less than the previous WHO estimates of 4 million in 1999 and 5.3 million in 1995 (Stanton et al. 2006). The SBR was estimated to be 23.9 per 1,000 (uncertainty interval 18.8–30.5 per 1,000). There was a fivefold difference in the SBRs between developing countries (25.5 per 1,000; uncertainty interval 20.1–32.5 per 1,000) and, developed countries (5.3 per 1,000, uncertainty interval 4.2–6.8 per 1,000). Estimated SBRs were reported for different parts of the world, although the world regions used in this analysis are not identical to those used in the PMR report: sub-Saharan Africa (32.2 per 1,000), south Asia (31.9 per 1,000), east Asia (23.2 per 1,000), west Asia (18.9 per 1,000), North Africa (18.6 per 1,000), Oceania (15.8 per 1,000), Latin America/Caribbean (13.2 per 1,000), Southeast Asia (12.7 per 1,000), and Eurasia (12.2 per 1,000). The two world regions with the highest SBRs combined were responsible for two-thirds of the world's stillbirths: 28% from sub-Saharan Africa and 40% from south Asia. Ninety-nine percent of stillbirths occurred in developing regions, and, 51% occurred in the four countries of India, China, Pakistan, and Bangladesh.

Neonatal Deaths

Four million infants out of the 130 million annual births die in the neonatal period (first 4 weeks after birth), giving a global NMR of 30 per 1,000 live births (Lawn et al. 2005). An eightfold difference in NMR between developing countries (33 per 1,000) and developed countries (4 per 1,000) has been reported. Consequently, 99% of neonatal deaths were estimated to occur in developing countries. The NMR and percentage of global neonatal deaths in six world regions have been reported as follows: Africa (44 per 1,000), Eastern Mediterranean (40 per 1,000), Southeast Asia (38 per 1,000), Western Pacific (19 per 1,000), Americas (12 per 1,000), and Europe (11 per 1,000). Two-thirds of neonatal deaths occurred in two regions: Africa and Southeast Asia. Countries in sub-Saharan Africa have the highest NMRs (majority over 45 per 1,000) especially in those countries plagued by civil war. However, countries in Southeast Asia have the greatest absolute number of neonatal deaths. The NMR and percentage of global neonatal deaths in the top 10 countries accounting for two-thirds of the world's neonatal deaths were as follows: India (43 per 1,000), China (21 per 1,000), Pakistan (57 per 1,000), Nigeria (53 per 1,000), Ethiopia (51 per 1,000), Bangladesh (36 per 1,000), Congo (47 per 100), Afghanistan (60 per 100), Tanzania (43 per 1,000), and Indonesia (18 per 1,000).

The four major causes of neonatal death globally were estimated to be infections (sepsis, pneumonia, tetanus, and diarrhea, 36%), prematurity (28%), asphyxia (23%), and congenital abnormalities (7%) (Lawn et al. 2006). Infection accounted for over 50% of neonatal deaths in countries with a high NMR of above 45 per 1,000, compared to 20% in countries with a low NMR of below 20 per 1,000, where tetanus and diarrheal illnesses were almost never a cause of neonatal death. The risk of neonatal death in high-NMR countries compared to that in low-NMR countries was estimated to be 11-fold for infection, 8-fold for asphyxia, and 3-fold for prematurity. The highest risk of death was reported on the first day after birth, primarily as a result

of intrapartum complications leading to asphyxia, contributing to the fact that three-quarters of all neonatal deaths occurred in the first week.

Problems and Obstacles

Perinatal Deaths

The availability of healthcare resources is a major problem. A 10-fold difference in PMR between developing and developed countries is frequently associated with a 10-fold difference in healthcare expenditure per capita. For example in the Asia–Oceania region, countries with the lowest PMR were also reported to have the highest ranking for healthcare expenditure per capita: Japan (US $1760), Australia (US $1600), New Zealand (US $1390), South Korea (US $860), and Singapore (US $750). In contrast, countries with the highest PMR were among the lowest ranking for healthcare expenditure per capita: India (US $84), China (US $74), Pakistan (US $71), Indonesia (US $56), and Nepal (US $41).

Lack of healthcare resources in a country is aggravated by the problem of maldistribution within the same country, especially in developing countries with already scarce resources. A large proportion of the limited healthcare budget reaches only the more privileged members of the community. It is not uncommon to find that 80% of the country's healthcare workers are serving 20% of the population who reside in relatively affluent urban areas. Conversely, only 20% of healthcare resources are available to 80% of the population who reside in impoverished rural areas. Even in emerging economies where the socioeconomic condition is rapidly improving, the gap between the rich and poor continues to widen. The "inverse care law" which states that the availability of good medical care tends to vary inversely with the need for it in the population served, is also the "inverse information law" when applied to the fetal and neonatal population. The communities with the highest PMR and number of perinatal deaths have also the least basic clinical information on these deaths, and the least research investment to evaluate cost-effective strategies to lower their PMR.

Stillbirths

Most population-based surveys and even WHO publications have not routinely included reports on stillbirths. Neither did the Millennium Development Goals and estimates of the global burden of disease feature stillbirths. Counting stillbirths is particularly problematic. On the one hand, they are unlikely to be registered in many parts of the world. On the other hand, live births that died early might be recorded as stillbirths for reasons such as failing to accurately assess the signs of life, avoiding blame in the review of the birth attendant's performance, reducing administrative work or funeral costs, or minimizing emotional trauma of the loss for the family. No uniformity exists in the definition of stillbirths, and fetal deaths from 20, 22, 23, 24, or 28 weeks of gestation have been used in surveys. Recent advances in perinatal–neonatal care have lowered fetal viability to 22 weeks in developed countries, prompting changes in the definition of fetal death. However, this phenomenon of increasing neonatal survival at 22–28 weeks of gestation is largely irrelevant in the majority of countries in the developing world. For the purpose of international comparison, the WHO has recommended the use of fetal death occurring from 28 weeks of gestation or from 1,000 g birth weight as the definition of stillbirth, that is, late fetal death during the last trimester of pregnancy.

Neonatal Deaths

The inequity between developing and developed countries has continued to worsen in recent years. The already lower NMRs in developed countries have been reducing at a faster rate compared to that in developing countries. Between 1996 and 2005, the percentage reduction in NMR was 29% in developed countries compared to only 8% in developing countries. Reduction in the global NMR is only possible when there is high coverage of perinatal services in high-mortality developing countries where the poorest people with the greatest risk live. Although only 2% of neonatal deaths occurred in developed countries, they have been the subject of extensive confidential audits and, if perinatal services were judged to be substandard, there would have been a public outcry. In contrast, there is a lack of basic epidemiological data on causes of neonatal death in 98% of deaths that occur in developing countries because of their inadequate vital registration coverage. Furthermore, most medical research projects, including randomized clinical controlled trials of perinatal–neonatal interventions, were conducted in developed countries where the smallest number of neonatal deaths occur. The work of identifying and implementing cost-effective interventions within developing countries with the highest burden of neonatal deaths has therefore been an extremely slow process.

Eighteen million newborn infants or 14% of births were estimated to be low birth weight, but they accounted for 60–80% of neonatal deaths. Most deaths in low birth weight infants, either in those who are moderately preterm or those born at term but who are growth-restricted in utero, are preventable without expensive high-technology interventions, but simply through extra attention to warmth, feeding, and prevention of sepsis. In spite of the known biological survival advantage of girls over boys in the neonatal period, there is no epidemiological evidence of this especially in south Asia and China where the practices of sex-selective abortion, female infanticide, and reduced care seeking for girls have been reported. The intrapartum risk factors of obstructed labor and malpresentation have been identified to carry the highest risk for early neonatal death. Unfortunately, 44% of women globally were estimated to deliver without a skilled attendant, and this figure might be up to 95% in the poorest of developing countries. More than 50% of neonatal deaths were reported to be associated with home birth in the absence of skilled care. The target to totally eliminate neonatal tetanus globally has been missed, and although it is now only responsible for 6% of neonatal deaths, it is a disease that is almost exclusively found within poor communities.

Strategies for the Future

Strategies that address inequalities within individual countries and between developing and developed countries are necessary before we can see a significant improvement in global perinatal health in this century. Currently, developed countries give less than half a percent of their gross national product (GNP) as foreign aid to developing countries. A target for governments of affluent countries facing up to their global responsibilities is to contribute at least 1% of their GNP to developing countries.

The paucity of accurate vital registration data from many countries, especially those from the developing world with high SBRs, poses the primary difficulty in estimating stillbirth numbers and their underlying causes. With continued advances in obstetric care, the SBR might improve, especially with intrapartum stillbirths, and this could lead to an increase in early neonatal deaths. Therefore it is mandatory to count both stillbirths and neonatal deaths in routine perinatal audits. Otherwise, our assessment would be incomplete and decision making and priority setting for the development of maternal and neonatal healthcare programs might be misguided. Most of the stillbirths in developing countries are avoidable, as evidenced by the low SBRs of 4 per 1,000 seen in some developed countries, compared to the high SBRs of 40 per 1,000 in the worst of the developing countries. Better counting of stillbirths and having information on the causes of stillbirths are important as a means to advocate for action and to prioritize preventive healthcare strategies. For example, some definable causes of stillbirths, such as syphilis in at-risk regions or communities, could be identified and effective preventive measures taken. However, experience in developed countries, has shown that even when extensive resources are available to investigate stillbirths, the cause of death might not be established in up to one-third of stillbirths. Ultimately, political will and financial investment in registering stillbirths and documenting their causes are required. This would facilitate development of maternal–fetal interventions targeted to reduce the SBR in that region or community. To complete the loop, systematic assessments could then be devised to monitor the effectiveness, equity, and costs of any perinatal initiatives, especially if they have been introduced in low-income countries with the weakest healthcare systems.

The Millennium Development Goal (MDGs) for child survival – to reduce mortality in children aged

below 5 years by two-thirds between 1990 and 2015 – will be impossible to meet without halving the NMR. Because childhood mortality after the neonatal period has been falling faster than neonatal mortality, an increasing proportion of early childhood deaths is now in the first month. It has been estimated that in the year 2000, 38% of all under-5 child deaths happened in the neonatal period.

There is a wrong perception that only expensive high-technology and facility-based neonatal intensive care can reduce NMR. Many neonatal deaths are preventable with low-level, low-cost community-based health care. Historically, the fall in NMR in England from 30 per 1,000 in 1940 to 10 per 1,000 by 1975 was associated with the introduction of free antenatal care, skilled attendance at childbirth, and availability of antibiotics. To prevent the 4 million annual neonatal deaths, it is necessary to first be able to accurately count them and second to know what is causing them in those settings where most neonatal deaths occur. An evidence-based review has been carried out on the efficacy and effectiveness of cost-effective interventions to reduce the global NMR from its existing level of 30 per 1,000 (Darmstadt et al. 2005). Sixteen interventions with proven efficacy for neonatal survival were identified: preconception (folic acid supplementation), antenatal (tetanus toxoid immunization, syphilis screening and treatment, pre-eclampsia and eclampsia prevention, malaria treatment, detection and treatment of asymptomatic bacteriuria), intrapartum (antibiotics for premature rupture of membranes, corticosteroids for preterm labor, detection and management of breech, labor surveillance for early diagnosis of complications, clean delivery practices), and postnatal (resuscitation of newborn infant, breastfeeding, prevention and management of hypothermia, kangaroo mother care, community-based pneumonia case management). These interventions have been combined into packages for scaling up in healthcare systems according to the three service delivery modes of outreach, community–family, and facility-based clinical care. The total cost of a package of maternal or neonatal interventions has been estimated to be less than the sum of the costs of each component evaluated separately. Furthermore, because of this synergy of costs, packages of interventions are more cost-effective than individual interventions. Therefore, it is important to implement maternal and neonatal interventions in parallel and to have effective integration of the different components of perinatal services. The development of regionalization of perinatal services that integrate primary, secondary, and tertiary levels of care has been shown to be effective in improving both the quality and the availability of essential services to a geographically defined region (Yu and Dunn 2004).

If 99% coverage of these 16 interventions could be achieved, an estimated 41–72% of neonatal deaths worldwide could be averted. Reliance on outreach and community–family services alone would achieve an 18–27% reduction in neonatal deaths, and the addition of facility-based clinical care would achieve reductions of over 50%. The aim to halve the global NMR is therefore an achievable goal using the three basic intervention packages. This target NMR of 15 per 1,000 would be similar to the NMR in today's developed countries back in the era immediately before the introduction of neonatal intensive care in these countries. In developing countries with weak healthcare systems and high NMRs, the emphasis must initially be on antenatal and postnatal care through family–community interventions that include health education to improve domiciliary neonatal care practices and care seeking for illness (Bhutta et al. 2005). Because effective, yet simple interventions are not reaching those most in need, there needs to be a systematic scaling up of neonatal care in countries where the coverage of interventions is low and inequity is high (Knippenberg et al. 2005). Reduction in NMR is less dependent on technology and commodities than on people with skills. Increased coverage depends on a commitment to increase the number of midwives and doctors, together with innovative approaches to retain trained staff in poor rural communities. In many of the world's poorest countries, even without developing expensive high technology, there is a need to double or triple the healthcare budget in order to halve the NMR. The cost per neonatal death averted has been estimated at about US $2000 (Martines et al. 2005). Although more than 10,000 newborn infants die every day in developing countries, estimates have suggested that up to three-quarters of these deaths could be prevented with low-technology interventions at an additional cost of less than US $1 per capita in these countries where the highest NMRs were seen.

Conclusion

Under-reporting of stillbirths remains a major challenge, especially in regions where most of the stillbirths occur. Improving the global database on stillbirths is an essential first step toward effective preventive action. There is a lack of reliable cause-of-death data for both stillbirths and neonatal deaths especially in developing countries with the highest mortality rates. Evidence-based reviews have shown that population-oriented outreach and community-oriented and family-oriented healthcare interventions are highly cost-effective for the promotion of perinatal health, but their current coverage is insufficient. When individual-oriented facility-based clinical services are added to these primary care services, up to 70% of neonatal deaths could be prevented provided they are implemented with high coverage where they are needed most. Governments need an overall strategy to promote perinatal health, and to work with donors to invest in well-integrated programs for maternal, neonatal, and child care.

Key Terms

Antibiotics	Intrapartum complications	Pre-eclampsia
Breastfeeding	Kangaroo mother care	Premature rupture of
Congenital abnormalities	Low birth weight	membrane
Cost-effective interventions	Malaria	Prematurity
Disparities	Millennium Development	Pre-term birth
Female infanticide	Goals (MDGs)	Reproductive loss
Folic acid supplementation	Neonatal mortality rate	Sex selection abortion
Gestational age	Newborn	Stillbirth rate
Gross national product	Obstetric care	Syphilis screening
Healthcare system	Perinatal mortality rate	Uncertainty interval
Infant mortality rate	Perinatology	
International comparison	Preconception	

Questions for Discussion

1 Define the following terms:

   a. Infant mortality

   b. Neonatal mortality rate

   c. Perinatal mortality rate

   d. Gestational age

   e. Live births

   f. Low birth weight

   g. Pre-term birth

2 Briefly discuss the major risk factors for perinatal mortality.

3 What factors account for the wide disparity in perinatal outcomes between high-income and low-income countries?

4 Sixteen interventions with proven efficacy for preventing neonatal survival have been identified in the literature. List any five of these and discuss in about 200 words, the challenges of implementing them in one low-income country of your choice.

References

Bhutta ZA, Darmstadt GL, Hasan BS et al. (2005) Community-based interventions for improving perinatal and neonatal health outcomes in developed countries: a review of the evidence. Pediatrics 115:519–617

Darmstadt GL, Bhutta ZA, Cousens S et al. (2005) for the Lancet Neonatal Survival Steering Team. Evidence-based, cost-effective interventions: how many newborn babies can we save? Lancet 365:977–988

Knippenberg R, Lawn JE, Darmstadt GL et al. (2005) Lancet Neonatal Survival Steering Team. Systematic scaling up of neonatal care in countries. Lancet 365:1087–1098

Lawn JE, Cousens S, Zupan J (2005) Lancet Neonatal Survival Steering Team. Neonatal survival 1. 4 million neonatal deaths: when? Where? Why? Lancet 365:891–900

Lawn JE, Wilczynska-Ketende K, Cousens SN (2006) Estimating the causes of 4 million neonatal deaths in the year 2000. Int J Epidemiol 35:706–718

Martines J, Paul VK, Bhutta ZA et al. (2005) for the Lancet Neonatal Survival Steering Team. Neonatal survival: A call for action. Lancet 365:1189–1197

Stanton C, Lawn JE, Rahman H et al. (2006) Stillbirth rates: delivering estimates in 190 countries. Lancet 367: 1487–1494

World Health Organization (WHO) (1996) Perinatal mortality. Maternal Health and Safe Motherhood Programme. Geneva: WHO/FRH/MSM/96.7

World Health Organization (2006) Neonatal and perinatal mortality – country, regional and global estimates. Geneva: World Health Organization. http://www.who.int/making_pregnancy_safer/publications/neonatal.pdf, cited 27 July 2008

Yu VYH (2003) Global, regional and national perinatal and neonatal mortality. J Perinatal Med 31:376–379

Yu VYH, Dunn PM (2004) Development of regionalized perinatal care. Sem Neonatol 9:89–97

Chapter 4
Maternal and Child Health in the Organization for Economic Cooperation and Development (OECD) Countries

Ian G. Child and John E. Ehiri

Learning Objectives After reading this chapter and answering the discussion questions that follow, you should be able to

- Discuss health and income inequality among the different member countries of the OECD and between OECD as a whole, and the rest of the world.
- Evaluate MCH issues in OECD countries in relation to structure and financing of health care, health status indicators, service delivery models, and social determinants.
- Analyze the different ways that maternal and child health services are organized and delivered in OECD member countries.

> **Box 4.1 OECD Member Countries**
>
> **North America:** Canada, the United States, and Mexico.
> **Western Europe:** Austria, Belgium, Denmark, Finland, France, Germany, Greece, Iceland, Ireland, Italy, Luxembourg, the Netherlands, Norway, Portugal, Spain, Sweden, Switzerland, Turkey, and the United Kingdom.
> **Former USSR members:** Czech Republic, Hungary, Poland, and the Slovak Republic.
> **Asia and Australasia:** Japan, The Republic of Korea, Australia, and New Zealand.

Introduction

This chapter focuses on MCH practices in countries that are members of the 30-nation Organization for Economic Cooperation and Development (OECD) with its headquarters in Paris, France (Box 4.1). It examines the different ways that maternal and child health services operate in member states of the OECD. The chapter begins with a brief overview of health and income inequity among the different member nations of OECD and between OECD as a whole and the rest of the world. It then discusses MCH issues in OECD countries from four perspectives, namely

- Structure and financing of health care: This section examines the typology and different healthcare financing mechanisms in OECD member nations, analyzing the relative importance of public funding, social programs, employer-supported health insurance, private insurance, and out-of-pocket payments in the various member nations. This section also examines the influence of different national social philosophies on the predominance of particular financing mechanisms as well as differences in healthcare expenditures and human resource capacities in the various member nations.
- Health status indicators: This section presents a comparative overview of maternal, infant, and child health indices, contrasting high performing nations with those that have poorer indices, and examining the role of differing economic and social factors.

I.G. Child (✉)
University of Alabama at Birmingham, USA

J.E. Ehiri (ed.), *Maternal and Child Health*, DOI 10.1007/b106524_4,
© Springer Science+Business Media, LLC 2009

- MCH service delivery models: This section examines variations in national approaches to antenatal care, using the United Kingdom, Germany, France, Australia, Sweden, Canada, and Japan as examples.
- Social determinants: This concluding section of the chapter discusses the relationships between biological and genetic causation, and the complex network of social, environmental, and behavioral determinants of health.

The authors highlight the puzzling fact that despite the multiplicity of prenatal and postnatal care approaches, technological improvements, and increased expenditure and intensity of care over the last 30 years, no significant improvement in the proportion of infants born with low birth weight has been observed in any high-income OECD country. The need for greater policy and programmatic attention to economic and social determinants of maternal and child health is emphasized.

Within the OECD, healthcare systems reflect a wide range of social philosophies and economic and political systems. Together, the OECD countries are home to 18% of the world's population but produce 80% of the world's economic output. Thirty-nine and fifty-one percent of the world's doctors and nurses, respectively, practice in OECD countries (WHO 2006). The United States is the only high-income nation that does not recognize universal health care as a right of citizenship and permits critical provider and insurance sectors to profit. The US healthcare expenditures are double the OECD average, yet fewer services are delivered to a younger population; 47 million persons are left uninsured, and life expectancy, infant mortality, and low birth weight outcomes are worse.

OECD grew out of the Organization for European Economic Cooperation (OEEC) created in 1948 with the support of the United States and Canada to consolidate the Marshall Plan for reconstruction of Europe after World War II (OECD 2008). As a counterpart to NATO, OECD took over from OEEC in 1961 with the mission of helping member governments to achieve sustainable economic growth while maintaining financial stability and contributing to the development of the world economy (OECD 2008). The OECD includes seven of the powerful G8 nations (Canada, France, Germany, Italy, Japan, Russia, the

United Kingdom, and the United States) – with average annual per capita national incomes which, in 2005, ranged from US $30,000 to US $44,000. The 11% of the world's population that live in the G8 nations produces 64% of the world's economic output. The World Bank classifies 29 nations with populations over 1 million as "high-income" countries (per capita gross national income (PC GNI) >US $10,066 in 2004). Twenty-three are OECD members. The six high-income, non-OECD members are Hong Kong, Singapore, Israel, and the oil-rich nations of Kuwait, Saudi Arabia, and the United Arab Emirates. Membership in the OECD is expanding. In the past 7 years, four former USSR nations, plus Mexico, Turkey, and South Korea became OECD members. Their 2005 per capita GDPs ranged from $4,700 in Turkey to $16,000 in South Korea. Five prospective members are Chile, Estonia, Israel, Russia, and Slovenia, and discussions are underway with the highly populated but middle-income nations of Brazil, China, India, Indonesia, and South Africa.

The OECD is a forum where member nations compare policy experiences and address the economic, social, and governance challenges of globalization. For example, within the OECD, the 23-nation Development Assistance Committee (DAC) is the principal body through which, if all countries honored promises to give 0.7% of their GDPs annually as aid for the poorest developing nations, approximately US $245 billion ($10^9$ in the US terminology) in aid would have been donated in 2007 (UNICEF 2007). In 2005, five countries, Denmark, Luxembourg, the Netherlands, Norway, and Sweden exceeded the promised 0.7% of GDP; at the opposite end of the scale, Italy, Greece, and the United States are ranked 20th–22nd in generosity with donations of slightly less than 0.2% of GDP (UNICEF 2007).

In many ways, this chapter is about the heterogeneity among high-income countries. The diverse ways in which different OECD nations' healthcare systems are structured, financed, and delivered reflect each member's unique history, culture, industry, social welfare, and political philosophies. It is not possible here to describe all members' health systems in detail and we, therefore, have selected seven to illustrate the different healthcare structures as they relate to MCH processes of care and outcomes. We address issues related to the prenatal period, infancy, childhood, and adolescence, where young people and families are considerably influenced by the social infrastructure and environmental determinants of health. OECD members have relatively better functioning healthcare systems and better health outcomes for their MCH populations than many middle- and low-income countries. It is thus germane to explore MCH practices within the OECD to determine whether there are lessons to be learned.

Several references are made in this chapter to commonly used economic and developmental terms, defined briefly in Box 4.2.

Box 4.2 Definition of Terms

Gross Domestic Product (GDP): The total final value of all goods and services produced by a nation in a given year.

Gross National Income (GNI): GDP plus income received from abroad such as a proportion of wages sent home, known as remittances, by foreign workers.

Purchasing Power Parity (PPP): A widely used conversion of GDP or GNI to compensate for recent exchange rate changes and for the equivalent purchasing power of a common market basket of household items in the nation.

Gini Coefficient (World Bank 2008): A measure of income inequality within each nation, where a value of 0 indicates perfect equality and a value of 1 indicates total inequality. Among OECD members, the United States has the biggest gap between the haves and the have-nots. The countries with the highest degrees of equality in 2004 were Sweden, Denmark, Finland, and Germany.

Freedom Index (Heritage Foundation 2008): Issued by Freedom House, it measures the relative degree of social and political rights and freedom of choice in 190 countries. Its annual report is widely relied upon by international policy makers in organizations such as the World Bank and IMF. Forty-seven countries were listed as "most free" and they included all OECD nations except Greece, Japan, and the Republic of Korea.

Corruption Index (Transparency International 2002): A widely referenced product of the Berlin-based company called Transparency International. It measures the degree to which corruption in the actions of local politicians and public officials is perceived in 12 surveys of businesspersons, international policy experts, and others. The index is a scale from 1 (most corrupt) to 10 (least corrupt) nations. Nordic countries, Australia, New Zealand, Singapore, and Switzerland are rated as the least corrupt. The United States was ranked 20th.

Human Development Index (HDI) (UNDP 2008): This covers 175 countries and is published annually by the United Nations. HDI is sometimes referred to as the "livability index" and is based on a composite measure of life expectancy, literacy, and standard of living. The five most livable OECD countries based on 2004 data were Norway, Iceland, Australia, Ireland, and Sweden.

Human Poverty Index (HPI) (United Nations 2005): There are two HPI indices. HPI-1 is designed for developing nations and is a composite measure of life expectancy, literacy, access to clean water, and proportion of appropriate weight children. HPI-2 is designed for high-income nations and is a composite of the probability of not surviving to 60 years of age, percent of adults lacking functional literacy skills, population in poverty (50% of median adjusted household income), and percent of population unemployed longer than 12 months. OECD countries with the lowest poverty index are Sweden, Norway, the Netherlands, Finland, and Denmark.

International Classification of Diseases (ICD): Endorsed by the WHO, this is the world's international standard diagnostic classification scheme. It is very widely used by governments for vital statistics recording, by healthcare providers for medical records and financial and billing systems, and by policy makers. Diseases, signs and symptoms, accidents and many other health problems are coded. The latest revision ICD-10 was released in 1994.

OECD in an Unequal World

In 2007, the world's population was 6.6 billion and produced a total income (GNI) of US $49 trillion (UNICEF 2007). The world is extremely heterogeneous and income is unevenly spread among, or within, nations (see Tables 4.1 and 4.2). The following key facts illustrate the degree of international inequality that exists: (a) 61% of the world's people live in the 11 largest countries (China, India, the United States, Indonesia, Brazil, Pakistan, Russia, Bangladesh, Nigeria, Japan, and Mexico), each of which has a population greater than 100 million residents (UNICEF 2007). Two of these countries, the United States and Japan, together are home to 6.6% of world's population but produce 42% of its income; (b) the 10 countries (the United States, Japan, Germany, the United Kingdom, France, Italy, Spain, Canada, Mexico, and South Korea) with the largest economies (all of whom are members of the OECD) have 70% of the world's economy but only 14% of the world's population; (c) 34% of the world's population resides in the 44 poorest nations (of the 44 poorest nations: 31 are in sub-Saharan Africa, 9 are in south/Southeast Asia, and 4 are in Central Asia) and have per capita incomes of less than US $2 per day and produce only 3% of its economic output. In 2004, China and India, respectively, had 20 and 17% of world's population and 4.8 and 1.7% of the world's economy. Tables 4.1 and 4.2 show key indicators for all 142 countries with populations of 1 million or more that publish data. Table 4.1 divides the countries into eight income groups: the first two rows correspond with the World Bank (WB) category of low-income nations; the third and fourth rows correspond with the WB low middle-income nations, the fifth and sixth rows with WB upper middle-income nations, and the seventh and eighth rows with WB's high-income category. Table 4.2 subdivides the countries by geographic area.

Life expectancy in Western Europe is approximately double that of the poorest countries in the world, where infant mortality rates are 20 times higher and maternal mortality rates are 75 times higher (OECD 2006). But economic and social inequality between nations is not the end of the story. There is sometimes more difference between MCH outcomes in different regions of the same country than there is between

neighboring countries. To explore the context, delivery, and status of MCH in OECD nations, the remainder of this chapter has been structured into the following sections: (i) structure and financing of healthcare systems; (ii) health status indicators – outcomes, processes, and resources; (iii) specific processes of MCH care in six countries; (iv) the relationships between biological and genetic causation, and the complex network of social, environmental, and behavioral determinants of health.

Structure and Financing of Health Care

Table 4.3 presents a summary of healthcare financing mechanisms in selected OECD countries. The five dominant financing mechanisms include the following:

Public taxation: Federal, state, county, or municipality government income taxation that creates a pool of cash (often called a general fund) out of which amounts to pay for services such as health, education, pensions, law and order, roads are allocated. Government has funding flexibility, typically defined by an annual budget, to direct general taxation funds toward these specific purposes and to place them under federal or state control. This approach is primarily used in Australia (state control), Canada (federal and provincial control), New Zealand (federal), Spain (federal and private), Sweden (counties), the United Kingdom (federal and regional), and the United States (States' control of Medicaid). These countries typically use a system of delegation of some authority and flexibility to define the "right" coverage for the populations of its regions together with strictly held global budgets to control operating and capital expenditure in each region.

Social programs: Federal, state, county, or municipality government taxes are specifically designated for health care and cannot be used for other purposes such as welfare, social security, subsidized housing, education, roads. This approach is primarily used in France, Italy, Japan, and the Netherlands. Some countries such as France have complex authority and control structures.

Table 4.1 Distribution of countries by per capita GNI groups (2004 data unless otherwise stated)

W B terminol	# countries	Per Cap income range	Popn millions	% Pop	Cum %	Average GNI/Cap	GNI/Cap PPP IMF	GNI $trillion	% GNI	Cum % GNI	Life exp	Inf mort / 000 bths	<5 mort /000	Matern mortal	MDs /000	GINI	Corrup 2006	Hum Dev Index
LI	25	<$400	406	6.4	6.4	$226	$1,188	92	0.2	0.2	48	100	160	975	0.12	0.347	2.4	0.420
LI	23	$400 - $825	1,810	28.4	34.8	$579	$2,812	1,049	2.6	2.8	61	66	95	536	0.56	0.359	2.5	0.531
LMI	14	$826 - $1,499	516	8.1	42.9	$1,153	$4,629	$595	1.5	4.3	68	31	41	218	0.73	0.346	2.7	0.710
LMI	24	$1,500 - $3,255	1,880	29.5	72.5	$1,814	$7,316	$3,411	8.5	12.8	71	27	31	91	1.06	0.404	3.2	0.715
UMI	14	$3,256 - $4,999	374	5.9	78.3	$3,680	$10,482	$1,376	3.4	16.2	66	23	28	92	2.57	0.385	3.9	0.763
UMI	14	$5,000 - $10,065	201	3.2	81.9	$6,724	$11,945	$1,352	3.4	19.5	75	16	19	55	2.23	0.284	4.3	0.782
HI	14	$10,066 - $29,999	277	4.4	85.8	$20,974	$25,681	$5,810	14.4	34.0	79	6	7	11	2.73	0.309	7.1	0.973
HI	14	$30,000 +	694	10.9	96.7	$37,222	$35,274	$25,832	64.1	98.1	79	5	6	13	2.68	0.305	8.4	0.947
	142	Countries pop >1mill	6,158	96.7	96.7	$6,417		$39,516	98.1	98.1								
	36	Pop <1 mill c GNI	11	0.2	99.5	$7,233		80	0.2	98.3								
	30	Pop < 1 or no GNI	174	2.7	99.7	Unk		Unk										
	208	Total above	6,343	99.7		$6,242		39,596	98.3									
		WB Grand total	6,365	100		$6,329		$40,282	100.0		67	54	79	400				

LI = low income; LMI = lower middle income; UMI = upper middle income; HI = high income

Table 4.2 Distribution of countries by geographic region (2004 data unless otherwise stated)

# countries	Region	Popn 000,000's	% Pop	Cum %	GNI/cap	GNI/cap PPP IMF	GNI $trillion	% GNI	Cum % GNI	Life exp	Inf mort /000 bths	<5 mort/ 000	Matern mortal	MDs /000	GINI	Corrup 2006	Hum Dev Index
16	Europe	395	6.2	6.2	$29,613	$29,459	$11,697	29.0	29.0	79	4	5	9	3.35	0.315	7.8	0.941
27	E. Central Asia	467	7.3	13.5	$3,358	$9,246	$1,568	3.9	32.9	69	23	27	54	2.92	0.291	3.5	0.766
4	E. Asia (high inc)	187	2.9	16.5	$30,482	$28,101	$5,700	14.2	47.1	81	4	4	13	1.87	0.356	7.6	0.926
10	E. Asia (low/mod inc)	1,796	28.2	44.7	$1,457	$6,590	$2,618	6.5	53.6	70	26	32	92	0.86	0.410	2.9	0.680
5	S. Asia	1,417	22.3	67.0	$598	$3,103	$848	2.1	55.7	63	63	85	518	0.57	0.351	2.6	0.592
9	Caribbean	51	0.8	67.8	$2,392	$5,497	$122	0.3	56.0	70	26	33	162	0.78	0.490	3.2	0.746
10	S. America	371	5.8	73.6	$2,952	$8,422	$1,095	2.7	58.7	72	26	28	211	1.45	0.532	3.7	0.792
3	N. America (NAFTA)	430	6.8	80.3	$32,082	$33,320	$13,795	34.2	93.0	77	11	13	32	2.39	0.410	6.4	0.906
15	N. Africa & Mid East	306	4.8	85.2	$3,336	$7,276	$1,021	2.5	95.5	71	31	38	132	0.89	0.379	3.8	0.719
41	Sub-Saharan Africa	714	11.2	96.4	$603	$2,119	$431	1.1	96.6	46	96	161	889	0.18	0.355	2.6	0.452
2	Australasia	24	0.4	96.7	$25,890	$29,880	$621	1.5	98.1	80	5	6	8	2.45	0.357	9.2	0.947
142	Countries pop >1 mill	6,158	96.7	96.7	$6,417		$39,516	98.1	98.1								
36	Pop <1 mill c GNI	11	0.2	96.9	$7,233		80	0.2	98.3								
30	Pop <1 mill or no GNI	174	2.7	99.7	Unk		Unk		98.3								
208	Total above	6,343	99.7		$6,242		$39,596	98.3									
	WB grand total	6,365	100		$6,329		$40,282	100.0		67	54	79	400				

Table 4.3 Healthcare financing mechanisms in OECD countries

	Financing				Providers	
		Public taxation			Primary care provider	
	Social	National	Regional	Private	Public	Private
Australia		Yes				Yes
Canada		Yes	Yes			Yes
Denmark		Yes			Yes	
France	Yes				Yes	Yes
Germany	Yes				Yes	Yes
Italy	Yes	Yes			Yes	
Japan	Yes				Yes	Yes
The Netherlands	Yes			Yes		Yes
NZ		Yes			Yes	Yes
Norway		Yes			Yes	
Spain		Yes				Yes
Sweden		Yes	Yes		Yes	
Swiss				Yes		Yes
The United Kingdom		Yes				Yes
The United States	Yes		Yes	Yes		Yes

Source: OECD (2006)

Health insurance: Direct payments by employees to health insurance funds that are largely independent of government and are typically negotiated by employers or unions. Examples are the sickness funds in Germany and the insurance companies in the United States.

Private insurance: Little government control of payments. In some countries, private insurance can offer full coverage. In others it may be used for comfort and convenience items such as hospital single rooms, or dental, ophthalmic, prescriptions, and long-term care. In Canada, private insurance may be used only for services not provided by government.

Out of pocket: Direct patient usage payments either as co-payments, deductibles, or entire charges for certain services are widely used in the United States but are not used in most high-income countries with strong social support philosophies. Out-of-pocket payments are sometimes sub-classified according to necessity, such as different classes of drugs in France.

In most countries, more than one financing mechanism is used. For example in the United States, Medicare (which covers citizens over 65 years of age and others of any age with long-term disabilities) funding is collected as a separate wage tax plus funds from general federal income tax.

Other US federal government plans include TRICARE (ex-military persons) and the excellent coverage for congresspersons and federal government staff. Coverage and purchasing is centrally regulated in similar ways to some European systems. Medicaid (for low-income populations) is jointly funded from state income taxes plus a varying proportion of matching financing by the federal government. The US state governments define the range of available treatment coverage and eligibility based on the patient's personal financial status. Individual states differ markedly in their eligibility and coverage criteria. Employers and employees pay a proportion of wages for health insurance coverage for themselves and, typically at an additional premium, for their families. Employers and unions choose from a number of competitive for-profit health insurance management companies or self-insure. In the United States, it is not mandatory that employers provide health insurance and many do not, particularly for part-time workers. The United States is the only country in the OECD that does not have a philosophy of universal health insurance as a fundamental right of citizenship and, in 2007, 47 million residents had no insurance and a further 25 million had inadequate insurance for at least a part of the year. It should be noted that some young and healthy employees in the United States prefer not to be insured and not to pay a proportion of their income for services they believe they will never need.

Different national cultures and social philosophies play a role in general citizen welfare in ways that go well beyond health and cover pensions, housing, food subsidies, and education – including higher education. However, when we comment on the "generosity" of a country like Sweden, whose government pays directly for health and social welfare programs, and has almost eliminated child poverty, it should be noted that this "generosity" is made possible by higher taxation and a culture in which it is a core value that the richer members of society should contribute to the well-being of the poorer members. Fig. 4.1 presents the relative tax

burden (the percentage that a nation's taxes are of that country's GDP) in selected OECD nations.

OECD healthcare expenditures and processes: Fig. 4.2 compares the per capita expenditure on health care (in US $ PPP) in a cross section of OECD nations. The US expenditure of $6,000 per capita is approximately double the OECD average but serves a comparatively younger population (on average, 15% fewer citizens over 65 years of age than some nations have), provides fewer services such as prescriptions (the data predate the Medicare Part D prescription plan), long-term care, dental and ophthalmic care (some, but not all, OECD countries provide these), and delivers fewer physician visits and bed-days per capita. This is accompanied by worse outcomes such as life expectancy,

TOTAL TAX REVENUE AS % OF GDP

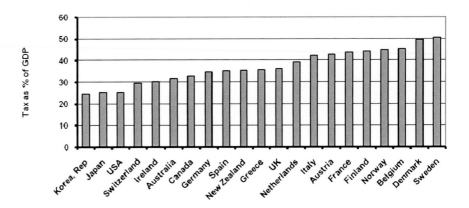

Fig. 4.1 Tax burden in selected OECD countries (2004). Source: OECD (2006)

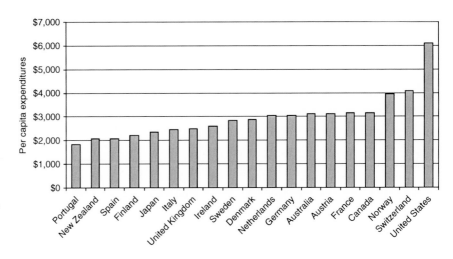

Fig. 4.2 Per capita expenditure on health care in 2004 US $PPP, OECD members. Source: OECD (2006)

infant mortality, and low birth weight. Some researchers question whether these statistics accurately and comparably represent the true situation. Some draw attention to possible problems with equivalent definition and rigor in the collection of comparative outcomes data in all countries (Howell and Blondel 1994). In 2000, the WHO ranked the US healthcare system in the 37th place but "informal opinion" ranks the United States between 15th and 20th among 30 OECD nations (WHO 2000). Countries (with populations > 1 million persons) that led the WHO ranking were France, Italy, Singapore, Spain, Austria, Japan, and Norway, and some question that order. A 2006 survey comparing adult healthcare experiences in seven nations (Australia, Canada, Germany, the Netherlands, New Zealand, the United Kingdom, and the United States) found wide national differences in access, after-hours care, coordination, and medical errors (particularly when patients saw multiple doctors; Schoen et al. 2006). The "United States stands out for its cost-related access barriers and less-efficient care" and "practices least use of electronic medical records" (Schoen et al. 2006). The United States ranked lowest in patient satisfaction but together with the German system was ranked highest in speedy access. Similarly, results from the Commonwealth Fund's National Scorecard report show that the US health system continues to fall short of what is attainable based on a survey of 19 industrialized nations (The Commonwealth Fund Commission on a High Performance Health System 2008). Across 37 core indicators of performance, the United States achieved an overall score of 65 out of a possible 100. Overall performance did not improve from 2006 to 2008. Access to health care significantly declined, while health system efficiency remained low (The Commonwealth Fund Commission on a High Performance Health System 2008).

A nation's population health status is dependent on a complex web of interconnected factors, of which the healthcare system is only one factor (see Chapter 5 on Health systems and MCH). Different countries have different philosophies regarding responsibility for, and provision of, health care for their citizens. Except the United States, all high-income OECD countries have had universal health insurance coverage for decades. In Germany,

however, residents with annual salaries over a specified level have a choice of opting out of public health insurance if they purchase private insurance that gives at least equivalent coverage. Approximately 10% of Germans opt for this. In the Netherlands, it is mandatory that the approximately 20–25% of residents earning more than a certain annual threshold level each year leave public health coverage and subscribe to private insurance.

No system is wholly accepted as perfect, and most countries have individual and common concerns. In general, annual healthcare expenditures in OECD members have grown at more than double the rate of GDP growth (111%) over the past 5 years. This ranges from 3% increase in Greece to >120% in France and Norway (OECD 2006) (Table 4.4). Two major population transitions that are common to most high-income countries may provide some explanation for this. First, fertility rates have slowed to or are below the replacement rate, and second, in general, populations live longer. As medical costs increase, the working population, who make contributions through wage and salary deductions, whether in general taxation or specific health and welfare contributions, will have an increasing load placed on them to support health care for the elderly and unemployed sectors of the population that do not pay for health care.

Health systems' human resources in OECD countries: Table 4.5 shows numbers of physicians, nurses, and nurse midwives per 1,000 population (WHO 2006). The number of physicians per 1,000 population is a useful but incomplete measure. Of at least equal importance are the following: (a) the average time ("face time") that patients spend in discussion with their physicians, (b) the content and quality of the information imparted, (c) the proportion of that time devoted to prevention, and (d) the written materials or web sources given to the patient. A study in the *British Medical Journal* compared the "face time" of patients in the United States, Australia, and New Zealand and found that Australian and New Zealand patients, respectively, had double and 50% more "face time" than the US patients (Bindman et al. 2007). The amount of time a patient spends with other caregivers in the practice (e.g., a prevention nurse) is clearly also important but was not included in this study.

Table 4.4 OECD gross domestic product (PPP) and health expenditure

WHO rank	Country	Year 2004 – all PPP					2000–2004			Other comparisons			
		Per cap GDP US$	PC GDP Index USA = 100	Tot. Health expend per cap	Health exp index USA = 100	Health expend as % GDP	Annual GDP PPP growth	Annual health exp growth	Difference % of GDP growth	Health empl wage Index	Gini coef (diff years)	Livability rank 2005	Corruption index 2006
21 countries with a per capita GDP PPP >US $20,000													
24	Australia	$32,573	82	$3,120	51	9.6	4.4%	6.8%	55	65	0.352	3	8.7
5	Austria	$32,519	82	$3,124	51	9.6	3.5%	4.0%	14	71	0.291	14	8.6
14	Belgium	$31,381	79	$3,260	53	10.4	4.2%	9.4%	124	72	0.330	13	7.3
22	Canada	$31,828	80	$3,165	52	9.9	3.3%	6.0%	82	72	0.326	6	8.5
26	Denmark	$32,304	81	$2,881	47	8.9	2.9%	4.9%	69	77	0.254	15	9.5
23	Finland	$29,778	75	$2,235	37	7.5	3.6%	6.8%	89	64	0.269	11	9.6
1	France	$29,945	75	$3,159	52	10.5	2.9%	6.6%	128	71	0.327	16	7.4
17	Germany	$28,816	72	$3,043	50	10.6	3.1%	3.7%	19	66	0.283	21	8.0
9	Greece	$21,586	54	$2,162	35	10.0	7.3%	7.5%	3	31	0.343	23	4.4
12	Ireland	$36,479	92	$2,596	43	7.1	6.0%	9.4%	57	61	0.343	4	7.4
2	Italy	$28,352	71	$2,467	40	8.7	2.4%	4.3%	79	51	0.360	17	4.9
6	Japan	$29,567	74	$2,340	38	7.9	3.2%	4.4%	38	69	0.249	7	7.6
43	Korea, Rep	$20,668	52	$1,149	19	5.6	6.0%	10.0%	67	39	0.316	25	5.1
10	The Netherlands	$32,978	83	$3,041	50	9.2	3.7%	7.8%	111	74	0.309	10	8.7
31	New Zealand	$24,744	62	$2,083	34	8.4	3.2%	6.8%	113	46	0.362	20	9.6
7	Norway	$40,715	102	$3,966	65	9.7	2.9%	6.5%	124	79	0.258	1	8.8
4	Spain	$25,875	65	$2,094	34	8.1	5.3%	8.4%	58	55	0.347	19	6.8
16	Sweden	$31,139	78	$2,825	46	9.1	3.5%	5.6%	60	77	0.250	5	9.2
3	Switzerland	$35,149	88	$4,077	67	11.6	3.6%	6.4%	78	102	0.337	9	9.1
11	UK	$30,822	77	$2,508	41	8.1	4.8%	7.8%	63	76	0.360	18	8.6
28	USA	$39,772	100	$6,102	100	15.3	3.5%	7.4%	111	100	0.408	8	7.3

Table 4.4 (continued)

WHO rank	Country	Year 2004 – all PPP					2000–2004			Other comparisons			
		Per cap GDP US$	PC GDP Index USA = 100	Tot. Health expend per cap	Health exp index USA = 100	Health expend as % GDP	Annual GDP PPP growth	Annual health exp growth	Difference % of GDP growth	Health empl wage Index	Gini coef (diff years)	Livability rank 2005	Corruption index 2006
7 countries with a per capita GDP PPP <US $20,000													
35	Czech Rep	$18,634	47	$1,361	22	7.3	6.4%	8.5%	33	35	0.254	6.5	4.8
51	Hungary	$15,948	40	$1,276	21	8.0	7.2%	10.5%	46	32	0.269	5.9	5.2
46	Mexico	$10,242	26	$662	11	6.5	3.0%	6.8%	127	14	0.495	n/a	3.3
37	Poland	$12,409	31	$805	13	6.5	4.6%	8.0%	74	22	0.345	n/a	3.7
8	Portugal	$18,125	46	$1,824	30	10.1	1.1%	3.0%	173	41	0.385	27	6.6
47	Slovak Rep	$14,060	35	$855	14	6.1	6.7%	9.4%	40	24	0.258	n/a	4.7
52	Turkey	$7,562	19	$580	10	7.7	2.8%	6.3%	125	8	0.436	n/a	3.8

Source: OECD 2006

Table 4.5 OECD resources and processes of care

WHO rank[1]	Country	MDs/ 000 popn.	Nurses/ 000 popn.	NMWs/ 000 popn.	MD consults/ capita	Acute bed-days/ capita	Ac beds/ 000 pop. '03 or '04	Ac bed % occup '03 or '04	Ac bed ALOS '03 or '04	Tot beds/ 000 2003	% measles immune 2004	% DPT immune 2004	% >65 Flu vacc 03 or 04	CTs/ 000,000	MRIs/ 000,000
	21 countries with a per capita GDP PPP >US $20,000														
24	Australia	2.38	9.35	n/a	6.0	1.0	3.6	70.6	6.1	3.8	94.0	92.3	79.1	n/a	3.7
5	Austria	3.34	9.29	0.20	6.7	1.8	6.6	79.0	6.2	8.3	88.0	83.0	n/a	28.5	14.9
14	Belgium	4.45	5.78	0.63	7.6	1.2	4.8	n/a	7.3	6.8	97.0	95.0	65.0	29.8	6.8
22	Canada	2.09	9.70	n/a	6.1	1.0	3.0	91.0	7.3	3.4	82.0	n/a	63.0	10.8	4.9
26	Denmark	2.90	10.26	0.22	7.5	n/a	3.3	85.0	3.6	4.0	96.9	95.0	50.8	14.6	10.2
23	Finland	3.16	14.32	0.76	4.2	0.9	3.0	74.9	4.8	n/a	81.0	n/a	46.0	14.2	14.0
1	France	3.38	7.27	0.26	6.7	1.0	3.8	74.9	5.6	7.7	97.3	98.0	68.0	7.5	3.2
17	Germany	3.37	9.72	0.10	n/a	1.8	6.6	75.5	8.9	8.7	88.0	97.7	48.0	15.4	6.6
9	Greece	4.32	3.80	0.17	n/a	n/a	3.8	n/a	n/a	4.7	93.3	88.0	n/a	n/a	n/a
12	Ireland	2.79	15.19	4.12	n/a	0.9	2.9	85.3	6.5	4.3	74.0	89.0	61.4	n/a	n/a
2	Italy	4.18	5.42	0.29	n/a	1.0	3.7	75.8	6.8	4.2	93.5	92.7	66.6	20.6	10.2
6	Japan	1.97	7.78	0.19	13.8	2.1	8.5	79.3	20.7	14.3	95.8	100.0	43.0	92.6	36.0
43	Korea, Rep	1.56	1.73	0.18	n/a	n/a	5.9	71.6	10.6	7.1	100.0	97.0	75.7	31.5	11.0
10	The Netherlands	3.12	13.61	0.12	5.3	n/a	2.8	68.0	7.4	4.8	95.0	98.0	73.0	n/a	n/a
31	New Zealand	2.20	7.59	0.52	3.2	n/a	n/a	n/a	n/a	n/a	87.1	n/a	49.2	12.1	3.7
7	Norway	3.09	14.62	0.49	n/a	0.9	3.1	86.4	5.2	3.8	96.0	91.0	n/a	n/a	n/a
4	Spain	3.17	7.38	0.15	9.5	0.8	2.8	79.2	6.9	3.4	99.9	96.6	68.6	13.3	7.7
16	Sweden	3.24	10.08	0.69	n/a	n/a	2.2	n/a	4.7	n/a	99.6	99.0	n/a	n/a	n/a
3	Switzerland	3.50	10.42	0.27	n/a	1.2	3.9	86.3	8.7	3.9	n/a	95.0	57.0	17.9	14.3
11	UK	2.23	11.78	0.61	5.3	1.1	3.7	84.4	6.6	4.1	96.4	91.5	71.0	7.0	5.0
28	USA	2.49	9.09	0.02	3.9	0.7	2.8	66.9	5.6	3.3	81.0	85.5	64.6	32.2	26.6

Table 4.5 (continued)

WHO rank[1]	Country	MDs/ 000 popn.	Nurses/ 000 popn.	NMWs/ 000 popn.	MD consults/ capita	Acute bed-days/ capita	Ac beds/ 000 pop. '03 or '04	Ac bed % occup '03 or '04	Ac bed ALOS '03 or '04	Tot beds/ 000 2003	% measles immune 2004	% DPT immune 2004	% >65 Flu vacc 03 or 04	CTs/ 000,000	MRIs/ 000,000
7 countries with a per capita GDP PPP <US $20,000															
35	Czech Rep	3.53	9.74	0.47	13.1	1.8	6.4	74.7	8.1	8.7	85.5	97.9	n/a	12.6	2.8
51	Hungary	3.26	8.65	0.20	12.6	1.7	5.9	76.6	6.5	7.8	82.0	99.8	37.9	6.8	2.6
46	Mexico	1.88	0.85	n/a	2.5	0.4	1.0	62.2	3.9	1.9	96.0	98.1	29.1	3.1	1.7
37	Poland	2.49	4.94	0.58	6.2	n/a	4.8	77.0	6.6	n/a	80.7	99.0	n/a	6.9	1.9
8	Portugal	3.28	4.18	0.08	3.8	0.8	3.0	70.5	7.0	3.6	97.0	97.8	n/a	12.8	3.9
47	Slovak Rep	3.18	6.77	0.27	11.9	1.4	5.9	69.1	7.7	7.2	85.0	99.3	22.9	8.7	2.0
52	Turkey	1.34	1.69	n/a	3.1	n/a	2.4	64.9	5.2	2.6	93.0	85.0	n/a	7.3	3.0

Source: Outcomes – OECD 2006. Personnel – WHO.
Key: AC = acute; ALOS = average length of stay
CT = computed tomography (CT) scan
MRI = Multiple Resonance Imaging

The number of nurse midwives is low in the United States, Germany, the Netherlands, and Spain. This has implications for pregnancy management and child care. Numbers of physician visits per capita are lowest in New Zealand, the United States, and Finland. Acute bed-days in the United States and Finland are low. Occupancy is lowest in the United States (67%, suggesting an oversupply of hospital beds); length of stay is lowest in Denmark, Sweden, and Finland.

Health Status Indicators

Maternal, infant, and child mortality in OECD countries: Table 4.6 shows a ranking of OECD countries based on a composite, unweighted index of life expectancy, infant mortality, under 5-year mortality, and maternal mortality.

The countries with the best indices are Sweden, Norway, and Finland. The bottom ranked countries are the United States, Mexico, and Turkey. Infant mortality rates fell steadily in all countries until the mid-end of the 1990s when they began to flatten (Fig. 4.3). In 1970, infant mortality rates ranged from the lowest rate of 11 per thousand births in Sweden to the highest rate of 28–29 per thousand births in Italy and Spain. By 2004, this range had declined in all countries from a low of 4 per thousand births in Sweden and Japan to a high of 7 per thousand births in the United States where rates also vary considerably according to race (UNICEF 2007).

Table 4.7 ranks major causes of infant mortality in the United States. We may now be approaching a natural limitation where only slight reductions in infant mortality rates can be anticipated in the future. Four Asian high-income countries (Hong Kong, Japan, Republic of Korea, and Singapore) and several North European countries have the world's lowest infant mortality rates of 3–4 per thousand births. Infant mortality rates in the United States still remain double the level of those countries. Infant mortality rates among African-American births (13.5 per thousand) are 2.4 times higher than among Caucasian births (5.7 per thousand) (Shen et al. 2005; CDC 2007). The US infant mortality rate among African-Americans is similar

to the general populations of Malaysia, Costa Rica, Sri Lanka, Bosnia Herzegovina, and Mauritius (World Bank 2008).

Pregnancy termination: In interpreting and comparing adverse pregnancy outcomes across OECD countries, one question that merits research is whether pregnancy termination and abortion regulations and practices have an impact on national pregnancy outcome statistics. Abortion is legal in all European countries except Ireland and Switzerland (unless the mother's life is in danger) but the regulations of individual nations vary markedly. For example, the gestational age limit for on-demand or unreviewed abortion in Belgium, Denmark, France, Germany, and Italy is 12 weeks but in Finland and the United Kingdom it is 24 weeks. In the Netherlands, abortion is available under 14 weeks free of charge under their federal insurance plan. The Scandinavian countries have the lowest infant mortality rates in Europe. These nations have the most open acceptance of abortion as a rightful choice for women. However, a study in 1999 showed that abortion rates in Scandinavia, Finland, the Netherlands, and England are slightly lower than the United States. Use of abortion in Southern European countries varies (Bindman et al. 2007). France and Italy have moderate use but Spain's use is lower. There is no indication (as there was not when oral contraceptives were introduced in the 1960s) of a strong tendency to follow the Catholic Church that condemns the practice. For example, abortion is available on demand in Italy where 99% of the population is Roman Catholic. In the United States approximately 20% of pregnancies are ended by surgical or drug-induced abortion (Henshaw et al. 1999). In some Northern European OECD countries as many as 60% of pregnancies where a high risk of congenital abnormalities has been detected are terminated, and clearly, this would have significant impact on infant mortality rates in those countries (OECD 2006).

Pregnancy outcomes: In comparison with low- and middle-income nations, maternal mortality and death of children between ages 1 and 4 years have a much lower incidence in high-income countries. Low numbers and statistical significance may limit their value as a comparative measure of MCH status among OECD nations. The percentage of

Table 4.6 OECD life expectancy & maternal and child outcomes, 2004 (ordered by the composite outcomes index)

WHO rank	Country	Popn. 000,000s	HE index USA = 100	Hum dev index	Life exp at birth	Inf mort/ 000	<5 mort/ 000	Mat mort[1]/ 00,000 bth	L B W %	C-sect % of bths	Composite outcome index[2]
16	Sweden	9.0	46	0.951	80.6	3.1	4	3	4.2	17.2	3.70
7	Norway	4.6	65	0.965	79.9	3.2	4	4	4.8	15.6	4.03
23	Finland	5.2	37	0.947	78.8	3.3	4	5	4.2	16.3	4.10
14	Belgium	10.4	53	0.945	78.9	4.3	5	n/a	n/a	n/a	4.65
2	Italy	57.6	40	0.940	80.0	4.1	5	3	6.7	37.0	4.66
35	Czech Rep	10.2	22	0.885	75.8	3.7	4	4	6.8	16.0	4.70
12	Ireland	4.0	43	0.956	78.5	4.9	6	3	5.0	21.8	4.74
4	Spain	42.7	34	0.938	80.5	3.5	4	4	7.1	23.6	4.87
9	Greece	11.1	35	0.921	79.0	4.1	5	2	8.6	n/a	4.91
17	Germany	82.5	50	0.932	78.6	4.1	5	4	6.9	26.0	4.97
3	Switzerland	7.4	67	0.947	81.2	4.2	5	4	6.3	25.7	4.98
5	Austria	8.2	51	0.944	79.3	4.5	6	4	6.8	22.1	5.24
24	Australia	20.1	51	0.957	80.6	4.7	6	5	6.3	29.7	5.39
8	Portugal	10.5	30	0.904	77.6	4.0	5	5	7.6	29.2	5.52
6	Japan	127.7	38	0.949	82.1	2.8	4	6	9.4	n/a	5.60
10	The Netherlands	16.3	50	0.947	79.2	4.1	6	7	5.4	13.6	5.61
22	Canada	31.9	52	0.950	80.0	5.3	6	6	5.8	24.7	5.70
1	France	60.2	52	0.942	80.3	3.9	5	8	6.8	17.8	5.81
26	Denmark	5.4	47	0.943	77.6	4.4	5	10	5.3	19.9	6.25
11	UK	59.8	41	0.940	78.7	5.1	6	7	7.5	21.9	6.45
37	Poland	38.2	13	0.862	75.0	6.8	8	5	6.1	n/a	6.53
31	New Zealand	4.1	34	0.936	79.2	5.0	7	10	6.1	22.2	6.93
51	Hungary	10.1	21	0.869	72.8	6.6	7	7	8.3	27.9	7.23
47	Slovak Rep	5.4	14	0.856	74.1	6.8	9	7	7.2	19.2	7.49
43	Korea, Rep	48.1	19	0.912	77.3	5.3	6	15	4.2	35.2	7.71
28	USA	293.7	100	0.948	77.7	7.0	8	10	8.1	29.1	8.32
46	Mexico	104.0	11	0.821	75.2	19.7	28	67	9.1	37.9	28.10
52	Turkey	71.8	10	0.757	71.2	24.6	32	n/a	n/a	n/a	28.30

Source: Outcomes — OECD 2006.
1. Maternal mortality = average of 2000–2004.
2. Based on 4 pregnancy outcome columns IM through LBW.

Fig. 4.3 Trend in infant mortality, OECD, 1970–2004. Source: OECD (2006)

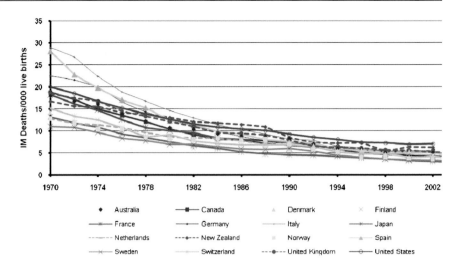

Table 4.7 Causes of infant mortality in the United States, 2003

Rank	18,893 neonatal deaths	R% of total	9,132 post-neonatal deaths	% of total
1	Short gestational and/or low birth weight	25.2	Sudden infant death syndrome	21.6
2	Congenital and chromosomal abnormality	21.2	Congenital malformation chromosome abnormality	17.7
3	Maternal complication of pregnancy	9.0	Unintended injuries	9.1
4	Newborn affected by complications of placenta, chord, or membranes	5.7	Disease of circulatory system	4.5
5	Newborn respiratory distress	4.1	Influenza or pneumonia	3.2
6	Bacterial sepsis of newborn	3.9	Homicide	3.2
7	Neonatal hemorrhage	3.4	Gastritis, duodenitis, non-infective enteritis, or colitis	3.1
8	Intra-uterine hypoxia or asphyxia	2.7	Septicemia	3.0
9	Atelectasis	2.3	Chronic respiratory disease	2.4
10	Necrotizing enterocolitis	1.9	Short gestational and/or low birth wt	1.1
	All other	20.7	All other	31.1

Source: CDC (2007). Note that 34% of the US post-neonatal deaths were as a result of SIDS, injuries, or homicide

babies born prematurely or with low birth weight provides a better comparative measure. A measure of appropriate weight for gestational age together with a national fetal growth curve is perhaps the best method of all. Low birth weight rates have not decreased significantly across OECD countries in spite of the advances in technology, clinical and social welfare interventions over the past three decades (US Department of Health and Human Services 2006). In eight countries (Australia, Canada, Denmark, Finland, New Zealand, Norway, Sweden, and the United Kingdom), low birth weight rates have remained flat or increased very slightly from 1970 to 2002 (Fig. 4.4) (OECD 2006).

In France, Germany, Italy, and the United States, rates of low birth weight have increased slightly and in Japan and Spain, they have increased significantly (Fig. 4.5). Ironically, Japan, the country with the lowest infant mortality rates, has the highest rate of increase in low birth weight and in 2004 had the highest absolute rate (9.5%) (OECD 2006).

The above findings suggest a need for research to determine (a) why, despite the clinical and social interventions of the past 30 years, low birth weight rates have not been reduced in any OECD nation, (b) whether the data are real or are an offsetting combination of a decrease in real mortality and an

Fig. 4.4 Low birth weight,
OECD, 1970–2003. Source:
OECD (2006)

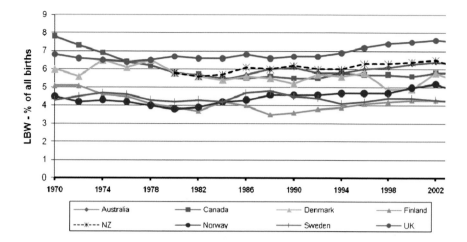

Fig. 4.5 Increasing rates of
low birth weight, selected
OECD countries. Source:
OECD (2006)

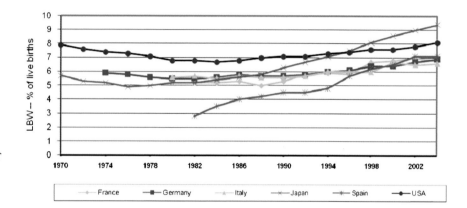

improvement in more complete and better defined
data collection and reporting, and (c) whether the
data represent the role of a mix of as yet unidentified
social influences.

Delivery of MCH Services

Provision of prenatal care services: There are four
fundamental issues relating to the provision of evidence-based prenatal care (also known in some
countries as antenatal care). These are as follows:
(i) who should deliver it to the patient – general
practitioner physicians, specialist obstetricians,
nurse midwives, or a team of caregivers including
both physicians and midwives; (ii) is there an
accepted standard number of prenatal care visits a
woman with a normal pregnancy should attend; (iii)

what should be the standard content of prenatal
care testing and advice and how can quality be
monitored; (iv) which countries have national clinical guidelines and what are they? The approaches
taken by many OECD countries are discussed
below.

(i) **Who should deliver prenatal care:** Before describing some of the contrasting processes of prenatal
care utilized in individual OECD nations, it is
useful to have an overall sense of the relative
numbers of healthcare professionals in each
country. As shown in Table 4.5, midwives play
a major role in Belgium, Finland, New Zealand,
Norway, Sweden, and the United Kingdom.
The lowest numbers of midwives are in the
United States (only 5,000 in the country as a
whole), followed by Portugal, Germany, the
Netherlands, and Spain.

(ii) **Standard number of prenatal care visits:** In the 1990s, the WHO published a general guideline for prenatal care and updated it in 2003 (OECD 2006). The WHO guideline recommends 12–16 prenatal care visits, which seems to have become the standard in a number of countries. However in the United Kingdom, the National Institute for Health and Clinical Excellence (NICE), an independent organization responsible within the National Health Service for providing evidence-based guidance, recommends 10 prenatal care visits for uncomplicated, first pregnancies and seven visits for second and subsequent pregnancies.

(iii) **Content of prenatal care visits:** As described below, some countries are very specific about recommended prenatal care content. Bernloehr and colleagues (2007) concluded that

… there are sufficient differences in national guidelines to produce gaps or an unnecessary, expensive and possibly harmful multiplication of tests for pregnant women.

Thirty-seven tests were reported by 25 nations, and of these, 23 are recommended by more than 12 countries (Table 4.8).

Only three tests were recommended by all 20 nations (maternal BP, blood group, and rhesus factor). Only one country recommended routine fetal

fibronectin, and only three recommended placental hormones or hemoglobinopathies. Nations with lower national incomes tend to recommend more tests than those with higher national incomes (OECD 2006).

Variations in National Approaches to Antenatal Care

It should be noted that in the future within Europe, greater standardization is likely to take place as a result of increasingly open borders and the overall European Union's basic aim of free movement of persons, capital, and goods, and services between countries. Nine countries no longer require passports to be shown for passage between them of residents of each country; inter-nation employment is encouraged; and freedoms for patients of country X to obtain medical care from a physician or hospital in country Y are growing (Bernloehr et al. 2007). In the following pages, comparisons of national practices are described for six countries (the United Kingdom, Germany, France, Australia, Canada, and Sweden) that have different structures and different attitudes toward the dissemination of national guidelines.

Table 4.8 Most frequently mentioned tests (23 tests mentioned by at least 50% of countries)

Physical	Technical	Laboratory
Blood pressure	Fetal heart auscultation	Alpha-fetoprotein (triple)
Body mass index	Abdominal ultrasound	Red cell antibodies
Fetal position	Transvaginal ultrasound	Blood group
Formal risk scoring		Gestational diabetes
Fundal height		Hemoglobin
Maternal height		Hepatitis B
Maternal weight		HIV
Vaginal examination		Lues
		Rhesus factor
		Rubella titer
		Bacteria in urine
		Glucose in urine
		Protein in urine

Source: OECD (2006)

The United Kingdom

The philosophy that health care is a right of all citizens is fundamental and the British National Health Service (NHS), formed in 1948, covers all legal residents. Care costs are paid from general taxes and cover a wide range of medical, ophthalmic, dental, psychiatric, long-term, and other services. Independent contractor general practitioners serve as gatekeepers and are paid a capitation fee for each patient on their "list" plus additional fees for preventive or other activities that are deemed beneficial. Patients choose their own physician and list sizes are limited to 2–2,500 patients except in unusual circumstances. Evidence-based guidelines exist for a wide range of clinical conditions and the one for management of pregnancy is described below. Hospitals, owned by National Trusts, are controlled by the central government via strictly enforced regional authority and individual hospital global budgets. Hospital physicians and specialists are salaried – as they are in most of Europe. Central purchasing of drugs, supplies, and equipment ensures the bargaining power of the entire country and prices for the same item are, for example, lower than in the United States. Total healthcare system costs per capita are less than half of those in the United States and British outcomes are somewhat better. Approximately 10–15% of residents are privately insured. Waiting list problems for elective surgery exist and some hospital facilities are in need of renovation. In the late 1990s and early 2000s the English parliament recognized that its cost control measures had been too severe and that NHS services were suffering. Hospital and clinic building programs were increased and waiting times reduced. However, ironically during the period of discontent, some outcomes improved slightly (early data). This may be similar to a recent report in the United States that shows that as a result of a large, on-going geographical study, the best outcomes were not necessarily linked to the areas where most funds were spent.

Approximately 10–15% of British citizens are covered by private insurance. One company, BUPA, is a global health and care organization, with members in nearly 190 countries worldwide. Nurse midwives play a significant role and several home visits both prior to and after delivery are a key component of the care plan (BUPA 2008). In the United Kingdom, the National Institute for Health and Clinical Excellence (NICE) published, in October 2003, a very detailed guideline entitled "Antenatal Care: routine care for the healthy pregnancy woman" which has been updated in 2008 (National Collaborating Centre for Women's and Children's Health 2008). Like many OECD nations over the past decade, this guideline emphasized a focus on "Woman Centered Care." NICE guidelines stress the need to inform and support pregnant women, explain their choices (including termination), communicate in written and electronic forms, set up a schedule of prenatal visits and procedures, and explain the woman's right to accept or refuse diagnostic testing or treatment. Parallel evidence-based guidelines for healthcare professionals explain the clinical thinking behind these recommendations. Women in the United Kingdom receive 6–9 months paid maternity leave and this is soon to be increased to 1 year.

NICE recommends 10 prenatal care visits for uncomplicated first pregnancies and seven visits for second and subsequent pregnancies. Screening recommendations and non-recommendations are given in Table 4.9. The specific processes of care recommended at each visit are described and several processes carried out in the past are specifically discouraged. Screening for Down's syndrome that gives a detection rate over 60% and a false-negative rate less than 5% (nuchal translucency integrated with serum tests at 11–20 weeks) is specifically recommended. An early ultrasound scan is

Table 4.9 Recommended prenatal screenings in the United Kingdom

Recommended	Not recommended
Gestational age (ultrasound)	Asymptomatic bacterial vaginosis
Anemia (first appointment and 28 weeks)	Cytomegalovirus
Proteinuria	Hepatitis C
Blood group and red cell alloantibodies	Streptococcus group B
Sickle cell and thalassemia	Toxoplasmosis
Structural abnormalities	Gestational diabetes mellitus
Down's syndrome	Cervical exam to predict preterm birth
Hepatitis B	Fetal fibronectin
HIV	Transabdominal scan at 36 weeks unless placenta extends over the os
Rubella	Fetal movement counting
Syphilis	Cardiotocography
Pre-eclampsia risk level	Routine ultrasound after 24 weeks
Fetal presentation at 36 + weeks	Umbilical artery Doppler ultrasound
Symphysis-fundal distance	Fetal heart auscultation unless requested by the patient

Source: National Collaborating Centre for Women's and Children's Health (2008)

recommended to determine gestational age [as opposed to the last menstrual period (LMP)] and to detect multiple pregnancies. Screening for gestational diabetes is discouraged.

Recommended appointment schedules are as follows:

Nulliparous women: <12 weeks, 16, 18–20, 25, 28, 31, 34, 36, 38, 40.

Parous women: <12 weeks, 16, 18–20, 28, 34, 36, 38.

Germany

Germany was the first country to introduce universal health care in 1883 (Murray 2006; WHO 2004). All citizens are covered but those with a salary over a certain moderate level can opt out and cover themselves – via private insurance. Approximately 5% of Germans do that (Murray 2006). Another 5% are government employees covered by a separate plan. Employers and employees make equal contributions from wages into a "social insurance fund." The fund is administered by approximately 200 not-for-profit "sickness funds" (down from 1300 in the 1990s), based on region and occupation, that contract with physicians and hospitals. The federal government pays fees for the unemployed or retired persons and retains oversight control of funds and providers. Satisfaction levels are high and waiting lists are among the lowest in Europe. Patients are free to choose general practitioners, specialists, and hospitals. There are approximately 50% more physicians per resident in Germany than in the United States or the United Kingdom and approximately 50% work from solo practices. Public health is not an important part of German health care.

France

The French healthcare system structure has changed little over the past two decades because generally there is a high degree of public satisfaction coupled with the circularity that it is structured to be resistant to change. Funding is a combination of employee and employer payroll taxes, property taxes, and social security contributions. It was ranked number 1 by the 2000 WHO multi-national comparison report (United Nations 2005). France is one of the only countries where a key part of their medical payment philosophy is to make the patient aware of the cost of treatment in a belief that this will reduce the "moral hazard" problem. This is accomplished by making the patient directly responsible for paying the provider bill, and then having the patient reimbursed, almost in full and fairly quickly, by the private or government payer. Any concerns the patient may have about the care received can be directly addressed to the physician at this time.

In 1971 a pregnancy management program change was made at a national level following a cost–benefit analysis that suggested that both short- and long-term cost savings would be realized if the incidence of preterm and low birth weight births could be reduced. The program involved a combination of (a) improvements in social welfare, (b) greater involvement of the patient in her own care planning, and (c) implementation of a clinical protocol for management of high-risk pregnancies and certain lifestyle changes. Nurse midwives do not play as significant a role in France as in other countries except for some home visits and community maternity clinics, particularly in economically disadvantaged areas. Whereas the focus of British policy has been on clinical guideline aspects of care specifically during pregnancy, the French approach, begun in 1971, was an ambitious national scale pregnancy management program focused on reducing social and work-related risk factors.

The French pregnancy management program concentrated on four coordinated interventions: (i) risk scoring, e.g., previous preterm birth or stillbirth (internationally, this is one of the few significant predictors of a future adverse pregnancy outcome), (ii) patient education about risk, (iii) reduction of physical activity and workplace stress, and (iv) self-assessment and self-management.

Simultaneously, some changes in the healthcare system were made. Since 1945, pregnant women had been financially induced to begin prenatal care during the first trimester under the care of a general practitioner. However the physicians were less than enthusiastic to participate and tended to refer women to out-patient maternity clinics where they either were seen by an obstetrician or by a midwife. The financial incentive to a woman was unaffected by whether she was seen by a physician or a midwife. This policy was instituted nationally in 1992 and a 12-year intervention measurement study known as the Haguenau Project was implemented in a fairly self-contained area in northeast France.

In reports published in 1985 (Papiernik et al. 1985) and 1986 (Papiernik et al. 1986), reductions in both preterm birth and low birth weight levels were reported over a period of 12 years (1971–1982) divided into three 4-year periods. In these three periods, low birth weight rates decreased from 4.6 to 4.0 to 3.8%, and preterm birth levels fell from 5.4 to 4.1 to 3.7%. Unfortunately, the OECD database used extensively in this chapter did not publish preterm birth rates or show low birth weight levels until 1982 (5.2%), then 1986 (5.3%), and annually thereafter. These OECD data show that low birth weight levels increased from 1988 (5.0%) to 1998 (6.8%). The results for the last period of the Haguenau Study and the OECD figures are not compatible and the reasons for this remain unknown at this time.

The French healthcare system is strongly connected with school health programs from age 5, and there is also a very active preschool health program. For many years, the French have used an adjunct to their medical records system called the *carnet de santé* which is an 80 page notebook issued at birth in which parents and physicians make notes on care, immunizations, treatments, developmental, and clinical observations so that a child's entire medical history is immediately available to the next caregiver. Confidentiality concerns have made the French slow to introduce electronic medical records. The carnet de santé is well accepted by both physicians and parents. The Japanese and Russian systems have a similar parent-held record.

Australia

The Australian prenatal care system is currently undergoing change. Until recently, there have been no comprehensive and nationally promoted prenatal care protocols. However, the concept of evidence-based medicine and guidelines is well accepted. Low infant mortality and low birth weight levels have placed Australia in the middle of the OECD ranking. A study published in 2002 showed that major hospitals that delivered more than 200 births/year vary as follows in their practices of six protocols (Hunt and Lumley 2002):

1. **Number of prenatal care visits:** Most hospitals (90%) seemed to have based their policies on a 1929 recommendation from the United Kingdom. This policy recommended 13 prenatal care visits (every 4 weeks up to the 28th, every 2 weeks from 29 to 36 weeks, every week from 37 to 40).
2. **Gestational diabetes mellitus screening:** Although widely known to be of questionable value, 90% of hospitals still recommended glucose challenge, glucose tolerance, HbA1c, and random blood sugar tests.
3. **Syphilis screening:** Ninety-two percent of hospitals recommended screening at the first visit.
4. **HIV:** Only 55% of hospitals recommended screening. Half of hospitals screen at-risk women and half screen all women.
5. **Hepatitis C:** Fifty percent of hospitals recommended screening even though evidence-based research questions the value. Two-thirds of women tested were "selected" as being at risk. The policy for hepatitis B is not known.
6. **Smoking cessation counseling:** Ninety percent of hospitals had no written guidelines.

Sweden

Nurse midwives play a significant role via geographically closely spaced community care centers. The centers were specifically designed to promote teamwork between different types of caregivers. Physicians were required to locate their offices in these centers. Much attention was devoted to restructuring the entire healthcare system during the 1990s following serious public and staff discontent with services, waiting times for surgery, escalating costs, dissatisfaction with global budgeting, lack of incentives for quality care, and poor morale among relatively low paid personnel. *Note*: the discontent took place at the same time that outcomes were improving and Sweden consistently ranks in the top three nations in indicators such as life expectancy, infant mortality, and low birth weight. The Swedish healthcare system is based on a fundamental policy of decentralization of management and control to 23 counties and 3 large municipalities. Numbers of physicians are a little higher than the often-quoted ideal of 3 physicians per 1,000 citizens and there are a high proportion of primary care physicians. Physicians are well trained, paid by government, work in community teams, and are willing to share responsibilities with nurses and other caregivers. School-based health services are an important component of child care. Hospitals are well equipped. Because the proportion of residents aged 65 and above (19%) is high in comparison with some other European countries and with the United States (13%) the average cost per patient is relatively high.

Swedish guidelines for prenatal care include a higher number of tests than the European average. In addition, special emphasis is now placed on offering women a choice of extensive genetic screening. All pregnant women must be given information on genetic screening and particular care is taken to be sure that women are made aware of their choices. Additional emphasis on screening is given to women aged 35 and over, and to women who have previously given birth to children with some impairment or who are known to be carriers of a hereditary disease. Screening for phenylketonuria (PKU), galactosemia, hyperthyroidism, and the adrenogenital syndrome is recommended.

Traditionally, for patients of all ages, screening has not been emphasized in Sweden. Decisions about the health of all members of a family are based more on family-centered observation arising from the close relationship between the entire family and community health centers staff. Sweden is a country with very advanced social and welfare programs – and a high taxation burden to pay for them. Child poverty has almost been eliminated. Per capita incomes are high and the Gini coefficient indicates low-income inequality – similar to Denmark, Finland, Japan, and Norway. The nations with the highest income inequality are Italy, Mexico, Turkey, and the United States.

Canada

The Canadian healthcare system is based on a combination of funding by the Federal government and each of the 10 provinces and 4 territories. The provinces and territories have considerable freedom to set their own priorities. The Federal Prevention of Low Birth Weight in Canada Report (Stewart et al. 1998) declared that "the prevention of low birth weight is the most important perinatal issue in Canada." Extensive guidelines are published for both patients and care givers. Most care is initially delivered by a primary care physician (PCP) who acts as a gatekeeper for specialist referral. Patients can elect to go directly to a specialist of their choice but must pay a small additional charge.

A central component of the federal guideline is extensive patient education in written and electronic media. Canada began its "E-health Program" in 1997 and now has at its core, a nationally common electronic patient medical record (Health Canada-Santé Canada 1999). Some parts of Canada are extremely remote and E-health permits patients to contact physicians and other caregivers from any home PC or hand-held device. For decades, Canada has had a stronger sense of the importance of social determinants and the concept of "population health." Extensive guidelines are available for physicians and also for patients. High emphasis is placed on "the fully informed patient and family." Health Canada–Santé Canada (HC-SC) boasts several general guidelines produced as a joint effort between the federal government and the Society of Obstetricians and Gynecologists. In addition they reference 27 specific guidelines on separate topics such as morning sickness, breech delivery, SIDS. They refer physicians to the Cochrane Library.

Japan

Japan has the highest life expectancy in the world and the lowest infant mortality. Its healthcare system covers everyone, and the very strong philosophy that an employer has a responsibility to its employees dominates the type of system. Typically, a doctor visit requires a 25–30% co-pay (the employer wants the employee to know the value of the services) and this usually is reimbursed. Many

Japanese hospitals are private but are contracted to employers who negotiate rates. Hospitals can seem to be an odd mix of older buildings and very modern equipment. Few ambulatory care physicians have appointment systems (first come, first seen). Until recently there were few pharmacies. Therefore, physicians dispensed medications and patients returned for refills. The average length of stay in hospitals in Japan is longer than in Europe and North America because often, patients live in small houses in which living rooms become bedrooms at night, making it difficult to accommodate a recuperating patient at home. Paradoxically, Japan, which has the lowest infant mortality rate among OECD nations (better than half the US rates), has the highest rate of increase in low birth weight levels.

Child Care in OECD Countries

The available evidence shows that the objectives of child care are fewer than two general headings, each with three components that, although perhaps worded differently, are common to most OECD nations (American Academy of Pediatrics 2000):

1. **Clinical health:**

   (a) Ensuring adequacy of nutrition, sleep, and exercise, in a safe, loving and caring, stress free, dual parent family, and immediate neighborhood environment.

   (b) Immunization and vaccination, recreational safety and injury prevention. Early, age-appropriate health education about risks of alcohol, drugs, sexual behaviors, and contraception. Collaboration with law enforcement to prevent sale and distribution of harmful substances to minors.

   (c) Early detection and clinical treatment of acute or chronic diagnoses and hearing or eyesight problems.

   (d) Milestones against which to continuously measure every child's physical, clinical, academic, behavioral, and social development.

2. **Mental, behavioral, and psychosocial health:**

   a. Special attention to ensure that children who fall behind in learning the basics of letters and numbers are not subject to ridicule when they do attend school.

   b. Fostering socialization with peers and adults. Respect for the rules of society, and the rights and duties of individuals. Discourage gang memberships and initiation ceremonies that are often a child's introduction to illegal substances or crime.

   c. Early detection, counseling, or treatment of clinical, social, and behavioral problems that impair personal learning and development and that disrupt the learning opportunities of peers and the dedication of teachers.

Several recent reviews have reconsidered how well-child care is delivered (Schor 2004). The ways in which these goals are implemented vary considerably and three conceptual differences emerge (Kuo et al. 2006). First, some countries do not formally take steps to link the care given to an individual child by different providers. Second, some countries do foster collaborative teamwork among the caregivers. And third, some countries, particularly in Northern Europe, encourage entire families to use the same primary care physician or community nurse, so that a holistic family picture plays a role in assessment of a child's health. Clearly the development of electronic medical records could have a major impact. The French do not discourage multiple physician care for the same child but back that up by the individual record called the *carnet de santé* described earlier. Electronic medical record systems that are increasingly widely used in some Northern European countries fill the same role. The United States lags behind Europe in its use of patient management computer systems.

The following comments illustrate the wide range of approaches adopted within the OECD. Some countries such as Germany, the Netherlands, and the United States rely heavily on physicians (general practitioners and/or pediatricians) operating from a clinical setting to treat the child as an individual. Child care in Denmark and Sweden is based on the concept of the same physician for the entire family. These countries feel that the relationship of a child within the context of the total family is important, while other countries such as Germany and the Netherlands do not. Physicians in Sweden tend to be opposed to routine screening and feel that the same results will be obtained by frequent observation of the whole family. Swedish physicians must be located in the same premises as other members of the healthcare team to encourage information sharing. Other systems in Europe and Australasia rely on treatment by a range of typically well-coordinated community and school personnel, including physicians, nurses, and home visitors. Some nations combine sick child care (referral to hospital in- or out-patient facilities, psychologist or psychiatrist care, or specialist pediatricians) with well-child care, some do not. Some are closely linked with schools, others are not. Some are based on clinics and others on numerous, geographically close, shared community centers. Some report to local or regional authorities: others to federal management. In Sweden, France, and Australia, well-child care, immunizations, prevention, and psychosocial counseling is largely the responsibility of public health or defined child health nurses. In France, home visits are not unusual and there are close health contacts with public pre-schools (beginning when a child reaches age 4). In Sweden, these functions come under county or municipality control. In Canada, Australia, and Denmark control flows from the region. In the United Kingdom and Spain, control is national where there is a federal, single payer, and a powerful drugs/supplies purchasing authority. In the United Kingdom and Holland, patients typically have a single, primary care provider, often for life, who acts as a gatekeeper making specialist recommendations when appropriate. In Germany, patients often retain the same primary care doctor but chose from many specialists. German pediatricians typically see children only up to age 6. There are complex arrangements for patient and service sharing between hospitals and ambulatory physicians. All give universal access with no co-pay or cost sharing.

We have earlier drawn attention to the extent of use of nurse midwives in Belgium, Finland, Norway, Sweden, and the United Kingdom, and for disadvantaged persons in France. The geographical areas served by these community centers are often located within walking distance of small concentrations of residents. All caregivers are encouraged to share impressions, even though they may not be fully formed, about a child's health, eye sight, hearing, dental needs, physical coordination, play patterns, and particularly his/her social interaction

with peers and with persons outside what might be the usual age group for friends. If asked, law enforcement and truancy officers can carefully add their comments in a spirit that is more aimed at prevention than punishment.

Social Determinants of Health

Finally, in order to design cost-effective prevention, early detection, and treatment interventions for any disease, we must first comprehend the deepest and most fundamental layers of causation. For example, race, widely accepted to primarily be a social rather than a biological construct, and poverty are often blamed. But what layers of causality lie beneath these phenomena? Pregnancy is a healthy condition that occasionally results in an adverse outcome. Our understanding of the etiology of adverse pregnancy outcomes is incomplete and more research into causes hidden in our external environments is much needed. In a 1998 study of low birth weight and preterm birth in the United States, Goldenberg (1998) made the following statement, which sadly is as true today as it was then: "Unfortunately, despite the utilization of ever increasing amounts of research and clinical care resources ... there is very little evidence that any intervention or practice has had a major impact on prevention of low birth weight. Neither medical/obstetric strategies, nor behavioral approaches have had a significant impact on the rate of preterm birth."

Our lack of complete knowledge is illustrated by two puzzling situations that raise fundamental questions for further research. First, in spite of the application of advanced technology, improvements in patient care, and increased resources spent on a wide range of public health and social welfare interventions over the past three decades, there has been no significant reduction in the rates of low birth weight in all of the world's richest nations. Second, the United States has infant mortality and low birth weight rates that are twice as high among African-American women as among Caucasian women, but with no disparity observed between Caucasian and Hispanic women. Black/white disparities in these two important outcomes have persisted in the United States in spite of medical and social efforts to reduce the gaps. Research into racial and ethnic differences in health care in Europe is scarce.

It is widely argued that the causes of health and illness among individuals, communities, regions/states, and entire countries go beyond biological and genetic factors and lie in a mix of (a) working, living, and psychosocial environments, (b) personal choices, life styles, and behaviors, (c) family and community support, (d) the psychology of inequality, (e) the social philosophy of government, and (f) each nation's healthcare system. In her paper on the complex web of causation, Krieger (1994) asks the key question "Has anyone seen the spider?" What is the response to this question within MCH? Is the response the same in all developed nations? It may well be that effective strategies for significant improvements in MCH indicators would benefit more from attention to the social determinants of health than from any specific clinical services. In a remarkably prescient report to the Canadian Parliament in 1967 (Lalande 1967), the Hon. Mark Lalande observed "…changes in lifestyles or social and physical environments would likely lead to more improvements in health than would be achieved by spending more money on existing healthcare delivery systems."

The impact on health of a broad range of social, economic, living and working environments, and lifestyle choice determinants is considerable and has been recognized since ancient Greek, Roman, and Chinese times. The current impetus was rekindled in the last quarter of the 20th century. McKeown (1979) in "The Role of Medicine: Dream, Nemesis or Mirage" proposed that social changes, improvements in housing, sanitation, nutrition, work conditions, and practices had greater effect on health status in Europe since the 1900s than specific medical interventions. Reports to the UK government such as the 1980 Black Report (Black et al. 1980) and the 1998 Acheson Report recognized the importance of social determinants and concluded that the traditional assumption that biology and genetics are the primary cause of disease in high-income economies is not correct. These major contributions all brought the relationship between socioeconomics and health into the political debate. Other reports in Canada (Romanow

2002), the United States (Institute of Medicine 2003), and undoubtedly many more in European and Asian publications hidden from many of us by language barriers are powerful reminders. We must never forget these factors that are so often ignored because they lie outside the daily practice of medicine. And we must always dig more deeply into the layers of causality until we find, as Marmot states, the "causes of the causes" (Marmot 2007). Finally, we should heed Strobino et al.'s (1995) admonition that "Public policy is frequently based on simplistic solutions to complex problems, often leading to failure and the belief that these problems are intractable."

Conclusion

- Everywhere except in the United States, universal health care (equal access to basic care for all citizens and legal residents based solely on clinical need and not on ability to pay, and funded by all) is considered to be a fundamental societal right. This philosophy has a redistributive cost to some; consequently, taxation levels in most countries are higher than in the United States. For-profit insurance companies, so dominant in the US healthcare system, play a considerably smaller role in the rest of the developed world.
- There is considerable variation among nations in the ways that health care is financed and delivered. The mechanisms used are of five types: (a) payment of providers by central or regional government out of a general fund from income taxes; (b) payment of providers by central or regional governments out of a fund specifically collected for health purposes; (c) payment of providers by independent health funds; (d) direct payment as premiums to private insurance companies; and (e) direct, out-of-pocket payment of providers by patients for all or part (co-payments) of services received. Some countries utilize several of these mechanisms for different sectors of society.
- No country's healthcare system is considered by its residents to be ideal in all respects and most

countries continually strive for improvement. Typical, macrolevel concerns are as follows: (a) increasing annual costs; (b) the cost of new technology; (c) the aging population and the corresponding decline in numbers of supporting workers. Fertility has declined in many countries in Europe to at or below replacement rates; (d) immigration and growing problems of social inclusion of minorities, many of whom do not speak the language of their adopted countries; (e) need to be responsive to the increasing expectations of patients; (f) uneven access and quality of care in different parts of the same country; (g) waiting lines for less urgent care; (h) maximizing the use of information technology; and (i) some countries are concerned that the balance between specialist and primary care physicians, and between urban and rural providers, is moving in the wrong direction.

- The highest life expectancy is attained in Japan, Switzerland, Sweden, Australia, France, and Spain. The lowest infant mortality rates are found in Japan, Finland, and Sweden and the lowest low birth weight rates in Finland, Sweden, and Norway. The rate of increase of low birth weight rates in Japan and Spain is puzzling. The fact that the United States is an outlier, with generally worse outcomes and higher costs may not so much be an indictment of the US healthcare system as it is a reflection of poverty, social, and behavioral determinants.

- The highest numbers of physicians per thousand population are in Belgium, Italy, and Greece, the highest proportions of nurses/1,000 are in Ireland, Norway, and Finland, and of midwives are in Finland, Norway, New Zealand, Belgium, Sweden, and the United Kingdom. The highest numbers of acute hospital beds per thousand population are in Japan, which has longer average length of stay (ALOS). Austria and Germany have the shortest surgery waiting times.

- Among countries other than the United States, there was little difference in percentage of GDP devoted to health care (9.2%), or the national healthcare expenditures per capita ($2,650). The United States spent 15.3% of

GDP or $5,700 per capita even though it has fewer residents aged over 65 years, offers fewer services (doctor visits, bed-days, and prescription coverage in 2003), leaves more than 45 million without health insurance coverage, and has poorer outcomes. The "face" time between a patient and physician is twice as long in Australia and 50% as long in New Zealand as in the United States.

- Total taxation levels as a percentage of GDP are on average 15% higher in Europe than in the United States, with Scandinavian countries and Finland being the highest. Generally, higher paid persons bear a proportionately higher taxation load in Europe than in the United States and welfare and other national goals such as higher education are heavily subsidized.

- Hospital physicians are often salaried and global budgets are widely used in Europe. The personal cost of medical education and the probability of litigation are lower everywhere than in the United States.

- Most European, Canadian, and Australian practices make greater use of computer technology such as universally accessible medical records and shared responsibility for care 24 h per day, 7 days per week.

- Some countries have very well-developed evidence-based guidelines for prenatal and early child care, others have not. Realization of the importance of behavioral and social determinants of health is better developed in some countries than others. The importance of prevention and early detection, and the concepts of population health are well established in Canada, Europe, and Australasia. Countries differ widely in their use of nurse midwives in community pregnancy management teams. In some countries, child care is closely integrated with schools.

- In the United States there is a twofold gap between infant mortality and low birth weight levels for Caucasian and African-American pregnancies.

- In Eastern Europe and Central Asia, falling outcomes of care, such as a drop in life expectancy, are a cause for concern.

Key Terms

Abortion	Gross national product (GNP)	Well-child care
Acute bed-days	Growth curve	Women-centered care
African-Americans	Haguenau project	World War II
After-hours care	Healthcare expenditure	Last menstrual period (LMP)
Antenatal care	Health insurance	Low birth weight
Asia	Health system	Low-income countries
Average length of stay	Healthcare systems	Marshall Plan
Behavioral determinants	Hemoglobinopathies	Maternal mortality
Behavioral health	Hepatitis C	Medicaid
Capitation fees	HIV	Medical errors
Caregivers	Human Development Index	Medicare
Carnet de santé	Human Poverty Index	Mental health
Caucasians	Immunization	Middle-income country
Causality	Incidence	National scoreboard
Child health nurse	Income inequality	North Atlantic Treaty
Child mortality	Inequality	Organization (NATO)
Corruption Index	Infant mortality	Northern European countries
Cost per capita	Insurance plan	Nulliparous
Development Assistance	International Classification of	Nurse midwife
Committee (DAC), G8	Diseases (ICD)	Occupancy rate
nations	Scandinavian countries	Out-of-pocket payment
Down's syndrome	School health programs	Out-patient maternity clinic
Economically disadvantaged	Smoking cessation	Parous
areas	Social influence	Patient satisfaction
E-Health Program	Social philosophies	Per capita income
Environmental; determinant	Social welfare interventions	Placental hormones
Evidence-based guidelines	South European countries	Political systems
Fertility rate	Specialist obstetricians	Postnatal care
Fetal fibronectin	Stillbirth, patient education	Pregnancy outcomes
Fetal growth curve	Sub-Saharan Africa	Prenatal care
Freedom Index	Sustainable economic growth	Prenatal care visits
Fundamental human rights	Syphilis screening	Pre-school
General practitioner physicians	TRICARE	Preterm birth
Gestational age	Trimester	Private insurance
Gestational diabetes	Under-5 mortality	Psychological health
Gini coefficient	Uninsured	Purchasing power parity (PPP)
Globalization	The United States of America	
GNP per capita	Weight for gestational age	
Gross national income (GNI)		

Questions for Discussion

1. (a) What is the OECD? (b) How did the OECD originate? (c) What was its mission?
2. It is said that healthcare systems in the different OECD countries are a reflection of each country's social, economic, and political philosophies. What does this mean?
3. What are social determinants of health? Using specific examples in relation to any OECD country, explain how social, environmental, economic, political, and lifestyle factors influence any four MCH indicators of your choice.
4. Despite the plethora of pre- and postnatal care approaches, technological improvements, increased expenditure and intensity of care over the past three decades, no significant improvements have been recorded for the proportion of infants born with low birth weight in any high-income OECD country. Why is this so? What are the implications of this phenomenon to low-income countries?
5. Define the following terms:

   a. Capitation
   b. Gross domestic product (GDP)
   c. Gross national product (GNP)
   d. Gross national income (GNI)
   e. Gini coefficient
   f. Human Development Index (HDI)
   g. Human Poverty Index (HPI)
   h. Life expectancy
   i. Per capita income
   j. Per capita expenditure
   k. Purchasing power parity (PPP)

References

Acheson D (1998) Independent inquiry into inequalities in health. Her Majesty's Stationery Office London, UK

American Academy of Pediatrics (2000) Recommendations for preventive pediatric healthcare. Elk Grove Village, USA: Author

Bernloehr A, Smith P, Vydelingum V (2007) National guidelines on antenatal care: a survey and comparison of the 25 member states of the European Union. European Clinics of Obstetrics and Gynecology 2, 213–222

Bindman AB, Forrest CB, Britt H et al. (2007) Diagnostic scope of and exposure to primary care physicians in Australia and New Zealand, and the US: cross sectional analysis of results from three national surveys. British Medical Journal 334(7606), 1261–1263

Black D, Morris JN, Townsend P (1980) Inequalities in health. London, UK: Penguin Books

BUPA (2008) Health insurance tailored for you. London, England: British Provident Association (BUPA). http://www.bupa.co.uk/, cited 13 July 2008

Centers for Disease Control and Prevention (2007) News report shows decline in stillbirths: racial disparities persist. http://www.cdc.gov/media/pressrel/2007/r070221.htm?s_cid = mediarel_r070221_x, cited 16 July 2008

Goldenberg R (1998) Low birth weight PORT – Patient Outcomes Research Team. Low birth weight in minority and high risk women. Agency for Healthcare Policy and Research, Washington, DC

Henshaw SK, Singh S, Haas T (1999) The incidence of abortion worldwide. International Family Planning Perspectives 25 (suppl), S30–S38

Heritage Foundation (2008) Index of economic freedom. http://www.heritage.org/Index/, cited 14 July 2008

Howell EM, Blondel B (1994) International infant mortality rates: bias from reporting differences. American Journal of Public Health 84(5), 850–852

Hunt JM, Lumley J (2002) Are recommendations about routine antenatal care in Australia consistent and evidence-based? Medical Journal of Australia 176(6), 255–259

Institute of Medicine (2003) The future of the public's health in the 21st century. Washington, USA: National Academies Press

Krieger N (1994) Epidemiology and the web of causation: has anyone seen the spider? Social Science and Medicine 39(7), 887–903

Kuo AA, Inkelas M, Lotstein et al. (2006) Rethinking well-child care in the United States: An international comparison. Pediatrics 118(4), 1692–1702

Lalande M (1967) A new perspective on the health of Canadians. Ottawa, Canada: Health Canada Publications

Marmot M (2007) Achieving health equity: from root causes to fair outcomes. Lancet 370(9593), 1153–1163

McKeown T (1979) The role of medicine: dream, mirage, or nemesis? Nuffield Provincial Hospitals Trust, London, UK

Murray JE (2006) The persistence of the health insurance dilemma. Social Science History 30(4), 465–477

National Collaborating Centre for Women's and Children's Health (2008) Clinical guideline # CG62. Antenatal care: routine care for the healthy pregnancy woman. National Collaborating Center for Women's and Children's Health. National Institute for Health and Clinical Excellence (NICE) and UK National Health Service (NHS). http://www.nice.org.uk/nicemedia/pdf/CG62FullGuidelineCorrectedJune2008.pdf, cited 26 November 2008

Organization for Economic Cooperation and Development (OECD) (2006) Health Data 2006. Paris: Organization for Economic Cooperation and Development

Organization for Economic Cooperation and Development (OECD) (2007) OECD Journal on Development: Development Co-operation Report 2007. www.oecd.org/dac/dcr, cited 14 July 2008

Organization for Economic Cooperation and Development (OECD) (2008) OECD – history. http://www.oecd.org/pages/0,3417,en_36734052_36761863_1_1_1_1_1,00.html, cited July 15 2008

Papiernik E, Bouyer J, Dreyfus J et al. (1985) Prevention of preterm births: a perinatal study in Haguenau, France. Pediatrics 76(2), 154–158

Papiernik E, Bouyer J, Yaffe K et al. (1986) Women's acceptance of preterm birth prevention program. American Journal of Obstetrics and Gynecology 155(5), 939–946

Romanow RJ (2002) Building on values. The future of heath care in Canada. Canada: Saskatoon

Schoen C, Osborn R, Huynh PT et al. (2006) On the front lines of care: primary care doctors' office systems, experiences, and views in seven countries. Health Affairs 25(6), 555–571

Schor EL (2004) Rethinking well-child care. Pediatrics 114(1), 210–216

Shen JJ, Tymkow C, MacMullen N (2005) Disparities in maternal outcomes among four ethnic populations. Ethnicity and Disease 15(3), 492–497

Stewart P, Sprague A, Niday P et al. (eds) (1998) Prevention of low birth weight in Canada: literature review and strategies. Technical Report. Toronto: Ontario Prevention Clearing-house Best Start Resource Centre. Sponsored by the Perinatal Education Program of Eastern Ontario

Strobino D, O'Campo P, Schoendorf KC et al. (1995) A strategic framework for infant mortality reduction: implications for "Healthy Start". The Milbank Quarterly 73(4) 507–533

The Commonwealth Fund Commission on a High Performance Health System (2008) Why Not the Best? Results from the National Scorecard on U.S. Health System Performance, 2008, New York, USA: The Commonwealth Fund. http://www.commonwealthfund.org/usr_doc/Why_Not_the_Best_national_scorecard_2008.pdf?section=4039, cited 15 September 2008

Transparency International (2002) Corruption Fighters Tool Kit. http://www.transparency.org/tools/e_toolkit/corruption_fighters_tool_kit_2002, cited 11 December 2008

UNICEF (2007) State of the world's children 2007. New York: UNICEF. http://www.unicef.org/sowc07/report/report.php, cited 28 July 2008

United Nations (2005) Human Development Report 2005 - Human Poverty Index for less developed countries (LDCs). New York: United Nations Development Programme (UNDP) http://www.un.org/special-rep/ohrlls/ldc/2005%20human%20poverty%20index.pdf, cited 14 July 2008

United Nations Development Programme (2008) Human Development Index (HDI). New York: United Nations Development Programme (UNDP) http://hdr.undp.org/en/statistics/indices/hdi/, cited 14 July 2008

United States Department of Health and Human Services (2006) Health, United States, 2006. Washington, DC: USA: United States Department of Health and Human Services (US DHHS), Centers for Disease Control and Prevention, National Center for Health Statistics. http://www.ncbi.nlm.nih.gov/books/bookres.fcgi/healthus06/healthus06.pdf, cited 18 July, 2008

World Bank (2008) Measuring Inequality.http://go.worldbank.org/3SLYUTVY00, cited 14 July 2008

World Health Organization (2000) The World Health Report 2000: Health Systems: Improving Performance. Geneva: World Health Organization

World Health Organization (2004) Health care systems in transition. Regional Office for Europe. http://www.euro.who.int/Document/E84991.pdf, cited 28 July 2008

World Health Organization (2006) World Health report 2006 – Working together for health. Geneva: World Health Organization. http://www.who.int/whr/2006/whr06_en.pdf, cited 28 July 2008

Chapter 5
Health System Impacts on Maternal and Child Health

Nancy Gerein, Andrew Green, Tolib Mirzoev, and Stephen Pearson

Learning objectives After reading this chapter and answering the discussion questions that follow, you should be able to

- Discuss elements of a health system and identify key differences between a health system and a healthcare system.
- Appraise the mechanisms by which the various elements of the health system interact to influence access, quality, and use of health services, and ultimately the health of mothers and children.
- Identify and analyze major challenges for the health systems in improving maternal and child health.
- Describe the role of the health system in achieving the Millennium Development Goals (MDGs) related to maternal and child health.

Introduction

A story: One evening, Margaret went into labor with her first child at her home, and summoned help from the traditional birth attendant in the village. By the next evening, no progress had been made, and Margaret's husband decided to take her to the health centre. He went to his relatives to borrow money and then spent an hour trying to hire a private car to travel to the health centre. When Margaret and her husband arrived at the health centre in the middle of the night, no doctor was on duty (he was away for training) but they were able to find the midwife at her

home after half an hour. However, the health centre had run out of the drugs required to help Margaret, who was by now bleeding heavily. Margaret and her husband traveled to the hospital in the nearest town, where they were asked to find a suitable blood donor. This took another hour, by which time Margaret and her baby were dead. The cause of death was listed as obstructed labor and hemorrhage. But was that the real reason the mother and child died?

Technical (or medical) knowledge exists to prevent the death of Margaret and her child. In fact, technical knowledge exists to provide health services that could respond to many, if not most, of the serious health problems affecting mothers and children. Often, however, barriers prevent those who need these effective health services, like Margaret, from receiving them. The responsibility for removing these barriers lies with the health system. This chapter focuses not on specific aspects of maternal and child health (MCH) but on the critical contribution that the wider healthcare system makes to MCH. It discusses the main elements of a healthcare system and examines key differences between a health system and a healthcare system. To present the contribution of the health system to maternal and child health in proper context, the chapter uses a conceptual model to characterize the different elements of the health system from both the biomedical and holistic perspectives. Components of the model including the healthcare system (health services delivery, resources and support systems, and governance), community inputs, and health-related services (e.g., water and sanitation, education and literacy, social services) are delineated. The mechanisms by which these various

N. Gerein (✉)
Nuffield Centre for International Health and Development, University of Leeds, England

facets interact to influence access, quality, and use of health services and ultimately the health of mothers and children are analyzed. Major challenges for healthcare systems in improving the health of mothers and children are discussed. The chapter concludes with a discussion of the role of the health system in achieving Millennium Development Goals (MDGs) related to maternal and child health and an examination of future policy and practice directions.

The healthcare system is the structure which supports the provision of necessary health services. It ensures that the right staff and materials are available in the appropriate place at the right time to allow utilization of health services by those in need. When working well, the healthcare system's presence is often largely ignored by health professionals. However, when the healthcare system fails to perform adequately, the consequences for the provision of MCH services can be severe. It is therefore important that health professionals are aware

of the major components of a healthcare system, and how the healthcare system should work effectively to maintain and improve MCH.

Conceptual Framework

Fig. 5.1 presents a framework that illustrates the relationships between MCH and the components of the health system. It differentiates between the *healthcare system* and the wider *health system*. The main differences between these two concepts originate from two broad interpretations of health:

- A *biomedical* or clinical interpretation, which refers mostly to physiological processes of an individual and delivery of health services.
- A wider *holistic* interpretation, which includes social determinants of health such as water supply, education, and social services.

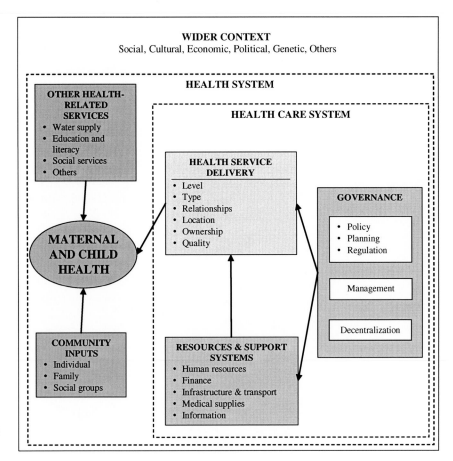

Fig 5.1 Relationships between MCH and the health system.
Source: Adapted from WHO (2000)

According to the World Health Organization (WHO), the health system comprises the following:

> ... all organizations, institutions and resources ...whose primary purpose is to improve health (WHO 2000).

The health system, therefore, reflects the wider holistic interpretation of health, which goes beyond the boundaries of the health sector to include *other health-related services*. Female literacy, for example, is a critical determinant of MCH, and indeed, of uptake of health care. While action on such factors is not usually the direct responsibility of the health sector, health professionals should be aware of these factors' importance in affecting the health of their patients and in seeking ways to get appropriate responses from the relevant sectors.

The biomedical interpretation of health fits perfectly within the boundaries of the healthcare sector, which is often referred to as the *healthcare system* or a system for *health service delivery*. The overarching aim of the healthcare system is to improve health. This is done primarily by expanding and improving the delivery of health services. *Community inputs* have an important role in improving and maintaining maternal and child health in many ways – including through the lifestyles that individuals adopt, through provision of informal care in the home, and through participation (either as individuals or as a community) in decisions about healthcare provision.

Also, MCH exists within a *wider context*. Social, cultural, economic, and political factors inevitably affect both health and the way the healthcare system operates. Although these factors may be outside the direct influence of the health system and wider public system, it is essential to recognize and, where possible, to respond to these factors. This chapter recognizes the importance of the wider health system, but focuses more on the biomedical interpretation of health to describe the impacts of the healthcare system on MCH.

Elements of the Healthcare System

Fig. 5.1 shows three broad components of the healthcare system: *health service delivery* (which is deliberately placed in the center of the framework), *governance*, *resources*, and *support systems*. These components broadly correspond to the conventional interpretation of the functions of the healthcare system, which are described by the WHO (2000) as follows: delivery of services (healthcare system), stewardship (governance), and financing and creating resources (resources and support systems) (Fig. 5.2).

As shown on the right side of Fig. 5.2, the main objective of the health system is to produce good health. Another objective is to ensure the fair financial contribution for health. Health services should also be "responsive" to the public's demands for quality in the non-medical aspects of health care, such as promptness in receiving care, privacy, and respectful communication. All of the components in

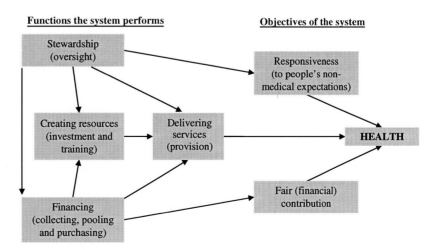

Fig. 5.2 Relationships between the functions and objectives of a health system. Source: WHO (2000)

Fig. 5.1 and their constituent elements combine in complex ways to meet the objectives of the health system. The next sections provide a broad overview of key elements and components from the system perspective.

Health Service Delivery

The purpose of the healthcare system is to deliver health services in the most effective and efficient way to address priority health needs. As such, the delivery of health services should be the centerpiece of the healthcare system. Health service delivery is a complex issue, requiring consideration of:

a) What types of health services are needed and at what level?
b) What relationships should exist between health services?
c) Where should health services be provided?
d) Who should own the health service institutions?
e) What level of quality should health services maintain?

Each question describes a characteristic of health services, which are discussed in the following sections. Remember, however, that these characteristics are closely related.

Types and Levels of Health Services

Within the healthcare system, a hierarchy of different levels of services exists, which is normally divided into three broad levels: primary, secondary, and tertiary.

- *Primary Health Care* (PHC) comprises a basic "package" of health services aimed at provision of essential health services at the community level. The term PHC is also used to refer to the philosophy that underpinned the Alma Ata Declaration of 1978 (WHO/UNICEF 1978) which sets out a series of principles for a health system. These principles were equity, community participation, appropriate technology, health promotion, and multi-sectoralism. Normally,

health service delivery at the PHC level includes facility-based out-patient services and outreach services performed at the community level. For MCH, such services should include antenatal and postnatal care, family planning services, child immunizations, treatment of common childhood illnesses (such as malaria, diarrhea, and upper respiratory infections), and health education around child care. Some PHC facilities may offer MCH in-patient services including normal deliveries, newborn care, and treatment for child malnutrition and severe infections. Basic diagnostic facilities such as laboratory facilities for diagnosing anemia and malaria should be part of such services. Health professionals working at the PHC level have general skills (such as community nurses, medical assistants, or general medical practitioners). In some health systems, the health centers or health posts which offer PHC also act as a "gateway" to secondary levels of care.

- *Secondary Health Care* includes more specialist diagnostic facilities and expertise, available on an out-patient and in-patient basis. Such facilities are usually provided at district hospitals which may have a supervisory and support role for PHC services. In addition to the MCH services offered at PHC, secondary health facilities should offer in-patient services for complicated deliveries and specialist newborn care.

- *Tertiary Health Care* is the most sophisticated level of health services where, for example, treatment for infertility takes place. Tertiary healthcare facilities are normally located at a regional or country level. This is the level where narrow specialization takes place, as well as training of health professionals. Tertiary health care is the most resource-intensive level of health services (both in terms of cost of health services and human resources).

The boundaries between the three levels can be fuzzy. For example, PHC services may be provided from the out-patient department of the district hospital. The examples of MCH services given above can be classified into three types:

- *Promotive services* include health education on topics to enable people to protect their health, e.g., practicing safe sex, avoiding smoking, feeding nutritious weaning foods to infants, and screening for diseases such as vitamin A deficiency and cervical cancer.

- *Preventive services* are provided to prevent health problems, e.g., family planning, immunization, clean water and sanitation to reduce diarrheal disease, and provision of vitamin and mineral supplements.
- *Curative services* are provided to treat existing illness, such as anemia and skin infections.

The PHC level is supposed to take a major role in providing promotive and preventive services, along with basic curative care. Secondary and tertiary levels tend to focus on curative services, but increasingly it is recognized that secondary and tertiary levels should provide promotive and preventive services alongside their traditional curative services. In many health systems, vertical disease control programs (e.g., voluntary counseling and testing centers for HIV/AIDS) will operate alongside the primary, secondary, and tertiary levels of service.

healthcare system, and lost opportunities for maintaining and improving health by not adopting a holistic interpretation of health.

Vertical integration is referral between different levels of health services, e.g., primary to secondary care (Murray and Frenk 2000). A well-functioning referral system is needed when health services are provided at more than one level. Effective referral is particularly important for emergency health care, as in the care of children with life-threatening malaria, or for women with obstetric complications (as shown in the story of Margaret). A well-functioning referral system should include a clear and effective distribution of roles and responsibilities (in this case, types of health services at each level), clear lines of communication (both between different levels of health services and between patients and healthcare providers), and adequate transportation for moving patients between levels. The referral system should also include feedback systems between the levels to ensure appropriate follow-up care for patients.

Relationships Between Health Services

How services relate to each other is a critical feature of a health system. An integrated approach, where planning, financing, and provision of all health services occur together, will benefit both patients and staff. Patients need to be able to move easily between types and levels of services according to their particular needs. For example, a pregnant mother might prefer to receive, in one visit to one facility, a combination of antenatal care, sexually transmitted infection testing, and immunization for her infant, rather than having to move to another facility or return another day. This type of referral is called *horizontal integration* (referral at the same level and between different programs). Non-integrated services (e.g., a clinic providing only HIV/AIDS treatment and care) may result from separately managed services which give priority to a particular program, with earmarked budgets, clear targets, and independent management structures. Such programs have advantages of having a clear technical focus to improve quality and ensure priority to particular health problems through earmarked resources. Disadvantages, however, include a greater management and administrative burden for the whole

Location of Health Services

The geographical location of health services clearly affects the ease of access for a population, and decisions should be based on factors including health needs, population densities, the transportation infrastructure, and the relative costs of services. Some healthcare systems have norms for the provision of different types of health services, reflected either in terms of time–distance (e.g., 2 h travel) or physical distance (e.g., 10 km). Historically, health services have tended to cluster in urban centers, leaving rural populations underserved. As urbanization becomes a growing phenomenon in populous countries such as China, India, and Nigeria, the peri-urban dwellers who often live in illegal shanty areas become the new underserved. One mechanism for providing care to remote or underserved populations is through outreach services. A common outreach service involves health staff traveling through villages to provide immunization to children. Outreach has been shown to improve immunization coverage, particularly to rural and poor populations (Bryce et al. 2003; Azubuike and Ehiri 1998).

Ownership of Health Service Institutions

Health care can be provided by either the public or private sector. The relative merits of these two sectors for MCH are subject to great debate. One argument is that the public sector is more likely to respond to patient need, whereas the private-for-profit sector's focus on income generation and profits may lead to inappropriate services, and a focus on better-off people in urban areas. In South Africa, for example, 75% of obstetric specialists work in the private sector (in which only 9% of women give birth) resulting in poorer quality services in the public sector for the other 91% of women giving birth (Parkhurst et al. 2005). An alternative argument is that the private sector has greater flexibility to manage MCH services and is therefore more responsive and attractive to patients.

These arguments are further complicated first by the extensive presence of non-governmental organizations (NGOs) who can be described as having motivations similar to the public sector, but with the ability to operate in a private manner. NGOs often operate in geographically remote areas and work on politically sensitive issues, for example, HIV/AIDS education for commercial sex workers and drug users. NGOs have also been important advocates for policy change for important issues such as reproductive rights. Second, the public and private sectors are becoming increasingly "mixed" and the boundaries between them are therefore blurred. For example, health professionals may work in both public and private services, and services may be contracted to the private sector by the public sector. Indeed, no "pure" public or private models of healthcare systems exist, and the relative involvement of both sectors is dependent on the wider political and economic context.

Quality of Health Services

Low-quality health services are unlikely to be effective. Services may suffer from a lack of or poorly trained and managed staff; from a lack of appropriate medical supplies or equipment or an inadequate physical environment. Perceived quality of services is a key driver behind the willingness of the public to use available health services. Therefore, a vital element of a health system should focus on assuring that there is adequate quality. Donabedian's (1980) structure/process/outcome model is a conventionally accepted framework for assessing and improving the quality of health services. According to this model

- *Structure* refers to the professional and organizational resources associated with the provision of care, such as staff qualifications, and infrastructure, equipment, and supplies.
- *Process* refers to the things that are done to, and for, patients by practitioners in the course of treatment.
- *Outcome* refers to the desired results from service delivery processes, which may include reductions in morbidity, disability, and improvements in the quality of life.

Quality assurance systems are an important element in the governance (stewardship) of health systems; they provide a systematic way of focusing on the quality of services and on the structure–process–outcome factors that produce quality. A quality assurance system includes the development of objectives for quality, setting, and communicating standards to staff and the public, developing indicators, collecting data to monitor compliance with the standards, and applying solutions to improve health care. Returning to the debate over public and private ownership of MCH services, what evidence is available on the quality of these two sectors? Patients may perceive quality as being high in the private sector, for example, due to the flexibility of opening hours, short waiting times, and increased personal attention from the healthcare provider. However, some studies have found that the quality of care from private-for-profit practitioners is technically worse, with poorer prescribing practices (over-medication, use of expensive rather than cheaper generic drugs), over-use of diagnostic tests, and neglect of preventive care. In maternal care, medically unnecessary (but lucrative) cesarean sections increasingly are common in Latin America and urban areas of Asia, even though they carry greater health risks to women and newborns, and may incur catastrophic expenditures for clients (Ravindran et al. 2005).

Governance

Governance (and the related term "stewardship") emerged in the late 1990s as a key concept for improving health systems. It refers to how decisions are made and how the health sector is regulated. Key questions around governance include the following:

- What are the underlying values of the healthcare system?
- Who makes decisions and to whom are the decision makers accountable?
- How transparent and inclusive is the decision-making process?
- How effective and efficient are the management and planning processes in identifying and responding to needs?
- How are different entities (individuals or institutions associated with the health system) brought together?
- What should the appropriate balance be between regulations in the form of control versus incentives?

One of the key values within the healthcare system is equity of access to healthcare services. This is particularly important for MCH as mothers and children are one of the most vulnerable groups of population:

> In Afghanistan, the differences [in the Maternal Mortality Ratio] were...striking, with mortality being 418 maternal deaths per 100,000 live births in the capital city of Kabul compared with 6,507 maternal deaths per 100,000 live births in the remote district of Ragh. ....In sub-Saharan Africa, the pooled estimate for urban areas is 447 maternal deaths per 100,000 live births compared with 640 maternal deaths per 100,000 live births in rural areas. Differences in physical access to obstetric care are likely to explain at least part of this variation. Other mechanisms might be involved, such as high prevalence of HIV or of unsafe abortion, or the poor quality of emergency obstetric care in hospitals (Ronsmans and Graham 2006).

During the 1990s, many countries reformed their health systems with particular emphasis on decentralization of management and greater roles for the private sector in service provision. This has raised other governance issues, for example, changing the role of national ministries of health from operational aspects of health services management to a more strategic policy making and regulatory role.

The importance of health policy, health planning and management, and the effects of decentralization are described below.

Health Policy, Planning, and Management

Health policy is a statement of intent by the central government as to the development of the health system. For example, a child health policy could include the following:

- Guidance for the planning, implementation, monitoring, and evaluation of health services for children, including goals and targets for children's health status and services
- Strategic approaches to achieve these goals and targets
- The types of services to be provided
- Human and financial resources needed
- Management and coordination of the services
- Research and information systems support needed
- The roles of the government, private sector, and communities in promoting and protecting child health

The development of policy can be thought of as a series of inter-related stages in the form of a cycle or a spiral (emphasizing an iterative nature). Being closely linked to politics, health policy making therefore involves complex power interactions between different individuals and groups with distinct values, ideologies, agendas, and practices (Buse et al. 2005). To be meaningful, health policy needs to be translated into services through the setting of plans and ultimately, the allocation of appropriate resources and budgets.

Health planning can be defined as follows:

> ...a systematic method of trying to attain explicit objectives for the future, through the efficient and appropriate use of resources, available now and in the future (Green 2007).

Health planning includes strategic and operational planning. *Strategic planning*, which is often seen as an integral part of health policy making, focuses on the priority direction for the development of a sector or a program. *Operational planning* focuses more on the shorter term technicalities of the planning process (such as the construction of new buildings or the provision of staff training programs) and should link into the regular recurrent budget.

Approaches to planning are often described as top-down or bottom-up. For *top-down*, the planning process occurs at the highest level (e.g., central government) with decisions (plans) being communicated to lower levels. The *bottom-up* approach emphasizes the involvement in the planning process, of actors at the local levels through assessment of health needs, identification of priorities and participation in decision making. As health policy making and planning should involve different actors to achieve the desired objectives, a balance between technical and political dimensions is needed. How this balance is achieved is critical to the success of the MCH system, and can be aided by ensuring that key stakeholders are consulted and feel "ownership" of policy-making and planning processes.

Health management is concerned with the best possible use of available resources to achieve health goals through the implementation of plans (Green and Collins 2006). Health management can be both general (managing an overall system) or related to specific resources used within the health system, in particular human resources, financial resources, infrastructure, and medical supplies. The decision-making processes involved in setting MCH policies and plans, and managing MCH services often have been neglected in healthcare systems. Such neglect results in poor policies, strategies, and services. Strengthening decision-making processes requires the active involvement of relevant actors from the health system, patients, communities, the appropriate use of evidence, and transparent and effective decision-making processes.

Decentralization

Decentralization has become a popular policy in many healthcare systems, but with varying results. Decentralization can be defined as follows:

A transfer of authority to make decisions, to carry out management functions and use resources. Focusing on

the public sector, it means the passing of these from central government authorities to such bodies in the periphery as local government, field administration, subordinate units of government, specialized authorities and semi-autonomous public corporations (Collins 1994).

Different forms of decentralization have been tried, with varying implications for health services. Two key forms are as follows:

- *Devolution* – the transfer of authority from the center to a multi-functional authority which may be seen as a separate lower level of government with its own legitimacy, authority, and sources of revenue.
- *Deconcentration* – the transfer of resources, responsibilities, and authority to a lower level with main line management control being maintained.

Decentralization can affect the provision of MCH services through different elements of the health system. On the plus side, decentralization can allow for better planning for local needs and greater financial allocation to these needs, improved availability of drugs and transport, more flexible and appropriate deployment of staff, and the generation of local funds. However, decentralization can also produce the opposite of these results, greater inequity between local districts, a reduction in the quality of services because of loss of the most experienced staff and other effects. Decentralization is a continual process, and with effective monitoring and decision-making systems and processes, and sufficient capacity within the healthcare system, improvements can be made.

Under a decentralized health system, therefore, local health managers could have greater influence over local health planning. With an effective Health Management Information System (HMIS) and evidence on the likely effectiveness of different intervention options, spending could be more closely matched to health needs. Ideally, local health managers could also receive inputs from local communities to make healthcare delivery more appropriate and strengthen community "ownership" of the healthcare system. But could such an approach work in practice? The Tanzania Essential Health Interventions Project applied such a package of affordable interventions in two districts in Tanzania in the late 1990s (de Savigny et al. 2004). This was credited to have resulted in a 40% reduction in child mortality over 5 years. This successful intervention is now being scaled up to the whole of Tanzania.

Resources and Support Systems

Resources and support systems are vital in underpinning the delivery of MCH services. For "frontline" professionals providing health services, resources and support systems may be taken for granted but is critical to the professionals' abilities to work effectively. As described in the next sections, crucial resources and support systems for MCH services include human and financial resources, infrastructure and transportation, medical supplies and information.

Human Resources

The healthcare system is very labor intensive and is dependent on a rich variety of professionals and other staff. A shortage of key staff may critically compromise the provision of quality MCH services. Staff shortages may reflect an overall national shortage or a geographical imbalance. In many countries, health professionals are concentrated in urban centers and in the private sector. In India, for example, the availability of midwives in rural areas was between 6 and 27% of the national norm (Koblinsky et al. 2006). Opportunities for MCH staff to emigrate to work in richer countries are increasingly attractive, leading to a current or impending crisis for the health system, especially in sub-Saharan Africa. High levels of HIV infection among health personnel also contribute, in some countries, to loss of health workers. For example, of all nurses lost from the public sector in Malawi and Zambia (two countries with high HIV prevalence rates) in the late 1990s, 40% were due to deaths (Schneider et al. 2006).

Staffing is an especially critical issue in maternal care. Delivery by a skilled attendant is argued to be one of the best ways to reduce maternal mortality (and it would also substantially reduce neonatal

mortality). Progress toward the Millennium Development Goal (MDG) (United Nations Development Programme 2003) to improve maternal health is monitored by the percentage of women whose delivery is managed by skilled personnel (midwives and doctors with appropriate training). For developing countries, the indicator increased from an estimated 43% in 1990 to 57% in 2005 (United Nations 2007).

As well as being available in sufficient numbers, human resources require skills, supplies, motivation, and good management, in order to provide health-improving services. What are the important considerations in planning and managing health staff? First, as initial training of health professionals takes several years, a long time is required to achieve shifts in professional staffing. Second, as priorities and services change, staff should be retrained periodically and equipped for new challenges. Integrated management of childhood illness (IMCI), for example, is a promising strategy for delivering essential child health interventions as discussed in Chapter 27. Consistent and high-quality implementation of IMCI has been hampered, however, due to very few health workers being trained in IMCI, lack of IMCI-trained supervisors, and high staff turnover (Bryce et al. 2003).

Third, being human, staff are very different to other "resources". They have personal circumstances, needs, and ambitions which have to be considered alongside the needs of the healthcare system. Unlike equipment, for example, staff cannot easily be redeployed elsewhere in the health sector. Furthermore, changes in priorities and health service approaches (for example, allowing midwives to provide safe abortions, instead of only doctors) may be resisted by professionals, and yet their agreement is critical to the success of any change in an MCH program.

The planning and management of human resources may be the most critical responsibility for planners and managers and yet has strangely been neglected by many healthcare systems. Issues involved in planning, developing and maintaining the maternal, newborn, and child health workforce are explored in greater detail in Chapter 28. The growing crisis in health human resources was also the focus of WHO's (2006) World Health Report.

Finance

Finance is, of course, the underpinning resource for all health services. All health systems have less finance than they would like, hence the need for clear priority setting. Health systems need to consider two broad issues related to health financing – how finance is raised (resource generation) and how it is allocated.

There are five broad approaches to generating resources (Green 2007):

(a) *User fees* collect a payment from the patient at the point of service delivery. Different types of user fees are possible: the main types being per case treated/ diagnosis; per duration (e.g., per bed-day); and per type of services (e.g., per consultation/prescription).

(b) *Private insurance* is a complement to user fees and provides a mechanism for pooling risk among a group. A fixed sum is prepaid to a private insurance company, which then covers all, or part, of any subsequent health costs.

(c) *Social insurance* is a public insurance system with risk pooling similar to private insurance. The key difference, however, is that the contributions by the employee and the employer are related to the level of income of the employee.

(d) *Taxation* generates revenue through a government system of taxes on income, goods, and businesses. The strength of general taxation is that it is compulsory and is usually not the responsibility of the health sector to administer.

(e) *Community-based financing* is increasingly popular and includes several of the above approaches, but implemented at the community level. A well-known example is the *Bamako Initiative* (Ridde 2003) which involves Revolving Drug Funds and is a variation of user fees with revenue retained at the community level.

Each approach has its advantages and disadvantages for MCH. Two important considerations are how the approach affects equity through affecting the accessibility of services by poorer groups and the risk of services being provided to raise income rather than to meet health needs. In most countries that have introduced user fees, the poorest population groups subsequently have reduced their use of MCH services (WHO 2006). When the South African public health system removed fees for services for pregnant women and children under 6, service use surged (Gilson and McIntyre 2005). This surge, however, resulted in health workers complaining of overwork and inadequate supplies and medicines, showing how elements of health systems are related. In China, diminished financial support from the government encouraged professionals to earn more income through curative medicine, over-use of diagnostic tests and technology (e.g., cesarean sections), and selling of medicines (Ravindran et al. 2005).

In theory, the social insurance approach to generating revenue encompasses the principles of equity (richer groups of the population pay more, thus covering some costs for the poorer groups). In practice, however, social insurance schemes involve a substantial management burden. A scheme needs a critical mass of employed individuals to be able to generate enough revenue; a reliable registration system; and willingness of employers to contribute toward the scheme. Community-based financing is argued to empower local communities to be involved in health-related decisions. In theory, risks are pooled and every community member has access to the services that are financed by the community-generated funds. In practice, many communities have marginal groups (such as women and children) for whom health-related decisions are made by more "powerful" members of the family or community (such as husbands or elders).

Infrastructure and Transportation

Appropriate physical structures and equipment, together with a functioning transport system, are essential for the provision of high-quality MCH services. It is important to tailor these features to the patterns of service delivery (e.g., transportation requirements for facility-based care are different from those of outreach services) as well as to the health needs of the local population. Transportation arrangements are particularly important for emergency health situations such as obstetric health care. An adequate communication system between patients and health facilities and between different levels of the healthcare system is paramount to making the referral system work effectively.

Medical Supplies

An adequate supply of appropriate medicines is needed for MCH care systems. Preventive (e.g., immunization) and curative (e.g., treatment of infections with antibiotics) interventions require a reliable supply of in-date and good-quality medicines. Medical supplies, however, can absorb a sizeable amount of a health service's operating budget. Good planning and management is therefore critical, with health system issues including

(a) The choice of medicines (selection of generic versus branded medicines)
(b) The use of an essential drug list which limits the use of medicines to an agreed list
(c) The purchase, distribution, and storage of medicines
(d) Rational prescribing practices by health providers

Information

How can policy be informed, and resources and delivery of health services planned and monitored, without relevant and up-to-date information? Within the health system, different types of information could be collected, including data on inputs, processes, and service delivery, and on the health status of the population. A Health Management Information System (HMIS) is concerned with routine collection, transmission, processing, analysis, and storage of health and health service-related data within the healthcare system. Some programs such as maternal health also establish their own vertical information systems to generate evidence for their own planning and decision making. The overall aim of an HMIS is to generate information to support decision-making processes, including monitoring and evaluation of health service delivery. This is easier said than done, however. Why do most HMISs in developing countries under-perform?

- Data are lacking in accuracy and reliability, which are related to the HMIS' capacity for data collection and processing.
- Information is not used at the appropriate level of the healthcare system, which is related to the system's organizational structure.
- Feedback mechanisms within and across the levels of the healthcare system are poor, which is related to the inter-relationships between the different levels.

How important is it to have a good HMIS, medical supplies, and a transportation system? In Arua District in Uganda in the 1990s, cases of childhood measles were increasing, despite an existing immunization program. District health managers identified and prompted improvements in the HMIS and cold chain (the system for maintaining a temperature controlled supply of vaccines). As a result, the number of measles cases reduced by three-quarters (Bryce et al. 2003).

Other Health-Related Services

Referring back to Fig. 5.1, health-related services provided in other sectors are equally important for MCH when taking the wider holistic interpretation of health. This has also been acknowledged in one of the key international policy statements, the MDGs, where health is included in non-health goals such as those related to poverty eradication and environmental sustainability (United Nations Development Programme 2003). Examples of health-related services include improving the socio-economic status of the population (e.g., poverty reduction initiatives) and interventions targeted at a particular group (e.g., female literacy). For example, in India, one study showed that deaths due to domestic violence were the second largest cause of death in pregnancy (16%), requiring a response from the police and judicial system, as well as health and social services (Ronsmans and Graham 2006). In child health, diarrhea is a leading cause of morbidity and mortality. Safe water supply, adequate sanitation, sufficient food supply, and personal and household hygienic practices all help to prevent childhood diarrhea, yet require work by many sectors of society outside of the healthcare system. Effective responses to multi-sectoral issues need to establish and maintain partnerships between the sectors, each of which has its own priorities and practices.

Community Inputs

If health systems focus entirely on the provision of services to people, this dangerously ignores the critical roles that these people have in the process of promoting and maintaining good health. These roles can be seen at several levels (Fig. 5.1). First, *individual and family behaviors* are vital in ensuring the survival, healthy growth, and development of children, through, for example, decisions to breast-feed babies, sleeping under bed-nets to prevent malaria, and drinking safe water. It is estimated that combining family–community care and out-reach care at 90% coverage could avert 18–37% of neonatal deaths in low-income countries (Darmstadt et al. 2005). Most of these deaths would be averted through care such as keeping new-borns warm, exclusive breastfeeding, aseptic cord care, and "kangaroo mother care" (a system of care for "particularly premature" newborns, focusing on skin-to-skin contact, exclusive breastfeeding, and support for the mother and infant) for low birth weight infants.

Much health care is provided informally within families through the purchase and administration of over-the-counter medicines. If the health service recognizes and values this home-based care, real opportunities are presented for support and improvement, while concurrently ensuring that individuals are able to access formal care when necessary. Up to 80% of deaths of children under 5 are estimated to occur at home without contact with health providers (Olumole et al. 2000), underscoring the importance of family and community care, as well as strengthened linkages between health services and communities. Second, decisions on using health-care services are made by individuals and families in the wider *social*, *cultural*, and *economic* contexts (Fig. 5.1). The influences of these contexts vary from the availability of cash to pay for health services or transport, the implications of time lost from

employment and domestic activities through attending health services, to household decision processes and wider cultural norms and beliefs about health and its determinants. In the story at the beginning of this chapter, for example, why did the husband make the decision that Margaret should attend the health center? In most societies, men have greater power than women in making decisions around family members' health behaviors, spending on health care, and accessing health care. Other factors that can affect a person's status, power, and access to resources within a society include age, social class, ethnicity, poverty status, and sexuality. Health systems often are ill-informed about these wider influences and yet they can be critical in ensuring that MCH services are used in a timely and appropriate way by all groups in society.

Communities also have the potential (if the process is managed appropriately) to be involved in the planning and delivery of services in response to the communities' own perceived needs. For example, community members can be involved in local management of staff or facilities or give views on how to improve the provision of services. The community members can also help health staff with immunization days and organizing well-baby clinics, or set up a system to transport emergency obstetric cases to hospital.

Conclusion

The MDGs are important international targets for development, particularly for the least developed countries of the world. Reaching the MDGs for MCH crucially depends on the performance of health systems. This is especially true of maternal and neonatal health which is particularly affected by health systems' attributes of access, quality, and responsiveness of care, and high utilization of key services such as antenatal care, routine and emergency delivery care, safe abortion care, family planning services, and immunization. The research literature has many examples of disease-specific MCH interventions with some evidence of effectiveness for small target groups (see Chapter 20 on Evidence-based MCH). Ensuring that interventions are sustainable, however, and have equitable public health benefits beyond a relatively small group, requires working with a robust, cost-effective, and responsive health system.

For maternal health, encouraging women to have their babies in facilities rather than at home, with the help of teams of skilled midwives and assistants, has been cited as the single largest measure to reduce maternal and neonatal mortality (Ronsmans and Graham 2006). This goal can conflict with cultural norms around birthing in the family home, and would require families to have easy access to health services offering (what families perceive as) high-quality and responsive delivery services. An effective referral system is needed to connect the different levels of the healthcare system, so that emergency obstetric care is available promptly. New communication technologies and community-run transport schemes potentially can improve the referral system, but the greatest challenge will always be the short time available between detecting and recognizing symptoms of an obstetric emergency and receiving appropriate treatment.

Child health (especially communicable and parasitic diseases, such as diarrhea, malaria, and worms) is also affected by elements of the health system such as access, quality, and use of healthcare services. After the neonatal period, however, other non-health system factors become more important, and child health is reduced by poverty, unclean environments, poor nutrition, low parental education, disempowered mothers, etc. These factors can hinder appropriate use of curative care. Scaling-up PHC along with a more multi-sectoral approach to deal with issues of poverty, environment, nutrition, and education underpins a sustainable improvement in child health. As discussed earlier, however, multi-sectoral work has its own challenge of involving all sectors effectively. Also, scaling up of any health intervention is a process with its own challenges. A small, focused intervention usually receives lots of attention, support, and can more easily identify, involve, and encourage community participation. A few motivated managers and staff can play key roles in ensuring the intervention works and is tailored to one, local context. All these enabling factors can easily dissipate when the intervention is scaled up to the regional or national level.

Strategies for the effective involvement of families, communities, and civil society organizations in the health system are needed so that optimal health practices become widespread, and services become available to and used by families. The value placed on motherhood and child bearing in many cultures means that families can be motivated to ensure that mothers and children do receive high-quality treatment.

The private sector is very important in providing MCH services in some countries – it needs to be regulated and supported to ensure that high quality is maintained. However, the private sector (both for-profit and NGOs) is very diverse, dynamic, and not well understood. Understandably, governments traditionally have focused on the public health sector. A clear need exists for research-based evidence on how to develop and sustain partnerships between health and other government sectors, and between the public and private health sectors.

A major bottleneck in scaling up the availability of health services, especially for maternity care, is the lack of adequate human resources. Training, deploying, and retraining skilled health workers, at primary, secondary, and tertiary levels, are key and are discussed elsewhere in this book (see Chapter 28). To work effectively, staff need adequate financing, medical supplies, equipment, and supportive and efficient management systems. All of these are critical areas for research aiming to identify and evaluate locally feasible ways to improve the availability and quality of MCH services. With regard to financing, cost-sharing approaches may be necessary to sustain and expand MCH programs, but the impacts on equity need to be compared to the resources generated. Much more research and experience with insurance schemes is needed, now that user fees have demonstrated such clear negative effects on equity of access to MCH services.

Monitoring of progress toward the MDGs is faced with several methodological challenges including unavailability, unreliability, and inconsistency of information from different contexts (Anonymous 2007). Furthermore, the development of new methods for measuring progress, especially in maternal health, is needed. Across all the topics identified for further research, involving policy makers and health managers in the research process, and ensuring that findings are communicated effectively, will help to ensure that research findings are used to inform improvements in MCH services. Researchers often state their desire to see their findings used to improve health services, but the researchers' working environments and capacity in knowledge transfer limit their abilities to make this happen.

In order to ensure all of the above, effective and inclusive decision-making processes for health policy making and planning are needed. Good governance of the health system should bring together professional, community, and management perspectives to seek solutions to the problems identified and to develop effective and sustainable MCH policies and plans. Evidence from communities, patient groups, and civil society organizations suggests they do want to be involved and have valuable evidence to inform the development of policy. However, policy making has historically been cited in the domain of central government, and government (central and local) and other actors need to develop new ways of thinking, capacity, and confidence to ensure an inclusive policy-making process.

Finally, it is important to note that good health care for mothers and their children will help to eradicate poverty. Many governments in developing countries face great difficulties in investing in the health sector to provide even the minimum packages of care at reasonable standards. Therefore, substantial long-term global support from other sources is needed to enable governments in developing countries to improve the performance of their health systems and make services available to all those in need.

Key Terms

Alma-Ata Declaration	Health education	Over-medication
Health system	Community nurses	Generic drugs
Healthcare system	Secondary health care	Monitoring and evaluation
Biomedical model	Tertiary health care	Health Information
Holistic model	Healthcare financing	Management System
Female literacy	Horizontal integration	(HIMS)
Antenatal care	Vertical integration	Private-for-profit providers
Postnatal care	Earmarked budget	Strategic planning
Family planning	Immunization coverage	Top-down
Child immunization	Referral system	Bottom-up
Newborn care	Emergency health care	Community ownership
Voluntary counseling and	Obstetric complications	Staff shortage
testing	Underserved	Sub-Saharan Africa
Integrated approach	Outreach services	Safe abortion
Decentralization	Feedback system	Children in difficult
Deconcentration	Follow-up care	circumstances
Devolution	Public sector, private sector	Bamako Initiative
Recurrent budget	Non-governmental	Taxation
Skilled attendant	organization	User fees
Human resources	Quality of health service	Private insurance
Financial resources	Ethnicity	Social insurance
Cesarean section	Poverty	Revolving Drug Fund
Low birth weight	Sexuality	Community-based financing
Regulation	Infrastructure	Social class
Social services	Social groups	

Questions for Discussion

1. Distinguish between a health system and a healthcare system.
2. Through what mechanisms can a health system influence maternal and child health status?
3. How does a holistic model of the health system differ from the medical/clinical model?
4. Distinguish between horizontal and vertical integration.
5. Using one MCH service as an example, e.g., infant and child healthcare services, describe Donabedian's Framework for quality of health services.
6. Discuss "governance" in relation to health systems management.
7. Write short explanatory notes (not more than a quarter of a page) to demonstrate your understanding of the meaning of health policy, health planning, health management, decentralization, devolution, and deconcentration.
8. List four common mechanisms for financing healthcare systems and discuss the advantages and disadvantages of each.

References

Anonymous (2007) Millennium development holes (Editorial). Nature, 446(7134), 347

Azubuike MC, Ehiri JE (1998) Action on low immunization uptake. World Health Forum, 19(4), 362–364

Bryce J, Arifeen S, Pariyo G et al. (2003) Multi-Country Evaluation of IMCI Study Group. Reducing child mortality: can public health deliver? Lancet, 362, 159–164

Buse K, Mays N, Walt G (2005) Making Health Policy. Open University Press, London

Collins CD (1994) Management and Organization of Developing Health Systems. Oxford University Press, Oxford

Darmstadt GL, Bhutta ZA, Cousens SN et al. (2005). Evidence-based, cost-effective interventions: how many newborns can we save? Lancet, 365(9463), 977–988

de Savigny D, Kasale H, Mbuya C (2004) Fixing health systems. International Development Research Centre, Ottawa

Donabedian A (1980) The Definition of Quality and Approaches to its Assessment Vol. 1. Health Administration Press, Ann Arbor, http://www.pubmedcentral.nih.gov/picrender.fcgi?artid = 1072233&blobtype = pdf, cited 13 July 2008

Gilson L, McIntyre D (2005) Removing user fees for primary care in Africa: the need for careful action. British Medical Journal, 331(7519), 762–765

Green A (2007) An Introduction to Health Planning for Developing Health Systems. 3rd Edition, Oxford University Press, Oxford

Green A, Collins C (2006) Management and planning. In: Merson M, Black R, Mills A (Eds.), International Public Health (553–594). Jones and Bartlet, Boston, MA

Koblinsky M, Matthews Z, Hussein J et al. (2006) Going to scale with professional skilled care. Maternal Survival Series 3. Lancet, 368, 1377–1386

Murray C, Frenk J (2000) A framework for assessing the performance of health systems. Bulletin of World Health Organization, 78(6), 717–731

Olumole D, Mason E, Costello A (2000) Management of childhood illness in Africa. British Medical Journal, 320, 594–595

Parkhurst JO, Penn-Kekana L, Blaauw D et al. (2005) Health systems factors influencing maternal health services: a four-country comparison. Health Policy, 73(2), 127–138

Ravindran TKS, Weller S, Moorman J et al. (2005) Public-private interactions in health. In: Ravindran TKS, de Pinho H (Eds.), The Right Reforms? Health Sector Reform and Sexual and Reproductive Health. Women's Health Project, University of the Witwatersrand, School of Public Health, Johannesburg, South Africa

Ridde V (2003) Fees-for-services, cost recovery, and equity in a district of Burkina Faso operating the Bamako Initiative. Bulletin of the World Health Organization, 81(7), 532–538

Ronsmans C, Graham WJ, Lancet Maternal Survival Series Steering Group (2006) Maternal mortality: who, when, where, and why? Lancet, 368(9542), 1189–1200

Schneider H, Blaauw D, Gilson L et al. (2006) Health systems and access to antiretroviral drugs for HIV in Southern Africa: service delivery and human resources challenges. Reproductive Health Matters, 14(27), 12–23

United Nations Development Programme (2003) Human Development Report: Millennium Development Goals: A Compact among Nations to End Human Poverty. Oxford University Press, New York

United Nations (2007) The Millennium Development Goals Report: Statistical Annex. United Nations, New York, http://mdgs.un.org/unsd/mdg/Resources/Static/Data/Stat%20Annex.pdf, cited 19 August 2008

World Health Organization (2000) World Health Report, Health Systems: Improving Performance. World Health Organization, Geneva, http://www.who.int/whr/2000/en/whr00_en.pdf, cited 13 July 2008

World Health Organization (2006) World Health Report 2006 – Working Together for Health. World Health Organization, Geneva, http://www.who.int/whr/2006/whr06_en.pdf, cited 13 July 2008

World Health Organization/United Nations Children's Fund (1978) The WHO/UNICEF Conference on Primary Healthcare, Alma Ata., World Health Organization, Geneva, http://www.euro.who.int/AboutWHO/Policy/20010827_1, cited 13 July 2008

Chapter 6
The Environment and Maternal and Child Health

Mary Ann Pass and Rebecca Pass

Learning Objectives After reading this chapter and answering the discussion questions that follow, you should be able to

- Discuss the characteristics of children that predispose them to greater risks of exposure to environmental hazards and to more lasting damage from such exposures.
- Identify and describe differences in environmental risks and outcomes for children in high- and low-income countries.
- Appraise the benefits of monitoring environmental health indicator data at the national, regional, and global levels.
- Discuss strategies for reducing environmental health threats to children at different levels – home, community, national, and global.

Introduction

> In affluent as well as in deprived populations, the most compelling socio-medical problems have their origin in the lasting and often irreversible effects of early environmental influences (Rene Dubos et al. 1966).

Our environment is a critical determinant of the health status of individuals and populations. Broadly defined, our environment includes both the Earth's thin layer of land, water, atmosphere and the man-made structures or modifications to the natural world in which humans live, work, and play. Differences in environmental resources, the built environment, and the degree of development lead to profoundly different environmental risks across geographic and economic regions of the world. In the poorest nations, environmental risks stem from unclean water, poor sanitation and human waste disposal, poor hygiene practices, water-, soil-, and air-borne diseases, crowded homes, and smoke from biomass cooking and heating fuels. In developed and developing nations, risks include atmospheric pollution from industry and power plants, chemical or petroleum pollution of groundwater, asbestos or lead contamination in houses, tobacco smoke, and injury from traffic accidents. This chapter will identify key contaminants and environmental risk factors that impact the health of women, children and adolescents.

The concept of *environmental health* in children encompasses all the external conditions, influences, and interactions between children and their environment as well as the effects of these interactions on their health. This broad view of environmental health includes the chemical, physical, and biological risks that cause or influence diseases in women and children. While environmental risk factors vary across regions of the world, children have characteristics that make them particularly susceptible to environmental hazards in all regions. The scope of environmental health is immense and the field of environmental health has profound implications for both human health and the sustainability of our ecosystem. As J.P. Grant, Executive Director of UNICEF (1992), asserted eloquently at the United Nations (UN) Conference on Environment and Development, "We must preserve our planet in order to nurture our children; equally, we must nurture our children if we are to preserve our planet."

M.A. Pass (✉)
University of Alabama at Birmingham, USA

J.E. Ehiri (ed.), *Maternal and Child Health*, DOI 10.1007/b106524_6,
© Springer Science+Business Media, LLC 2009

In less developed countries, environmental health risks are particularly profound. Social, economic, and environmental risks combine to create a triple burden for mothers and children. Poverty, poor nutrition, environmental pressures, and displacement caused by such forces as climate change or conflict precipitate more exposure to environmental health threats. These threats also erode household stability and weaken public health infrastructure, thereby exacerbating health outcomes. While health workers have made dramatic progress in control of vaccine preventable diseases and diarrhea, their work has uncovered the need for even more attention to the control of the underlying social and environmental contributors to these diseases. Children in the poorest regions die from the "usual" conditions of childhood, but at higher rates than seen elsewhere in more developed or protected environments.

International Recognition of Children's Environmental Health

Increased understanding of the linkages between diseases in children and their underlying environmental risk factors has fostered international recognition of children's environmental health issues over the past decades (Box 6.1).

Box 6.1 A Chronology of Children's Environmental Health

1776 Percival Pott, a London doctor, notes incidence of scrotal cancer in young chimney sweeps, in what is generally considered to be the first linking of cancer to environmental hazards.

1904 J.L. Gibson of Queensland, Australia is the first to recognize paint as the source of lead poisoning among children.

1953 Mercury Linked to Nervous System Damage in Developing Fetus. Grain contamination in Sweden in 1953 demonstrates the devastating effect of high-dose prenatal exposure to mercury and its derivative methyl mercury to the developing nervous system. Other historic incidents of mercury poisoning include: contaminated fish in Minimata, Japan in 1958; pollution in Nugota, Japan in 1965; grain contamination in Iraq in 1971; and grain contamination in New Mexico in 1972. These incidents illustrate the extreme vulnerability and susceptibility of the fetus to mercury.

1970 The enacting of the Clean Air Act in the US eliminates the worst sources of air pollution and leads to health-based standards. Similar legislation is adopted across the developed world.

1970s Regulations to reduce lead in motor fuel in Europe and the US.

1984 First evidence of long-term effects of low-level lead exposure (Needleman et al. 1984).

1990 US Environmental Protection Agency (EPA) and International Life Sciences Institute (ILSI) sponsor conference on Similarities and Differences Between Children and Adults: Implications for risk assessment, one of the first scientific symposia on children's health issues (ILSI 1992).

1993 National Academy of Sciences (NAS) report highlights the pesticide exposure of infants and children through food and food consumption (NAS 1993). Report points to large gaps in our knowledge.

1996 Food Quality Protection Act passed in the US, partly in response to the NAS report. Act requires that children's special needs be taken into account in setting pesticide standards.

1997 President Clinton issues Executive Order on Children's Environmental Health and Safety (US Environmental Protection Agency 1997a). EPA sets up Office of Children's Health Protection (US Environmental Protection Agency 1997b). The G8 issues a Declaration on Children's Environmental Health (G8-Group 1997).

2000 EPA publishes a strategy for future research and a first set of indicators on children's environmental health issues (EPA 2000).

2002 International Conference on Environmental Threats to the Health of Children, held in Bangkok; Major reviews of scientific literature published by European Environment Agency (WHO 2002a,b) and Danish Environmental Protection Agency (2002). Children's health a key issue at Johannesburg World Summit (United Nations 2002).
Source: Children's Environmental Health Network (2008); Sharpe (2002)

In 1989, the UN Convention on the Rights of the Child declared that children have universal rights to safe, healthy, and clean environments that are fundamental to their ability to thrive. The International Network on Children's Health, Environment and Safety (INCHES – http://www.inchesnetwork.net/) – a global network of people and organizations interested in promoting the protection of children from environmental and safety hazards – was established in 1998 as a coordinating structure for organizations and individuals involved with children's environmental health. Members include national and international professional associations, research and policy institutes, advocacy organizations, universities, parents' and children's organizations, national and intergovernmental agencies, and individuals (INCHES 2008; Bistrup and van den Hazel 2008). The First International Conference on Children's Environmental Health held in Bangkok in 2002 strongly affirmed "that all children should have the right to safe, clean and supportive environments that ensure their survival, growth, development, healthy life and well-being" (Suk 2002). Delegates at this conference recognized both the traditional risks from poor housing and insanitary conditions and the "new" environmental exposures from chemicals and byproducts of development. They realized that these "new" exposures present increasing risks to children and that these risks are exacerbated by poverty, poor education, and malnutrition. The conference recommended stronger programs for recognition, assessment, and understanding of environmental influences on children's health. Participants pledged "to collaborate in promoting children's health through protection from environmental threats" (Suk 2002).

Currently, the Millennium Development Goals (MDGs) provide the overarching international policy and development framework that addresses the threats to health from adverse environmental conditions. Integral to the MDGs is an understanding that the health of the environment and environmental sustainability is intrinsically linked to human health. Progress on environmental health is required for attainment of many of the UN Millennium Development Goals, particularly Goal # 1 to eradicate extreme poverty and hunger, Goal # 4 to reduce child mortality, and Goal # 6 to combat HIV/AIDS, malaria, and other diseases. Considerable interaction exists between progress toward these MDGs and Goal # 7 to ensure environmental sustainability, access to safe water, improved sanitation and waste disposal, and reduction in the use of solid fuels. In turn, progress toward additional goals will facilitate progress on environmental health, for example, Goal # 2 – targeting universal primary education for both girls and boys is critical for successful health promotion, improved hygiene, and community development. Goal # 3 which targets reduction in gender disparities and empowerment of women will allow women to become involved in making healthy choices regarding their environment and that of their children. Their achievement depends on the ability of the MDGs to spawn research-based policies that recognize the unique susceptibility of children to environmental health threats and engender action to improve environmental sustainability.

The Unique Vulnerability of Children

The statement that "children are not little adults" is the fundamental principle behind the need for more attention to, and better understanding of, children's environmental exposure. Developmentally, physically, and behaviorally, children are at higher risk from environmental hazards. Children's bodies develop rapidly both physically and intellectually.

These spurts may be compromised by undernutrition – a lack of macro- and micro-nutrients often exacerbated by diarrheal diseases – or exposure to harmful substances. Children have higher metabolic rates; they eat more, drink more, and breathe more in relation to their body size, increasing the exposure to harmful substances when reported as a proportion to body mass. In addition, elements characteristic of children's body composition (the proportion of water, fat, protein, and mineral) further intensifies the toxicity of some environmental hazards on their systems compared with those of adults. Yet, a child's immature organs and systems lack competence to detoxify and excrete potentially hazardous compounds. Children have smaller airways, increasing the hazardous effect of agents that cause mucosal irritation and airway narrowing. Finally, children's behaviors and relation to their physical surroundings can expose them to greater transmission risks – from the hand-to-mouth conduct of toddlers that carries infections to dust inhalation while crawling and exploring. With neither the life experience to identify and avoid potential risks nor the ability to alter their surroundings, children are vulnerable to danger and dependent on the knowledge and habits of caregivers and the customs and beliefs of their family and community (Louis et al. 2006).

Children not only bear a disproportionate share of the disease burden from environmental hazards, but also experience more profound, lasting damage from environmental exposure. "Windows of susceptibility" exist during periods of a child's life, when a brief exposure to a toxicant can permanently alter the structure and function of an organ. Distinct life stages have been defined by dynamic processes at the molecular, cellular, organ, system, and organism level (Louis et al. 2006). Exposures to hazards prenatally can contribute to complications of pregnancy, stillbirth, and birth defects. However, the potential result of an insult prenatally or even in early childhood may not become apparent until years later in the course of a child's development, particularly the development of his neurological system (Landrigan et al. 2004; Louis et al. 2006; Gauderman et al. 2004). Simultaneous exposures to environmental threats may combine to further exacerbate health outcomes. Co-morbidities, such as upper respiratory tract infections, diarrhea, HIV/

AIDS, and malaria, perhaps coupled with prematurity or low birth weight, could lead to stunting, poor developmental outcomes, or death. A child's distinct developmental stage at the time of exposure, along with the intensity of the exposure, and the toxicity of a substance shape the severity of the environmental health impact and may be pivotal to the outcome of the illness.

The World Health Organization (WHO) used the Delphi method to quantify global environmental risk and published results from a panel of experts in its 2006 report *Preventing Disease through Healthy Environments*. The report found that 23% of global deaths and 24% of the global burden of disease in disability-adjusted life years (DALYs) are attributable to environmental exposures and risks related to climate change (Prüss-Üstün and Corvalán 2006). While experts acknowledge that different methods exist for calculating exposure and risks, they agreed that the risks are highest among children 0–14 where the proportion of deaths attributed to modifiable environmental factors reached 36% by some estimates. Among children, those under the age of 5 years are most vulnerable to environmental conditions. This subgroup of children is estimated to bear 40% of global environmental disease risk although it represents only 10% of the total population (Prüss-Üstün and Corvalán 2006).

Environmental Risks – Different Risks, Different Outcomes

Communities, states, and regions of the world vary markedly in environmental risks and associated health outcomes, creating huge disparities in child health. Pneumonia, diarrheal diseases, and malaria, the top three causes of child death worldwide, all have underlying environmental causes and disproportionately impact children in developing countries. In the cases of diarrheal disease and lower respiratory infection, the poorest WHO regions experience a level of disease attributable to the environment 120–150 times higher than the wealthier regions (Prüss-Üstün and Corvalán 2006). The total number of healthy life years lost per capita as a result of environmental factors was 15 times higher in developing countries than in the more developed countries (Prüss-Üstün and Corvalán 2006). By contrast, studies have found little overall difference between developed and developing countries in the fraction of non-communicable disease attributable to the environment (Prüss-Üstün and Corvalán 2006).

Infants, young children, and their mothers often share risks because they inhabit the same environmental spaces for most of the day, particularly in resource-poor countries. In most high-income countries, mothers tend to be separated earlier from their children. In these situations, the environments of both mothers and children may be influenced more by income level, residential location, parental education, occupation, and community exposures to smoke, heavy metal toxins (arsenic, lead, and mercury), or industrial chemicals. Specific environmental risks to children include household and industrial chemicals, air pollution, lack of clean water, and insanitation (Prüss-Üstün et al. 2008).

Use of Chemicals

Industrial and agricultural byproducts of development and increased food production may enable development but also pose health threats to children. Agricultural chemicals are the major source of poisoning among children and highly dangerous when used without knowledge of safe handling practices (Gordon et al. 2004). Children may be exposed to agricultural chemicals directly or through their parents. Parents may of necessity take children with them to work into the fields where they may be directly exposed to agricultural chemicals through work or play. Outside of homes in poorer countries, women carry out a major role in non-mechanized, subsistence farming. As a result, they have an increased likelihood of physical contact with pesticide or chemical effluent. Whether contaminated from agricultural exposure to pesticides and herbicides or from mining, smelting, or lead industries, clothing worn by parents poses contamination risks to children.

In high-income countries, children may not have direct or indirect contact with agricultural chemicals. However, many chemicals are marketed for use in the home despite inadequate safety data. Families often have choices regarding their use of these household chemicals. Nevertheless some items commonly found around the house have serious toxicity. These items include household cleaners, solvents, glues, fragrances, cosmetics, certain plastics, paints, auto products, and yard and garden products. In the United States the National Institute of Health has a web site for consumer information on household products, http://householdproducts.nlm.nih.gov/index.htm. Unfortunately, even where risks are known, lack of global product safety standards may insufficiently protect households from toxic exposure. Product recalls of items from toys to candles with lead added to candlewicks are common. Labels required in developed regions may not be present in developing countries, may not be translated into local languages or, because of the literacy levels in the local population, may not be understood (Gordon et al. 2004).

Industrial chemicals also commonly impact children's health. Some fat-soluble chemicals are of particular concern because they persist in the environment and accumulate in the food chain through a process called bioaccumulation. These chemicals are called persistent organic pollutants or POPs. Studies in toxicology, a field of health concerned with the effects of chemicals on living organisms, have linked the fire retardant polybrominated diphenyl ethers (PBDEs) to poor health outcomes. Other POP chemicals are industrial byproducts such as dioxins, furans, and polychlorinated biphenyls (PCBs). Known as endocrine disrupters, PCBs, plastics and additives to plastic including phthalates, polyvinyl chloride (PVC), and bisphenyl A (BPA) are also of increasing concern because of their potential effects on children's development (Rogan and Ragan 2007).

The European Union (EU) currently has the most stringent chemical regulatory programs. Under the policy, Registration, Evaluation, and Authorization of Chemicals (REACH), chemical producers have the responsibility for safety testing (Foth and Hayes 2008). Unfortunately, storage and manufacturing of chemicals are increasingly being shifted to the regions of the world that are less likely to develop, implement, and enforce environmental regulation. The Organization for Economic Co-operation and Development (OECD 2001) estimated that by the year 2020, nearly one-third of the world chemical production will take place in non-OECD countries and that global output will be 85% higher than it was in 1995. In 2006, the International Conference on Chemical Management finalized a Strategic Approach to International Chemicals Management or SAICM and urged member states to take action on chemical safety and build the capacity for dealing with chemical incidents. They partnered with OECD to make chemical safety information available through the OECD's electronic "chemportal" (http://webnet3.oecd.org/echemportal/).

Air Pollution

Both indoor and outdoor air pollution cause respiratory illnesses in children. As many as 60% of acute respiratory infections (ARI) are related to environmental conditions including air pollution (Prüss-Üstün and Corvalán 2006). Indoors, exposure to air pollutants can be 60 times greater than exposure outdoors. In homes in less developed countries, poor indoor air quality is among the greatest risks to child health. Biomass fuels or coal may be the cheapest or only fuels available to families. Because women and children spend more time in the home, they are disproportionately affected by poor indoor air quality. However, all homes using biomass fuels do not have the same level of particulate matter. Dasgupta et al. (2006) reported significant variation in the quality of indoor air and particulates among households in Bangladesh. Household exposure is strongly affected by structural arrangements: cooking locations, construction materials, and ventilation methods. The poorest, least educated households had twice the pollution levels of relatively high-income households.

By contrast, regions with reliable electricity, natural gas, or kerosene have comparatively low levels of childhood respiratory disease. However, exposure to tobacco smoke in homes is still a significant threat. In families where an adult smokes tobacco, children are exposed to increased risks for otitis media, respiratory infection, worsened asthma, sudden infant death, fires, burns, childhood behavioral problems, and impaired physical and intellectual development (Prüss-Üstün 2006). Exposures in childhood to air pollution and widely distributed environmental contaminants are increasingly linked to pediatric morbidity from asthma, cancers, obesity, and earlier age of onset of diabetes, endocrine and sexual disorders, and neuro-developmental disorders such as autism (Woodruff et al. 2004).

Inhabitants of large cities throughout the world deal with the highest levels of air pollution. An estimated 1.1 billion people worldwide breathe air that is considered unhealthy, and those in developing countries are exposed to a much greater concentration of small particulates (UNEP 2002). Industry, transportation, and household fuels are major pollution sources. Burning of trash as a means to dispose of waste in urban environments in less developed countries is another significant source of air pollution with dioxins, furans, and heavy metals. In high-income countries, pollution from transportation and industry remains a problem. Children riding on school buses are exposed to toxins and particulate counts 5–10 times higher than levels outside the bus (Behrentz et al. 2005). School bus diesel exhaust is associated with a host of respiratory problems and is classified as a likely carcinogen. Despite clean air regulatory activities in high-income countries, it is estimated that 24% of the US children live in counties where one or more air pollutants exceed standards (EPA 2006). In Europe, air pollution is second to injury as an environmental burden of disease (Valent et al. 2004). In both high- and low-income countries, there is consistent association between long-term exposure to smoke and particulate matter and poor respiratory health in children. Ironically, many of these exposures to unhealthy air derive from the rapid expansion of industry and technology that developing regions seek.

Lack of Clean Water and Sanitation

Diarrheal disease is the second most important cause of child mortality worldwide. Approximately 80–90% of diarrhea cases are related to environmental conditions, specifically to contaminated water and food, and to inadequate sanitation. Childhood diarrheal diseases can stem from lack of clean water for drinking, cooking, and preparation of weaning foods. Sewage runoff, inadequate wastewater treatment, and inadequate sanitation all contaminate water supplies. In resource-poor countries, mothers who work in subsistence farming have a high likelihood of contact with unclean water in streams and irrigation ditches or exposure to animal feces. Women and girls are often disproportionately responsible for collecting clean water. Often traveling long distances, they are exposed to potential environmental contaminants and may pay the opportunity cost of attending school. Lack of education regarding basic hygiene and sanitation threatens both mothers and children in their care.

Pathogens in water supply include viruses, bacteria, intestinal parasites, and parasitic protozoan. While diarrheal diseases claim the largest number of children's lives among the water-related environmental health threats, schistosomiasis, dengue fever [http://www.cdc.gov/ncidod/dvbid/dengue/index.htm#history], malaria, and West Nile Virus [http://www.cdc.gov/ncidod/dvbid/westnile/] are also serious health hazards. Mostly affecting parts of Africa and South America, schistosomiasis is contracted from swimming or bathing in lakes, rivers, and ponds contaminated by freshwater snails that carry the *Schistosoma* parasite [http://www.dpd.cdc.gov/dpdx/html/schistosomiasis.htm]. Malaria, dengue fever, and West Nile Virus all involve disease cycles dependent on mosquitoes for transmission. An estimated 90% of malaria cases in children occur in sub-Saharan Africa where ineffective water resource management, irrigation, or sanitation strategies, along with environmental degradation that increases runoff and produces standing water, amplify the transmission of these vector-borne diseases (UNEP 2002).

Expected to aggravate existing environmental threats and usher in new environmental health threats, climate change will place further burden of disease on those areas of the world least able to adapt to new conditions. Deforestation can cause further depletion of water resources, erosion, and flooding due to runoff, as soils are no longer able to absorb the same amount of rainfall. The expected incidences of extreme drought and flooding that threaten fragile ecosystems will likely create habitat suited to the pathogens that cause water-borne diseases. Disease vectors of water-borne diseases will

likely follow temperature bands both latitudinally and altitudinally, as conditions conducive to their transmission spread. Poor regions where people's livelihoods depend on subsistence farming, particularly in areas of sub-Saharan Africa, are considered the most vulnerable to climate change with least adaptive capacity (UNEP GEO 2007). Poor children and families may lack access to the resources necessary to adapt to their environment or to move. Those families that do move may face environmental risks associated with large population migrations. The 0–4 years age group bears the heaviest burden of death from factors related to drought, flooding, and changing disease patterns accompanying global climate change (Prüss-Üstün and Corvalán 2006).

Environmental Health Indicators

Environmental health indicators enable health professionals and policy makers to quantify environmental health status of the population and gauge the impact of environmental risks discussed above. Indicators are essential to identifying the most critical problems, establishing a baseline by which to measure trends, and assessing the efficacy of interventions. The development, tracking, and monitoring of regional indicators for children's environmental health also assist in focusing attention on specific regional needs and comparing health status across regions.

Through conferences, workshops, and publications, the WHO (2008) has promoted the development of region-specific environmental health indicators for children (Briggs 2003). Each region is to define their critical exposures and to identify their specific needs for the measurement of the environmental conditions that lead to health disparities. The indicators can be compared and used for tracking progress in each region. Kyle et al. (2006) suggested that indicators include both measures of environmental contamination, studies of the body burden, and the morbidity from specific diseases. Gordon et al. (2004) developed an atlas to display selected environmental challenges for each region. The WHO web site for the indicators is given below. Some examples of regional exposure indicators are

Box 6.2 Environmental Health Indicators

Sample Environmental Health Exposure Indicators
- Households without basic services for water supply, sanitation, and hygiene
- Households using biomass fuels or coal as the main source of heating and cooking
- Households in which at least one adult smokes tobacco on a regular basis
- Mean annual exposure of children aged 0–4 to atmospheric particulate pollution
- Living in proximity to heavily trafficked roads
- Living in homes with a source of lead exposure

Sample Environmental Health Outcome Indicators

- Mortality rate for children aged 0–4 years of age due to acute respiratory illness
- Diarrhea mortality rate in children aged 0–4 years

Sample Environmental Health Policy Indicators

- Attributable change in the number of households lacking basic services
- Attributable change in atmospheric pollutant concentrations
- Attributable change in numbers of household relying on biomass fuels or coal as the main source of heating and cooking.

shown in Box 6.2 (http://www.who.int/ceh/indica tors/indicators2003/en/index.html).

The goal is to use indicators to craft policy interventions to both improve access to basic environmental health measures and reduce disparities in health, particularly differences seen between urban and rural health in all countries. Such interventions must start at the community level. In communities, in contrast to what is seen in a controlled scientific or laboratory setting, complex combinations of exposures are the norm rather than the exception. Because biological processes are complex, symptoms may be variable, knowledge of the exposure

and its effect is limited, and combinations of environmental exposures are particularly difficult to study. Animal studies are expensive and may not be reliable as conditions are difficult to reproduce in a laboratory. Children can respond in only so many ways to whatever mix of toxins presented. Effects from co-exposure may be additive or interactive. Community risk assessment must factor in the complex web of environmental risks, the health threats resulting from these risks, and their potential effect on children.

Briggs used the multiple exposures multiple effects (MEME) (Fig. 6.1) model to show that health effects in children can be traced back to many different environmental exposures and any one particular environmental risk can often lead to a wide range of health effects. In this model, the relationship between environmental exposure and health outcome is rarely based on simple direct relationships. Instead, complex interrelationships between both exposures and health outcomes are affected by contextual conditions such as social, economic, or demographic factors (Briggs 2003).

Historically, community risk assessment has been based on a population-oriented exposure model. In this model, risk was traced back to an identified exposure "source" and quantified based on the variables related to that source. For example, risk from a smokestack or factory might be based on its geographical location, toxin produced, release rate of toxin, rate of dispersion, and other measures that are time and place bound. Children move through different communities over their course of development. More recently, the US EPA developed a framework to guide risk assessment for children that considers children's critical developmental stages and discussed the complexities of the exposure assessment and data collection. A change from prior EPA risk assessment, their so-called person-oriented model recognizes the existence of multiple independent sources, all of which could contribute to total exposure to a chemical or mixture of chemicals. Kyle et al. (2006) reviewed these efforts and concluded that the person-oriented exposure for children better characterizes the individual and life stage of interest along with the applicable exposure sources than population-oriented exposure assessment.

Fig. 6.1 Multiple exposures multiple effects (MEME) model. Source: Briggs (2003)

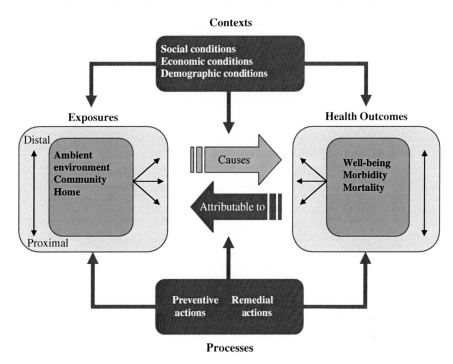

Prevention – Policy Action

In both high- and low-income countries, environmental health policy frameworks must be linked to an assessment of pertinent environmental health threats and the social, economic, and political conditions that enable these threats to persist. Children from the most disadvantaged families are at greatest risk from environmental hazards; yet, it is precisely these families that may be least able to afford safe environments. Environmental injustice is a term used for targeted placement of environmental risks in resource-poor communities. The US Environmental Protection Agency (2005) defines Environmental Justice as follows:

> The fair treatment and meaningful involvement of all people regardless of race, color, national origin, or income with respect to the development, implementation, and enforcement of environmental laws, regulations, and policies. Fair treatment means that no group of people, including a racial, ethnic, or a socioeconomic group, should bear a disproportionate share of the negative environmental consequences resulting from industrial, municipal, and commercial operations or the execution of federal, state, local, and tribal programs and policies. Meaningful involvement means that: (1) potentially affected community residents have

an appropriate opportunity to participate in decisions about a proposed activity that will affect their environment and/or health; (2) the public's contribution can influence the regulatory agency's decision; (3) the concerns of all participants involved will be considered in the decision making process; and (4) the decision makers seek out and facilitate the involvement of those potentially.

Environmental injustice recognizes that communities with the least resources bear the biggest burden of health disparities. Poor families need assistance in working with local authorities and the private sector in order to participate in decision making and ensure development and implementation of prevention and intervention programs. Coalitions of family, community, government, and aid groups are crucial to promote adoption of rules, minimum safety standards, and policies and practices that value child health and empower families.

At Home

A safe environment for children starts at home where they typically spend the bulk of their time.

Basic measures such as improved housing, avoidance of biomass fuel smoke, breastfeeding, safe food and water, oral rehydration, and hand washing protect children, enhance health and delay exposure to potentially toxic compounds. Access to safe water is often listed first in importance among environmental indicators for children, particularly during weaning. Promoting breastfeeding practices is crucial for early childhood survival. Extended breastfeeding delays the risk of disease from unclean water and offers the infant a critical period of protection for growth and development. The survival benefit of breastfeeding is most pronounced in poor environments (Ehiri and Prowse 1999). Education of mothers and families can improve child health and survival. Educational materials should reflect the practical and cultural needs of the community. The incidence of diarrhea can be reduced when mothers boil water for drinking and supplemental food preparation for their babies. In situations where fuel for cooking is in short supply, households may, in a bid to save energy, prepare large quantities of food in advance and then store it until needed (Ehiri et al. 2001). The potential for microbial contamination and growth of pathogens (and thus diarrhea) increases in the absence of facilities for monitoring food temperature and for properly storing leftover foods as is often the case in many low-income countries. Hand washing is a simple but effective way of blocking fecal–oral disease transmissions (Ejemot et al. 2008; Clasen et al. 2007). Williams et al. (1994) identified time-honored health promotion strategies for families including hygiene in the home, how to build homes and keep them clean, proper ventilation, the water supply, the kitchen, the latrine, and the elimination of stagnant water. Unfortunately, as reported by Carpenter et al. (2006), prevention strategies often take a back seat to more fundamental issues of safe food.

In the Community

Schools and daycare centers can also provide parents with culturally relevant information about the special vulnerability of children to environmental threats. The WHO (Pond et al. 2007) guidelines promote development of curricula to identify region-specific environmental health-related problems and list strategies to involve children in the solutions. Schools can also serve as sites for community education on key issues of community development, safe water and sanitation facilities, waste management, air quality and ventilation, safety, vector control, and personal hygiene. Health and development specialists can help communities to launch focused actions that are key to recognition of problems, development of strategies to address specific problems, and implementation of policy and programmatic changes to protect children. The WHO has promoted basic preventive strategies in their Integrated Management of Childhood Illness (IMCI), details of which can be found in Chapter 27. IMCI includes a community component that focuses on preventive health services and community-based strategies that can shift the focus toward primary prevention.

National Concerns

Children's environmental health cannot be just a concern of health agencies. Multi-sectoral involvement is critical for sustainable action to reduce environmental threats to the health of women and children. Research studies and best practices need to be made available to policy makers within and outside of governments. Most important would be policies to improve air and water quality, regulate and control chemicals, remove lead from gasoline, paints, water pipes, and ceramics, and to provide smoke-free environments in all public buildings. Non-governmental groups and the media can give high priority to efforts to safeguard children's health, and disseminate information on environmental health issues and potential solutions.

Policies must also map the environmental health risks of a particular country or region. In low-income countries, access to clean water, provision of adequate sanitation, and improvement of air quality are critical. In places without access to basic health care and sufficient food, these efforts must be linked with measures to achieve food security and further access to primary health care. Control of water resources to combat breeding grounds of vector-borne diseases must also be implemented. Since a 2002 meeting of the WHO Regional Committee for Africa, African countries have been developing national strategic plans to address negative health outcomes and environmental degradation, "inter alia." National Environmental and Health Action Plans, or NEHAPS, are country-by-country collaborations between governments, NGOs, and technical experts to propose solutions to environmental health problems, as a component of national development agendas. Implementing interventions in an integrated fashion will assist efforts toward better health care and environmental sustainability (UNEP 2008).

Access to safe water in high-income countries is complex as public water supplies face costly regulation and testing requirements. For example, in the United States under the Safe Drinking Water Act, the EPA defines maximum contaminant levels for 90 pollutants out of some 700 organic, inorganic, biological, and radiological contaminants detected in public water supplies around the country. Community water treatment is a multiple-step and costly process of physical treatment, including sedimentation, coagulation, and filtration, and disinfection or chlorination with continuous monitoring of quality. Contaminant occurrence in public drinking water systems is highly variable depending on water source, surface or ground water, and well depth (Barnes et al. 2008). In low-income countries, where piped water is available, routine testing for water safety is costly and not feasible for many communities where bacterial contamination, increased salinity, and products of agricultural run-off are common.

Extreme drought may cause resource, food, and water scarcity, while rise in sea level could cause flooding in heavily populated low-lying regions of the world. Both of these changes could lead to intensified conflict over environmental resources and population migration, both of which could have a serious impact on maternal and child health. In addition, global climate change and natural disasters can contribute to undernutrition and the spread of infectious disease, and quickly wipe out hard-earned health gains. Deforestation and environmental degradation cause soil erosion, pollute streams with sediment and debris, reduce biodiversity, change patterns of vector-borne disease transmission, and alter host–pathogen interactions. In today's context of transportation and global trade, infectious diseases can travel quickly from low-income countries and impact the health of people in high-income countries. There have also been instances of high-income countries dumping toxic waste in low-income countries that cause catastrophic health damages to vulnerable populations, including women and children. Participation by all nations is crucial for early warning systems, disease surveillance networks, and global problem solving. To be successful, action must take place at the community, national, and international levels and recommendations of scientific research must be reflected in political decision making. Increasingly, policies of Corporate Social Responsibility call for polluting parties to manage the impact of their own externalities – pollution and potential hazardous byproducts – on communities (BPH 2007). Table 6.1 describes the sources, exposures, and public health impacts of nine key pollutants.

Global Concerns

Some environmental threats to human health truly transcend political boundaries. While some air pollution concentrates relatively close to the source, greenhouse gases emitted through polluting activities affect climate globally. Atmospheric concentrations of carbon dioxide from increased energy production and unsustainable global consumption are at historically high levels and are considered a major contributor to global climate change.

Priorities for Research

Specific research priorities include the impact of multiple exposures, the impact of chemicals specifically on children, and the health effects from an ever-increasing number of chemical compounds. Policy responses to chemical threats in high-income countries too often are late responses to identified toxicity in children and fragmented across different countries. Australia was among the first countries to ban lead from paint following an epidemic of lead

Table 6.1 Common environmental exposures

Air pollution: Indoor	Air pollution: Outdoor	Arsenic
Overview: Crowded, poorly built or poorly ventilated homes increase risk of chronic exposure to smoke from biomass fuel, tobacco, dust, and animal allergens	*Overview:* Very large urban areas commonly struggle with poor air quality. Specific chemical mixtures vary by proximity to industrial sources and automobile exhausts, geography, wind patterns, temperature, and time of day	*Overview:* Some regions have high concentrations of arsenic in soil, water, and food – particularly seafood. Arsenic can be released by mining and smelting, from hazardous waste sites, and during volcanic activity
Source: Combustion products contain thousands of health-damaging substances and particles. The smallest particles are the most dangerous because they can carry other pollutants on their surface and penetrate to the deepest levels of the lung. The smoke from cured tobacco contains up to 4,000 different chemicals, some of which are carcinogenic. Other noxious agents such as lead, arsenic, carbon monoxide, cadmium, formaldehyde, nitrogen and sulfur oxides, pesticides, nitrosamines, hydrocarbons, molds, or cleaning fluids can accumulate in indoor air	*Source:* The US EPA monitors outdoor air for six "criteria" pollutants including ozone (O_3), a potent irritant present in urban smog, sulfur dioxide (SO_2), carbon monoxide (CO), several nitrogen oxides (NO_x), lead, and particulates. In addition, 188 "air toxic" substances are recognized. This group contains volatile hydrocarbons, heavy metals, solvents, and combustion byproducts such as dioxin. Exhaust from automobiles or diesel engines is major hazards. Fuel vapors contain volatile organic compounds (VOCs) that react with sun to produce ozone. Most cities in the developing world lack regulation of outdoor air quality	*Source:* Drinking water is the most common source of arsenic risk, particularly in Asian regions such as Bangladesh and China. Tube wells bored into naturally occurring ore such as arsenopyrite lead to mobilization of arsenic. The WHO has set a standard for arsenic in water of less than 10 ppb and recommends that all wells be tested for arsenic. In other regions, arsenic has been used as a pesticide. Copper chromium arsenate has been used as a wood preservative and in the industrial production of semiconductors and other electronic components
Exposure: An estimated 50% of the world's population and 70% of population of Africa, south and Southeast Asia uses biomass fuels for cooking and heating. Use of solid fuels is still prevalent in poorer regions within developed countries	*Exposure:* Children are exposed to air pollutants during outdoor play and in transportation. Ambient lead levels are highest near urban roadways. Toxins in smog can accumulate in airway secretions and become ingested	*Exposure:* Arsenic is ingested through water, food, or inhaled. Where water levels are known to be high, water for drinking can be purified through special filtration systems. A major concern for children is outside play in contaminated soil
Toxicity: Smoke irritates the mucous membranes of the eyes, nose, throat, and respiratory tract. It contributes to allergies, asthma, lower respiratory disease, chronic obstructive pulmonary disease, and cancers	*Toxicity:* Outdoor air pollution is a respiratory system irritant, increasing risks of asthma, respiratory infection, and certain cancers. Health impacts from acute exposures may be reversible, but extended exposure is associated with long-term reduction in lung function and increased risk of chronic obstructive lung disease	*Toxicity:* Children are less able than adults to detoxify arsenic. Symptoms differ with acute or chronic exposure and impact almost every organ. Arsenic is associated with hyperpigmentation and sores of the skin, kidney, and liver, and respiratory effects, cancers of the skin, bladder, liver and lung
Public Health Implications: Even in developed nations, mean 24-h concentrations of particulates in indoor air may exceed by a factor of 2–60 health and safety standards for air pollution levels defined by OECD nations. Improved stoves, chimneys, housing, and education are beneficial (Gordon et al. 2004)	*Public Health Implications:* Smog reduction is a critical priority in all countries, rich and poor. Despite regulation in the United States, 58% of children reside in counties that exceed limits for ozone. In addition, 19% of the US children reside in counties that exceed particulate standards (EPA 2005)	*Public Health implications:* In addition to toxicity listed above, the cancer risk from arsenic at this level exceeds 1 in 10,000, leading to calls for even lower standards. Developing countries may lack the regulatory structures in place for testing and detoxification (Gordon et al. 2004)
Endocrine disruptors	**Fluoride**	**Lead**
Overview: Endocrine disruptors are a diverse group of chemicals that mimic or modify the action of endogenous hormones. They are	*Overview:* Fluoride is beneficial for prevention of oral health cavities and is added to water supplies in small amounts in the developed	*Overview:* Lead has many uses and has been recognized as a toxin for centuries, but only recently has the special vulnerability of children to

Table 6.1 (continued)

Air pollution: Indoor	Air pollution: Outdoor	Arsenic
typically slow to degrade in the environment and accumulate in biological tissues. They are toxic to plants, fish, animals, and humans	world. Unfortunately, when humans are exposed to the element through coal ores or ground water in excessive amounts, it is toxic	the neuro-developmental toxicity at very low doses been accepted
Source: This group of toxins includes well-known pollutants like DDT, dioxins, furans, and PCBs. Other group members include certain pesticides such as Aldrin, Chlordane, Dieldrin, Endrin, Heptachlor, Hexachlorobenzene, Mirex, and Toxaphene; compounds in fire retardants such as polybrominated diphenyl ethers (PBDEs) and phthalates which are used in plastics	*Source:* Fluoride exists naturally in soil and groundwater in some regions. It is added to water in small amounts to prevent dental disease	*Source:* Lead is still used in pipes, batteries, ceramics, and some paints. It is still used as an additive in some fuels despite being phased out in the developed countries for automobiles. It is also found in some jewelry and toys in excessive concentrations
Exposure: These compounds are most commonly ingested through fatty food and milk, including breast milk. These agents are of special concern in developing countries where children can be simultaneously exposed to both pesticides and infectious pathogens when their immune systems are already compromised by other factors such as malnutrition	*Exposure:* Children can be exposed to excessive amounts of fluoride through drinking water contamination. In China, the burning of fluoride-rich coal increases fluoride exposure through air pollution	*Exposure:* Children are most often exposed through inadvertent contamination of paint from old houses, food, natural medicines, glazed ceramics, battery recycling, lead pipes for water supply and in emissions from smelters. Proximity to traffic is a risk in areas where leaded gas is still used
Toxicity: In very small doses disrupters may mimic or block hormones, interfere with normal growth and development, cause sterility, lower sperm counts, impair nervous system development, lower intelligence, and contribute to behavioral abnormalities, childhood leukemia, lymphoma, CNS cancers, breast cancer, and compromised immune function (Rogan and Ragan 2007)	*Toxicity:* At higher exposures fluoride produces a condition known as fluorosis. It destroys teeth, accumulates in developing bones, and can lead to crippling skeletal damage. Fluorosis is endemic in 25 countries. Toxicity is related to levels of exposure and nutrition status, particularly intakes of calcium, vitamins A and C	*Toxicity:* Acute exposure causes life-threatening encephalitis with irreversible neurological sequelae. Low lead levels can reduce IQ, cause learning disabilities, poor school performance and violent behaviors. Lead use is still prevalent in many parts of the world
Public Health Implications: Reduction of these chemicals is critical. The Stockholm Convention (UNEP 2001) seeks the elimination or restriction of production and use of industrial chemicals, pesticides, and unintentionally produced POPs, such as dioxins and furans	*Public Health Implications:* There is a need for resources and improved technology to monitor fluoride and to remove it from water where levels are excessive, and reduce childhood fluoride exposures (Gordon et al. 2004)	*Public Health Implications:* Reducing exposure depends primarily on governmental action restricting lead in gasoline and paint, and vigilance in monitoring of consumer products. The urban poor remain at greatest risk for exposure (Gordon et al. 2004)
Mercury	**Nitrates**	**Pesticides (or agrochemicals)**
Overview: Mercury exists in certain ores and fossil fuels. Elemental mercury is less toxic than organic mercury compounds like methyl mercury. Mercury is used in fluorescent lights, thermostats, and thermometers, in science and chemistry lab equipment and electrical systems	*Overview:* Nitrogen is an atmospheric component essential for biological processes. It requires "fixation" before use by plants as ammonium. Used globally for improved crop yields, nitrogen fertilizer can contaminate water supplies through runoff. Sodium nitrite is added to cured meats as a preservative	*Overview:* Over 900 insecticides, herbicides, fumigants, and repellents are in use worldwide. Important classes include organophosphates, carbamates, pyrethrums, glyphosate (Roundup), organochlorines (Lindane), and insect repellents N, N-diethyl-3-methylbenzamide (DEET).

Table 6.1 (continued)

Air pollution: Indoor	Air pollution: Outdoor	Arsenic
Source: Levels of mercury in air, land, and water increase with industrialization. Contamination occurs with mining, smelting, industrial discharges, or waste incineration. Coal-fired power plants are significant sources of emissions. Mercury is released into the air, falls to the ground in rain, becomes deposited in rivers, lakes, and streams, and then is converted to harmful forms by bacteria	*Source:* Children are exposed to excessive nitrates from food or drinking water. Infants less than 4 months of age are at particular risk from nitrates in regions where contaminated water is used to prepare formula. Shallow and poorly constructed wells in rural areas are at great risk of nitrate contamination and are unlikely to be adequately monitored	*Source:* Agriculturally, pesticides are used to increase crop yields and decrease pests. Domestically, they are used in insect control products, pet shampoos, lice shampoos, and community mosquito abatement products. While potentially toxic, pesticides are of critical importance in control of mosquitoes and other disease-carrying vectors
Exposure: The most common exposure is from eating contaminated fish. Methyl mercury, the most toxic form, accumulates in biological tissues, particularly fish or animals at the top of the food chain. Concern exists for island communities dependent on fish for subsistence	*Exposure:* Nitrate levels in drinking water increase with the increase in use of nitrogenous fertilizers, intensive livestock operations that produce large amounts of animal waste, substandard human septic systems, and municipal waste streams	*Exposure:* Absorption is through the skin or through ingestion of contaminated food. Farm workers and their families are particularly at risk. In poor rural populations where men, women, and children all work and live in close proximity to fields and orchards where chemicals are applied and stored, safe use policies may be most needed and most lacking
Toxicity: Methyl mercury is a potent neurotoxin that can cause brain damage and developmental disorders in fetuses and children. Childbearing women in the United States are warned against eating too much of certain types of fish. Chronic exposure to methyl mercury may cause cancer or damage other organs	*Toxicity:* Nitrates can be converted to nitrites in the intestinal tract. The nitrites react with iron to produce a condition in infants called "blue baby syndrome" or methemoglobinemia where the hemoglobin is incapable of carrying oxygen	*Toxicity:* Each pesticide class has differing symptoms. Whereas acute exposure can lead to death or serious illness, long-term exposure increases disorders of development and the reproductive system, disrupts the immune and endocrine systems, impairs nervous system function, and leads to certain cancers
Public Health Implications: Some nations have taken steps to regulate the inadvertent release of mercury and to reduce the production and uses of mercury (Gordon et al. 2004)	*Public Health Implications:* Adequate monitoring of intensive agricultural production systems, such as feed lots and chicken and hog farms is needed to ensure better disposal of production waste	*Public Health Implications:* Two-thirds of pesticide deaths occur in the developing world where excessive exposure is related to inappropriate use, poor environmental management, and lack of policies for education and regulation (Gordon et al. 2004)

poisoning in children in Queensland. Limits on release of mercury from factories developed in part because of the devastating effects of methyl mercury poisoning in Japan. In their report on pesticides, the National Research Council in the United States (NRC 1993) identified inadequate safeguards against exposure to pesticides in children's diets and expressed concern regarding the special vulnerability of children to environmental toxins. They noted that acceptable tolerance levels for pesticides were developed based on the residual amounts that might exist safely in food for general adult consumption. Prior guidelines did not consider the particular vulnerabilities of children and their greater risk of negative health effects. Furthermore, tolerances did not address inadvertent exposure unrelated to food. The NRC report recommended that a new approach to risk assessment be developed for the unique effects of the toxins in children.

However, research on the vulnerability of children to toxins and risk assessment regarding the effects of toxins in children is still insufficient. While pesticides have received some degree of public health attention, other chemicals have never been studied for toxicity. In the last century's chemical revolution, over 80,000 chemicals were produced for various industrial and consumer uses. In the report, *Toxic Ignorance*, Roe et al. (1997) identified gaps in the most basic testing data available for more than 70% of the top-volume commercial use chemicals in the United States. Following this report, the US Environmental Protection Agency (EPA) in 1998 identified almost 3,000 high production volume chemicals (HPV) representing 3% of all industrial chemicals. Only 7% of the HPV chemicals had a full set of basic toxicity data, while 43% of HPV chemicals had no test data. EPA developed a voluntary testing program, the results of which have been summarized by Dennison (2007). Despite industry sponsorship of approximately 2000 chemicals, many chemicals remain without sponsors and without adequate testing data. The chemicals without sponsors have been referred to as "orphans" and continue to be produced in high volume amounts without complete, publicly available safety data. New chemicals are added to the HPV list every year.

In many instances, the scientific community lacks tools, resources, and biological markers to clearly define safety for children as a specific population subgroup. Despite the attempt of new models to understand multiple exposures in children, scientific studies on multiple exposures and their impact on children's environmental health remain limited. A study in Eastern Europe followed children living near historical non-ferrous smelters and found evidence of subtle effects on children's renal and nervous systems from exposure to a mixture of heavy metals even though there was no clear evidence of a threshold effect

(de Burbure et al. 2006). The bioaccumulation of persistent pollutants and the impact on children's neurodevelopment are particularly troublesome and only partly understood.

Children might be exposed to multiple agents that have a common toxic effect, and estimates of exposure and of risk could be improved by allowing and accounting for simultaneous exposures. Likewise information is needed on the differences in acute and chronic effects of specific agents. In 2000, the United States initiated a longitudinal study, the National Children's Study, to determine the environmental influences on children's health and development from birth until age 21. Approximately 100,000 children are to be followed with measures of certain biological, chemical, physical, genetic, social, psychological, cultural, and geographical factors. There is great hope that this will provide a valuable resource in the field (NRC and IOM 2008).

Precautionary Principle

Advocates for children believe that when the health and safety of children is potentially at risk, public health personnel must take action to investigate, to intervene, and to reduce potential risk following the *precautionary principles approach*. This precautionary principle requires that scientific uncertainty should not postpone preventive measures. Supporters say a precautionary approach is comparable to the action of John Snow in 1854 who removed the Broad Street pump handle in London to slow a cholera epidemic, when the exact cause of the outbreak was still being debated. Key components of the precautionary principle include (i) taking preventive action in the face of uncertainty, (ii) shifting the burden of proof to the proponents of an activity, (iii) exploring a wide range of alternatives to possible harmful actions, and (iv) increasing public participation in decision making. Past failures to take adequate action in a timely manner are chronicled in a report of the European Environmental Agency, *Late Lessons from Early Warnings* (Harromoës et al. 2001). The report documents delays in recognition of health and environmental toxicity from use of benzene, asbestos, endocrine disruptors such as polychlorinated biphenyls (PCBs), diethylstilbestrol (DES), organochlorine compounds, and the impact of halocarbons on the ozone layer.

Appraisal of Relevant Themes

The poorest children aged 0–4 with their compounded risks from poverty, undernutrition, and socioeconomic disadvantage are almost always the group most vulnerable to environmental hazard. Improvements in housing for poor families, basic environmental hygiene measures such as safe water, adequate sanitation, and safe air are measures to significantly reduce morbidity and mortality among the most vulnerable. However, newer risks, such as our lack of understanding of risk from chemicals and toxins in our increasingly technological world, threaten all children. Our clinical and public health knowledge has lagged far behind the development, distribution, and regulation of the chemicals. The long latent period between exposure, intervention, and recognition of a child's developmental outcome complicates study of the effect of environmental hazards on children. Our collective actions toward environmental sustainability will determine the survival of all of our children.

Conclusions

- Mothers and children living in different regions, urban or rural, very underdeveloped or highly developed communities, are exposed to vastly different environmental risks. The environmental risks in the developing regions from unclean water, sanitation, and human waste disposal are well described in the literature (Genser et al. 2008; Ezzati et al. 2005). The man-made pollutants and other environmental determinants of health present new challenges. In high and low-income countries alike, air

pollution, accidental and deliberate release of industrial waste, petroleum and chemical effluent pollution of water tables are major concerns in urban areas. Agricultural chemical pollution from fertilizer, insecticides, and herbicides leaching into streams and rivers particularly affects rural areas. In the poorer countries, crowded homes with indoor air polluted by smoke from biomass cooking and heating fuels are difficult to change as improvements in the environment may be limited by socioeconomic and cultural factors.

- Children are uniquely vulnerable as a result of their early physical and intellectual developmental processes and their immature immune systems. Children are not small adults. As our future, they deserve our protection and investment.

- Community health workers and peer groups can advise families, neighborhoods, and communities about hazards to children and work to develop resources, infrastructure, and to promote policies to protect and to improve conditions. Where resources are limited, wise investments are most crucial.

- The use of global and regional indicators and measures such as the MDG's promotes awareness and allows the monitoring of progress in meeting specific environmental goals to reduce disparities and provide safer communities for women and children.

- More research is needed to improve our understanding of the levels at which environmental chemicals and toxins interact to impact children's growth and development. Safer and sustainable development strategies that acknowledge and address health and developmental concerns are critical to our future.

- Global health leaders and the international business communities in nations with weak regulations must recognize the risks posed when industries are located close to residential neighborhoods and emit chemical and radiological pollutants and accept social responsibility. Environmental pollution is a global issue as it does not recognize geographical, political, or economic boundaries.

Key Terms

Air pollution	Environmental Protection Agency	Natural disasters
Arsenic	Environmental resources	National environment and health plans (NEHAPs)
Asbestos	Environmental risk factors	Neuro-developmental disorders
Asthma	Environmental pressures	Non-communicable diseases
Autism	Environmental sustainability	Obesity
Benzene	Environmental threats	Outdoor air pollution
Biodiversity	Exposure	Paints
Biphenyl A (BPA)	Extreme poverty	Persistent organic pollutants (POPs)
Breastfeeding	Fragrances	Person-oriented model
Cancers	Freshwater snails	Pesticides
Carbon dioxide	Furans	Phthalates
Chemical effluent	Glues	Plastics
Chemical revolution	Greenhouse gases	Pneumonia
Climate change	Groundwater	Pollution
Community risk assessment	Heavy metals	Polybrominated diphenyl ethers (PBDEs)
Contaminants	Herbicides	Polychlorinated biphenyls (PCBs)
Convention on the rights of children cooking and heating fuels	High-income countries	Polyvinyl chloride (PVC)
Corporate social responsibility	High production volume chemicals (HPV)	Population-oriented exposure
Deforestation	HIV/AIDS	Precautionary principle
Deforestations	Household cleaners	Sanitary conditions
Dengue fever	Hygiene practices	Sanitation
Diabetes	Indoor air pollution	Schistosomiasis
Diarrhea	Industrial chemicals	Sewage
Diethylstilbestrol (DES)	International Network on Children's Environmental and Safety (INCHES)	Solvents
Dioxins	Lead	Tobacco
Drought	Low-income countries	Toxicant
Early warning systems	Lower respiratory tract infection	Unclean water
Ecosystem	Malaria	Vector-borne diseases
Empowerment	Mercury	Ventilation
Endocrine disruptors	Millennium Development Goals	Water-borne diseases
Environmental degradation	Multiple exposures multiple effects (MEME)	West Nile Virus
Environmental hazards		
Environmental health		
Environmental health impact		
Environmental influences		
Environmental justice		

Questions for Discussion

1. Distinguish between leading environmental health risk factors for children in low income countries, and children in high income countries.
2. Why are children at greater risk of exposure to environmental health risks and to more damaging effects of environmental hazards than adults?
3. What are environmental health indicators? Give examples of any five of such indicators. Of what value are environmental health indicators in ensuring a safe environment for children?
4. Define the following terms:

   a. Environmental justice.
   b. Precautionary principle.

5. What are the implications of environmental justice and the precautionary principle for the promotion of children's environmental health?

References

Barnes KK, Kolpin DW, Furlong ET et al. (2008) A national reconnaissance of pharmaceuticals and other organic wastewater contaminants in the United States – I. Groundwater Science of the Total Environment, 402(2–3), 192–200

Behrentz E, Safin LD, Winer AM et al. (2005) Relative importance of school bus-related microenvironments to children's pollutant exposure. Journal of the Air and Waste Management Association, 55(10), 1418–1430

Bistrup ML, van den Hazel P (2008) About Inches, International network on children's health, environment and safety, http://inchesnetwork.net/about.html, cited 20 October 2008

Board on Population health and public health practice (BPH) (2007) Global environmental health in the 21st century: From governmental regulation to corporate social responsibility. Washington, D.C.: National Academies Press. http://books.nap.edu/catalog.php?record_id = 11833, cited 31 August 2008

Briggs D (2003) Making a difference: Indicators to improve children's environmental health. Geneva: World Health Organization, http://www.who.int/phe/children/en/cehin dicsum.pdf, cited 31 August 2008

Carpenter DO, El-Qaderi S, Fayzieva D et al. (2006) Children's environmental health in central Asia and the Middle East. International Journal of Occupational and Environmental Health, 12(4), 362–368

Children's Environmental Health Network (2008) Chronology of Children's Environmental Health. http://www.cehn.org/Chronology.html, cited December 26, 2008

Clasen T, Roberts I, Rabie T et al. (2007) Interventions to improve water quality for preventing diarrhea, The Cochran Collaboration, http://www.cochrane.org/reviews/en/ab004794.html, cited 31 August 2008

Committee on Pesticides in the Diets of Infants and Children (1993) Pesticides in the Diets of Infants and Children, National Research Council (NRC). Washington, D.C.: National Academies Press, http://www.nap.edu/openbook.php?isbn = 0309048753, cited 31 August 2008

Danish Environmental Protection Agency (2002) Children and the Unborn Child: Exposure and susceptibility to chemical substances – an evaluation, Environmental Project 589, Danish Environmental Protection Agency. www.mst.dk/udgiv/publications/2001/87-7909-574-7/html

Dasgupta S, Huq M, Khaliquzzaman M et al. (2006) Who suffers from indoor air pollution? Evidence from Bangladesh. Health Policy and Planning, 21(6), 444–458

de Burbure C, Buchet J, Leroyer A et al. (2006) Renal and neurologic effects of cadmium, lead, mercury, and arsenic in children: Evidence of early effects and multiple interactions at environmental exposure levels. Environmental Health Perspectives, 114(4), 584–590

Dennison RA (2007) High Hopes, Low Marks: a final report card on the high production volume chemical challenge. New York: Environmental Defense. http://www.edf.org/documents/6653_HighHopesLowMarks.pdf, cited 31 August 2008

Dubos R, Savage D, Schaedler R (1966) Biological Freudianism, lasting effects of early environmental influences. Pediatrics, 38:789–800

Ehiri JE, Prowse JM (1999) Child health promotion in developing countries: the case for integration of environmental and social interventions? Health Policy and Planning, 14:1, 1–10

Ehiri JE, Azubuike MC, Ubbaonu CN et al. (2001) Critical control points in the preparation and handling of complementary foods in eastern Nigeria. Bulletin of the World Health Organization, 79:5, 432–433

Ejemot RI, Ehiri JE, Meremikwu MM et al. (2008) Hand washing for preventing diarrhoea. Cochrane Database of Systematic Reviews, Issue 1. Oxford, England: John Wiley & Sons Ltd

Environmental Protection Agency (1997a) Presidential Task Force on Environmental Health Risks and Safety Risks to Children. Executive Order 13045: Protection of Children from Environmental Health Risks and Safety Risks. Environmental Protection Agency. http://yosemite.epa.gov/ochp/ochpweb.nsf/content/whatwe_executiv.htm, cited December 26 2008

Environmental Protection Agency (1997b) Children's health Protection. EPA Office of Children's Health Protection. http://yosemite.epa.gov/ochp/ochpweb.nsf/content/homepage.htm, cited December 26 2008

Environmental Protection Agency (2000) America's children and the environment: a first view of available measures. EPA Report # 240-R-00-0006. Environmental Protection Agency, 2000

Environmental Protection Agency (2005) Environmental Justice Smart Enforcement Assessment Tool. September. U.S. Environmental Protection Agency Office of Enforcement and Compliance Assurance. http://www.epa.gov/

compliance/resources/policies/ej/ej-seat-112905.pdf, cited December 26, 2008

Environmental Protection Agency (2006) Children's Environmental Health: 2006 Report. http://yosemite.epa.gov/ochp/ochpweb.nsf/content/CEH06_Final.htm/$File/CEH06_Final.pdf, cited 31 August 2008

Ezzati M, Utzinger J, Cairncross S et al. (2005) Environmental risks in the developing world: exposure indicators for evaluating interventions, programmes, and policies. Journal of Epidemiology and Community Health, 59(1), 15–22

Foth H, Hayes A (2008) Concept of REACH and impact on evaluation of chemicals. Human and Experimental Toxicology, 27(1), 5–21

G8-Group (1997) Declaration of the Environment Leaders of the Eight on Children's Environmental Health. http://yosemite.epa.gov/ochp/ochpweb.nsf/content/declara.htm, cited December 26 2008

Gauderman WJ, Avol E, Gilliland F et al. (2004) The effect of air pollution on lung development from 10 to 18 years of age. New England Journal of Medicine 9;351(11): 1057–67

Genser B, Strina A, dos Santos LA et al. (2008) Impact of a city-wide sanitation intervention in a large urban centre on social, environmental and behavioural determinants of childhood diarrhoea: analysis of two cohort studies. International Journal of Epidemiology, 37(4), 831–840

Gordon B, Mackay R, Rehfuess E (2004) Inheriting the World: The atlas of children's health and the environment. Geneva: World Health Organization. http://www.who.int/ceh/publications/atlas/en/index.html, cited 31 August 2008

Grant JP (1992) Address to the United Nations Conference on Environment and Development. In Children in the new millennium: environmental impact on health (p. 12), United Nations Environment Programme, United Nations Children's Fund and the World Health Organization, (2002) http://www.unep.org/ceh/children.pdf, cited 20 October 2008

Harromoës P, Gee D, MacGarvin M et al. (Eds) (2002) Late lessons from early warnings: the precautionary principle 1896–2000. Copenhagen: European Environment Agency, Environmental Issue Report No. 22. 2001. ISBN 92 9167 323 4. Catalogue no. TH-39-01-821-EN-C http://reports.eea.europa.eu/environmental_issue_report_2001_22/en/Issue_Report_No_22.pdf, cited 31 August 2008

International Life Sciences Institute (1992) Similarities and differences between children and adults: implications for risk assessment. International Life Sciences Institute, 1992. www.ilsi.org

International Network on Children's Health, Environment and Safety (INCHES) (2008). About INCHES. http://inchesnetwork.net/about.html, cited December 26 2008

Kyle AD, Woodruff TJ, Axelrad DA (2006) Integrated assessment of environment and health: America's children and the environment. Environmental Health Perspectives, 114(3), 447–452

Landrigan PJ, Kimmel, CJ, Correa A et al. (2004) Children's health and the environment: Public health issues and challenges for risk assessment. Environmental Health Perspectives, 112(2), 257–265

Louis GB, Damstra T, Díaz-Barriga F et al. (2006) Principles for evaluating health risk in children associated with exposure to chemicals, Environmental Health Criteria 237. Geneva: World Health Organization. http://www.who.int/ipcs/publications/ehc/ehc237.pdf, cited 31 August 2008

National Academy of Sciences (1993) Pesticides in the diets of infants and children. National Academy of Sciences

National Research Council and Institute of Medicine (2008) The National Children's Study Research Plan: A Review. Panel to Review the National Children's Study Research Plan. Committee on National Statistics, Division of Behavioral and Social Sciences and Education. Board on Children, Youth, and Families and Board on Population Health and Public Health Practice, Institute of Medicine. Washington, D.C.: The National Academies Press. http://www.nap.edu/catalog.php?record_id=12211, cited 20 October 2008

Needleman H, Rabinowitz M, Leviton A et al. (1984) Relationship between prenatal lead exposure and congenital anomalies. JAMA, 251, 2956–2959

Organization for Economic Co-operation and Development (OECD) (2001) Environmental outlook for the chemicals industry. Paris: OECD. http://www.oecd.org/dataoecd/7/45/2375538.pdf, cited 31 August 2008

Pond KP, Kim R, Carroquino M et al. (2007) Workgroup Report: Developing Environmental Health Indicators for European Children: World Health Organization Working Group. Environmental Health Perspectives, 115(9), 1376–1382

Prüss-Üstün A, Corvalán C (2006) Preventing disease through healthy environments, toward an estimate of the environmental burden of disease. Geneva: World Health Organization. http://www.who.int/quantifying_ehimpacts/publications/preventingdisease/en/index.ht, cited 31 August 2008

Prüss-Üstün A, Bonjour S, Corvalán C (2008) The impact of the environment on health by country: a meta-synthesis. Environmental Health, 27(7). http://www.pubmedcentral.nih.gov/articlerender.fcgi?artid=2276491 cited August 5, 2009

Roe D, Pease W, Florini K et al. (1997) Toxic ignorance. New York: Environmental Defense http://www.edf.org/documents/243_toxicignorance.pdf, cited 31 August 2008

Rogan WJ, Ragan NB (2007) Some evidence of effects of environmental chemicals on the endocrine system in children. International Journal of Hygiene and Environmental Health, 210, 659–667

Sharpe M (2002) In harm's way: children's environmental health. Journal of Environmental Monitoring, 4, 92–98

Suk WA (2002) Beyond the Bangkok statement: research needs to address environmental threats to children's health. Environmental Health Perspectives, 110(6), A284–A286

United Nations Environmental Program, Global Environmental Outlook (2007) http://www.unep.org/geo/geo4/report/GEO-4_Report_Full_en.pdf, cited 19 October 2008

United Nations Environment Programme, United Nations Children's Fund and the World Health Organization (WHO) (2002) Children in the new millennium: environmental impact on health, http://www.unep.org/ceh/children.pdf, cited 20 October 2008

United Nations Environment Program (UNEP) (2001) Stockholm Convention on Persistent Organic Compounds. Stockholm Conventions. Geneva: Stockholm Convention. Available at: http://chm.pops.int/Portals/0/Repository/convention_text/UNEP-POPS-COP-CONVTEXT-FULL.English.PDF cited August 5, 2009

Valent F, Little D, Bertollini R et al. (2004) Burden of disease attributable to selected environmental factors and injury among children and adolescents in Europe. Lancet, 363, 2032–2039

Williams CD, Baumslag N, Jelliffe DB (1994) Mother and child health, delivering the services 3rd ed. New York: Oxford University Press

Woodruff TJ, Axelrad DA, Kyle AD et al. (2004) Trends in environmentally related childhood illness. Pediatrics, 113(4), 1133–1140

World Health Organization (2002a) Children's Health and Environment: a review of evidence. Environmental Issue Report 29, European Environment Agency and WHO Regional Office for Europe, 2002. Available at http://reports.eea.eu.int, cited December 26, 2008

World Health Organization (2002b) Children in the New Millennium: Environmental impact on health. Geneva: World Health Organisation. www.who.int/peh/ceh/, cited December 26, 2008

World Health Organization (2008) Children's Environmental Health Indicators http://www.who.int/ceh/en/index.html, cited 31 August 2008

Part II
Politics, Power, and Maternal and Child Health

Chapter 7
Impact of Wars and Conflict on Maternal and Child Health

Emmanuel d'Harcourt and Susan Purdin

Learning Objectives After reading this chapter and answering the discussion questions that follow, you should be able to

- Analyze the nature of modern conflicts, and emerging trends.
- Summarize the impact of conflicts on the health and well-being of women, children, and adolescents.
- Develop a causal model to explain the pathways by which conflicts affect maternal and child health.
- Discuss the relationship between war and poverty.
- Identify and discuss strategies for mitigating the impact of wars on women, children, and adolescents.

Introduction

This chapter presents an overview of the nature and emerging trends in modern conflicts. With examples of recent and current conflicts around the world, the chapter examines the impact of conflict on the health and well-being of women, children, and adolescents, including direct trauma, malnutrition, displacement, rape, increased vulnerability to infectious diseases, and adverse obstetric conditions. The relationship between war and poverty is examined. Using a causal model, the chapter analyzes the pathways by which conflict affects maternal and child health, including food insecurity, economic collapse, decline in habitat,

E. d'Harcourt (✉)
International Rescue Committee, New York, USA

diversion of public spending, destruction of infrastructure, and loss of qualified personnel. Strategies for mitigating the impact of conflict on maternal and child health are discussed, including how to respond to immediate needs in acute, complex emergencies, provision of routine care in non-routine conditions, primary health care, and post-conflict healing and rebuilding.

It is impossible to improve global maternal and child health without addressing the issue of violent conflict. Modern conflict – including war between states, civil war, and insurgencies – has had a devastating impact on the health of women and children, and is getting worse. The civilian share of war deaths has gone from an estimated 53% in World War I and 60% in World War II (Keegan 1999, 1997) to more than 98% in the 1998–2004 war in the Democratic Republic of Congo (Coghlan et al. 2006, 2008). Conflict can cause an immediate and extreme rise in the crude mortality rate, and in many modern conflicts, mortality remains elevated for years after the official end of the war (Coghlan et al. 2006, 2008). Unfortunately, most of the civilian victims of modern conflict are women and children. In Congo, for example, an estimated 45% of all excess deaths during the conflict period were of children under the age of 5 (Coghlan et al. 2006, 2008). Worldwide, war is strongly associated with poor maternal and child health. Of the 20 countries with the world's highest child and maternal mortality, 13 have recently emerged from violent conflict or are still experiencing conflict (Table 7.1).

These countries represent a tiny proportion of the world's population, but account for one-fifth of the 10 million preventable child deaths annually (Fig. 7.1). Another 2 million preventable child deaths occur in

J.E. Ehiri (ed.), *Maternal and Child Health*, DOI 10.1007/b106524_7,
© Springer Science+Business Media, LLC 2009

Table 7.1 Countries with the highest child mortality and conflict status

	Country	Conflict status		Mortality	
		Recent	Current	Children <5*	Maternal**
1	Sierra Leone	α		282	2,000
2	Angola	α		260	1,700
3	Afghanistan		α	257	1,900
4	Niger			256	1,600
5	Liberia	α		235	760
6	Somalia		α	225	1,100
7	Mali			218	1,200
8	Chad		α	208	1,100
9	DR Congo		α	205	990
10	Equatorial Guinea			205	880
11	Rwanda	α		203	1,400
12	Guinea-Bissau	α		200	1,100
13	Côte d'Ivoire		α	195	690
14	Nigeria			194	800
15	Central African Republic		α	193	1,100
16	Burkina Faso			191	1,000
17	Burundi	α		190	1,000
18	Zambia			182	750
19	Ethiopia	α		164	850
20	Swaziland			160	370

*Deaths per 1,000 live births;
**Pregnancy-related deaths per 100,000 live births
ªCountries with recent or current conflict are shaded
Source: UNICEF (2006)

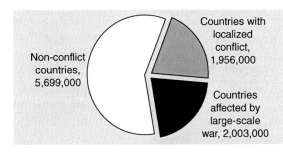

Fig. 7.1 Total annual child deaths in conflict and non-conflict countries. Source: Zwi et al. (2006)

countries such as Nigeria, which have not had war recently, but have substantial localized conflicts. The impact of war on maternal and child health goes beyond the deaths of women and children. Stunted growth, chronic infection, and obstetric fistula are just some of the serious but non-fatal consequences of conflict on women and children worldwide (Coghlan et al. 2006, 2008).

Conflict can impact maternal and child health to different degrees (Fig. 7.2). In Rwanda, the impact was dramatic but relatively short-lived: child mortality increased by 25% during, and in the aftermath of the genocide, but 10 years later, it improved back to baseline. In Sierra Leone, there was no recorded spike in child mortality. However, one of the hallmarks of maternal and child deaths in conflict-affected countries is that they are rarely recorded; over a decade of civil war, child mortality remained stagnant when other equally poor but more peaceful countries, such as Mali, experienced a continuing improvement in child survival. Within countries, regions in which conflict is most intense have much higher mortality than peaceful areas. This was documented most clearly in a 2004 mortality survey in the Democratic Republic of Congo (Coghlan et al. 2006). The Congo survey, conducted by the International Rescue Committee and the Burnett Institute (Coghlan et al. 2006), sampled 19,500 households in an effort to understand the impact of conflict on mortality.

The results showed the effect the Congo war had on overall mortality (Fig. 7.3), and specifically on children. Areas with violence had a rate of 6.4 deaths per month, per 1,000 under-5 children, as compared to 3.1 in zones in which no violence was reported. This

Fig. 7.2 Child mortality rate, 1960–2002, in three sub-Saharan African countries

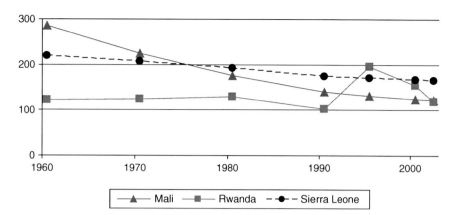

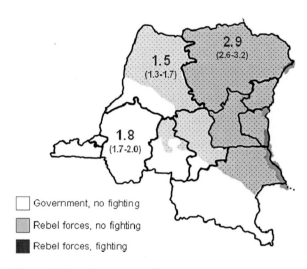

Fig. 7.3 Mortality and conflict in DR Congo. Numbers represent crude mortality rates, expressed in deaths per month per 1,000 people. Numbers in parenthesis represent confidence intervals. Source: Coghlan et al. (2006)

survey was not designed to examine the impact of war on women specifically, but other reports have documented widespread violence against women, as well as high rates of fistulas attributed to trauma and to inadequate obstetric care, in the eastern zones of DR Congo where fighting had been most intense (USAID 2006).

The Changing Nature of Conflict

The nature of conflict in the world has changed significantly since the end of the Cold War. In the past 1000 years, nearly all wars were conducted by, and

between, nation states. Many wars today, even if they are about resources, are cast as identity conflicts, in which warring factions are divided by personal characteristics such as religion and ethnicity (Smyth 2002). One dramatic effect of identity conflict is the deliberate targeting of civilians. Propaganda and other forms of hate speech fuel ethnic or religious hatred. This hatred, coupled with the breakdown in social fabric and collective trust, pushes combatants to inflict harm, not on an opposing army but on a despised people – including women and children, who form more than half of the population.

In some cases, such as the genocides in Rwanda and the former Yugoslavia, children and women were deliberately targeted so that the hated group could not reproduce itself. Strategies that were traditionally used to attack a military opponent, such as infrastructure destruction, are now used primarily to hurt civilians. Combatants inflict physical damage not only on air bases, but on civilian infrastructure such as clinics, schools, and family homes, with the deliberate intent of harming a group of people, rather than crippling a military opponent. In Bosnia, the religion and ethnicity of a family could be determined by the distinct construction of their home. Opposing forces used this knowledge to attack "enemy" houses (Purdin 1996).

Increasingly, even wars begun by states are becoming complicated by identity conflicts. In Afghanistan, the invasion by the Soviet Union eventually evolved into a civil war between Pashtun- and Farsi-speaking tribes; in Iraq, the collapse of the regime as a result of war between nation states, has led to a civil conflict based on religious differences.

Unfortunately, identity conflicts are challenging to resolve. Negotiation and compromise are more difficult when enmity is linked to personal characteristics. Furthermore, many such conflicts are led not by one government but by a variety of groups, which may fight each other as well as a common enemy. In Burundi, for example, a peace agreement was delayed by several years because, although the war was ostensibly between two ethnic groups, each group was divided into many smaller factions and militias, each with its own agenda and geographic base.

Other trends have also contributed to making war more deadly for women and children. The surge in the global small arms trade has made weapons such as semi-automatic rifles much cheaper – in some cases as little as $20 a piece – allowing groups such as ethnic militias to equip combatants in ways that, in the past, only states could. A militia member can now, in minutes, wipe out a family with a machine gun and destroy a clinic with a couple of grenades. In some areas, such as the Karamoja region in Uganda, the flood of small arms has turned traditional conflict with spears into a much deadlier operation.

Another devastating trend has been the recruitment of children for combat and other combat-related duties. Children are easier to recruit and more expendable if they die; they are easier to train, condition, and more defenseless. Children are used as combatants, porters, domestic workers, and sexual objects. There has been some outcry, but little effective action by the United Nations or by its member states to stop the practice. The enrollment of children in conflict has many negative consequences for maternal and child health, including direct harm to the children themselves through combat injury, sexual assault, psychological trauma, HIV infection, the harm that the children are forced to inflict on civilians, including their own communities, high risk of pregnancy for recruited girls, and high rates of infant mortality for the children they bear. Some examples of recent conflicts that illustrate this phenomenon are presented hereunder.

Somalia: In Somalia, the saying goes: "Myself against my family, my family against other families of my clan, my clan against all other clans, and all the Somalis against the rest of the world." In practice, as in many other civil conflicts around the world, it is the first two or three components of this saying which best describe the daily reality.

Many years of intense identity conflict in Somalia have devolved it into a country that is more a collection of feudal fiefdoms than a nation state.

Sudan: The Sudanese people endured a long-running civil war between the mostly Muslim north and the predominantly Christian south of the country. The war had a religious dimension, but many observers felt the root of the conflict was the systematic hostility of a regime that views itself as Arab toward compatriots who saw themselves and were seen as "black Africans." This explanation has been buttressed by the current conflict in Darfur, where the Sudanese government has led a proxy war primarily targeting civilians who are both Muslim and black African. In both cases, the government, in waging ethnic war against its own citizens, has used local ethnic divisions: in South Sudan, the government took advantage of hostility between the Dinka and other southern tribes, and within Dinka sub-tribes; in Darfur, the government has armed and financed local Janjawid militias against the Fur and other tribes.

Afghanistan: In the past, the conflict in Afghanistan took place in the context of the Cold War between the United States and the Soviet Union, then against the surge of Islamic fundamentalism. Today, the conflict in Afghanistan is primarily internal, between different warlords that are all Afghan and Muslim. Many of the hostilities have an ethnic undertone, with loyalty to one or another warlord based on ethnic background.

Conflict and Maternal and Child Health

Understanding the exact mechanism by which conflicts affect maternal and child health is no academic exercise. It is an essential step for the public health and human rights community as we try to protect women and children affected by conflict and to prevent the conflicts in the first place. There are in fact, not one but many links. These are summarized in Fig. 7.4 and in the following paragraphs.

Direct injury: First, and most obviously, combatants target children and women, killing and injuring them intentionally. Rape in particular has become a systematic weapon of war in places such as Congo and the former Yugoslavia. In Rwanda,

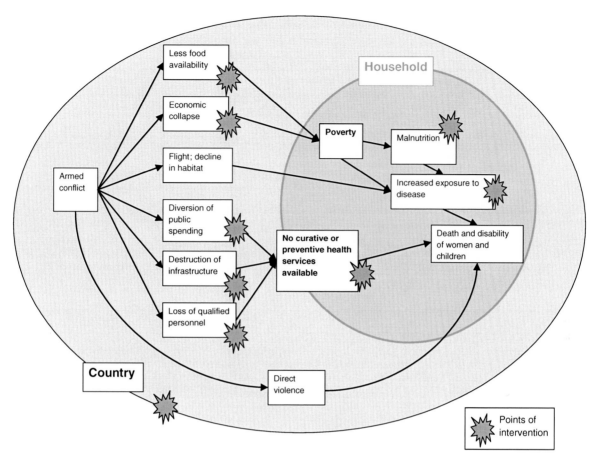

Fig. 7.4 A causal model for the impact of conflict on maternal and child health

militias deliberately targeted children, so that "they don't grow up to be rebels and fight us." (Human Rights Watch 1999a). These direct injuries to women and children, while devastating and by no means rare, represent a small portion of the burden of conflict. Of the millions of deaths for Eastern Congo recorded in the International Rescue Committee's 2004 mortality survey (Coghlan et al. 2006), only 1.3% were from direct violence. Over two-thirds of these victims were men. Adult men were almost 5 times more likely than women and 16 times more likely than children to die of direct violence.

Impaired food availability: War affects food availability in different ways. In agricultural societies, insecurity stops farmers from going to their fields to tend crops. Traders stop bringing necessary inputs, such as seeds and tools. Many families move closer to population centers for protection (as militias maneuver through less populated areas), losing

agricultural self-sufficiency in the process. In many places, such as Congo, combatants – both rebels and regular army – loot civilian fields and food stores for their own survival. In Sierra Leone, the population reported that during the war, most of their rice was harvested and eaten by soldiers (Human Rights Watch 1999b). To compound these problems, relief agencies often cannot deliver food aid to conflict areas. Children and women, who in many areas already have much higher rates of malnutrition prior to conflict, suffer the brunt of the added malnutrition and the attendant morbidity and mortality.

Economic collapse: Even in non-agricultural areas, economic activity plummets in times of conflict, leading to a decline in the standard of living. Traders flee, markets close; there is a sudden stop in outside investments. On a national level, governments in conflict zones often spend less to build their economies, diverting resources to military purposes, a loss made more acute by the accompanying reduction in international aid. To make matters worse, governments often lose their ability to collect taxes and other revenue in conflict zones, as in Liberia and Sierra Leone, where the near totality of the diamond trade went underground during the peak war years (United Nations 2001). As with food availability, poor economic performance translates into impaired maternal and child health status, as families lose the ability to buy food, live in more precarious and disease-prone environments, and can no longer afford medical care.

Displacement: Displacement is the most immediate consequence of conflict for millions of refugees and internally displaced people and has a dramatic impact on health. Children separated from their parents are much more likely to die. Even when families can stay together, children and women are at high risk as the normal community networks that provide safety and care are disrupted. Sometimes the passage itself, on foot over long distances, endangers the health of women and children, exposing them to physical exhaustion, extreme temperatures (both heat and cold), disease vectors, and malnutrition. In Eastern Congo, many children suffered broken bones when they fell while running, at night and over uneven terrain, from looting militias. Children and pregnant women sleeping outside are particularly vulnerable to malaria. The lost boys of Sudan (United Nations High Commission for Refugees [UNHCR] 2001), a group of South Sudanese children (mostly, though not exclusively, boys), were decimated as they walked across East Africa, vulnerable to malnutrition, exposure, wild animals, and their worst enemy – armed human beings. Displacement can also cause devastating psychological trauma. Even when displaced people reach the comparative safety of a refugee camp – where mortality rates are relatively low – they are vulnerable to abuse, particularly women and children.

Loss of health services: Health services in conflict areas decline precipitously. In some cases, as in Eastern Sierra Leone in the 1990s, they disappear altogether. In others, such as Eastern Congo, services continue but are provided on a strictly cash-for-service basis, excluding many women and children. Services decline for three major reasons. First, governments, which in many cases were already

spending too little on health services, divert public spending away from health to finance weapons and ammunition. Second, the service infrastructure is destroyed as health centers are razed by bombardments or grenades, hospitals are looted or used for housing by displaced people, and equipment deteriorates beyond repair. Third, qualified health workers become rare as nurses, doctors, and other agents flee for their lives, migrate to more stable areas in which they can provide for their families, or are killed. In Cambodia, for example, educated personnel were especially targeted for death and imprisonment. Whatever the reason, in areas where diarrhea, pneumonia, malaria, and obstetric complications kill many women and children even in peacetime, losing access to medical care inevitably means that more women and children die. This effect is compounded by the concurrent loss of preventive health services. In times of conflict, preventive interventions that have saved millions of lives, such as immunizations, vitamin A supplementation, and insecticide-treated bednets, become less available, leaving women and particularly children more vulnerable.

Of the three factors discussed above, economic collapse and the loss of health services are particularly devastating because their impact is felt for years after the end of hostilities. In South Sudan for example, 3 years after a peace accord was signed, the absence of roads and clinics, an economy still in a battered shape, and the near-total absence of qualified health workers meant that most of the population did not have access to any health services; an obstetric complication in this setting could be a death sentence. In Eastern Sierra Leone, 6 years after the end of the war, the diamond trade has fully resumed, but public clinics are still not adequately funded, and there have been no systematic efforts to distribute mosquito nets. As a result, infectious diseases which would have been prevented or treated in a non-conflict setting kill thousands of children. Likewise, obstetric complications such as hemorrhage or obstructed labor, which would have been dealt with in a clinic or hospital, become deadly. For example, in Sierra Leone thousands of children die each year of malaria that could have been saved by a net costing less than $10; this is in sharp contrast to nearby Senegal, which has been largely at peace and has made great strides in the fight against malaria (United Nations 2007a). In an indirect but very real way, a pregnant woman dying of postpartum hemorrhage in South Sudan or a child dying of cerebral malaria in Sierra Leone are victims of conflict – the most common face, in fact, of suffering in twenty first century conflicts.

Mitigating the Impact of Conflict

When conflict occurs, as it sadly continues to do, there is much that can be done to reduce the enormous burden it imposes on women and children. Over the last decade, the maternal and child health response in acute emergencies has improved considerably as agencies have learned from past failures and successes. Measles was the leading cause of mortality in humanitarian emergencies in the 1980s, but is now much less common thanks to early and widespread immunization (CDC 1992). There is a growing body of best practices and written standards. Elements of an effective response to the impact of violent conflict include the following:

Acute complex emergencies: responding to immediate needs: Where people are displaced, governments, agencies, and other parties can work quickly to establish safe camps with essential services, including curative and preventive health care. To be effective, relief needs to follow the best practices outlined in the Sphere Guidelines [http://www.humanitarianinfo. org/darfur/uploads/sphere/Sphere%20Handbook_ full.pdf] which include standards on the provision of water, food, shelter, and health services in emergencies (The Sphere Project 2004). For children in developing countries where the vast majority of conflicts occur and where most of the maternal and child mortalities from conflict occur, this will include systematic vaccination for measles. For women, immediate needs are outlined in the Minimum Initial Service Package (MISP), which includes prevention of HIV transmission, assuring access to emergency obstetric care, preventing and managing the consequences of sexual violence, and planning for more comprehensive reproductive health services as the crisis situation becomes more stable.

In addition to these universal actions applicable to nearly all emergencies, Sphere Guidelines mandate that public health workers in acute emergencies

identify and respond to specific threats in a given context. In 1994 for example, in the space of a few days, a million Rwandese refugees fleeing the genocide crossed the border into Goma, in Eastern Democratic Republic of Congo (then Zaire), settling on the shores of Lake Kivu, a seasonal reservoir of cholera. In the absence of any other option, the refugees used the lake for all their water needs. Within days, over 50,000 people had died in a blazing cholera epidemic (CDC 1996; Goma Epidemiology Group 1995). In retrospect, public health practitioners have recognized that the most effective way to prevent and mitigate the epidemic would have been to add chlorine to water collection containers at lakeside until adequate amounts of clean water could be transported throughout the refugee settlements. Because speed is so important in acute emergencies, the United Nations and private organizations working in emergencies pre-stock emergency kits in warehouses strategically located near places where emergencies are likely to occur. These kits include basic supplies and medicines to meet the needs of people for days to weeks.

Unfortunately, even with pre-packaged kits and efforts to prepare for and anticipate conflict crises, timely access is often a difficult issue. Emergency aid groups were able to provide some shelter and health care within days to refugees fleeing from Darfur into neighboring Chad, for example, but were much more limited in their ability to provide basic services to people displaced from their villages within Darfur itself.

Chronic complex emergencies: providing routine care in non-routine conditions: Many violent conflicts last months or years. Some of the affected population is displaced, many are not. Some of the displaced cross an international border and are recognized as refugees (United Nations 1951); others stay within their country and are described as internally displaced persons (United Nations 1998). Some displaced persons are in camps; most are not. In some cases, conflict is nearly continuous. South Sudan experienced fighting for most of the second half of the twentieth century; the Democratic Republic of Congo, the Darfur region of Sudan, and Northern Uganda are areas in which fighting has become chronic. Humanitarian workers have a choice of alternative strategies to improve maternal and child care in these contexts. One approach is to continue the type of programming implemented in acute conflicts, accessing short-term funding, focusing on providing basic inputs such as medicine, with many services performed by expatriate and other outside providers, and concentrating on traditional emergency interventions such as mass immunization campaigns and feeding centers for malnourished children.

Increasingly, however, humanitarian agencies are taking a different approach, with programming that combines some features of acute emergencies, such as the provision of key supplies and the elimination of user fees, with attention to some of the longer-term needs of the population, such as training and other forms of capacity building. In the Democratic Republic of Congo, for example, non-governmental organizations (NGOs) have begun to address family planning. Family planning may not be a needed life-saving activity in an acute emergency, but it is an appropriate focus for chronic emergencies. First, in conflict as in non-conflict periods, thousands of women wish to exercise their right to make reproductive choices, including the choice to not become pregnant; second, family planning is a highly effective way to decrease both maternal and child mortality; last, but not least, family planning services are feasible in chronic emergencies and can be offered in many of the same channels through which other health interventions are offered, including clinics and community-based providers.

Even when they are addressing longer-term needs and using more development approaches, maternal and child health workers operating in chronic emergencies may need to adapt their methods. In the Democratic Republic of Congo, for example, humanitarian agencies took a more development approach to supporting health clinics, including training providers and setting up revolving drug funds, but have had to make provisions for re-stocking health centers that were looted by combatants. To the extent possible, humanitarian organizations and other external actors should bring low-value assets rather than lootable assets. This can often be achieved in maternal and health programs without compromising impact. Activities such as vaccination programs or preventive health education can achieve concrete results without exposing centers to looting. Even when drugs are provided, the drugs most effective in helping

mothers and children, such as zinc for diarrhea or ergometrine to stop postpartum hemorrhage, are less likely to interest looters.

In some cases, approaches considered "developmental," such as the use of community health workers to provide care, may actually be well adapted for conflict areas. In Northern Uganda, for example, community-based workers stocked with several months of medicines have been able to continue to provide basic care even when clinics were destroyed.

Primary health-care provision in camps: Maternal and child health programming in camps, as in chronic emergencies, combines features of emergency actions with those of long-term development. New arrivals often need services for acute needs: young children, for example, may need therapeutic feeding for malnutrition and almost always need catch-up immunizations. At the same time many people, whether refugees or internally displaced people, remain in camps for months and years. As their situation stabilizes, agencies offer longer-term programming, including training, household-level health education, and prevention. For this reason, camps often have much lower mortality than surrounding areas or the areas from which camp residents fled.

Post-conflict healing and rebuilding: The impact of conflict on women and children is felt for years after hostilities cease. There is much that can be done to mitigate that impact. In the early post-conflict period, governments and NGOs should rebuild the infrastructure, such as health clinics, and replace equipment or supplies that have been destroyed or looted. At this time, it may also be helpful to provide salary support, either directly or through institutions, to attract health workers into what are often remote places with harsh working conditions. The early post-conflict period is also a time to begin thinking about rebuilding not only clinics but also systems – reporting systems, human resource systems, and logistics systems. Although this work is less glamorous and harder to explain to donors and the public than direct provision of services, it ultimately will have more impact on the health of women and children.

Even in this early period, it is important to work with local institutions, such as district-level Ministry of Health offices or local NGOs, building their capacity to manage and provide services. This can be difficult, in part because these institutions can be extremely short-staffed and have limited financial and organizational capacity and in part because NGOs may have been used to the flexibility of working on their own in the acute emergency phase. In the long term, however, work done to build local institutions, from the very start, is likely to help as much or more than the direct provision of supplies and services.

The late post-conflict period starts months after the end of hostilities and can last more than a decade. In some cases, NGOs may no longer need to supply all the necessary inputs; in others, such direct support may be necessary for years. In all cases, donors and agencies should be developing ways to sustain primary care services. In this period, NGOs and donors should be working with local institutions to develop and improve the systems they have begun to work on in the immediate post-conflict phase. Health services may play a crucial role in the late post-conflict period. A functioning health system and the availability of high-quality basic health services at little or no cost can create goodwill and help legitimize a new government by showing evidence of its competence. Although this is still a hypothesis, and there are little hard data on whether health services in practice do help to stabilize a country, the possibility is credible enough that donors are increasingly willing to support basic health-care provision as an element of their "fragile states" policy (USAID 2005).

It is important to note, however, that even in post-conflict settings, or in more developmentally oriented chronic conflict programming, there may be important differences between work in conflict and non-conflict countries. In conflict countries, rebuilding health services requires direct investment, a form of assistance that cannot be easily diverted, and a higher ratio of external project financing.

The rights-based approach: Conflict in the twenty first century is marked by massive violations of human rights. Humanitarian aid workers, whether working in maternal and child health or in other areas, need to respond to these violations. They can do so at various levels. Most immediately, they can redress the violation of the right to health by helping to provide health services. They can work with community-based institutions, building the capacity of local groups to monitor and improve respect for

basic human rights. For example, some NGOs are working with local leaders and women's groups to raise awareness about gender-based violence and to implement locally designed solutions (IRC 2004). Humanitarian workers can shine a spotlight on the abuses they see firsthand and work to decrease the impunity which is a major factor in the epidemics of sexual abuse and other human rights violations. In some cases, testimony on the abuse of human rights they have witnessed is the most powerful action humanitarian workers can take.

Conflict-sensitive and "do-no-harm" programming: Even with the best of intentions, combatants or civilians may perceive humanitarian work as helping one side of the conflict or having other negative effects. Health program managers need to analyze the conflict situation in which they operate and the implications of their projects on fighting factions, politicized communities, and the dynamics of conflicts in their areas. For example, an NGO may open a health center near an army base. If the center is used – or looted regularly – by soldiers, the NGO may be seen, by outsiders as well as by a resentful local population, as in fact supporting continued conflict. Where possible, the workers and beneficiaries of development projects should be drawn from across conflict lines. In some situations there may be a case for bypassing governments, in particular when operating through governments which lend support to abusive regimes.

Preventing Conflict

The surest way to protect women and children from conflict is to prevent the conflict from ever happening in the first place. Prevention is difficult, because it requires attention to the complex problems of remote countries, and the news media rarely cover wars that have not yet happened. There is little reward to the effort – few Nobel Prizes have been given for preventing wars. It is, however, clearly the best way to care for the millions of women and children who live in areas of the world where conflict might flare up again. Preventing conflict means promoting the conditions that make conflict less likely, including good governance, economic development, and equity. When conflict is brewing, advocacy can help to bring attention from outside nations and put pressure on potential combatants. Public health workers can play an important role, because they often work in countries before conflict breaks out and because they work at the field level and may have learned to understand the complex realities of rural and urban communities in potential conflict countries. To be effective, however, it is essential that they share their unique perspective and knowledge with others, including political advocates, human rights lobbyists, and journalists. In conflict prevention as in maternal and child health, foresight and teamwork are essential to success.

Advocacy

Advocacy is a powerful tool and often the most powerful way for humanitarian aid workers and other concerned citizens to help women and children in conflict areas. There are several ways to advocate. NGO personnel who work directly in conflict sites can witness, to the media, decision-makers in their countries or others about the abuses they have seen. Advocates can also participate in decisions about how aid is given out and other policy decisions that affect conflict countries. Such policy issues can range from export bans for conflict diamonds and fair-trade laws to structuring economic reform packages that are sensitive to the needs of conflict-affected populations. Economic reform packages that include major cutbacks in government spending may have devastating humanitarian impacts – and be economically ill-advised, especially in immediate post-conflict areas where public investment is needed after years of neglect. Whatever the issue, real progress on a large scale will only be possible if the voices and interests of women and children in conflict areas are heard and taken into account in national and international policy decisions. Thus advocacy is an important element of maternal and child health work.

Millennium Development Goals (MDGs) and Countries in Conflict

Conflict-affected countries are more likely to stay poor, and poor countries are more likely to experience conflict. Civil wars have been shown to occur most often in poor and slowly growing countries. And, as demonstrated in the foregoing discussion, when they do occur they inflict enormous hardship. World Bank models (Djankov and Reynal-Querol 2007) show a profound relationship between the poverty of a nation and its chances of having a civil war. A country where the average person survives on less than $1 per day has a predicted probability of war (at some point over the next 5 years) of 15%, even if it is otherwise considered an "average" country (Gagain 2006). This probability of war reduces by half for a country with GDP of $600 per person; and countries with per person income over $5,000 have a less than 1% chance of experiencing civil conflict (Gagain 2006). Although none of the Millennium Development Goals (MDGs) specifically addressed conflict, goals 3–5 (promote gender equality and empower women; reduce child mortality; improve maternal health) deal with maternal and child health. Indeed, countries in conflict are more likely to be poor and to stay poor, which is an obstacle to reaching any of the MDGs. They are particularly less likely to reach the MCH-related MDGs because of the profound negative impact of war on women and children. Countries at war will need more resources if they are to achieve the MDGs. Countries which have experienced protracted conflict such as Afghanistan or the Democratic Republic of Congo will require particularly large assistance to achieve parity among non-conflict states when aiming to achieve the Millennium Development Goals – whether economic or health indicators are measured.

In weak states, evaluation of progress toward the MDGs should take account of progress toward achieving the goals at a provincial or smaller level rather than at a national level only. In states where ethnic, regional, or religious divisions run deep, MDG reports should take note of the ways in which MDG policies address the concerns of these different groups and not simply the national attainment of the goals. Countries emerging from conflict such as Liberia have established MDG teams and produced interim reports (United Nations 2007b). Such reports from post-conflict settings illustrate the distance yet to be traveled by some of the world's poorest countries.

Conclusion

Conflict is a significant cause of maternal and child morbidity and mortality. As conflict has evolved, combatants deliberately target civilians, both through direct violence and through the destruction of essential services. Women and children, whose well-being depends on health services, particularly in pregnancy and early childhood, have felt the greatest impact. Concurrently, the public community, both internationally and within affected countries, has adapted its response and become more effective at mitigating the effect of conflict on the health of women and children. This response has included more effective humanitarian action, adapted to the varied contexts in which conflict occurs, as well as advocacy, to help avoid conflict in the first place. The international public health community is increasingly recognizing that mitigating and preventing conflict is essential to achieving the Millennium Development Goals.

Key Terms

Abuse	Conflict-sensitive	Humanitarian emergencies
Acute complex emergencies	programming	Identify conflict
Acute emergencies	Darfur	Immunization
Adverse obstetric condition	Democratic Republic of Congo	Insecticide-treated bednets
Advocacy	Destruction of infrastructure	Insurgencies
Afghanistan	Diamond trade	Insurgents
Airbase	Dinka tribes	Internally displaced people
Arab	Direct injury	International Rescue
Black Africans	Displacement	Commission
Bombardment	Do-no-harm programming	Iraq
Bosnia	East Congo	Islamic fundamentalism
Burnett Institute	Economic collapse	Janjawid militias
Burundi	Enemy	Lake Kivu
Cambodia	Ethnic divisions	Loot
Camps	Ethnicity	Loyalty
Catch-up immunization	Family planning	Machine guns
Child mortality	Farsi-speaking tribes	Malaria
Chlorine	Feudal fiefdoms	Mali
Cholera	Food aid	Malnutrition
Christian	Food insecurity	Maneuver
Chronic emergencies	Fur tribes	Maternal mortality
Civil war	Genocide	Militia
Civilian victims	Goma	Millennium Development
Clan	Grenades	Goals (MDGs)
Cold war	Hate speech	Minimum Initial Service
Combat injury	Hatred	Package (MISP)
Combatants	Hemorrhage	Muslim
Conflict	HIV infection	Nation state
Conflict zones	Hostilities	Obstetric care
Conflict-affected countries	Human rights	Obstetric complications

Obstetric fistula	Semi-automatic rifles	United Nations High Commission for Refugees (UNHCR)
Obstructed labor	Sexual assault	
Pashtun-speaking tribes	Sierra Leone	
Post-conflict period	Small arms	United States
Post-conflicts rebuilding	Soldiers	Violence against women
Postpartum hemorrhage	Somalia	Vitamin supplementation
Propaganda	Soviet Union	Vulnerability
Proxy war	Sphere Guidelines	War
Psychological trauma	Standard of living	Warlords
Rape	Sudan	Weapon of war
Rebels	Surge	Weapons
Refugees	Trauma	World War I
Regular army	Uganda	World War II
Relief agencies	United Nations	Yugoslavia
Religion		Zaire

Questions for Discussion

1. The nature of conflicts in the world has changed significantly since the end of the Cold War. Briefly explain what you understand by this statement. What are some of the consequences of identity conflicts? Why are they difficult to resolve?

2. Summarize in 150 words, the relationship between poverty and wars.

3. Discuss some of the maternal and child health implications of recruiting children for combat and combat-related duties.

4. Draw a causal diagram to illustrate the pathways by which conflicts affect the health and well-being of women, children, and adolescents.

5. What are chronic complex emergencies? Summarize key strategies for addressing them.

References

Centers for Disease Control and Prevention (CDC) (1992) Famine-affected, refugee, and displaced populations: recommendations for public health issues. Morbidity and Mortality Weekly Report 41(RR-13)

Centers for Disease Control and Prevention (CDC) (1996) Morbidity and mortality surveillance in Rwandan refugees – Burundi and Zaire, 1994. Morbidity and Mortality Weekly Report, 45(05), 104–107

Coghlan B, Brennan RJ, Ngoy P et al. (2006) Mortality in the Democratic Republic of Congo: a nationwide survey. Lancet, 367(95040), 44–51

Coghlan B, Ngoy P, Mulumba F et al. (2008) Mortality in the Democratic Republic of Congo: an ongoing crisis. http://www.theirc.org/resources/2007/2006-7_congomortalitysurvey.pdf, cited 22 January 2008

Djankov S, Reynal-Querol M (2007) The Causes of Civil War. World Bank Policy Research Working Paper 4254 (WPS4254), June 2007. The World Bank, Washington DC, http://www-wds.worldbank.org/external/default/WDSContentServer/IW3P/IB/2007/06/15/000016406_20070615144341/Rendered/PDF/wps4254.pdf, cited 22 January 2008

Gagain JR (2006) Millennium Development Watch: The Dominican Republic as a pilot project. United Nations Chronicle 4(XLIV). http://www.un.org/Pubs/chronicle/2006/issue4/0406p74.htm, cited 22 January 2008

Goma Epidemiology Group (1995) Public health impact of Rwandan refugee crisis: what happened in Goma, Zaire, in July, 1994? Lancet, 345(8946), 339–344

Human Rights Watch (1999a) Leave none to tell the story: genocide in Rwanda. http://www.hrw.org/reports/1999/rwanda/, cited 6 June 2008

Human Rights Watch (1999b) Sierra Leone rebel abuses spreading. http://www.hrw.org/english/docs/1999/12/06/sierra8922.htm, cited 22 January 2008

International Rescue Committee (2004) 2004 Annual Report. http://www.reliefweb.int/library/documents/2004/irc-anurpt-31dec.pdf, cited 22 January 2008

Keegan J (1997) The Second World War. Pimlico Publishers, London

Keegan J (ed.) (1999) The First World War. Pimlico Publishers, London

Purdin S (1996) Personal observation

Smyth L (2002) Identity-based conflicts: a systemic approach. Negotiation Journal, 18(2), 147–161

The Sphere Project (2004) Humanitarian Charter and Minimum Standards in Disaster Response. Geneva: The Sphere Project. www.sphereproject.org, cited 20 July 2008

United Nations (1951) Convention relating to the status of refugees. Adopted on 28 July 1951 by the United Nations Conference of Plenipotentiaries on the Status of Refugees and Stateless Persons convened under General Assembly resolution 429 (V) of 14 December 1950.   http://www.unhchr.ch/html/menu3/b/o_c_ref.htm, cited 20 July 2008

United Nations (1998) Guiding Principles on Internal Displacement United Nations E/CN.4/1998/53/Add.2. http://www.unhchr.ch/html/menu2/7/b/principles.htm, cited 20 July 2008

United Nations (2001) Conflict diamonds. http://www.un.org/peace/africa/Diamond.html, cited 22 January 2008

United Nations (2007a) At a glance: Sierra Leone. http://www.unicef.org/infobycountry/sierraleone_39463.html, cited 22 January 2008

United Nations (2007b) Liberia: MDG Profile. http://www.mdgmonitor.org/factsheets_00.cfm?c = LIB&cd = , cited 23 January 2008

United Nations Children's Fund (UNICEF) (2006) State of the World's Children, 2006. http://www.unicef.org/sowc06/pdfs/sowc06_fullreport.pdf, cited 22 January 2008

United Nations High Commissioner for Refugees (UNHCR) (2001) David vs. Goliath. Refugees, 1:122, 14

United States Agency for International Development (USAID) (2005) Fragile States Strategy. http://www.usaid.gov/policy/2005_fragile_states_strategy.pdf, cited 22 January 2008

United States Agency for International Development (USAID) (2006) ACQUIRE Project. Traumatic Gynecologic Fistula: a consequence of sexual violence in conflict settings. Report of a meeting held in Addis Ababa, Ethiopia, September 6–8 2005.http://www.engenderhealth.org/ia/swh/pdf/TF-Report-English.pdf, cited 22 January 2008

Zwi AB, Grove NJ, Kelly P et al. (2006) Child health in armed conflict: time to rethink. Lancet, 367(9526), 1886–1888

Chapter 8
The Impact of Globalization on Maternal and Child Health

Sarah Wamala

Learning Objectives After reading this chapter and answering the discussion questions that follow, you should be able to

- Discuss the meaning and features of globalization.
- Evaluate how globalization directly affects maternal and child health through changing occupational roles of women, evolution of food production, preparation, and consumption patterns, and migration (including migration of health professionals).
- Analyze how globalization indirectly affects maternal and child health through limitations in the provision of care as a consequence of such economic policies as privatization, international trade agreements, and structural adjustment policies (SAPs).
- Propose potential public health policies and measures to reduce the impact of globalization on the health of women, children, and adolescents.

Introduction

This chapter presents an overview of how globalization and our increasingly interlinked world affect the lives and health of women and children. It begins with an analysis of globalization's impact on the provision of care through privatization and such international policy mechanisms as the Structural Adjustment Programs (SAPs),

which many writers believe has deepened poverty around the world. It then examines how globalization directly affects the health and livelihoods of women through changing occupational roles, evolution in food production, preparation and consumption patterns, and migration. It concludes with the investigation of possible public health and policy responses and examines the extent to which the Millennium Development Goals contribute to the alleviation of the adverse impacts of globalization on the health of women and children.

Contrary to popular opinion, globalization is not a new phenomenon (Frenk and Gómez-Dantés 2002). The forces of trade, migration, war, and conquest have historically bound people from distant places together. As Frenk and Gómez-Dantés (2002) observed, the expression "citizen of the world" was coined by the Greek philosopher Diogenes in the 4th century BC. There is consensus however, that the pace, range, and depth of integration have intensified over the past two decades. As never before, the consequences of actions that take place far away show up, literally at our doorsteps (Frenk and Gómez-Dantés 2002). Globalization is a term with multiple, contested meanings. For the purposes of this chapter, it is defined as "a process of greater integration within the world's economy through movements of goods and services, capital, technology and labor, which increasingly leads to economic decisions being influenced by global conditions" (Jenkins 2004). Thus, the concept of globalization is linked to the rise of transnational corporations (TNCs) and the associated internationalization of production, distribution, and consumption of goods and services. It is

S. Wamala (✉)
Swedish National Institute of Public Health, Forskarens väg 3., SE-831 40 Östersund, Sweden

J.E. Ehiri (ed.), *Maternal and Child Health*, DOI 10.1007/b106524_8,
© Springer Science+Business Media, LLC 2009

the process whereby national and international policy-makers promote domestic deregulation and external liberalization (Cornia 2001). Globalization gained momentum as a policy paradigm in the 1980s with the adoption of domestic deregulation, trade liberalization, and privatization policies that allow cross-border acquisitions by multinational firms (Cornia 2001; Dollar 2001). The process intensified in the 1990s with the removal of barriers to international trade, foreign direct investments (i.e., investments by foreign companies, such as construction of production facilities, buildings, machinery, and equipment), and short-term financial flows (Cornia 2001). Foreign direct investment (FDI) has been on the rise around the world since the 1970s. Table 8.1 presents information on FDI in developing economies from 1990 to 2006. In India, for example, incoming FDI has grown from 1.705 billion in the 1990s to 16.881 billion in 2006 and from 1.9% of the GDP to 8.7%. There is debate regarding the impact of globalization on health and the quality of life of people. However, empirical results on links between globalization and specific health outcomes are limited (Kawachi and Wamala 2006a). The impact of globalization has been debated in terms of both its positive (Dollar 2001; 2004) and its negative impacts (Rabbani et al. 2006).

Proponents of globalization believe that it creates new jobs and can lead to transfer and infusion of innovative technologies, management strategies, and workforce practices. Foreign direct investment is also argued to have expanded women's employment opportunities and hence, their economic autonomy (Dollar 2004). Globalization is believed to have aided the international transfer of reproductive technologies, such as contraception. The close integration of societies, particularly through telecommunications and the Internet, has mobilized the international women's movement. In arguing the case for the health benefits of globalization, Dollar (2001) also observes that the economic integration made possible by globalization is a powerful force for raising the incomes of poor countries. Within the past two decades, several large developing countries have opened up to international trade and foreign direct investment (e.g., China, India, and Vietnam). They have recorded more impressive economic growth rates than some rich countries. Dollar (2001) also observed that there is a tendency for income equity to increase in countries that have embraced trade liberalization and foreign direct investments. Dollar and Kraay (2001) attribute the increasing income equity to rising average incomes in, for example, China and India. The perception is that economic growth, brought about by globalization, contributes directly to improvements in the health status of the poor in less developed countries (especially women and children) through improvements in nutrition (Hawkes 2005), increased education of females, better maternal health, and lower child mortality (Filmer and Pritchett 1999).

Magnussen et al. (2004) argue that pro-growth macroeconomic, labor, and social policies widen income inequity and significantly disadvantage the poor and less privileged, particularly women and children. Such policies have the tendency to provide better opportunities to those with resources and high levels of education, while large segments of the population without these assets are unlikely to benefit and may in fact become casualties of the economic transition. As Lee (2004) argues, the

Table 8.1 FDI flows

FDI flows (millions of dollars) Developing economies					As a percentage of gross fixed capital formation			
	1990–2000	2003	2004	2005	2006	1990–2000	2004	2005	2006
Inward flow	130,722	178,699	283,030	314,316	379,070	9.3	12.9	12.6	13.8
Outward flow	52,836	45,372	877,301	837,194	1,215,789	7.9	10.1	92.	11.8
World economy									
Inward flow	495,399	564,078	742,143	945,795	1,035,852	7.8	8.5	10.4	12.6
Outward flow	492,622	560,087	877,301	837,194	1,215,789	7.9	10.1	9.2	11.8

Source: UNCTAD (2007)

health impacts of globalization are simultaneously positive and negative and vary according to factors such as geographical location, sex, age, ethnic origin, education level, and socioeconomic status.

Effect of Globalization on Maternal and Child Health

The relationship between globalization and health is complex. The analyses require conceptual frameworks that define links and mechanisms by which globalization impacts health in relation to context, social structure, history, and politics. A number of conceptual frameworks have been suggested (Huynen et al. 2005; Woodward et al. 2001; Labonte and Torgerson 2002). In one example, Huynen et al. (2005) proposed a framework that identifies the main determinants of population health (Table 8.2) and relates them to main features of the globalization process (Table 8.3).

Figure 8.1 provides an example to aid in understanding the interaction of these mechanisms.

Pinpointing the effects of globalization at the institutional, economic, sociocultural, and ecological

Table 8.2 Determinants of population health

Level/Nature	General Determinants	More Detailed Determinants
Contextual level		
Institutional	Institutional	Governance structure
	Infrastructure	Political environment
		System of law
		Regulation
Economic	Economic infrastructure	Occupational structure
		Tax system
		Markets
Sociocultural	Culture	Religion
		Ideology
		Customs
	Population	Population size
		Structure
		Geographical distribution
	Social infrastructure	Social organization
		Knowledge development
		Social security
		Insurance system
		Mobility and communication
Environmental	Ecological settings	Ecosystems
		Climate
Distal level		
Institutional	Health policy	Effective public health policy
		Sufficient public health budget
	Health-related policies	Effective food policy
		Effective water policy
		Effective social policy
		Effective environmental policy
Economic	Economic development	Income/wealth
		Economic equity
	Trade	Trade in goods and services
		Marketing
Sociocultural	Knowledge	Education and literacy
		Health education
		Technology
	Social interactions	Social equity
		Conflicts

(continued)

Table 8.2 (continued)

Level/Nature	General Determinants	More Detailed Determinants
Environmental	Ecosystem goods and services	Travel and migration Habitat Information Production Regulation
Proximal level		
Institutional	Health services	Provision of and access to health services
Economic	–	–
Sociocultural	Lifestyle	Healthy food consumption patterns Alcohol and tobacco use Drug abuse Unsafe sexual behavior Physical activity Stress coping Child care Lifestyle-related endogenous factors (blood pressure, obesity, cholesterol levels)
	Social environment	Social support and informal care Intended injuries and abuse/violence
Environmental	Food and water	Sufficient quality Sufficient quantity Sanitation
	Physical environment	Quality of the living environment (biotic, physical and chemical factors) Unintended injuries

Source: Huynen et al. (2005)

Table 8.3 Features of globalization

Feature	Characteristics
New global governance structure	Globalization influences the interdependence among nations as well as the nation state's sovereignty leading to (a need for) new global governance structures
Global markets	Globalization is characterized by worldwide changes in economic infrastructures and the emergence of global markets and a global trading system
Global communication and diffusion of information	Globalization makes the sharing of information and the exchange of experiences around common problems possible
Global mobility	Global mobility is characterized by a major increase in the extensity, intensity, and velocity of movement and by a wide variety in "types" of mobility
Cross-cultural interaction	Globalizing cultural flows result in interactions between global and local cultural elements
Global environmental changes	Global environmental threats to ecosystems include global climate change, loss of biodiversity, global ozone depletion, and the global decline in natural areas

Source: Huynen et al. (2005)

determinants of population health, the model demonstrates that the globalization process mainly operates at the contextual level, while influencing health through its more distal and proximal determinants (Fig. 8.2).

The effects of globalization on the health of women and children can also be characterized at the national, community, and individual levels. Figure 8.3 demonstrates how globalization impacts health-related policies, agriculture, social spheres, and the provision and funding of healthcare services at a national level. These national factors, in turn, influence capabilities, cohesiveness, social fragmentation, entitlements, endowments, resources, and

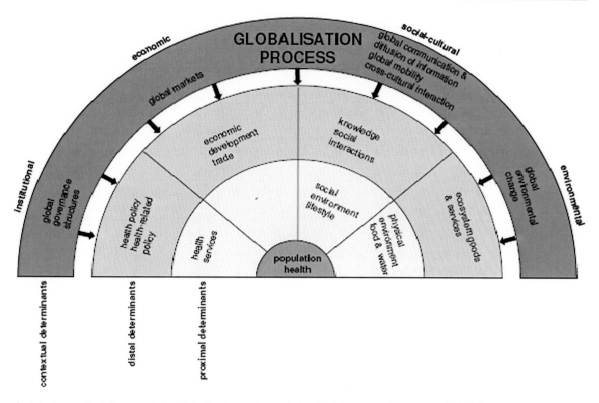

Fig. 8.1 Conceptual framework for globalization and population health. Source: Huynen et al. (2005)

services at the community level. These influences at national and community levels consequently impact women's occupational roles and household food and nutrition security, ultimately affecting maternal and child health.

Several trends affected by an increasingly global economy demonstrate the convergence of globalization and MCH: the privatization of healthcare and public services, Structural Adjustment Programs (SAPs and public health services), changing occupational roles, food production, preparation and consumption, and migration. These are examined in more detail in the following paragraphs.

Globalization and Commercialization of Healthcare and Public Services

The objective of the General Agreement on Tariffs and Trade (GATT) signed by 23 nations in 1947 was to promote and regulate the liberalization of international trade through rounds of trade negotiations.

The Uruguay Round of Multilateral Trade Negotiations (1986–1994) led to the Marrakech Agreements, which established the World Trade Organization (WTO) and extended the rules governing commercial relations between trading partners to several new areas that were previously excluded from trade liberalization. These include agriculture, services, investment measures, and the protection of intellectual property rights (Supakankunti et al. 2001). Thus, the WTO is one of the major features of globalization. It exerts its influence on the globalization process through health and health-related policies (Figs. 8.11 and 8.22). Its aim is economic growth and stability based on free markets and minimum governmental interference. It deals with the rules of trade between nations at a global or near-global level. It describes itself as an organization for liberalizing trade – a forum for governments to negotiate trade agreements and a place for them to settle trade disputes. Where countries have faced trade barriers and wanted them lowered, these negotiations have helped to liberalize trade (World Trade Organization 2008). WTO's membership includes 151 nation states (as of

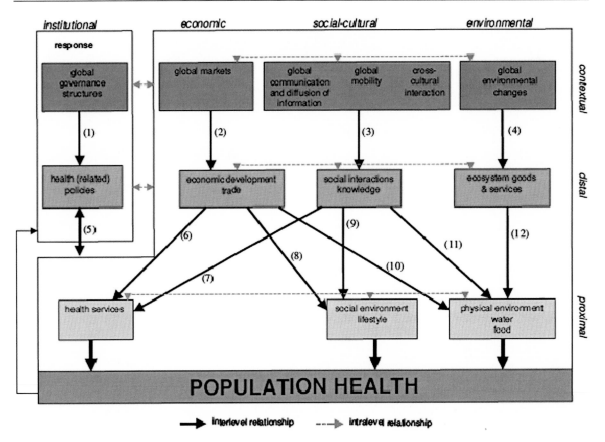

Fig.8.2 Conceptual framework for globalization and population health: the role of contextual, distal, and proximal factors. Source: Huynen et al. (2005)

Fig.8.3 Effects of globalization on maternal and child health: a conceptual framework

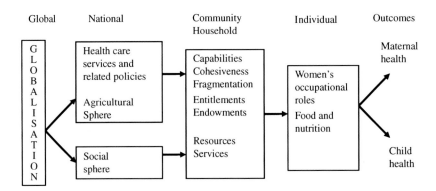

July 27, 2007) and voting is based on democratic terms. However, the transnational corporations that are represented on all significant advisory committees decide detailed policies and set the WTO's agenda. Low-income developing countries who constitute two-thirds of the organization's membership, have a weak bargaining position at the WTO

committees in the presence of these transnational corporations that desire expanded private enterprise involvement in the increasingly important service sectors. These sectors include telecommunications, transport, distribution, postal, insurance, environment, tourism, entertainment, and leisure services. The main problematic services are those managed by the public health sector namely healthcare, social services, education, and housing. The WTO's focus on the service industry reflects the sector's growing commercial importance. As such, WTO trade agreements have been described as a bill of rights for corporate business, not for nations (AFSC 2006).

In 1994, a comprehensive new treaty on intellectual property rights known as the Agreement on Trade-Related Aspects of Intellectual Property Rights (TRIPS), was established within the framework of the WTO. Later, this would have significant impact on global health. The treaty established minimum universal standards in all areas of intellectual property with the intention of implementing these standards globally through a strong enforcement mechanism. The treaty requires all WTO member countries to adopt minimum standards of protection for patents, trademarks, copyrights, and other intellectual property rights in their laws. Any member country failing to bring its patent law into conformity with the TRIPS agreement, if challenged by another member country, is subject to WTO's dispute settlement system, and sanctions can be imposed in accordance with WTO procedures. TRIPS requires universal patent protection for any invention in any field of technology. Accordingly, this affects pharmaceuticals, which many countries had previously excluded from patent protection in order to produce drugs at reduced prices. Although TRIPS has significant implications for public health, it was negotiated with little or no participation from public health authorities (Ehiri and Anyanwu 2004). As part of its obligations, it sets forth to protect inventions including the following:

- recognizing patents for pharmaceuticals without distinction between imported and locally produced products;
- granting patent protection for at least 20 years from the date of application;
- limiting the scope of exemptions from patent rights;
- enforcing patent rights through administrative and judicial mechanisms;
- compulsory protection against unfair commercial use of data submitted for the marketing approval of new pharmaceutical products.

Patents are supposed to contribute to the generation of funds for research and development of new drugs, but implementation of TRIPS without regard to the technological and financial limitations of resource-poor countries has had the following negative implications for public health in these countries (Correa 2001) and on the health of the poor, especially women and children:

- Patent holders, usually large pharmaceutical firms in industrialized nations, can exclude direct competition and charge higher prices for patented medicines than would have been expected in a competitive market.
- Life-saving drugs can become unaffordable (e.g., the cost of antiretroviral drugs is above the reach of most individuals and families in sub-Saharan Africa where HIV/AIDS poses a significant challenge to health and development).
- Poor countries are excluded from the benefits of protection for inventions because they lack the scientific infrastructure and the capital needed for research and development since the high costs and the need for economies of scale place the development of patentable pharmaceuticals beyond their reach.
- Pharmaceutical companies that invest in research and development focus mainly on diseases likely to yield the highest return for their shareholders. Such diseases of the poor that have more debilitating consequences for women and children, e.g., malaria and tuberculosis, are not considered priorities.

The application of TRIPS has caused serious problems to developing country producers of generic drugs such as India and Brazil and to importers of these drugs such as South Africa and Kenya. In Côte d'Ivoire, one of West Africa's wealthiest countries, only about 500 of the estimated 1,000,000 people infected with HIV/AIDS receive drug treatment. Even though the Ivorian and French governments subsidize over half of the cost, the drug regime still costs $1–$10 a month on average while the average monthly wage is only about $50 (Pompey 1999).

Various regional trade zones of the world (e.g., North Atlantic Free Trade Agreement (NAFTA) and the European Union (EU)) have rules which can facilitate privatization in relation to service provision and insurance schemes. In addition, national government leaders in a number of developed and developing countries frequently use privatization as a policy instrument to reduce the financial burden of the public sector. Their decisions are encouraged by global institutions such as the World Bank and International Monetary Fund (IMF) through mechanisms such as Structural Adjustment Programs (SAPs) discussed in the next section.

Structural Adjustment Programs (SAPs) and Public Services

Another marked feature of globalization is the privatization of public services. This was initiated with the argument of improving effectiveness and efficiency of publicly managed institutions and agencies – e.g., electricity corporations, water corporations, financial institutions, factories. Structural Adjustment refers to a set of policy advice that is given to developing countries by international agencies, mainly the World Bank and the International Monetary Fund, in order to enhance economic growth through macroeconomic stability and elimination of market distortions. The World Bank and IMF recommend SAPs to indebted poor countries as a means of achieving economic recovery. Developing countries, who implement the recommended policies, receive grants or loans from donor agencies for this purpose.

While national governments have a social responsibility to ensure access to basic amenities such as water, energy, and essential services, many opt to promote privatization with the belief that it facilitates market competition and efficiency (Gleick 2000). Private owners of public sector services are often dominated by transnational corporations (TNCs) with long-term contracts (even up to 50 years) and limited knowledge of local conditions. TNCs may set price policies that do not match local demands and capabilities. As a result, privatization of energy and water in sub-Saharan Africa, Latin America, and Central and Eastern Europe (Olivera and Lewis 2004; Gleick 2000) has resulted in limited access for local populations due to prohibitively high prices. In this example, the government does not provide services, the population cannot afford services provided by the private sector, and there is a resulting lack of access to basic infrastructure.

The implications for public health are clear. Improved access to basic public services such as safe water and energy is the key to improved child health in poor regions of the world. A large number of women and children in many poor countries walk several miles in search of water and firewood. Substantial research literature describes the effects of the Structural Adjustment Programs (SAPs) that integrated African countries into the global economy in the 1980s (De Vogli and Birbeck 2005). SAP measures such as domestic deregulation, privatization, fiscal austerity, and marketization of social services, combined with deeper liberalization and integration in specific sites such as Export Processing Zones (EPZs), reflected and reinforced the more fundamental changes in the organization of production and the distribution of wealth and risk under globalization (UNCTAD 1993).

After two decades of field studies and contests concerning the impacts, it is now accepted that the overall effects of these policies in Africa, in relation to social development and poverty, has been negative (Mkandawire 2005). There is evidence for negative health outcomes of deepening liberalization, commercialization, cost recovery in health and essential services, weakening community and public sector authority in health, increased food insecurity associated with changes in trade, and increased control of food markets by a limited number of buyers (FAO 2004a). An equally substantial body of research literature demonstrates that globalization's negative health effects have not been gender-neutral and that women have experienced some of the greatest negative consequences in health and caring burdens (Afshar and Barrientos 1998).

Globalization and Changing Occupational Roles

In spite of the fact that women's participation in the labor force increased particularly in the era of globalization (1980s and 1990s), a large proportion of women's unpaid work still goes unnoticed (United Nations 2005a). In many cases, while women's participation has increased, men's has fallen. Thus a phenomenon of "masculinization of unemployment" has occurred. An increasingly large underclass of younger men who cannot find work is observed in many poor countries. High unemployment rates and redundancy among men have contributed to increased alcohol consumption, unrest, and drug abuse which accelerate violence against women and children (UN 2005a).

"Feminization of employment" has occurred due to a number of explanations. One explanation is that the global labor force has become more female due to a greater demand for women workers in sectors of the economy related to globalization, such as export sectors (UN 2005b). Notable examples are low-skilled manufacturing, such as garments, footwear, and electronic products. These new export processing industries depend heavily on women workers, many of whom are young, rural immigrants. In fact, in countries where SAPs were introduced there are higher women's participation rates (Cagatay and Ozler 1995). Another explanation is that more women must now work to ensure family survival due to declining real wages and the increased monetary cost of subsistence, resulting from the SAP cutbacks in public services and subsidies. It should be noted that women's increased participation in the labor force brings increased opportunities to women, but the effects have not all been positive. Women's employment is associated with seasonal, unpaid, casual wage labor, long working hours, and generally poor working conditions (Loewenson 1999).

Changes in Food Production, Preparation, and Consumption

Globalization has an impact on healthcare through changes to livelihoods of small-scale farmers, an anticipated rural–urban migration, and changes to nutrition and food security. Globalization in the form of trade liberalization, increased economic growth, improved communication, improved information flows, and technology is expected to increase access to better food and cheap food supplies (FAO 2004b). Forces of globalization on the other hand can endanger food production and security (Hawkes 2005). It should be noted that in spite of the changes in the manufacturing sphere, a majority of the population depends on agriculture

for food. About 90% of the developing world's poor live in Asia and sub-Saharan Africa and about 75% of those live in rural areas. These people depend on agriculture for their daily existence. Yet, more than two-thirds of total exports from poor developing countries are agro-based commodities. Agricultural growth is therefore crucial to their livelihood. The globalization of agricultural markets brought about by trade liberalization and worldwide changes in markets and marketing channels poses special challenges for small-scale farmers and poor areas of developing countries.

It is known that women are responsible for 80% of food production in Africa, including the most labor-intensive work, such as planting, fertilizing, irrigating, weeding, harvesting, and marketing (FAO 2004b). However, changes in the agricultural sector wrought by globalization are widening gender inequalities. The focus of support on export production can include a bias toward larger scale farms, at the expense of support for small holders. These small holders are often women farmers, many of whom produce food for local, domestic markets. Women may become cheap laborers for more export-orientated commercial farming concerns. The only alternative for rural women is to migrate to urban centers to seek employment.

The attainment of food security and subsequent food consumption and nutrition patterns here take on another dimension (Hawkes 2005; McMichael 2005). Poor nutrition (under- or overnutrition) has substantial impacts on health. In Africa, this is marked in the context of poverty and HIV/AIDS, where the household workforce is decreased (Chopra 2004). Globalization has led to global expansion of agricultural trade and finance. It can also prevent fluctuations in food supply, by enabling developing countries to import food at adequate and stable prices. Improved market access for these countries can increase agricultural exports, thereby increasing foreign exchange. Raising the level of income and employment among low-income rural families increases the amount of food poor people can afford and protects them from higher food prices in the event of domestic market shortages.

Globalization has accelerated urbanization and changes in food preparation, choices, and consumption. It has created a shift in the structure of diets from traditional, low-cost diets rich in fiber and grain to high-cost diets that include greater proportions of sugars, oils, and animal fats (FAO 2004a). The local staple foods with rich nutrients have been replaced by high-carbohydrate foodstuffs from fast food restaurants. These include fried chicken, beef burgers, pizzas, potato chips, and soft drinks, among others. All of these foods have high proportions of oil, salt, and sugar that are higher in calories than other foods. Because higher socioeconomic status (SES) in many low-income countries is often associated with western lifestyle including food choices and behaviors, high SES individuals buy food from westernized fast food restaurants. In fact, a large number of people with high SES in the developing countries are overrepresented among people who suffer from obesity, hypertension, and type 2 diabetes. This is an epidemiological transition which many western industrialized countries bypassed in the beginning of the 19th century.

In many poor countries, a phenomenon of "street foods" in a takeaway style has also risen due to increased urbanization, coupled with low wages. Street foods account for 70% of the total calorie intake of the urban low- and middle-income groups. The choice of food depends mainly on SES. Many low- and middle-income households buy food from vendors to save on the cost of food ingredients and cooking fuel, save preparation time, and try new foods. The type of foods served by street food vendors include rice, stiff porridge from maize flour, plantains, maize cooked with beans, fried potato, cassava, sweet potato, chips, roast and fried chicken, and roast meat. There is often a lack of hygiene and proper handling methods associated with the preparation of street foods. This results in microbial contaminants that contribute to diarrhea and intensify other diseases, particularly among children and pregnant women. As many households adapt to street foods, wisdom and knowledge about traditional food preparation is forgotten between generations. This could lead toward worse nutritional problems in the future.

Globalization and Migration

Globalization has led to an increased number of women who migrate as potential participants in the labor market and principal breadwinners for their families. The United Nations estimates that women accounted for 48% of migration. However, the ratio of women to men migrating may be even larger in some parts of the world, for example, in sub-Saharan Africa and some Asian countries. Globalization has contributed to "feminization of migration" resulting in more women from poorer developing countries migrating to find paid employment. This can cause these women to be economically and socially independent of their own cultures. This cultural isolation is detrimental to their health and that of their children. While the increased availability of affordable migrant providers of care for young children, elderly parents, and disabled relatives has enabled women in wealthier countries to join or remain in the workforce (Ehrenreich and Hochschild 2004), migrant women themselves are often exposed to poor employment conditions. The poor conditions for a large domestic workforce of women from poor to wealthy countries have been well documented (Loewenson 1999; UNCTAD 1993; Ghosh 2003).

Migrant women often lack knowledge about their rights and entitlements and about healthcare access. This often negatively influences health. Poor health is intertwined with adverse social, economic, and institutional factors (e.g., sexually transmitted infections and being subject to gender-based violence) that affect low-wage earners and their families. These conditions have major policy implications in the host countries. In addition, the migration of women for work results in the fragmentation of the household structure, family dynamics, and social support mechanisms (Afshar and Barrientos 1998). In many poor countries women have the primary role in child upbringing. Thus, their migration leaves a vacuum in child care. Women's absence may create a care deficit for their children and disabled or elderly relatives. A common scenario is that women migrate from poor to rich countries to work as nannies and leave their children in their hometowns to be taken care of by another nanny (often a young girl) from a poorer family in a nearby rural area.

Thus, a large number of children grow up without the care of their parents. Wisdom of women is not passed on to their children. This leads to fragmented culture and lack of traditions which may have negative consequences on children's self-esteem, sense of coherence, and well-being. Because of fragmentation in household support and care mechanisms, more girls practice sex at earlier ages. Economic hardships force many women and girls into commercial sex work or transactional sex (entering into relationships with older and wealthier men in exchange for money). This increases their risk and vulnerability to HIV/AIDS and other infectious diseases, teenage pregnancies, poverty, and deteriorated maternal and child health (UNICEF 2005). Nearly 60% of HIV-infected individuals in sub-Saharan Africa are women, and the proportion rises to 75% among young people 15–24 years of age in the region. This process continues in a vicious cycle as the breakdown of their families further provides the motivation for family members to emigrate.

Migration of Healthcare Professionals

There is evidence that health workers are emigrating from Africa at an increasing rate to areas like Western Europe, North America, New Zealand, and Australia (Kuehn 2007; Connell et al. 2007; Stilwell et al. 2004). For instance in 2001 Zimbabwe lost about 30% of its newly graduated nurses to the UK and other countries. Within the European Union, marked migration of health workers from eastern and central Europe has been observed. Migration of health professionals has been attributed to low salaries, poor facilities, poor working conditions, and limited career development opportunities. Consequently, health service provision has been adversely affected, especially in remote regions. There is a global phenomenon of shortage of healthcare professionals. In spite of this fact, migrant health workers do not often end up working in healthcare in destination countries. Even those who succeed to do so often take lower-level jobs, such as medical assistants instead of working as physicians. This is an enormous waste of both national economic resources and individual resources that are put into training health professionals.

Policy Responses and Achieving the Millennium Development Goals (MDGs)

A global response to the world's main development challenges and to the calls of civil society, the MDGs promote poverty reduction, education, maternal health, gender equality and aim to combat child mortality, HIV/AIDS, and other diseases. The World Health Organization (WHO) plays an important role in reaching the MDG targets and the global health governance (Bonita et al. 2006). However, other global institutions such as the WTO, the World Bank, and the IMF have the potential to influence global health through economic policies (Fidler 2002). The MDGs have now become the central focus of development policy nationally and internationally and are regarded as a potentially powerful policy tool to further the agenda of improving maternal health and reducing child mortality. Thus, the relationship between globalization and the MDGs, especially goals 4 (reduce child mortality) and 5 (improve maternal health), gives key insight into the relationship between existing and changing economies and MCH.

Goal 4: Reduce Child Mortality

Target: To reduce by two-thirds the mortality rate among children under 5 years between 1990 and 2015.

Indicators:

(i) Under-5 mortality rate
(ii) Infant mortality rate
(iii) Proportion of 1-year-old children immunized against measles

The MDG report (2005) has shown small improvements in child survival. For example, in 1960, more than 1 in 5 children in the developing regions died before age 5. By 1990, the rate was down to 1 in 10 children. Such progress gave hope that child mortality could be cut by a further two-thirds by 2015. But advances slowed in the 1990s. Only Northern Africa, Latin America, the Caribbean, and South-East Asia have maintained a rapid pace toward progress. The progress has been attributed to increased economic growth, better nutrition, and access to healthcare services. However, unequal progress toward the MDGs by country and by region underscores variations in socioeconomic conditions and other local social policies. Africa has been highlighted in the monitoring of MDGs for several reasons. Almost half of all deaths among children under the age of 5 occur in sub-Saharan Africa. This increased mortality has been associated with weak health systems, conflicts, and AIDS. The same region has not benefited from the positive effects of globalization in relation to increased economic growth and decreased poverty. In fact, sub-Saharan Africa is the only region in the world where the number of poor people (living on less than $1 per day) has increased since 1990 (Melanovic 2002).

In Africa and elsewhere, poverty is a substantial determinant of child mortality and survival. There is a close link between a country's Gross Domestic Product (GDP) and child survival. Countries with high GDP have lower child mortality and vice versa. Basic public health services such as safe water, better sanitation, and good nutrition are major determinants. Other determinants such as education for girls and mothers are also of great importance and save children's lives. Having said this, in the light of the globalization era, privatization of basic services such as water and energy may not enhance child health. Children in developing countries suffer and die from a comorbidity of disease and adverse conditions. Just five diseases (pneumonia, diarrhea, malaria, measles, and AIDS) account for half of all deaths in children under the age of 5. In spite of the fact that preventive and treatment measures for these diseases are inexpensive and feasible, there are no committed efforts to combat these diseases. The question is "Why?" Local governments are unwilling or unable to make political commitments to social and public health policies that combat these diseases. On the other hand, globalization and its features leave limited space for national policies and political decisions (Labonte 2003).

In terms of undernutrition and hunger, however, globalization can play either a positive or a negative role. Of the world's 6 billion people, about 800 million do not have enough to eat. Africa has the largest number of chronically hungry people – hunger and undernutrition have worsened, despite improvements in other regions (FAO 2004b). In addition, food security (which is the ability of individuals to consume sufficient quantity and quality of food to meet their daily needs) has deteriorated in many households in Africa, particularly those that are headed by females. Improving nutrition will continue to be a challenge. If the MDG of reducing child mortality is to be achieved, other major determinants, particularly access to basic public health services, should be met. For example, public services should not be included in General Agreement on Trade in Services (GATS) and national governments should be given more space for policy actions.

Goal 5: *Improve Maternal Health*

Target: To reduce the maternal mortality ratio by three-quarters between 1990 and 2015.

Indicators:

(i) Maternal mortality ratio
(ii) Proportion of births attended to by skilled health personnel

The chances of dying during pregnancy or childbirth over a lifetime are as high as 1 in 16 in sub-Saharan Africa, compared with 1 in 3,800 in the developed regions of the world. This lifetime risk could substantially be reduced if women had the family planning services they need. Once a woman is pregnant, it is essential that she has good medical care and access to emergency obstetric care facilities in the case of unexpected complications.

The MDG report 2005 shows that countries with already low levels of maternal mortality have made further progress, but reductions in the worst affected regions require additional resources to ensure that the majority of births are attended to by doctors, nurses, or midwives. These medical personnel might be able to prevent, detect, and/or manage obstetric complications. However, globalization has resulted in migration of health professionals from low- to high-income countries. This means that the majority of women are less likely to be attended to by trained healthcare personnel. The issue of migration of health professionals calls for a global partnership to agree on common actions for policies and guidelines for ethical recruitment of health professionals. Thus, MDG 8 (develop a global partnership for development) provides a good opportunity for such common policies (Lee et al. 2004). In addition, features of globalization can be used to develop immigration policies of developed countries that facilitate movement at the same time as incorporating mechanisms to enhance economic growth in developing countries. For example, this could be done by establishing bilateral agreements and standardizing GATS commitments.

In addition, universal and equitable access to reproductive healthcare is essential for improved maternal health. However, this improvement is hampered by privatization of healthcare services, which limits access as a result of high costs. This limitation occurs particularly among the most vulnerable poor populations, most of which are women and children.

Conclusion

Many features of globalization pose a threat to women's health. For example, economic migration from poor to richer countries enhances women's

earning power, but also exposes them to the threat of exploitation and discrimination (Ehrenreich and Hochschild 2004). While some forms of reproductive technology, such as antenatal ultrasound, have contributed to improved maternal and child health in relation to early detection of illnesses, they are prone to abuse, such as when they are used to assist sex-selective abortion (Kohli 2005). These positive and negative impacts of globalization must be considered within their specific contexts: globalization's benefits and drawbacks are unequally distributed among different regions, countries, and communities (Kawachi and Wamala 2006b). For instance, the declines in extreme poverty in East Asia are offset by large increases in poverty in sub-Saharan Africa, Eastern Europe, and Central Asia, as well as a pattern of stagnation in Latin America and the Caribbean (Kawachi and Wamala 2006a). Women constitute a large proportion (70%) of poor people and there is a large proportion of children living in poverty (Gakidou et al. 2007). It remains to be seen whether the MDGs, including the global commitment and partnership, will contribute to improved maternal and child health in the era of globalization.

Key Terms

Agriculture	Foreign direct investment (FDI)	International Monetary Fund (IMF)
Bill of rights	Gender	International trade
Citizens of the world	Gender inequality	Internet
Contextual determinants of health	Gender-based violence	Marrakech Agreements
Copyrights	General Agreement on Trade in Services (GATS)	Migrants
Cross border acquisition		Migration
Deregulation	General Agreements on Tariffs and Trade (GATT)	Millennium Development Goals
Distal determinants of health	Globalization	Multinational firms
Economic growth rate	Gross Domestic Product (GDP)	North Atlantic Trade Agreement (NAFTA)
Economic integration		
Economic transition	Hunger	Patent
Employment	Import	Patents
Export	Indebted poor countries	Pharmaceuticals
Export processing zones (EPZs)	Intellectual property rights	Privatization
Feminization		Pro-growth policies

Proximal determinants of health	Trade liberalization	United Nations Conference on Trade and Development (UNCTAD)
Small-scale farmers	Trademarks	
Social fragmentation	Trade-Related Aspects of Intellectual Property Rights (TRIPS)	Uruguay Round of Multilateral Trade Negotiations
Street foods		
Structural Adjustment Policy (SAP)	Transnational corporation (TNCs)	World Bank
Telecommunications	Undernutrition	World Trade Organization

Questions for Discussion

1. What is globalization? List six features of globalization and their characteristics.
2. Using the framework proposed by Huynen et al. (2005), discuss the determinants of population health at the contextual, distal, and primal levels.
3. List any two global macroeconomic policies associated with globalization and discuss how their implementation indirectly impacts on maternal and child health.
4. Discuss any three pathways by which globalization directly effects maternal and child health.
5. In what ways can the Millennium Development Goal targets serve as a tool for monitoring and addressing the impact of globalization on maternal and child health?

References

Afshar H, Barrientos S (1998) Women, Globalization and Fragmentation in the Developing World. Palgrave

American Friends Service Committee (2006) World Trade Organization (WTO) http://www.afsc.org/trade-matters/trade-agreements/WTO.htm, cited 20 March 2008

Bonita R, Irwin A, Beaglehole R (2006) Promoting public health in the twenty-first century: the role of the World Health Organisation. In: Kawachi I, Wamala S (Eds.) Globalization and Health. Oxford University Press

Cagatay N, Ozler S (1995) Feminization of the labor force: the effects of long-term development and structural adjustment. World Development 23(11), 1883–1894

Chopra M (2004) Food security, rural development and health equity in Southern Africa, EQUINET Discussion Paper 22.South Africa: Ideas Studio

Connell J, Zurn P, Stilwell B et al. (2007) Sub-Saharan Africa: beyond the health worker migration crisis? Social Science and Medicine 64(9), 1876–1891

Cornia GA (2001) Globalization and health: results and options. Bulletin of the World Health Organization 79(9), 834–841

Correa CM (2001) Health and intellectual property rights. Bulletin of the World Health Organization 79(5), 381

De Vogli R, Birbeck GL (2005) Potential impact of adjustment policies on vulnerability of women and children to HIV/AIDS in Sub-Saharan Africa. Journal of Health Population Nutrition 23(2), 105–120

Dollar D (2001) Is globalization good for your health? Bulletin of the World Health Organization 79(9), 827–833

Dollar D (2004) Globalization, Poverty, and Inequality Since 1980. Washington DC: World Bank Policy Research Working Paper 3333 (June 2004)

Dollar D, Kraay A (2001) Trade, Growth and Poverty. Finance and Development. 8:3. http://www.imf.org/external/pubs/ft/fandd/2001/09/dollar.htm Washington, DC: International Monetary Fund (IMF), cited 14 April 2008

Ehiri JE, Anyanwu E (2004) The role of international agencies in health policy and practice in less developed countries. In: Kamel R, Lumley J (Eds.) Textbook of Tropical Surgery, pp. 85–88. London: Westminster Publishing Ltd.

Ehrenreich B, Hochschild A (Eds.) (2004) Global Woman: Nannies, Maids, and Sex Workers in the New Economy. New York: Metropolitan Books

Fidler D (2002) Global Health Governance: Overview of the Role of International Law in Protecting and Promoting Global Public Health. London: Centre on Global Change and Health, London School of Hygiene and Tropical Medicine

Filmer D, Pritchett L (1999) The impact of public spending on health: does money matter? Social Science and Medicine 49, 1309–1323

Food and Agricultural Organization (FAO) (2004a) The state of food insecurity in the world. Rome: Food and Agricultural Organization. http://www.fao.org/docrep/008/a0200e/a0200e00.htm, cited 17 March 2008

Food and Agricultural Organization (2004b) Globalization of Food Systems in Developing Countries: Impact on Food Security and Nutrition. Rome: Food and Agricultural Organization. http://www.fao.org/docrep/007/y5736e/y5736e00.htm, cited 17 March 2008

Frenk J, Gómez-Dantés O (2002) Globalization and the challenges to health systems. BMJ 325(7355), 95–97

Gakidou E, Oza S, Vidal Fuertes C et al. (2007) Improving child survival through environmental and nutritional interventions: the importance of targeting interventions toward the poor. JAMA 298(16), 1876–1887

Ghosh J (2003) Exporting Jobs or watching them disappear? Relocation, employment and accumulation in the world economy. In: Chandrasekhar CP, Ghosh J (Eds.) Work and Well-Being in the Age of Finance. Muttukadu Papers 1. New Dehli: Tulika Books

Gleick PH (2000) The World's Water 2000–2001: The Biennial Report on Freshwater Resources. Washington, DC: Island Press

Hawkes C (2005) The role of foreign direct investment in the nutrition transition. Public Health Nutrition 8, 357–365

Huynen MMTE, Martens P, Hilderink HBM (2005) The health impacts of globalization: a conceptual framework. Globalization and Health 1:14. http://www.globalizationandhealth.com/content/1/1/14, cited 21 July 2008

Jenkins R (2004) Globalization, production, employment and poverty: debates and evidence. Journal of International Development 16(1–12)

Kawachi I, Wamala S (Eds.) (2006a) Globalization and Health. Oxford University Press

Kawachi I, Wamala S (2006b) Poverty and inequality in a globalizing world. In: Kawachi I, Wamala S (Eds.) Globalization and Health. Oxford University Press

Kohli HS (2005) Ultrasound scanning in pregnancy: the hope and the shame. National Medical Journal of India 16(6), 332–333

Kuehn BM (2007) Global shortage of health workers, brain drain stress developing countries. JAMA 298(16), 1853–1855

Labonte R (2003) Dying for Trade: Why Globalization can be Bad for our Health. Ontario, Canada: The CSJ Foundation for Research and Education. http://www.social-justice.org, cited 21 July 2008

Labonte R, Torgerson R (2002) Frameworks for analyzing the links between globalization and health. Draft report to the World Health Organization. Saskatoon: SPHERU, University of Saskatchewan

Lee K (2004) Globalization: what is it and how does it affect health? Medical Journal of Australia 180(4), 156–158

Lee K, Walt G Haines A (2004) The challenge to improve global health: financing the Millennium Development Goals. Lancet 291, 636–638

Loewenson R (1999) Women's occupational health in globalization and development. American Journal of Industrial Medicine 36, 34–42

Magnussen L, Ehiri J, Jolly P (2004) Comprehensive versus selective primary healthcare: lessons for global health policy. Health Affairs (Millwood) 23(3), 167–176

Melanovic B (2002) True world income distribution, 1988 and 1993: first calculation based on household surveys alone. Economic Journal 112(1), 51–92

McMichael P (2005) Global development and the corporate food regime. In: Buttel FH, McMichael P (Eds.) New Directions in the Sociology of Global Development, pp. 265–300. Amsterdam: Elsevier/JAI

Mkandawire T (2005) Targeting and universalism in poverty reduction. Social Policy and Development. Programme Paper No. 23. United Nations Research Institute for Social Development, Geneva. http://www.un.org/docs/ecosoc/meetings/2005/docs/Mkandawire.pdf, cited 21 July 2008

Olivera O, Lewis T (2004) Cochabamba! Water war in Bolivia. Cambridge: South End Press,

Pompey F (1999) AIDS-Cote de Ivoire: Ivoirians derive little benefit from low-cost AIDS programme. Agence France-Presse. http://ww2.aegis.com/news/afp/1999/AF990929.html, cited 16 March 2008

Rabbani F, Shaikh B, Wamala S (2006) Living with globalisation: a menace or a chance? Journal of Pakistan Medication Association 56(4), 195–196

Stilwell B, Diallo K, Zurn P et al. (2004) Migration of healthcare workers from developing countries: strategic approaches to its management. Bulletin of the World Health Organization 82(8), 559–636

Supakankunti S, Janjaroen WS, Tangphao O et al. (2001) Impact of the World Trade Organization TRIPS agreement on the pharmaceutical industry in Thailand. Bulletin of the World Health Organization 79(5), 461–470

United Nations (2005a) The Millennium Development Goals Report. New York: UN. http://unstats.un.org/unsd/mdg/Resources/Static/Products/Progress2006/MDGReport2006.pdf, cited 19 March 2008

United Nations (2005b) What part do women play in world economic activity? Their contribution still not fully captured by official statistics. In: The World's Women 2005: Progress in Statistics. New York: United Nations

United Nations Conference on Trade and Development (UNCTAD) (1993) Export processing zones: selected country experiences: study by the UNCTAD Secretariat. Geneva: United Nations

United Nations Conference on Trade and Development (UNCTAD) (2007) World Investment Report 2007. www.unctad.org/fdistatistics, cited 20 March 2008

United Nations Children's Fund (UNICEF) (2005) The State of the World's Children 2005. New York: United Nation's Children's Fund

Woodward D, Drager N, Beaglehole R et al. (2001) Globalization and health: a framework for analysis and action. Bulletin of the World Health Organization 79(9), 875–881

World Trade Organization (2008) Understanding the WTO: Basics – what is the World Trade Organization? Geneva: World Trade Organization

Chapter 9
Gender Equity: Perspectives on Maternal and Child Health

Rachel Tolhurst, Joanna Raven, and Sally Theobald

Learning Objectives After reading this chapter and answering the discussion questions that follow, you should be able to

- Explain terminologies commonly used in the gender and health literature, including sex, gender, gender roles and relations, women's health gender analysis, gender equity, gender mainstreaming, gender divisions of labor, gender norms, gender identity, and bargaining positions.
- Use specific examples to illustrate how gender influences maternal, infant, and child health status and access to health care.
- Analyze the importance of mainstreaming gender into global health at the policy, health provider, and community levels.
- Identify current gaps in knowledge and priorities for future research and practice.

Introduction

This chapter introduces the concepts of gender equity and gender power relations. It begins with definitions of such key concepts as sex, gender, gender roles and relations, women's health and gender analysis, gender equity, gender mainstreaming, gender divisions of labor, gender norms and identities, bargaining positions, as well as access to and control over resources. It then illustrates how these concepts interact to influence and shape maternal,

infant, and child health status and access to health care. The chapter presents an exposition on the importance of understanding and mainstreaming gender into global health policies and programs, using cross-cutting approaches that consider the role of socioeconomic determinants, effectiveness, sustainability, participation, accountability, and multisectoral approaches. The importance of gender mainstreaming at the policy, health provider, and community levels is discussed. The chapter concludes with an examination of current gaps in knowledge and priorities for future research and practice.

A number of key concepts are integral to the concept of gender inequities in maternal and child health (MCH) (Box 9.1), and these must be understood in the context of place and time. Though they may appear to be "natural," gender roles are socially constructed rather than biologically determined. Because societies are different, and because every society develops and changes its practices and norms over time, gender roles and relations are neither fixed nor universal. In general, however, the social, economic, and cultural ramifications of gender roles and relations have significant impacts on the health status of women, infants, and children as well as on their access to care. While gender roles and responsibilities vary across societies, they are rarely equally balanced. Women and men generally do not have equal access to money, information, power, and influence. In almost all societies, what is perceived to be masculine is more highly valued than what is perceived to be feminine, and families and communities treat women, men, girls, and boys differently. Gender roles and relations therefore involve the exercise of power.

R. Tolhurst (✉)
International Health Research Group, Liverpool School of Tropical Medicine, Pembroke Place, Liverpool, L3 5QA, England, UK

J.E. Ehiri (ed.), *Maternal and Child Health*, DOI 10.1007/b106524_9,
© Springer Science+Business Media, LLC 2009

Box 9.1 Key Concepts and Definitions in Gender and Maternal and Child Health

Sex: Biological differences between women and men.

Gender: Characteristics of women and men that are socially and culturally determined.

Gender roles: Activities and responsibilities assigned to women and men.

Gender relations: Interactions between women and men and their underlying structural and institutional influences.

Women's health: Historically, a discipline that focused on biomedically defined health needs, specific to women's biological or sexual makeup.

Gender analysis: Contemporary approach to studying gender that looks at all health issues in order to understand the ways in which gender roles and relations impact every aspect of women's and men's, girls' and boys' health, and to promote gender equity.

Gender equity: Allocation of fair shares between the genders, rather than "equality" which implies allocation of equal shares.

Gender mainstreaming: Policy response to gender inequities that integrates a consideration of gender at every stage of health-care planning and provision.

Gender-sensitive policies: Policies that consider and meet the priorities and needs of different groups of women and men.

Gender division of labor: Different activities assigned by society to women and men at home and at work.

Productive roles: Paid work or the production of goods for subsistence or sale.

Reproductive roles: Domestic tasks including cooking, cleaning, and caring for children and sick people.

Community management roles: Participation in various tasks associated with managing community organizations or maintaining community services.

Gender norms: Implicit guidelines for the capacities, characteristics, roles, and social behavior for men and women, including their expected social and spatial mobility, their sexual behavior and openness about sexuality, their parental roles, and the acceptability of violent behavior.

Bargaining Power: The extent to which women and men can act in order to protect their own and their children's best interests in the case of a conflict with another's interests.

Access to and control over resources: Women's and men's ability to use and control resources such as money, transport, time, information, political power, and influence.

Sexual and reproductive health rights: Women's rights to control their fertility and sexual interactions, rights to safe abortion services, and freedom from sexual coercion and violence for women, men, girls, and boys.

Triple burden: Term used when women bear the responsibility of productive, reproductive, and community management roles.

Unequal gender roles and relations influence many aspects of women's and men's health, including relative health status, vulnerability to illness, access to preventative and curative measures, quality of services received, and burden of ill-health on family members. It is important to note that gender inequalities work mostly to the disadvantage of women, but also sometimes to the disadvantage of men. Because of the interaction between gender inequity and such other forms of social disadvantage as class, race and ethnicity, not all women or men experience gender-related health inequity in the same way. Consequently, the impact of gender roles and relations on individuals' health status and health-care access varies.

Historically, the discipline of women's health focused on biomedically defined health needs, such as those related to pregnancy. In contrast, the contemporary "gender analysis" approach seeks to understand the ways in which gender roles and relations impact on every aspect of health, in order to address related inequities and promote gender equity. In a health context, equity is concerned with achieving a system that gives everyone a fair and equal opportunity to attain their fullest health potential. The goal of health equity is to raise the health status of the population as a whole and minimize differentials in health status throughout the population. This requires actively recognizing and addressing the structures and processes that give rise to health differentials and gender inequities. Gender mainstreaming is the main policy response to gender inequities agreed to in global health. It is a commitment toward ensuring gender sensitivity in health systems, by integrating a consideration of gender at every stage of health-care planning and provision.

Gender analysis considers aspects of gender roles and relations in any given context. A key aspect of gender roles is "gender division of labor," or the work roles that societies assign to women and men. These include "productive," "reproductive," and "community management" roles (Gender and Health Group LSTM 1999). Generally, productive work is done by both women and men, but it is seen as men's work. Though women produce goods and services and often earn money, men usually have preferential access to such productive resources as land, tools, capital, and jobs and can earn higher wages. On the other hand, reproductive work is mainly done by women. Women may work less hours in "productive work" due to their "reproductive" work. "Community management" roles are often sex segregated. Men may be more involved in decision making about the use of community resources, while women are more likely to be involved in the day-to-day management of the resources. In many societies, women fill parts of all three roles, while men are involved in one or two. This tendency has led to the concept of the "triple burden" borne by women.

Women often have less "bargaining power" than men to act to protect their own interests or those of their children in the case of a conflict, including the ability to make decisions, command resources and, at times, influence the behavior of others. This is partly because of gender norms that recognize men as decision makers, but also because women are often in a poorer negotiating position because of their greater social and economic vulnerability if their relationships break down. Education, control over resources, and other socioeconomic factors can increase women's bargaining power. Women's agency or enhanced bargaining power is positively correlated with many aspects of women's and children's health (Lule et al. 2005).

Gender Perspectives on Maternal and Child Health

Social norms and behaviors based on gender affect maternal and child health throughout the life cycle, from preconception through old age. Figure 9.1 illustrates some of the negative health impacts of gender inequities in the specific context of South Asia.

Inequity in nutrition: Much of the inequity at the various levels shown in Fig. 9.1 can be attributed to the low value placed on girls' and women's well-being. This low value may have several dimensions, including the perceived burden of girls to their parents and traditional beliefs that differentiate between the needs of boys and girls. The undervaluing of girls often leads to lower access to key resources such as food and health care. In some contexts, girls may receive less food or even less nutritious food than boys and boys may also be given better treatment for illnesses. Malnutrition during childhood can have severe consequences in later life. Maternal undernutrition is prevalent in many regions. For example, in south-central Asia, more than 10% of women aged between 15 and 49 years are of short stature (shorter than 145 cm); and in most countries of sub-Saharan Africa, south-central and south-eastern Asia, more than 20% of women have very low body mass index (Black et al. 2008).

In adolescence, increased biological need may interact with low nutritional status to produce particular risks for anemia and malnutrition. Girls' nutritional needs increase in early adolescence because of the growth spurt associated with puberty and the onset of menstruation. The status of girls within the family and community may also be at its lowest during adolescence. Inadequate diet during

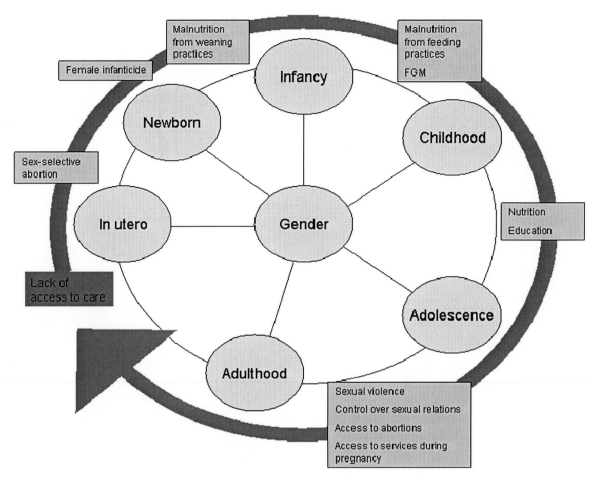

Fig. 9.1 Gender influences on women's health across the life cycle. Source: Fikree et al. (2004)

this period can jeopardize girls' health and physical development, with lifelong consequences. For example, skeletal growth is delayed by malnutrition, and since a smaller pelvis can prolong labor and obstruct deliver, this can pose serious risks during childbirth. Adolescence sets the stage for health and nutritional status in the later years. Once pregnant, women are particularly vulnerable to anemia. This may result both from a lack of access to resources, and the unequal allocation of resources between genders, or cultural practices specific to one gender. In some contexts, there are taboos against pregnant women eating certain foods, such as animal protein, that could reduce the risk of anemia. Maternal short stature and iron deficiency anemia increase the risk of death of the mother at delivery and account for at least 20% of maternal mortality (Black et al. 2008).

Marriage, Pregnancy, and Sexuality in Adolescence

Pregnancy in adolescence is common in many contexts. Because of its significant health considerations, a chapter (21) has been dedicated to it in this book. Here, we will discuss those dimensions of gender relations that contribute to high instance of pregnancy in adolescence. In some societies, the low value accorded to daughters and the perception that they are a financial burden to parents supports the gender norm of early marriage and pregnancy. The equation of female status with marriage and motherhood puts pressure on adolescent girls to prove their fertility as early as possible in some contexts. Girls' education is often not seen as a priority because of the perception that a role as a wife and mother does not require education, or that a daughter will marry into another family so that her family of birth will not gain from the investment. In addition, girls are often withdrawn from school to care for sick family members.

The lower educational status of girls lowers opportunities for independence, leaving girls to look for economic and social support from men. Girls who become pregnant while in school often lose the opportunity to continue their education. Girls may seek abortions from informal providers in order to avoid expulsion. Adolescent girls are also vulnerable to coerced sex, rape, and abuse, often lacking the power and confidence to refuse or resist unwanted advances. A study in Central African Republic found that 22% of women reported that their first sexual experience was rape (Chapko et al. 1999). Early marriage may also be seen as a practice that helps maintain the gender norm of male control over female sexuality. The gender norm that unmarried women, and particularly adolescents, should not be sexually active, limits girls' access to information and services that would help them protect their reproductive health.

Gender and Sexual Relations in Adulthood

Gender identities, norms, roles, and relations at household, community, national, and international levels all influence women's ability to protect their own sexual and reproductive health. Many women lack the bargaining power necessary to negotiate safe sex because they rely on sexual relationships for social and economic security or survival. This reduces their ability to choose whether, when, and how they have sex or use contraceptives, posing the risks of unwanted pregnancy, sexually transmitted infections, and vulnerability to sexual violence. Gender norms for men often emphasize risk taking, placing pressure on men to seek multiple partnerships, and reducing their interest in safe sex. These gender-based norms around sex are also key factors in family planning decisions and the use of contraceptives, particularly of male-controlled methods. Religious and cultural prescriptions around fertility control can also reduce women's rights to decide whether and

when they have children. In many societies, there is strong pressure on women to bear children, as motherhood secures social and economic status. Women are often vulnerable to divorce, abandonment, or are forced to put up with a polygamous marriage if they are perceived as infertile. In addition, women may not be the decision makers in having children. However, high fertility is associated with high levels of maternal mortality, both because more pregnancies mean more chance of pregnancy-related death and because pregnancy-related risks increase after the third child (Aliyu et al. 2005). Women who cannot choose whether to have children are denied a level of control over their own health.

Lack of power over sexual interactions and fertility can lead to unwanted pregnancy, and a proportion of women will seek abortions. For an in-depth discussion of abortion, refer to Chapter 11 of this book. Gender norms that deny rights to safe abortion services are a contributor to maternal mortality. Even when pregnancy termination is permitted, services are often not available to the full extent permitted by the law or are not accessible to certain women, such as young, unmarried women. Under such circumstances, women may resort to unsafe abortions. Each year, there are an estimated 19 million unsafe abortions worldwide, most in low-income countries. As a result, around 68,000 women die each year, making unsafe abortion a significant cause of maternal mortality (Singh et al. 2007). The consequences of unsafe abortion are greater in Africa, with nearly half of all deaths due to unsafe abortion.

Gender, Health Promotion, and Health-Seeking Behavior in Pregnancy

Gender norms and identities, divisions of labor and control over resources all influence women's willingness and ability to protect their own health and seek preventive and curative health care in pregnancy. In many countries, women continue with their full heavy workload right up until labor and resume work shortly after giving birth. Women's low control over work burdens prevents them from taking sufficient rest pre- and post-labor. This often leads to delays in seeking health care for themselves and their children (Azubuike and Ehiri 1998). Women's low control over household resources often translates into low decision-making power to seek health care. Where resources for care seeking are controlled by men, women may need to convince others of the seriousness of their illness to seek care. In some settings, men have little understanding of the risks associated with pregnancy and delivery but have decision-making power over the use of household resources for health services. In addition, women are often socialized to regard their own discomfort as unworthy of complaint, so may not seek care for danger signs in pregnancy.

Social restrictions on women's movement may also reduce their autonomy to seek care. For example, in Northern Nigeria, the *purdah* system may mean that a husband has to accompany his wife to use services and she may not be able to access services in his absence (Oxaal and Baden 1996). Gendered attitudes toward maternity-related problems in some communities may also limit access to care. For example, in some African societies, prolonged labor may be ascribed to marital infidelity and assistance may be withheld until the woman confesses to this (Oxaal and Baden 1996). If women do seek health care, they must give up time that they would normally spend on household chores such as caring for children, collecting water and fuel, cooking, doing agricultural work, and engaging in other employment. A study in Zaire showed that 13 out of 20 maternal deaths occurred during the first 5 months of planting and harvest, when women were reluctant to go to the hospital because of the need for them to work in the fields (Oxaal and Baden 1996).

Gender-Based Violence

Widespread physical violence and abuse against women results from a range of aspects of gender inequality, including women's limited bargaining positions in the family and broader community, men's perceived right to dominate women and gender norms that define masculinity as physically tough (Oxaal and Baden 1996). Available evidence shows that at least one in five women has been physically or sexually abused by a man at some stage in her life (DFID 1999). Present throughout the life cycle, from sex-selective abortion of female fetuses and female infanticide due to son preference, through child marriage and coerced sexual initiation, gender-based violence persists in adulthood through rape and physical and psychological abuse (DFID 1999). The abuse of women has an impact on many aspects of their lives, including their psychological well-being, bodily integrity, public participation, autonomy, sexual pleasure, and the well-being of their children (DFID 1999). Rape, the threat of violence, and sexual coercion can lead to unwanted pregnancies and unsafe abortions, and sexually transmitted diseases, including HIV infection, with consequent effects on maternal and child health (DFID 1999).

Gender-based violence is a significant and overlooked cause of maternal death (Heise 1993). A study in the United States found that one in six pregnant women experienced violence (Oxaal and Baden 1996). Women beaten during pregnancy are four times more likely to have a low birth-weight baby and twice as likely to miscarry. Fatal injuries may also be inflicted on the mother (DFID 1999). Young unmarried mothers may be particularly vulnerable to violence and even murder in some societies. One abiding problem related to gender-based violence is the practice of female genital mutilation (FGM) (see Chapter 10). Often referred to as "female circumcision," FGM comprises all procedures involving partial or total removal of the external female genitalia or other injury to the female genital organs whether for cultural, religious, or other nontherapeutic reasons (Jones et al. 2004). This practice affects an estimated 80 million women worldwide. It doubles the maternal death rate and increases the risk of stillbirth several times. FGM can cause obstructed labor and intense distress during labor (Jones et al. 2004).

Impact of Gender on Maternal Health Care

Gender affects maternal health care from the community level or "demand side" and from the health services or "supply side". At the community level, several factors already mentioned limit women's access to health care. Gender divisions of labor, gender norms and identities, access to and control over resources, and limited autonomy and bargaining positions within the family and community limit poor women's ability to use health-care services including during pregnancy or delivery (Afsana et al. 2007). The amount of time, money, information, and authority for decision making that women have determines their opportunities to use preventive and curative services during pregnancy, delivery, and the postnatal period. Women often do not have access to adequate transportation to health facilities or the cash to pay for it. They have to negotiate for transportation with men, other family members, or elders in the community. Lack of transportation can cause delays in emergency situations (see Margaret's story in Chapter 5). Absolute and relative poverty can pose a serious barrier to women's demand for and access to health care.

On the health system services, or "supply side," obstetric, abortion, and family planning services often do not respond to client's needs and rights (Kim and Motshei 2002). Patterns of social and gender discrimination that shape society as a whole influence the rights of women and men in the health system and shape the maltreatment of patients and their families (Freedman 2003). Gender norms in national and international policies may exacerbate the effect of gender norms within the household. Politically, at international and national levels, women's rights to control their bodies remain a battleground between religious conservative alliances and the radical vision of social change laid out at the landmark conferences on population policy in Cairo (1994) and women in Beijing (1995).

The goal of access to reproductive health services for all individuals of appropriate ages was removed in development of the Millennium Development Goals (MDGs), due to pressure from a US-led alliance of social conservatives. In some countries, legal or regulatory restrictions prevent groups of women, such as adolescents and unmarried women from using family planning services (Oxaal and Baden 1996). In Northern Nigeria, policy requires men's consent for women to obtain contraceptives, and in Lesotho, women's husbands and families have a "legal and cultural right" to deny them family

planning services (Oxaal and Baden 1996). Conversely, the gender norm that family planning is a woman's responsibility means that family planning services in many countries are focused on female-targeted methods such as intrauterine devices, injectables, contraceptive pills, and female sterilization. Services rarely target male decision makers or support women to negotiate the use of these methods.

Some providers may show judgmental and negative attitudes toward women, and especially toward poorer, more vulnerable groups of service users (Kim and Motshei 2002). A study of health-seeking behavior by pregnant women in southern Malawi found that the attitudes and behavior of providers were barriers to many women using services due to the real risk they posed to women's lives (Tolhurst et al. 2008). Acute human resource shortages and poor conditions of service for health workers are contributory factors toward ill-treatment of clients by health providers. The availability of female health professionals may have a strong influence over whether women use services in some contexts. In some cultures, the custom that women should not be seen by males except for close relatives after puberty translates into unwillingness to see a male doctor. In Northern Nigeria, for example, both women and men were opposed to female patients being treated by male physicians (Prevention of Maternal Mortality Network 1992). In contrast, in Ghana, there is a perception that older male physicians were more competent than younger or female doctors (Prevention of Maternal Mortality Network 1992).

Often, services that could address poor women's gendered needs are not provided, such as confidential and quality counseling and testing services, provision of antiretroviral therapy, STI screening and treatment, abortion and postabortion services (Mayhew 1996). Health systems seldom include women in making decisions about health service provision, and there are limited opportunities for women (especially poor women and their families) to influence the way that health services are provided. In addition, women's demand for health care is likely to be affected more than men's by rising costs, including user fees and under the table payments. In Nigeria, user-fee introduction reduced use of maternity care, with hospital deliveries falling by

46% over 5 years and maternal mortality increasing by 56% (Tinker and Koblinsky 1993).

Impact of Gender on Child Health Status and Health-Care Access

Gender roles and relations impact directly on children's health and indirectly through the position and power of their mothers and fathers. Even before birth, the availability of new technology for determining the sex of fetuses may lead to sex-selective abortion and risk for female fetuses due to strong gender norms that value sons. In many countries in Asia, the male to female birth ratio has increased, with far-reaching social implications. Maternal mortality can be affected by health system responses to sex selection. To respond to the practice of sex-selective abortion, a hospital in Gujarat, India, stopped providing abortion services. Some women sought abortions from traditional birth attendants. Consequently, maternal deaths due to complications increased (Oxaal and Baden 1996).

Women are the principal providers of care and nourishment during the most crucial periods of childhood development. However, low resources are allocated to childcare in most societies because it is associated with women's work. Health services perpetuate this association by targeting women as caregivers of children. Health promotion campaigns are directed toward women, ignoring other potential caregivers in the household such as fathers. The gender division of labor and the resulting labor burdens for women also potentially decrease the efficacy of interventions for child survival. Women may not have the time to utilize life-saving technologies and child-care approaches (Leslie 1989). Difficulty in taking time off work was one of the main reasons given by women for not attending a vaccination clinic in Nigeria (Azubuike and Ehiri 1998).

Women's relatively low ability to control resources reduces their opportunity to prevent and treat illness for their children. Women tend to allot a larger proportion of their income than men to the basic needs of the family but they may not have access to resources to provide sufficient nutrition,

buy appropriate medicines, or seek formal health care. In addition, studies have noted that fathers have more decision-making power than mothers about where and when their children should be treated. However, such dynamics vary subtly in the degrees and types of decision-making power available to women and cannot be seen as universal. Other factors such as women's educational status and position within the household structure may interact to influence their decision-making power.

Interaction Between Gender Equity and Other Socioeconomic Determinants

As discussed in the introduction, gender differences and inequalities interact with other forms of social disadvantage or socioeconomic determinants such as age, class, ethnicity, and education status to affect health experiences and health outcomes.

Ethnicity

Ethnicity and caste affect women's maternal health in both resource-poor and resource-rich contexts. For example, a study in the United States found that from 1940 to 1990 maternal mortality was consistently higher for black women than for white women (Oxaal and Baden 1996). Black women were three times more likely than their white counterparts to die from maternal causes. Possible explanations for this difference include unequal access to and use of health-care services and disparities in the content and quality of care. Studies indicate that black and white pregnant women may be given different advice and differential access to technology. In Nepal, the utilization of emergency obstetric care varies by caste. One study found that in mountainous areas, high-caste men were unwilling to transport *Dalit* (lowest caste) women to hospital (Neupane 2004). A study in Ghana showed that women preferred to travel further, and face higher opportunity costs, to see providers who were the same ethnic group as them (Prevention of Maternal Mortality Network 1992). This preference was related to the concept of "social distance" between providers and clients which in West Africa consists of differences in language, behavior, and expectations. Hence a provider from the same ethnic group was perceived as having a smaller "social distance" and worth traveling the extra distance for.

Geographic/Regional Variations

The extent of discrimination against girls may vary significantly within one country or region. For example, in some parts of India, there is evidence of greater malnutrition among girls whereas this is not observed in other regions. Cultural and religious practices and levels of poverty influence discrimination. Gender, poverty, and geography also intersect to affect women's birth experiences with direct implications for maternal and child morbidity and mortality. In Malawi, poorer, less educated and rural women are more likely to die in childbirth because of lack of access to services and a skilled attendant (Mann et al. 2006). The poorest 10% of women are nearly twice as likely as the richest 10% to deliver at home or be assisted by a TBA; rural women with no school education are nearly four times as likely to be assisted in delivery by a TBA (Mann et al. 2006).

Factors that cause poorer and rural women to have less access to skilled attendant at delivery can be categorized as follows (Thaddeus and Maine 1994):

- Delays in the decision to seek care;
- Delays in arrival at point of care;
- Delays in provision of adequate care.

In each type of delay, gender roles and relations intersect with poverty to affect access to resources and bargaining power. In rural areas, large distances that women must travel to seek care and the relative lack of skilled staff in rural health centers make delay in arrival at point of care and delay in provision of adequate care particularly problematic.

Disability

Disadvantage and discrimination due to disability interact with gender relations to produce particular vulnerabilities for women and children living with disabilities worldwide (see Chapter 18 for discussion on disabilities and MCH populations). Women with disabilities comprise 10% of all women worldwide, and yet, their reproductive health and rights are all too often neglected (Center for Reproductive Rights 2002). The sexuality and reproductive rights of women with disabilities and the basic rights of children with disability are rarely recognized by society or health policy (Smith et al. 2004). A generalized assumption that women with disabilities will not be sexually active, and not require reproductive health services, leads to increased vulnerability to sexually transmitted infection including HIV (Smith et al. 2004). Health professionals are often ill-trained to counsel women with disabilities regarding contraception or pregnancy (WHO 2001). Women with disabilities are also likely to encounter various financial, logistical, and physical barriers to accessing safe motherhood and reproductive health services, including the lack of assistive devices and suitable and affordable transportation (Smith et al. 2004). Women with disability are more likely to be concentrated in the poorer sections of society due to a lack of socioeconomic opportunities, and are therefore, likely to have low financial access to care.

Advocacy for Gendered Approaches

Much of the literature on gender and maternal and child health comes from a gender equity or rights-based perspective. The central argument is that gender and power shape vulnerability to disease and access to health care, and that women, regardless of economic position, age, residence, religion, etc., have a right to good maternal health services. However, advocacy efforts must also link these rights-based arguments to practical concepts used in policy, such as effectiveness and sustainability. For example, it could be argued that if gender roles and relations at community and health service levels are ignored, maternal health services will remain inaccessible to poor rural women, undermining both the effectiveness and sustainability of service provision. Likewise, both the effectiveness and sustainability of maternal health services are brought into question if service provision does not reflect the needs of different groups of women.

Advocacy efforts also benefit from linking arguments for better service provision for women to key frameworks or goals at international and national levels. For instance, *Poverty Reduction Strategy Papers* frame debates in many resource-poor contexts and often highlight the need for better maternal and child health. It can be argued that ignoring gender inequities and power differentials leads to ineffective health policies and programs and reduces the likelihood of achieving MCH-related MDGs. For example, it is widely recognized that improvements in maternal education and women's control over income will be important in efforts to reach MDG Goal number 4, which aims to reduce, by two-thirds, between 1990 and 2015, the under-five mortality rate (World Bank 2003).

Multisectoral Approaches

Gender impacts on maternal and child health are problems to be addressed both within and beyond the health sector. A more holistic approach to women's general and reproductive health-care needs may be necessary to create the kind of quality of care in health services necessary to increase women's access (Oxaal and Baden 1996). For example, there is a need to strengthen partnerships with the transport sector to address maternal health. Multisectoral action, including public–private partnerships and NGO involvement to alleviate transportation barriers to maternal and child health care, has the potential to raise the status of maternal, infant, and child health in resource-limited settings. Recognition of this challenge is the impetus behind the work of "Riders for Health" a nongovernmental organization (NGOs) whose mission is to ensure that health workers in Africa have access to reliable transportation so they can reach the most isolated people with regular and predictable health care (http://www.riders.org/about.aspx)

Working with education and employment sectors is also important. Low access to education for girls is a pathway to low maternal status and poor health. Employment that provides status and fulfillment is a factor encouraging the limitation of family size. Low paid, informal, and insecure work does not demonstrate the same effect (Oxaal and Baden 1996). Thus, gender norms and divisions of labor that limit

women's opportunities to carry out satisfying productive work also reduce the chances of improved maternal health. Partnerships with the Ministry of Education and other stakeholders should strengthen a focus on sexual, reproductive, and maternal health in educational curricula and offer increased training and employment opportunities for women.

Gender Mainstreaming in Policy and Practice

From the above analysis, we conclude that many different but interrelated dimensions of gender roles and relations impact on maternal and child health, including gender divisions of labor, gender norms and identities, women's bargaining positions, and access to and control over resources. These dimensions impact women's health status over their life cycle as well as the quality of health care they are able to access for themselves and for their children. Ignoring these issues in the design and delivery of maternal and child health services is a problematic and dangerous oversight. Gender mainstreaming is the agreed approach to addressing gender issues in policy and practice. The following sections explore the main components of a gender mainstreaming approach in maternal and child health policy and practice within and beyond the health sector, at policy, health service, and community levels.

Gender mainstreaming is the strategic policy approach to promoting gender equity agreed upon in the Platform for Action published by the Beijing Conference on Women in 1995. The Beijing Platform for Action states that "Governments and other actors should promote an active and visible policy of mainstreaming a gender perspective in all policies and programs so that, before decisions are taken, an analysis is made of the effects on women and men, respectively" (Beijing Platform for Action 1995). As the policy of gender mainstreaming is interpreted in practice, implementation strategies have been varied. However, there are some commonly identifiable elements. First, the approach should focus on gender equity as a goal and include a range of complementary initiatives. A focus on gender generally implies working with men as well as women as beneficiaries of change and as catalysts for change. Secondly, gender mainstreaming generally focuses on organizations as well as their work, including attention to gender equality within the structure, culture, and staffing of organizations. Women as well as men should participate in decision making at all levels, so that the interests of women as well as men can be integrated into mainstream priorities, policies, and programs. Finally, "mainstreaming" implies emphasizing the responsibility of all staff in organizations such as the health sector to ensure a gender equity perspective, rather than designating this responsibility to "women's units" (Theobald et al. 2005).

A gender analysis of the specific inequities in relation to maternal and child health in any given context should form the basis of a gender mainstreaming approach. Gender analysis frameworks can stimulate those involved in health policy and planning or community development to identify how gender roles and relations may affect planned projects or interventions. An example of a gender analysis framework focusing on health is given in Fig. 9.2. The first key question in the framework aims to identify gender differences and patterns in who becomes ill and asks why this may be. The second question stimulates a consideration of how women and men respond to ill-health – for example, how easily they can utilize health services. To answer these questions, we need to consider the various aspects of gender roles and relations, including women's and men's interactions with the environment, their activities (gender division of labor), their bargaining positions, and access to, and control over, resources, and gender norms. We also need to consider these at several levels, including the household, community, health services, and national/international levels. Finally we need to consider interactions with other social divisions and inequalities, including ethnicity, class, age, and religion.

Gender analysis should be used to develop policies and interventions appropriate to gender roles and relations in a specific context. However, there are some key goals that are agreed to internationally. Following the conferences on population policy in Cairo of 1994 and on women in

Fig. 9.2 Gender analysis framework. Source: Gender and Health group, Liverpool School of Tropical Medicine (1999)

Key questions	Aspects of gender	Levels of analysis and interactions with other socio-economic factors
Why do different groups of men and women suffer from ill-health? **How are men and women's responses to ill-health influenced by gender?**	How does the ENVIRONMENT influence who becomes ill? How do the ACTIVITIES of men and women influence their health and responses to illness? How do the relative BARGAINING POSITIONS of men and women influence their health and responses to illness? How does access to and control over RESOURCES influence the health of men and women and their responses to illness? How do GENDER NORMS influence health and responses to illness?	Households Communities Available health services Influence of states/markets/international relations Consider how the situation of women and men may differ across different social groupings (e.g. race, class, age, religion)

Beijing of 1995, the international consensus on population and reproductive rights has shifted from an emphasis on reducing fertility through improving women's status, advocating female education and employment, to the promotion of gender equality and women's empowerment (Oxaal and Baden 1996). This approach takes a more holistic view of women's health and well-being rather than providing for women only in terms of potential or actual motherhood. Key to this strategic approach are the concepts of sexual and reproductive health and rights. Sexual and reproductive rights include women's rights to control their fertility and sexual interactions, rights to safe abortion services, and freedom from sexual coercion and violence for women, men, girls, and boys.

A key component of a gender mainstreaming approach is advocacy for policies, services, and resource allocations to establish the sexual and reproductive rights of women, men, boys, and girls and to ensure that they are met. This goal requires intersectoral collaboration to improve women's bargaining power and access to and control over resources. Policies must aim to improve maternity rights, increase girls' access to education, improve women's equitable access to productive resources, and encourage men's increased contribution to reproductive work, including caring for children. Ensuring sufficient resource allocation nationally and internationally to guarantee the availability and accessibility of good quality, patient-centered maternal and child health care, including obstetric services, requires committed advocacy for improving geographically equitable provision of services. Policy-level approaches to improve access to services include removing user charges, including services in social- or community-based health insurance schemes, and providing free emergency transport to services.

The activity of organized women's groups is important for realizing reproductive health and rights worldwide. Involving such groups in policy and its implementation is a key strategy for improving both participation of, and accountability to, different groups of women. Such groups can lobby for relevant legal changes, greater commitment and resources to be given to safe motherhood, and they can engage in dialogue with health service providers over quality of care issues on behalf of patients

(Oxaal and Baden 1996). At the level of health sector practice, an important approach to improving the quality and gender sensitivity of maternal and child health-care services is working together in partnership with health workers. Participatory gender sensitivity training for health workers has the potential to enable them to drive change from the bottom up. An example is the Health Workers for Change program, which aimed to address the interpersonal aspects of quality of care through a series of workshops (Fonn and Xaba 2001). The workshops included sessions that enabled health workers to critically analyze provider–client relations, to become sensitized about how gender relations may impact on health and on provider–client relations, and to assess whether interventions to improve this aspect of quality could be developed by health-care workers themselves. Research shows that the workshops enabled health workers to reflect on women's disadvantage and the impact this has on their experiences of health care and to identify training needs to enable them to respond to this more positively (Fonn and Xaba 2001). Training health workers in a participatory approach can enable services to become more client and gender sensitive and therefore more effective (Khanna et al. 2002). However, such "bottom-up" approaches are likely to require resource allocation and a supportive policy to create sustainable change.

It is also important to promote gender equity in maternal and child health at the community level, or "demand side." At this level, two important strategic approaches are (1) involving men in reproductive and child health in ways that support women's rights and preferences and (2) encouraging broader gender-sensitive community participation in maternal and child health programs. The past decade has seen the emergence of programs to encourage men to take a more active role in reproductive health services. Most have focused on involving men in family planning services, but there are examples of initiatives focusing on broader maternal and child health issues such as those aiming to encourage men to accompany their pregnant wives to antenatal care appointments, or to improve their parenting skills (de Koning et al. 2005). By raising awareness of male partners about obstetric issues, these programs aim to improve maternal health outcomes. There is evidence that educating male partners and increasing male involvement in women's maternal health can lead to improved antenatal care attendance and discourage home deliveries (Nanda et al. 2005).

There is also some experience of the involvement of men in programs for the prevention of mother to child transmission (PMTCT) of HIV/AIDS and joint couple approaches to HIV voluntary counseling and testing (VCT). In pilot projects for PMTCT, male involvement was found to be important for the acceptance and uptake of antiretroviral treatment (de Koning et al. 2005). VCT programs that counsel couples in which one person is HIV positive have been shown to be significantly more effective than individual counseling in preventing transmission between partners (The Voluntary HIV-1 Counseling and Testing Study Efficacy Group 2000). However, involvement of men can threaten women's rights and autonomy if it is not conducted with a focus on gender. Relatively few programs take into account gender equity when addressing men's involvement in reproductive health services and even fewer have been evaluated (de Koning et al. 2005). Consulting and involving women in shaping interventions to improve male involvement is likely to be an important approach to prevent inadvertently threatening women's interests or positions.

Gender-sensitive community participation in programs that may improve maternal and child health outcomes includes involving women and men in the development of "birth preparedness plans," holding advocacy workshops and health forums and creating women's action groups. Some studies have successfully employed behavior change strategies to mobilize both women and men in communities to improve "birth preparedness," including awareness of signs of emergency obstetric complications and motivating families to seek services. Behavior change communication strategies use various reinforcing messages through multiple channels to target both men and women (Afsana et al. 2007). When combined with "top-down" action to improve obstetric care services, facilitating women's groups to take action can improve resources and support available to women. Supporting local women to influence decision-making processes may lead to increased prioritization of women's health needs.

Research Priorities

Despite widespread recognition that gender inequalities are an important influence on maternal and child health, there are surprisingly few published studies examining the influence of gender on maternal and child health and health services. To date, there is an insufficient evidence base for many potential approaches to addressing gender inequities. For example, there is insufficient research conducted on ways to enhance the role of men in improving maternal and child health, as well as a lack of assessment of gender sensitivity of existing programs for the involvement of men. There is a clear need to further develop participative and accountable maternal and child health services. Gendered approaches to participation and accountability that aim to recognize and address the multiple needs of different groups of women and men and power relations in "communities" and health systems will arguably lead to more gender equitable, efficient, and sustainable services.

Additional future research should both incorporate a context-specific gender analysis of maternal and child health and services and then evaluate the process and outcome of approaches to improve gender equity in different contexts. Research must address gender-related barriers to the delivery of quality maternal and child health care. Researchers must assess approaches to improve the gender sensitivity of providers and evaluate ways to provide incentives for change. In addition, further research is needed on the gender division of labor imbalance and decision-making inequities, in order to propose successful gender-sensitive approaches for involving men in reproductive and child health. Finally, there is an urgent need to improve access to reproductive and maternal and child health services for the most vulnerable groups of women, including the very poor, unmarried women, HIV positive women, and adolescents. Both process and outcome evaluation of approaches will enable researchers to grasp the broader impacts of interventions on gender equity in society.

Conclusion

In order to improve the gender equity, sustainability, and efficiency of MCH services, there is an urgent need to pay greater attention to the multiple ways in which gender roles and relations affect maternal and child health. This means gender mainstreaming in policy and practice, and innovative action, grounded in the reality of different country and regional contexts to address gendered barriers to access of quality services at both the health service (provider side) and community (demand side) levels.

Key Terms

Access to and control over resources	Gender identity	Psychological abuse
Advocacy	Gender norms	Purdah
Autonomy	Gender relations	Rape
Bargaining positions	Gender role	Religious practices
Beijing conference	Gender-sensitive policies	Reproductive roles
Birth preparedness plans	Gender-based violence	Safe sex
Cairo conference on population policy	Gendered attitudes	Sex determination
	Intrauterine device	Sex-selective abortion
Caste	Male-controlled family planning methods	Sexual and reproductive rights
Community management roles		
Contraceptive pills	Male–female birth ratio	Sexual coercion
Cultural practices	Marital infidelity	Sexuality
Dalit	Marriage	Social change
Educational status	Masculine	Social distance
Female genital mutilation	Maternal mortality	Stillbirth
Female sterilization	Maternity care	Traditional beliefs
Feminine	Millennium development goals	Traditional birth attendants
Fertility control	Motherhood	
Gender	Multisectoral approaches	Triple burden
Gender analysis	Polygamous marriage	Undervaluing
Gender analysis framework	Poverty	Unsafe abortion
Gender discrimination	Power relations	Vulnerability
Gender division of labor	Productive roles	Women's health
Gender equity	Prolonged labor	Women's rights

Questions for Discussion

1. Discuss how the traditional women's health approach differs from the more contemporary gender analysis approach.
2. Using specific examples, distinguish between gender analysis and gender mainstreaming.
3. It is said that unequal gender roles and relations influence many aspects of women's and men's relative health status, vulnerability to illness, access to, and quality of, care and the burden of ill-health on family members. In a short essay of not more than 200 words, discuss what you understand by this statement.
4. Discuss the impact of gender on maternal health care from the perspective of the community ("demand side") and the health system ("supply side").
5. Using specific examples, discuss the importance of involving men in health-care program for women, infants, and children.

References

Afsana K, Rashid SM, Chowdhury AMR et al. (2007) Promoting maternal health: gender equity in Bangladesh. British Journal of Midwifery, 15(11): 721

Aliyu MH, Salihu HM, Keith LG et al. (2005) Extreme parity and the risk of stillbirth. Obstetrics and Gynecology, 106(1): 446–453

Azubuike MC, Ehiri JE (1998) Action on low immunization uptake. World Health Forum 19(4): 362–364

Beijing Platform of Action (1995) The United Nations Fourth World Conference on Women. http://www.un.org/womenwatch/daw/beijing/platform/health.htm, cited 2 February 2008

Black RE, Allen LH, Bhutta ZA et al. (2008) Maternal and child under nutrition: global and regional exposures and health consequences. Lancet, 371(9608): 243–260

Center for reproductive rights (2002) Reproductive rights and women with disabilities: A human rights framework. Briefing paper. http://www.reproductiverights.org/wn_humanrights.html, cited 2 February 2008

Chapko MK, Somsé P, Kimball AM et al. (1999) Predictors of rape in the Central African Republic. Health Care Women International, 20(1): 71–79

Department for International Development (DFID) (1999) Gender Equity Mainstreaming Internet Resource: Gender and Health. Department for International Development, UK (DFID). http://www.siyanda.org/docs_gem/index_-sectors/health/gh_coretext.htm, cited 2 February 2008

de Koning K, Hawkes S, Martin Hilber A (2005) Integrating sexual health interventions into reproductive health services: Programme Experience from developing countries. World Health Organization, Geneva

Fonn S, Xaba M (2001) Health workers for change: developing the initiative. Health Policy and Planning, 16(1): 13–18

Fikree, Fariyal F, Omrana P (2004) Role of gender in health disparity: The South Asian context. British Medical Journal, 328(7443): 823–826

Freedman L (2003) Strategic advocacy and maternal mortality: moving targets and the millennium development goals. Gender and Development, 11(1): 97–108

Gender and Health Group, Liverpool School of Tropical Medicine (1999) Gender and Health Guidelines. http://www.liv.ac.uk/lstm/hsr/gg.html, cited 2 February 2008

Heise L (1993) Violence against women: the missing agenda. In: Koblinsky M, Timyan J and Gay J (eds.), The Health of Women. Westview Press, Oxford

Jones SD, Ehiri JE, Anyanwu EC (2004) Female genital mutilation in developing countries: an agenda for public health response. European Journal of Obstetrics, Gynecology and Reproductive Biology, 116(2): 144–151

Khanna R, de Koning K, Khandekar S et al. (2002) The role of research in sensitizing auxiliary nurse midwives to a women-centered approach to healthcare in Mumbai, India. In Cornwall A and Welbourn A. (eds.), Realizing Rights: Transforming Approaches to Sexual and Reproductive Well-Being, Zed Books, London, New York

Kim J, Motshei M (2002) Women enjoy punishment: attitudes and experiences of gender violence among primary

healthcare nurses in rural South Africa. Social Science and Medicine 54(8): 1243–1254

Leslie J (1989) Women's time: a factor in the use of child survival technologies. Health Policy and Planning, 4(1): 1–16

Lule E, Ramana GNV, Ooman N et al. (2005) Achieving the Millennium Development Goal of Improving Maternal Health: Determinants, Interventions and Challenges. World Bank Health, Nutrition and Population Discussion Paper. http://siteresources.worldbank.org/HEALTHNUTRITIONANDPOPULATION/Resources/281627-1095698140167/LuleAchievingtheMDGFinal.pdf, cited 2 February 2008

Mayhew S (1996) Integrating MCH/FP and STD/HIV services: current debates and future directions. Health and Policy Planning, 11(4): 339–353

Mann G, Bokosi M, Sangala W (2006) Why are pregnant women dying? An equity analysis of Maternal Mortality in Malawi. Malawi Medical Journal, 18(1): 32–28.

Nanda G, Switlick K, Lule E (2005) Accelerating Progress towards Achieving the MDG to Improve Maternal Health: A Collection of Promising Approaches. World Bank Health, Nutrition and Population Discussion Paper. http://siteresources.worldbank.org/HEALTH-NUTRITIONANDPOPULATION/Resources/281627-1095 698140167/NandaAcceleratingProgresswithCover.pdf, cited 2 February 2008

Neupane S (2004) Evaluation of Community Based Safer Motherhood Emergency Funds. Nepal cited in United Nations Millennium Development Project Taskforce on Child Health and Maternal Health (2005)

Oxaal Z, Baden S (1996) Challenges to women's reproductive health: maternal mortality, BRIDGE Report No 38, Report prepared at the request of the Social Development Department, Department for Overseas Development (DFID). UK: Institute of Development Studies, Brighton. http://www.bridge.ids.ac.uk/reports/re38c.pdf, cited 2 February 2008

Prevention of Maternal Mortality Network (1992) Barriers to Treatment of Obstetric Emergencies in Rural Communities of West Africa. Studies in Family Planning, 23(5): 279–291

Singh S, Shah IH, Standing H (2007) The high cost of unsafe abortion. Id21focus report. http://www.id21.org/focus/unsafe_abortion/art00.html, cited 2 February 2008

Smith E, Murray SF, Yousafzai AK (2004) Barriers to accessing safe motherhood and reproductive health services: the situation of women with disabilities in Lusaka, Zambia. Disability and Rehabilitation, 26(2): 121–127

Thaddeus S, Maine D (1994) Too far to walk: maternal mortality in context. Social and Science and Medicine, 38: 1091–1110

Theobald S,.Tolhurst R, Elsey H (2005). Engendering the bureaucracy? Challenges and opportunities for mainstreaming gender in Ministries of Health under Sector Wide Approaches. Healthy Policy and Planning,.20(3): 141–149

Tinker A, Koblinsky M (1993) Making Motherhood Safe. World Bank, Washington, DC

Tolhurst R, Theobald S, Kayira E et al. (2008) I don't want all my babies to go to the grave: Perceptions of pre-term birth in southern Malawi. Midwifery, 24(1): 83–98

Voluntary HIV-1 Counseling and Testing Study Efficacy Group (2000) Efficacy of voluntary HIV-1 counseling and testing in individuals and couples in Kenya, Tanzania, and Trinidad: a randomized trial. Lancet, 356(9224): 103–112

WHO (2001) Rethinking care from the perspective of disabled people; conference report and recommendations WHO Disability and Rehabilitation team. http://whqlibdoc.

who.int/hq/2001/a78624.pdf. Last checked 22/05/06, cited 2 February 2008

World Bank (2003) Gender Equality and the Millennium Development Goals. World Bank Gender and Development Group, Washington, DC

Chapter 10
Harmful Traditional Practices and Women's Health: Female Genital Mutilation

Sarah Windle, Chuks Kamanu, Ebere Anyanwu, and John E. Ehiri

Learning Objectives After reading this chapter and answering the discussion questions that follow, you should be able to

- Identify and discuss the origin, types, and prevalence of female genital mutilation (FGM).
- Critically appraise factors that help to perpetuate the practice of FGM globally.
- Review the immediate and long-term consequences of FGM and discuss the various approaches for caring for victims.
- Analyze opportunities for prevention activities targeted at local practitioners of FGM, parents, at-risk adolescents, health and social workers, governments, religious authorities, the civil society, and the community.

Introduction

This chapter examines the impact of harmful traditional practices on maternal and child health, using female genital mutilation (FGM) as a case study. Beginning with a brief overview of harmful traditional practices, the chapter discusses relevant terms, definitions, and types of FGM. First, the origin and prevalence of FGM are explored. Second, the health consequences and issues related to care of victims are discussed, and finally, factors contributing to FGM are critically analyzed. The chapter examines the policy and practice options for eliminating FGM and reviews examples of

interventions in order to identify the best practices for prevention. Recognizing that there is no simple solution to the problem, the chapter argues that interventions for preventing FGM should be non-directive, culturally sensitive, and multifaceted to be of practical relevance. Such interventions should not only motivate change but should also provide alternative options and help communities to establish the practical means by which change can occur. Potentially effective prevention interventions targeted at local practitioners of FGM, parents, at-risk adolescents, health and social workers, governments, religious authorities, the civil society, and communities are presented. According to the United Nations (2008), harmful traditional practices are those practices that are based on cultural values and beliefs, but which are harmful to a specific group within the culture (typically women and/or children). These traditional practices are often longstanding and benefit some, or all, of the community, but violate the rights of vulnerable populations. They include FGM, forced feeding of women, early marriage, early pregnancy, taboos or practices that prevent women from controlling their own fertility, nutritional taboos and traditional birth practices, son preference and its implications for the girl child (United Nations 2006), and female infanticide. Males are typically the main beneficiaries of harmful traditional practices, as these practices often lead to loss of female control over sexuality, economic dependence, and political subordination.

Harmful traditional practices have been very slow to change over time, particularly given past national and international reluctance to confront problems that are "cultural" in nature (United Nations 2008). In addition, longstanding practices are often continued by custom and social

S. Windle (✉)
Department of Maternal and Child Health, University of Alabama at Birmingham, USA

J.E. Ehiri (ed.), *Maternal and Child Health*, DOI 10.1007/b106524_10,
© Springer Science+Business Media, LLC 2009

reinforcement, perpetuated even by those who have themselves been victimized. In this chapter, FGM is used as a case study in order to examine the history, causes, prevalence, consequences, and prevention of a harmful traditional practice. FGM encompasses all procedures involving partial or total removal of external female genitalia or other injury to the female genital organs for cultural, religious, or other non-medical reasons (WHO 1995). The term FGM does not refer to sex reassignment surgery or genital modification of intersexuals.

Different terms are interchangeably used to describe the act of female genital mutilation. Opponents of this practice use the term FGM, while groups who support and practice this ritual tend to use the term female circumcision (FC). Some authorities argue that the term female circumcision results in an unwanted association between male and female circumcision (UNICEF 2005a). Some United Nations agencies use the term "female genital mutilation/cutting" wherein the additional term "cutting" is intended to reflect the importance of using non-judgmental terminology with practicing communities. Both terms emphasize the fact that the practice is a violation of girls' and women's human rights (WHO 2008a).

The term mutilation not only establishes a clear distinction from male circumcision but also emphasizes the gravity of the act as a violation of the human rights of women and girls, and thereby helps promote national and international advocacy toward its abandonment (UNICEF 2005b). In 1990, this term was adopted at the third conference of the Inter-African Committee on Traditional Practices Affecting the Health of Women and Children (IAC) in Addis Ababa (Shell-Duncan and Hernlund 2000). In 1991, the World Health Organization recommended that the United Nations UN adopt this terminology and it has subsequently been widely used in UN documents (United Nations 2002). In communities where this practice is entrenched, the term FGM is viewed as judgmental with the intention of demonizing certain cultures, religions, and communities. Against this background, the term female genital cutting (FGC) has increasingly been used to avoid alienating communities and to show more sensitivity toward individuals who have undergone some form of genital excision (WHO 1996). FGM is the preferred term for policy makers and human rights advocates working to protect girls and women from the practice (WHO 1998).

FGM was first subdivided into four types in 1995 when it became apparent that classification was necessary for measurement, medical management, and research. The WHO further classified FGM into seven subtypes in 2007 in order to better capture clinically significant variations within types (Table. 10.1). The extent of genital cutting typically

Table 10.1 Classification of FGM

WHO modified typology (2007)	WHO typology (1995)
Type I: Partial or total removal of the clitoris and/or the prepuce (clitoridectomy)	**Type I:** Excision of the prepuce, with or without excision of part or the entire clitoris.
When it is important to distinguish between the major variations of Type I mutation, the following subdivisions are proposed: **Type Ia**, removal of the clitoral hood or prepuce only; **Type Ib**, removal of the clitoris with the prepuce.	
Type II: Partial or total removal of the clitoris and the labia minora, with or without the excision of the labia majora (excision).	**Type II:** Excision of the clitoris with partial or total excision of the labia minora.
When it is important to distinguish between the major variations that have been documented, the following subdivisions are proposed: **Type IIa**, removal of the labia minora only; **Type IIb**, partial or total removal of the clitoris and the labia minora; **Type IIc**, partial or total removal of the clitoris, the labia minora, and the labia majora.	

(continued)

Table 10.1 (continued)

WHO modified typology (2007)	WHO typology (1995)
Note also that, in French, the term "excision" is often used as a general term covering all types of female genital mutilation.	
Type III: Narrowing of the vaginal orifice with creation of a covering seal by cutting and appositioning the labia minora and/or the labia majora, with or without excision of the clitoris (infibulation). When it is important to distinguish between variations in infibulations, the following subdivisions are proposed: **Type IIIa,** removal and apposition of the labia minora; **Type IIIb,** removal and apposition of the labia majora.	**Type III:** Excision of part or all of the external genitalia and stitching/narrowing of the vaginal opening (infibulation).
Type IV: Unclassified: all other harmful procedures to the female genitalia for non-medical purposes, for example, pricking, incising, scraping, and cauterization.	**Type IV:** Unclassified: pricking, piercing, or incising of the clitoris and/or labia; stretching of the clitoris or labia; cauterization by burning of the clitoris and surrounding tissue; scraping of tissue surrounding the vaginal orifice (angurya cuts) or cutting of the vagina (gishiri cuts); introduction of corrosive substances or herbs into the vagina to cause bleeding or for the purpose of tightening or narrowing it; and any other procedure that falls under the broad definition of female genital mutilation.

Source: WHO (2008)

increases from Types I to III, with Type IV representing unclassified varieties of FGM. Type I (clitoridectomy) is the partial or total removal of the clitoris and/or the prepuce (Figs. 10.1 and 10.2). Type II (excision) is partial or total removal of the clitoris and the labia minora, with or without excision of the labia majora (Fig. 10.3). Type III (infibulation) is the narrowing of the vaginal orifice with the creation of a covering seal by cutting and appositioning the labia minor and/or labia majora with or without excision of the clitoris (Fig. 10.4). Type IV (unclassified) is all other harmful procedures done to the female genitalia for non-medical purposes, for example, pricking, piercing, incising, scraping, or cauterization (Fig. 10.5) (WHO 2008b).

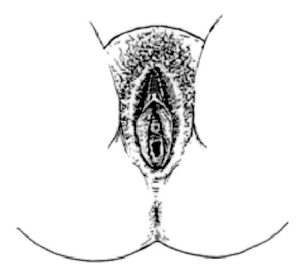

Fig. 10.1 Clitoridectomy (Type 1a). Source: WHO (2001a)

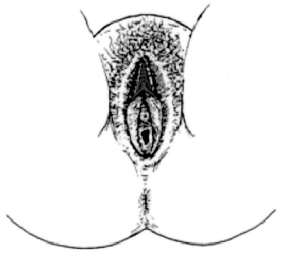

Fig. 10.2 Clitoridectomy (Type 1b). Source: WHO (2001a)

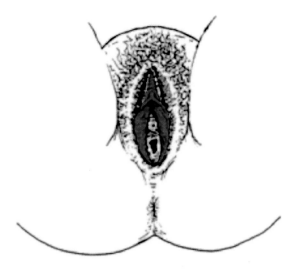

Fig. 10.3 Excision (Type IIb). Source: WHO (2001a)

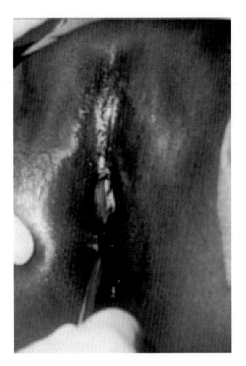

Fig. 10.4 Infibulation (Type III). Source: WHO (2001a)

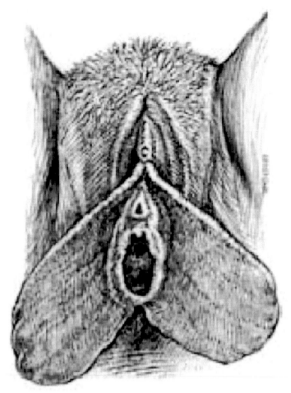

Fig. 10.5 Stretching of the Labia Minora (Type IV - Unclassified). Source: WHO (2001a)

Origin and Prevalence

FGM probably has multiple origins (Odoi 2005; Hathout 1963; Hosken 1992). However, the best documentation suggests that this practice began in ancient Egypt where the people believed in bisexuality of the external genitalia (Fourcroy 1983; Skaine 2005). FGM has been discovered on ancient Egyptian mummies dating from 200 BC (Hathout 1963; Barstow 1999; Skaine 2005). The custom was then presumably retained and spread throughout Mesopotamia and the Islamic countries. The presence of FGM in other regions is also recorded. For instance, in Europe, some Russian and Romanian religious sects kept the ritual in order to ensure perpetual virginity (Worseley 1938). Clitoridectomy was practiced fairly extensively in the English-speaking world during the 19th century for the treatment of diverse medical conditions like nymphomania, prevention of masturbation, hysteria, epilepsy, melancholia, and insanity (Sanderson 1981).

The WHO (2008) estimates that between 100 and 140 million women and girls have undergone FGM (Types I, II, and III) worldwide. Annually, 3 million girls (mostly under 15 years old) undergo genital mutilation (WHO 2006). Most women with FGM live in one of the 28 African or Middle Eastern countries where FGM is practiced (Fig. 10.6). FGM is also practiced in some areas of Asia and

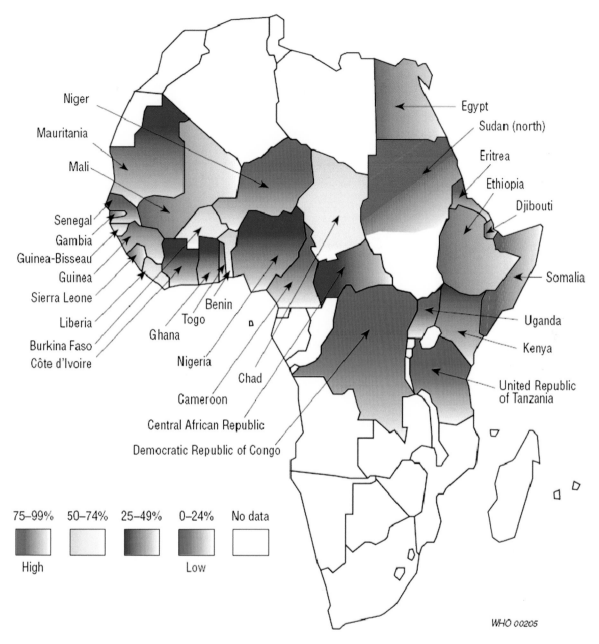

Fig. 10.6 FGM prevalence by country. Source: WHO (2001a)

South America (WHO 2006, 2008a). As shown in Tables 10.1 and 10.2, the prevalence of FGM varies greatly within and between countries, although two countries (Egypt and Ethiopia) account for nearly half of all women who undergo FGM worldwide (WHO 2006).

The characteristics of girls and women who are subjected to FGM vary greatly. The strongest predictor of risk for FGM is ethnicity (WHO 2008b), which explains how FGM can occur in isolated groups in non-practicing regions. For instance, in Indonesia and Malaysia, FGM is fairly common among the country's Muslim women (U.S. Department of State 2001), while overall prevalence is low. It also explains the increase in the practice of FGM in the United States, Canada, Australia, and

Table 10.2 Countries where FGM has been documented

Country	Year	Estimated Prevalence of Female Genital Mutilation in girls and women ages 15–49 years (%)
Benin	2001	16.8
Burkina Faso	2005	72.5
Cameroon	2004	1.4
Central African Republic	2005	25.7
Chad	2004	44.9
Cote d'Ivoire	2005	41.7
Djibouti	2006	93.1
Egypt	2005	95.8
Eritrea	2002	88.7
Ethiopia	2005	74.3
Gambia	2005	78.3
Ghana	2005	3.8
Guinea	2005	95.6
Guinea-Bissau	2005	44.5
Kenya	2003	32.2
Liberia*		45.0
Mali	2001	91.6
Mauritania	2001	71.3
Niger	2006	2.2
Nigeria	2003	19.0
Senegal	2005	28.2
Sierra Leone	2005	94.0
Somalia	2005	97.9
Sudan, northern (approximately 80% of total population in survey)	2000	90.0
Togo	2005	5.8
Uganda	2006	0.6
United Republic of Tanzania	2004	14.6
Yemen	1997	22.6

*The estimate is derived from a variety of local and sub-national studies (Yoder and Khan 2007)
Source: WHO (2008)

Europe as a result of international migration. In particular, France has migrant populations from Benin, Chad, Guinea, Mali, Niger, and Senegal, and the United Kingdom often receives immigrants from Kenya, Nigeria, and Ghana. In the 1970s, refugees from Eritrea, Ethiopia, and Somalia carried the practice of FGM into Norway, Sweden, and Switzerland (WHO 2006).

Ethnicity also affects the type and timing of FGM. Worldwide, approximately 90% of FGM is of Types I, II, or IV, with the remaining 10% being Type III. Country-level comparisons show wide variation in the extent of tissue cut. For example, despite having a similar prevalence of FGM (82 and 79% respectively), Sudan and Senegal differ by type. Type III accounts for 86% of FGM in the Sudan, while in Senegal, the majority of FGM (68%) is Type II, with the prevalence of Type III at only 1% (Table 10.3). Age at FGM also differs significantly among countries (WHO Study Group 2006). In Egypt 90% of FGM is performed between ages 5 and 14. In Ethiopia, Mali, and Mauritania, 50% of FGM is performed on those under 5 years old and in Yemen, 76% of FGM is performed on those less than 2 weeks old (WHO 2006). FGM may also be performed on women at significant life stages, such as at the time of marriage, pregnancy, or childbirth (WHO 2006).

Table 10.3 Distribution of FGM status and total FGM by country

	No FGM	FGM I	FGM II	FGM III	Total
	No (%)				
Burkina Faso	938 (19%)	1097 (23%)	2172 (45%)	609 (13%)	4816
Ghana	1841 (60%)	353 (11%)	867 (28%)	33 (1%)	3094
Kenya	1681 (40%)	865 (21%)	1201 (29%)	420 (10%)	4167
Nigeria	646 (12%)	3369 (63%)	1310 (24%)	41 (1%)	5366
Senegal	733 (21%)	837 (24%)	1850 (54%)	29 (1%)	3449
Sudan	1332 (18%)	335 (5%)	371 (5%)	5463 (73%)	7501
Total	7171 (25%)	6856 (24%)	7771 (27%)	6595 (23%)	28393

Source: WHO Study Group (2006)

There are also additional distinctions between the practice of FGM in urban versus rural areas. However, this finding may be partly attributable to the distribution of certain ethnic populations. In general, the prevalence of FGM is lower in urban areas. The Population Reference Bureau (PRB 2001) found this to be true in all countries surveyed except Sudan and Burkina Faso (Fig. 10.7). Other than patterns of ethnic settlement, this may be due to higher general education and greater availability of information about the practice in urban areas (PRB 2001). In all countries, approval of FGM was lower in urban compared with rural areas (Fig. 10.8).

The Population Reference Bureau (RPB 2001) also found that education status directly correlates with the likelihood of a woman undergoing FGM (Fig. 10.9). Women with primary or no school education are more likely to have experienced FGM than women with secondary or higher school education, although this is reversed in some countries (Burkina Faso, Sudan, and Yemen). This is not to suggest that the education of a woman decreases her likelihood of undergoing FGM, because FGM in the vast majority of cases occurs before school age. Education is correlated with a family's socioeconomic status, and higher SES may lessen the societal influence on the family's perception of the necessity of FGM (for instance, in order for their daughters to find husbands). Urban and more educated women are less likely to believe that men prefer women who have undergone FGM or that FGM is an important part of religious practice. Religion alone does not affect the prevalence of FGM, as prevalence varies by religion and country together, likely pointing again to the cultural origins of the practice (Table 10.4).

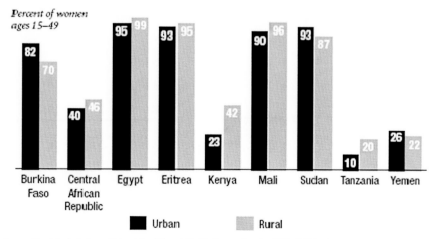

Source: Special tabulations of Demographic and Health Survey data for 1989–2000 by Principia International, Inc. (Chapel Hill, NC) and published data from ORC Macro (Calverton, MD).

Fig. 10.7 Prevalence of FGM by urban or rural residence. Source: PRB (2001)

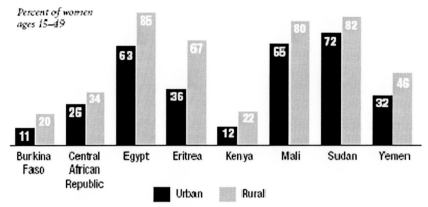

Note: No data on attitudes are available for Tanzania.
Source: Special tabulations of Demographic and Health Survey data for 1989–2000 by Principia International, Inc.
(Chapel Hill, NC) and published data from ORC Macro (Calverton, MD).

Fig. 10.8 Women who support FGM, by urban or rural residence. Source: PRB (2001)

Fig. 10.9 Prevalence of FGM by education level. Source: PRB (2001)

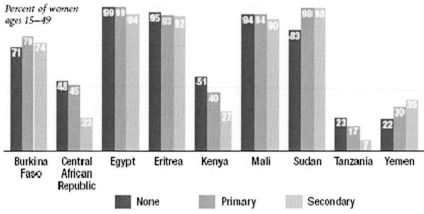

Note: In Egypt, primary education refers to primary incomplete.
Source: Special tabulations of Demographic and Health Survey data for 1989–2000 by Principia International, Inc.
(Chapel Hill, NC) and published data from ORC Macro (Calverton, MD).

Table 10.4 Prevalence of FGM by religion and country

	Muslim		Christian		Traditional/Other	
Country	% Surveyed	% Circumcised	% Surveyed	% Circumcised	% Surveyed	% Circumcised
Burkina Faso	56	78	27	66	17	61
Central African Republic	9	50	90	43	2	42
Egypt	95	98	5	88	-	-
Eritrea	38	99	62	92	-	-
Kenya	5	28	92	38	3	31
Mali	91	94	3	85	6	90
Sudan	98	90	2	47	-	-
Tanzania	31	14	57	19	12	22

Source: Special tabulations of Demographic and Health Survey data for 1989–2000 by Principia International, Inc. and published data from ORC Macro. Data for Yemen are not available.
Source: PRB (2001)

Health Consequences

Numerous negative health outcomes have been attributed to FGM. These include the immediate physical consequences as well as urinary, gynecological, psychological, and obstetrical complications (WHO 2000a). Given the dubious legality and sensitive nature of FGM, incidence of these complications is likely to be under-reported. Surgeons may be motivated to hide complications originating from it and, in communities where FGM is practiced, discussion about genital conditions may be embarrassing to the woman (Odoi 2005).

Acute complications are those that occur at the time of FGM. Performance of the procedure in unsterile conditions may cause cellulitis, clitoral gangrene, and sepsis (Nour 2004; Dirie and Lindmark 1992). Other acute complications include severe pain, hemorrhage, acute urinary retention, and death (Odoi 2005; Dirie and Lindmark 1992; Jones et al. 2004). FGM performed during pregnancy may result in the formation of fistulae, as well as pregnancy complications from hemorrhage or infection (WHO 2000a).

FGM may result in recurrent urinary tract infections. For women with Type I or Type II FGM, injury may affect the urethral meatus at the time of the procedure or subsequently during labor and delivery. Meatal stricture, obstruction, or periurethral tears may result from such trauma. For women with Type III FGM, the urethral meatus may be blocked by the infibulated scar, which can lead to accumulation of urine and menstrual blood, thereby creating a favorable environment for ascending bacterial infection into the urinary tract (Nour 2004; Dirie and Lindmark 1992; Eke and Nkanginieme 2006). Signs and symptoms may include slow urinary stream, straining, and urinary retention. Relief may be obtained by surgical opening of a urethral stricture or defibulation (Odoi 2005; Agugua and Egwuata 1982). Urinary retention during labor appears to be particularly common in women with Type III FGM and catheterization often cannot occur without defibulation (WHO 2000a).

Gynecological complications include the formation of cysts, chronic pelvic infection, and gynatresia. Epidermal inclusion cysts at the site of excision of the clitoris may grow as large as 18 cm in diameter (Hathout 1963; Agugua and Egwuata 1982). Chronic pelvic infection may result from the progression of acute infection at the time of performing FGM (Rushwan 1980) or the accumulation of vaginal secretions and urine, especially after Type III FGM. Other pelvic infections include recurrent vaginal candidiasis, trichomoniasis, and bacterial vaginosis (Larson and Okonofua 1999; De Silva 1989). FGM was found to be the most common cause of gynatresia (obstruction of part of the genital tract) in eastern Nigeria (Ozumba 1992). Such gynatresia have resulted in the formation of calculi in the vulva and posterior vaginal fornix (Ozumba 1992; Shandall 1967; Verzin 1975).

Sexual dysfunction in the form of dyspareunia (pain during intercourse) or even apareunia (inability to have intercourse) following Type III FGM has been reported by several authors (Odoi 2005; Hathout 1963; Shandall 1967). Urethral coitus resulting from apareunia and misdirected efforts at sexual intercourse has also been reported (Lawson 1967). Other sexual complications that can occur include anorgasmia and coital bleeding. An association between primary infertility and Type III FGM has recently been established. The likely mechanism is via ascending infections occurring after the procedure, causing damage (inflammation and scarring) to the fallopian tubes which leads to infertility later in life (Larson and Okonofua 1999; Almroth et al. 2005).

FGM may also put women at increased risk for contracting HIV (Brady 1999). The WHO and the International Federation of Gynecologists and Obstetricians (FIGO) have hypothesized reasons for this presumed link (Kun 1997), including the increased risk of inflammation and bleeding at coitus in genitally mutilated women and subsequent disruption to the genital epithelium and exposure to blood, abrasions in men attempting vaginal penetration, increased risk of hemorrhage in childbirth due to obstructed labor and tearing of vaginal and perineal scar tissue and the consequent increased need for blood transfusion, use of unsterilized instruments in the performance of FGM, and the practice of the more risky anal intercourse as a substitute for painful vaginal intercourse (Kun 1997; Rushwan 2000; Jones et al. 2004; Braddy and Files 2007).

Some authors have suggested that the most serious adverse effect of FGM is the mental and psychological agony that the victim goes through (De Silva 1989; Lightfoot-Klein and Shaw 1991). This is in part because these complications do not manifest outwardly as the physical complications do and are hardly addressed (Odoi 2005). Given the wide variation in age at which FGM is performed (WHO 2006), it is likely that psychological effects from the initial act of FGM will vary among women. These may include fear of having sexual intercourse, posttraumatic stress disorder, chronic anxiety, and depression. These complications are a consequence of the procedure and the short- and long-term physical complications that follow (Odoi 2005; Braddy and Files 2007; Morris 2006). During pregnancy, women may have fear of pain from pelvic examinations, tearing of the infibulation scar, of delivery due to the small size of the vaginal opening, and of incorrect suturing following birth (WHO 2000a). Immigrants to countries with low prevalence of FGM may have concerns about the knowledgeability of the healthcare provider with respect to FGM and fear of cesarean section, episiotomy, or perineal repairs because of lack of provider knowledge (WHO 2000a).

A recent perspective study by the WHO has highlighted a substantial contribution of FGM to morbidity and mortality in women of reproductive age (Box 9.1). This study revealed that women who undergo FGM are at substantially higher risk for cesarean section, postpartum hemorrhage, episiotomy, extended hospital stay, resuscitation of the infant, and inpatient perinatal death compared with women who have not undergone FGM (WHO Study Group 2006; Morris 2006).

Women who were subjected to FGM as neonates, children, at puberty, or at marriage (as opposed to during the pregnancy) are more likely than women who did not have FGM earlier in life to experience obstructed labor. Obstructed labor can be severe and directly relates to maternal and fetal mortality (WHO 2000a). Type III FGM clearly presents a mechanical barrier to delivery, but even Types I, II, and IV FGM can result in scarring and stenosis of the vaginal and vulval tissue from previous infection, inflammation, or the formation of

---

Box 9.1 Complications of FGM

1. **Medical**
   Acute urinary tract infections
   Recurrent urinary tract infections
   Local sepsis at site of operation
   Septicemia
   Transmission of viral infections (HIV, HBV)

2. **Surgical**
   Keloids
   Epidermal inclusion cysts
   Injury to the urethral meatus
   Injury to the rectum
   Hemorrhage and shock

3. **Gynecological**
   Vulval adhesion
   Gynatresia
   Hematocolpos
   Vulval/vaginal calculi
   Acute/chronic PID
   Primary infertility
   Vesicovaginal fistula (VVF)
   Rectovaginal fistula (RVF)

4. **Sexual**
   Dyspareunia
   Apareunia
   Anorgasmia
   Coital bleeding
   Urethral coitus

5. **Obstetric**
   Increased risk of cesarean section
   Postpartum hemorrhage
   Increased risk of perineal laceration and anterior episiotomy
   Increased risk of prolonged/obstructed labor
   Increased perinatal morbidity
   Increased inpatient perinatal death
   Increased risk of puerperal sepsis

6. **Mental and psychological**
   Posttraumatic stress disorder
   Chronic anxiety
   Chronic depression

vulval adhesions that can obstruct labor (WHO 2000a). A reduced vaginal opening may make assessment difficult, complicating antenatal and intrapartum care (WHO 2000a).

Sequelae to obstructed labor from FGM include fetal distress and death (WHO Study Group 2006; WHO 2000a). Episiotomy and perineal tears are common and these may lead to an increased incidence of postpartum hemorrhage (WHO 2000a). Obstructed labor may require the use of instruments or cesarean section for delivery (WHO Study Group 2006; WHO 2000a). Maternal death from improperly treated obstructed labor, postnatal infection, and vesicovaginal/rectovaginal fistulae (from prolonged pressure of the fetal head during delivery) is of particular significance for women who have had Type III FGM (Verzin 1975; Laycock 1950; Kelly and Hillard 2005; WHO 2000a).

Caring for FGM Patients

Women who have undergone FGM should be treated with sympathy, kindness, and in a non-judgmental way in order to avoid barriers to effective communication (Odoi 2005; Braddy and Files 2007). Prior knowledge of type of FGM, complications, or any previous pelvic examination will be of help in anticipating and managing complications in labor. Outside pregnancy, tight vaginal orifice resulting from Type III FGM may hinder proper pelvic examination and sexual intercourse. Defibulation should be performed anytime on patients' request, anytime infibulation is detected, after counseling and consent from the patient, or when she marries. During pregnancy, elective defibulation after counseling and obtaining consent should be done. This permits a proper pelvic examination anytime during pregnancy should the need arise and also a proper assessment of progress in labor. It also reduces the risk of prolonged labor.

Defibulation should be done early in the second trimester so as to allow for wound healing before labor. For pregnant women who present late in the third trimester, partial defibulation should be done early in labor in order to permit proper pelvic examination. Full defibulation should be deferred to late

second stage as the fetal head distends the vulva. Defibulation at this time has several advantages – minimal blood loss and reduced risk of trauma to the urethral meatus as the external urethral meatus tends to be displaced away from the fusion by the fetal head. Also the line of fusion of the vulva is highlighted following full stretching by the fetal head (Odoi 2005; Braddy and Files 2007; RCOG 2002). A woman who previously had Type III FGM may request for reinfibulation after vaginal delivery. This should be discouraged because of the long-term complications associated with infibulation. Counseling and advice against reinfibulation should be offered (Odoi 2005; Nour 2004; Braddy and Files 2007).

Factors Contributing to the Practice of FGM

There are numerous factors that contribute to the perpetuation of FGM. The WHO (1999) created a "mental map" highlighting the broad basis for FGM within communities, including some of the social, religious, and aesthetic reasons for continuation of the practice and community enforcement mechanisms (Fig. 10.10). These reasons vary in prevalence and strength across regions. Common themes include attitudes and beliefs regarding gender roles and ethnic identity, religion as justification, the perceived necessity of FGM for marriage and chastity, and the economic dependence of women.

FGM practices are deeply entwined with ethnic identity. This constitutes an important obstacle to change (Jones et al. 2004). In many communities FGM is so entrenched that it is the social norm rather than the exception (Jones et al. 2004). In some instances, one must be physically altered to be perceived as a true woman (Gruenbaum 2001). FGM may mark the transition from girlhood to womanhood. In such communities, elaborate ceremonies and lessons on the role of a wife and mother are often part of the procedure. However, it is important to remember that in most cultures FGM is performed at such an early age that it cannot be defined as a transition into womanhood (Gruenbaum 2001).

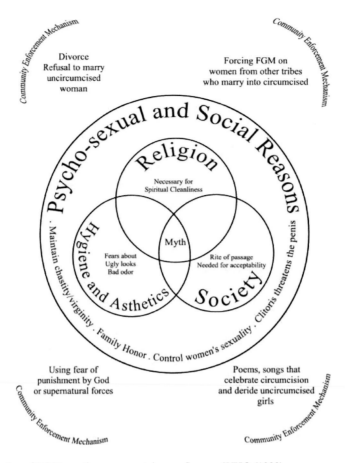

Fig. 10.10 Why the practice of FGM continues: a mental map. Source: WHO (1999)

While religion itself does not influence the prevalence of FGM (PRB 2001), the interaction of religion and culture may lead to religious justification of FGM. For example, "Sunna" refers to what the prophet Mohammed has said or done. In some Islamic communities where FGM is prevalent, the practice of excision of the prepuce of the clitoris (Type I) is referred to as "Sunna." This has led to the erroneous perception that FGM is closely tied to Islam. However, FGM is not a religious practice as it predates the arrival of both Christianity and Islam in Africa and FGM is not known in many Muslim countries (Jones et al. 2004; Gruenbaum 2001; Shell-Duncan and Hernlund 2000; Elmusharaf et al. 2006; Lockhat 2004; Rahman and Toubia 2000; Henrieka and Dhar 2003).

Virginity at the time of marriage and fidelity after marriage are vitally important in many cultures that practice FGM. In these cultures, FGM is clearly associated with chastity (Jones et al. 2004;

Gruenbaum 2001; Balk 2000). In a society where mutilation is perceived to protect virginity and virginity is directly linked to marriageability, we can begin to understand why mutilation might be viewed as an important step to realize future marriage (Gruenbaum 2001). Such communities also believe that excision of the clitoris or its prepuce (Type I) helps to curb sexual desire in the woman which ensures chastity after marriage. Furthermore, infibulation (Type III) is thought to increase sexual pleasure for the man by creating a tight vaginal orifice (Odoi 2005; Worseley 1938; Jones et al. 2004; Gruenbaum 2001; Toubia and Sharief 2003; Toubia 1994).

FGM is common in communities where marriage and motherhood are essential to the social and economic security of women. In such settings, a decision to forgo FGM can have negative consequences (Braddy and Files 2007). Women must rely on their husbands to provide for them in their reproductive years and their children to care for them in their old age (Jones et al. 2004). As a result, women themselves are often the strongest advocates of the practice because they believe it will ensure important benefits (marriage and security) for their female children (Braddy and Files 2007; Jones et al. 2004; Gruenbaum 2001; Dorkenoo 1996; Gerais and Bayoumi 2001).

Implications for Policy and Practice

Interest in curtailing the practice of FGM has increased in the past 20 years. Although the political and legal environment toward the practice has become more hostile, this awareness has yet to translate into measurable changes in prevalence (Jones et al. 2004). Identifying the most effective and appropriate strategies for eliminating FGM is among one of the most bitterly contested issues surrounding the practice (Larson and Okonofua 1999). Simple educational campaigns dealing with the health consequences of genital mutilation have not been as effective as was once expected (De Silva 1989). Program planners assumed that once people realized the dangers associated with FGM, the practice would be immediately abandoned; unfortunately, this has not been the case. Although education about health risks is an important component of change, intervention programs that do not address the causes of FGM will not be effective in ending the practice (Dirie and Lindmark 1992; De Silva 1989).

Since female genital mutilation is a highly sensitive and culturally embedded practice, it is critical for program strategies to be based on community values, customs, and roles of interaction (De Silva 1989). Those introducing prevention interventions must be familiar with the settings in which their programs will be implemented (Verzin 1975). Significant formative research should be done not only on the prevalence and type of FGM practiced in the area but also on the community perceptions and relevant importance of the practice within the culture. Better understanding of the practice within the community and culture where the program is being implemented makes the intervention more salient to the target audience. This gives the

program credibility and increases its effectiveness. According to the WHO (De Silva 1989), "communities need to play a central role in any initiative" targeting FGM. The alternative ritual program implemented by the Mandeleo Ya Wanawake organization (MYWO) in Kenya is an example of a highly successful intervention that involved the community in the planning and implementation of the intervention. MYWO involved the community by seeking their help in developing a conceptual framework for the problem in their community, designing and exploring the feasibility of the program, and implementing the program (De Silva 1989).

It is important for FGM prevention programs to be non-directive. While education about the harmful effects of FGM is important, the program should not seek to force communities to end the practice. Past directive approaches have been seen, with good reason, as imperialist attempts by "outsiders" to meddle in cultural issues they do not fully understand (Dirie and Lindmark 1992). These programs have not only failed to eliminate the practice but may also have actually created more resistance to change among some groups (Dirie and Lindmark 1992; De Silva 1989). A more appropriate goal for intervention programs is to seek to educate people about human rights and the health consequences of FGM and to be available to help the communities change when they determine they are ready to do so (Nour 2004; De Silva 1989). The history of FGM among the Sabiny people in the Kapchowra district of Uganda illustrates the importance of a non-directive approach. Efforts to stop the practice among the Sabiny began with the arrival of Christian missionaries in the district in the 1930s and 1940s. Sixty years of education, health risk communication, and awareness-raising campaigns yielded little success (De Silva 1989). In fact, the Sabiny community was so offended with arrogant "outsiders" passing judgment on their culture and traditions that one campaign program was actually linked to a dramatic increase in the number of girls who underwent FGM (De Silva 1989). This disturbing increase led to the creation of the Reproductive, Education and Community Health (REACH) project, which was designed with involvement from the local community. REACH's framework allows the Sabiny people to determine the process by which they will change harmful practices, and at what pace and how the changes will occur (De Silva 1989).

The success of this type of non-directive strategy, termed a "sensitive persuasive" approach by the WHO (De Silva 1989), has been highlighted in a program in Senegal, in which communities were involved in a year-long educational intervention that taught human rights and women's health with emphasis on the risks and dangers of FGM (Lawson 1967). The results have been impressive. In Senegal, 708 villages, representing 13% of the country's population that observed the practice, have made public declarations abandoning FGM. The remarkable thing about the results, as the program planners noted, was that the program never asked people to stop FGM. "Usually, participants come to the decision to abandon the practice on their own" (Lawson 1967). The decision to end the practice must be made by the people of practicing cultures themselves if there is to be real and lasting change.

Given that FGM is a problem with many causes, programs addressing the issue must have many facets to be effective. Eradication of a deeply entrenched practice like FGM cannot be accomplished through a singular approach (Almroth et al. 2005). Program implementers must focus their strategies on understanding and addressing the core values, myths, and enforcement mechanisms that support the practice (De Silva 1989). A successful program must not only motivate the community to change, but it must also provide alternative options and the means through which the anticipated change can occur. Intervention efforts should target several different groups, including practitioners of FGM, parents, at-risk adolescents, heath and social welfare professionals, religious leaders and other authoritative figures, relevant government institutions, and the civil society. These preventive approaches are described in the following sections. More details regarding best practices in FGM prevention can be found in the World Health Organization's (1999) publication entitled "FGM programmes to date: what works and what doesn't: a review."

Practitioners of FGM

Despite the fact that the number of urbanized parents who take their daughters to healthcare providers to undergo FGM is increasing, the practice is still being performed predominantly by "traditional female excisors" (De Silva 1989). The performance of FGM is considered a skill and the women who perform it are paid for their work. Educational programs teaching these women the health risks associated with FGM are needed. After having the opportunity to learn about the harmful effects of mutilation, these women should be offered the opportunity to be trained in an alternative skill. Without offering retraining to circumcisers, the women would have no way to financially support themselves and it would be unlikely that they would stop practicing their trade. While retraining efforts would vary slightly depending on the local infrastructure and needs, these women could be retrained as village health workers or birth attendants. The retrained women could then begin to work toward solving the most pressing problems facing their communities, such as communicable diseases and malnutrition. In addition to providing skilled workers to combat growing health problems, many of which are of greater immediate concern than FGM, retraining traditional circumcisers would allow these women to retain their place of importance and respect in the society without continuing the practice of FGM (De Silva 1989).

More than a third of responding agencies surveyed during a WHO program evaluation thought that alternative income and retraining programs for excisors were very effective strategies (De Silva 1989). Programs such as the one in Ghana that retrained circumcisers to become birth attendants initially yielded positive results (Laycock 1950). Other programs utilizing this strategy have resulted in a large percentage of circumcisers stopping the practice temporarily or, in some cases, permanently (Jones et al. 2004). However, used in isolation, this approach has proven ineffective since it does not reduce the demand for FGM in the community (Jones et al. 2004; De Silva 1989; Laycock 1950). Retraining of circumcisers must be done in conjunction with community education if retraining efforts are to foster lasting change.

Parents

Parents of children and adolescents are a second important target audience for change efforts. Among this group, the motivation to continue the practice of FGM is predominantly social conformity. Parents fear that if they do not follow the status quo, their daughters will suffer because they are considered unmarriageable. Parents do not have their daughters undergo FGM because they do not love them; they have them undergo the practice because they love them. They may perceive this to be the best way to ensure their daughters' future safety and happiness (Rushwan 1980). Successful programs must help provide a system where the prospect of marriage exists for girls who have not undergone FGM. Programming for parents should provide education about the health consequences and human rights aspects of FGM. Parents should be introduced to the idea that not all cultures practice genital mutilation. At the end of the educational phase, families who are ready to embrace change should be encouraged to form a pledge society (Kelly and Hillard 2005).

The value of the pledge society approach has been demonstrated through its success in ending foot binding in China in the early 1900s (Kelly and Hillard 2005). Foot binding involved tightly wrapping the feet of young girls after bending the toes under the feet, forcing the sole of the foot to the heel. Girls who underwent foot binding matured with tiny feet, perhaps only 5 in. in length. Although foot binding was painful and caused lasting health problems for women, its practice was perpetuated with the belief that it ensured the honor of the family and the virtue and marriageability of the young woman (Kelly and Hillard 2005). Like FGM, foot binding was an entrenched cultural practice that had existed for thousands of years when intervention programs began (Rushwan 1980). Foot binding eradication efforts included not only education about negative health consequences of the practice but also the formation of associations of parents who pledged not to have

their daughters' feet bound and not to let their sons marry young women with bound feet (Larson and Okonofua 1999; Kelly and Hillard 2005).

Pledge societies operate on the principle that change is desired, but not carried out because of the social consequences associated with it. Applied to the issue of female genital mutilation, this means that some parents have their daughters undergo FGM not because they support the practice but because they fear other families will not allow their sons to marry a young woman who has not undergone the procedure. Parents of daughters joining the pledge society would vow not to have their daughters undergo FGM; parents of sons joining the society would pledge to allow their sons to marry these girls. This creates a new "marriage market" for those who choose not to practice genital mutilation. Parents of daughters are guaranteed that their children will have marriage opportunities if they do not undergo FGM and what seems to be the greatest perceived barrier of ending the practice is eliminated (Rushwan 1980).

The Population Reference Bureau (Shandall 1967) attributed much of the success of the Senegal-based Tostan program to this type of approach which "enables people to agree collectively to stop the practice so that no one family stands out or no one person becomes socially stigmatized and thus unmarriageable." Public declaration programs appear to have been responsible for the rapid and total abandonment of FGM in several villages in Senegal (Laycock 1950). The pledge society approach has proven successful because it takes into account the fact that "discontinuation of FGM is largely a matter of social rather than individual change" (De Silva 1989).

At-Risk Adolescents

Another target group for intervention should be children and adolescents considered "at risk" for female genital mutilation practices. Young people are an important target for intervention because they tend to be less attached to cultural traditions and more easily influenced with sound arguments about the harmful effects of FGM than older members of the same community (De Silva 1989). Interventions geared toward reaching adolescents are of especially critical importance in cultures and communities that closely link initiation with FGM (Larson and Okonofua 1999). Programs for adolescents should be intensely culturally sensitive and should offer education while incorporating cultural practices and values whenever possible. For example, in a society where group seclusion during and after FGM is common, the alternative transition ritual might involve the girls leaving their community to participate in the educational program. If community or family celebrations are part of the FGM tradition, these celebrations could be held when the young woman finishes the alternative program.

Although the details of this type of intervention will vary from culture to culture, the girls should be provided with information not only about FGM practices and health consequences but also practical knowledge of basic health care. Family planning, reproductive rights, HIV/STDs, and child health practices would be possible topics to address. A second part of the educational program should provide the young women with knowledge of relevant cultural practices and traditions, such as what is expected of a wife and mother within the community. Ideally, the FGM alternative program provides a way for communities to keep cultural ideals and values without keeping the harmful practice of FGM. While help from cultural outsiders might be needed in the planning stages, this program should be implemented entirely by people inside the community. "Wise women" of the culture trained in basic health care should become the instructors for the educational program. The alternative teaching ritual has the potential to empower the older women by emphasizing their status and authority while empowering the young women by emphasizing the importance of the role they are taking in their culture, as well as the importance of the culture itself. Girls initiated into similar programs report that the training raised their self-esteem (Laycock 1950). The young women also develop a support system through the program that strengthens and helps them adjust to the changing roles they are expected to fill in their communities (Laycock 1950).

The most well-known example of an alternative ritual program currently in progress is a project based in Meru, Kenya, in which several communities have organized events which they call "Ntanira na Mugambo" (circumcision through words).

This is a ceremony that includes a week-long program of counseling, training, and provision of information to young women. It ends with a "coming of age" celebration that involves music, dancing, presents, and feasting (Lightfoot-Klein and Shaw 1991; Braddy and Files 2007). This program is reported to have prevented over 1000 FGM procedures in its 8 years of operation (Larson and Okonofua 1999). Although the long-term success of the alternative ritual approach has not been fully evaluated, recent reports from Kenya suggest that it is a promising strategy, especially when used in conjunction with other approaches (De Silva 1989; Lightfoot-Klein and Shaw 1991). An important aspect of Ntanira Na Mugambo is the flexibility that arises from the ability to stress various components in response to community characteristics. The success of this program has also been linked to the involvement of the entire family, community, and the inclusion of a male motivation component.

Health, Social, and Economic Sectors

The increasing medicalization of FGM mandates further research and creation of sensitization and training programs for nurses, midwives, and other health professionals (WHO 2001). Exploration of the use of religious leaders and other authoritative figures in the society, including law enforcement officials, as agents of change for harmful traditional practices like FGM is needed. It is also important that governments utilize many strategies, including establishing government departments or ministries to look after women's issues, strengthening safe motherhood initiatives, improving the knowledge and skills of health and social workers, and collaborating with non-governmental organizations (NGOs) and the private sector (RCOG 2002). The World Health Organization has produced several training materials (WHO 2000b, 2000a, b) that would serve as a useful resource for programs that seek to enhance the skills of health workers in addressing FGM. Health, social, and economic sectors should cooperate and collaborate in order to empower women in the areas of education, social status, and technology. Many governments have already made commitments at the UN Special Session on Children (Gruenbaum 2001) to end FGM in their countries. What is urgently needed is for these governments to establish the foundation for change recommended by the WHO (De Silva 1989) which includes the establishment of strong and capable institutions that implement anti-FGM programs at the national, regional, and local levels; support for FGM elimination with positive policies, laws, and resources; mainstreaming of FGM prevention issues into national reproductive women's health and literacy development programs; training of staff who can recognize and manage the complications of FGM; coordination with non-governmental agencies; and support for advocacy that fosters a positive policy and legal environment, increased support for programs, and public education (De Silva 1989). This foundation will not only ensure cross-cultural feasibility of the public health actions proposed in this chapter but will also result in meaningful reduction of the practice of FGM and thus its impact on women in these nations.

In addition, governments should demonstrate political commitment through policies that address poverty, nutrition, adolescent health, violence against women, and sexual abuse. Strategies to foster active dialogue and engagement of national institutions, including the media, religious institutions, and the civil society, to openly confront FGM and to ensure that women and families who choose not to undergo FGM are not discriminated against must be identified and utilized. Teachers, social workers, and community groups that interact with families must be encouraged to play significant roles in preventing FGM through active education and advocacy. The following are abridged versions of the case studies selected by the Population Reference Bureau (2006) to represent examples of successful interventions for FGM.

The Navrongo FGM Experiment

Between 1999 and 2003, efforts were made to hasten the elimination of FGM in a portion of the Kassena-Nankana district of northern Ghana and to determine which strategies were the most effective in reducing the practice. This is a rural area where

the practice of FGM was long-standing and the prevalence of FGM among girls aged 15–19 years was 34%. Although FGM had been illegal since 1994, the practice was still socially condoned as a rite of passage ritual for adolescent girls. Interventions involving a community participation approach were used in three communities with a fourth community as a comparison group. One intervention community participated in FGM education activities including group discussions, videos, clinic and school-based education, anti-FGM song and drama competitions, and radio programs. Another intervention community participated in livelihood and development activities including learning skills such as crafts and marketing, reproductive health education, and culturally relevant skills such as preparation of traditional dishes. The third intervention community participated in a combination of both programs.

Controlling for age, marital status, religion, and education, the community participation and education intervention compared with the control group was associated with a 93% decrease in the incidence of FGM and the combined community participation/education/skills intervention was associated with a 94% decrease in the incidence of FGM. The community participation and development activities showed a decrease in the incidence of FGM that was not significant. Survival analysis determined the percentage of girls who had not undergone FGM at age 15 at the start of the study and still had not at age 19. The incidence of FGM was found to be similar in all three intervention groups and nearly 4% higher in the control group (Fig. 10.11). Reported challenges were that the baseline prevalence of FGM was lower than expected (necessitating expansion of the study area) and that some girls who had initially reported having undergone FGM denied it in future surveys. Reversal of FGM status was determined to not bias the results, as it occurred similarly across all groups.

Intrahealth International in Ethiopia

This intervention's objectives were to identify current knowledge, attitudes, and practices regarding FGM, develop the capacity of community leaders to

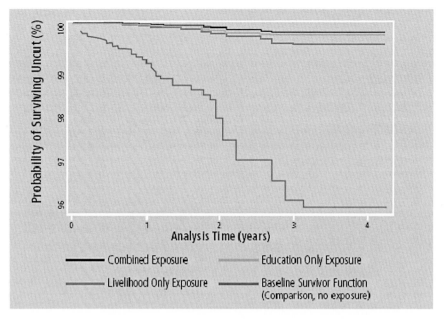

Fig. 10.11 Survival analysis: the probability of not undergoing FGM over time. Source: PRB (2006)

advocate against FGM, increase knowledge and change attitudes of community members about FGM, and to monitor and evaluate the impact of the interventions. The prevalence of FGM in Ethiopia in 1998 was 73% and a study in 2003 indicated a trend toward less extreme forms of FGM. Of girls undergoing FGM, 50% occurred before age 1 and 88%

occurred before age 10. The practice is supported with religious justification, a belief that FGM makes women better wives, by the idea that it protects a daughter's reputation and marital prospects, and even by the idea that it is necessary to stop the clitoris from growing. Three areas were selected for intervention because of their higher than average prevalence

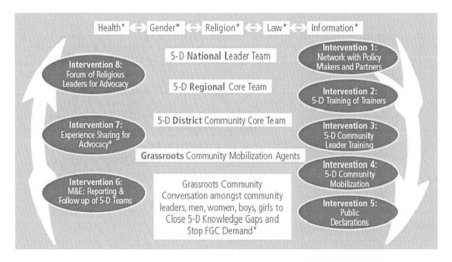

Fig. 10.12 A 5-dimensional approach to eliminating FGM in Ethiopia. Source: PRB (2006)

rates: Oromia (90%), Somali (99%), and Harari (94%).

This intervention took a five-dimensional approach to reducing FGM (Fig. 10.12). These dimensions were health, gender, religion, human rights/law, and information. Activities included engaging and empowering community leaders with education, advocacy, communication skills, mobilization of the community through reducing knowledge gaps, initiating discussion, and formulating grassroots action plans. Activities resulting from community mobilization included

- public demonstrations;
- anti-FGM arts (drama, music, etc.);
- traditional ceremonies such as the slaughtering of sheep; and
- anti-FGM declarations.

Multimedia were used in the form of pamphlets, televised drama, and radio announcements. A forum of religious leaders was held to discuss FGM and reach consensus on public banning of the practice. Project successes were measured through qualitative data only. They include legislation that made FGM illegal, a consensus of 83 national and religious leaders to criminalize and ban FGM, the participation of 4,200 community members in the intervention, public promises to stop performing FGM by 7 well-known practitioners in the community, and 2,252 community members publicly agreeing to ban FGM. Additional successes include the support of various religious leaders, continued coverage of the intervention by the media, and adoption of the project dimensions by local organizations. Feedback from the project suggests that its strengths were

community participation, coverage of FGM in multiple dimensions, transfer of the project to local stakeholders, multimedia training aids, focus on ending demand for FGM, encouraging community discussion and bridging gaps between social groups, respecting the social–cultural context of the practice, and working with local personnel and knowledge bases as well as other organizations.

Tostan Community Empowerment Program

Tostan is an NGO in Senegal and Guinea, where the overall prevalence of FGM in women (15–49) in 2005 was 28.2 and 95.6%, respectively. The areas in Senegal in which Tostan worked often had prevalence rates above 90%. Over the past decade, it is estimated that Tostan had 60 participants in each of 2,000 villages. The Tostan approach is based on the social convention theory of FGM which argues that FGM is practiced mainly to ensure community membership. On this basis, abandonment of the practice would be fairly rapid if it were a collective decision. Tostan conducted over 200 education sessions over a 2- to 3-year period. These sessions covered democracy, human rights, responsibilities, problem-solving methods, hygiene and health (including discussions on early marriage, childbearing, sexually transmitted infections, FGM), literacy, math, and management skills. The approach emphasized the underlying essential components of credibility of information, belief that people will make good

Table 10.5 Attitudes of men and women toward FGM

	Baseline	Intervention Group		Comparison Group	
		Endline Participant	Non-participant	Baseline	Endline
Women (n)	576	333	200	199	200
□ Approve of FGC	72	16*	28*	89	60*
□ Will cut daughters in the future	71	12*	23*	89	54*
Men (n)	373	82	185	184	198
□ Will cut daughters in the future	66	13*	32*	78	56*
□ Prefer a woman who has been cut	–	20	40	–	63

*$p < 0.05$
Source: PRB (2006)

decisions when they are informed, learner-centered, holistic, practical, and respectful of cultural learning practices. It also used an "organized diffusion" strategy, whereby participants shared what they had learned by choosing another person to teach.

The Tostan intervention was unique in that it did not explicitly target FGM. The inclusion of a session on FGM explicitly was only done after participants requested it. When two communities initially decided in 1997 to end FGM, the spread of the movement was largely due to the efforts of an Iman (an Islamic religious leader) who was concerned that girls from these villages would not be able to intermarry with other areas that had not abandoned FGM. He took it upon himself to speak with members of the surrounding communities also about ending the practice. This resulted in the first public declaration of FGM abandonment in 1998.

The Tostan approach has been evaluated by outside organizations a number of times. One evaluation found that the intervention resulted in increased knowledge of FGM, decreased the proportion of girls under age 10 who were undergoing FGM, and decreased approval of FGM and intent to subject daughters to the practice (Table 10.5). Another evaluation concluded that FGM and forced/child marriages had been abandoned in 83% of communities visited (22 of 24), and literacy/education classes were well attended. Other evaluations confirmed positive changes in attitudes, knowledge, and health practices, abandonment of FGM in project villages, and greater discussion about FGM in non-project villages. As of July 2006, Tostan estimated that as a result of its work, FGM was ended in 1,748 communities (33% of communities that practiced FGM in Senegal in 1997).

Conclusion

Many observers of the FGM controversy have asked whether such a complicated and entrenched cultural practice can ever be successfully changed. The answer to this question is a resounding "Yes" (Dirie and Lindmark 1992; Jones et al. 2004; Rushwan 1980). However, evidence shows that this can only be achieved through gradual persuasion, sensitization, and community education on human rights and health aspects of FGM, as well as efforts to change socioeconomic factors that perpetuate the practice. Women need to be provided with avenues for the expression of their social status approval and respectability, other than FGM. Mere repression through legislation has not been successful (Morris 2006) since people will only stop practicing FGM when they are presented with a safe alternative that preserves their culture and protects the welfare of their daughters (Rushwan 1980). Even now, individuals and families are challenging laws banning FGM practices in spite of the great risks (Dirie and Lindmark 1992; Rushwan 1980). Societies have proven to be open to interventions to end FGM when the community is included in program planning and implementation (Jones et al. 2004; De Silva 1989). Change has already begun. The ancient practice of FGM, which currently undermines the health of millions of the world's women, will eventually come to an end.

Key Terms

Acute urinary retention	Female genital mutilation	Perineal repairs
Adolescent health	Female genitalia	Periurethral tear
Alternative ritual	Female infanticide	Piercing
Anorgasmia	Fertility	Pledge societies
Anti-FGM songs	Fistula	Postpartum hemorrhage
Apareunia	Foot binding	Posttraumatic stress disorder
Ascending bacterial infection	Forced feeding	Prepuce labia minora
At-risk adolescents	Gender	Pricking
Bacterial vaginosis	Genital excision	Public declaration programs
Beliefs	Genital modification	Recurrent urinary tract
Calculi	Female circumcision	infection
Catheterization	Girl child	Reinfibulation
Cauterization	Gynatresia	Religious leaders
Cellulitis	Harmful traditional practice	Sensitive persuasive
Cesarean section	Hemorrhage	approach
Christianity	Human rights	Sepsis
Chronic anxiety	Hysteria	Septicemia
Chronic pelvic infection	Infection	Sex reassignment surgery
Circumcisers	Infibulated scar	Sexual abuse
Clitoral gangrene	Infibulation	Sexual dysfunction
Clitoridectomy	Infibulations scar	Sunna
Clitoris	Insanity	Tostan program
Coital bleeding	Islam	Traditional birth practices
Coming of age	Keloids	Traditional female excisors
Cultural outsiders	Labia majora	Trichomoniasis
Cultural values	Male circumcision	Unsterilized instruments
Custom	Marriageability	Urethral coitus
Defibulation	Masturbation	Urethral meatus
Depression	Meatal stricture	Urinary retention
Dyspareunia	Melancholia	Urinary tract infection
Early marriage	Menstrual blood	Vaginal candidiasis
Early pregnancy	Ntanira na Mugambo	Vaginal orifice
Epidermal inclusion cysts	Nutritional taboos	Violence against women
Episiotomy	Nymphomania	Virginity
Ethnicity	Obstetric complications	Vulnerable populations
Fallopian tubes	Organized diffusion	Vulval adhesion
Female control over sexuality	Painful vaginal intercourse	Wise women
Female genital cutting	Perineal laceration	Ya Wanawake

Questions for Discussion

1. Identify and describe the four types of FGM.
2. Discuss any two factors that influence the practice and type of FGM in developed and less developed countries.
3. Distinguish between acute and gynecological complications of FGM.
4. It is said that educational campaigns that provide information on the health consequences of FGM have not been effective. In an essay of about 250 words, discuss reasons for the failure of such programs.
5. Using a table to structure your response, produce at least one strategy for preventing the practice of FGM at the following levels – local practitioners of FGM, parents, at-risk adolescents, health and social workers, governments, religious authorities, the civil society, and communities. Cite the evidence base of each preventive recommendation you identify.

References

Agugua NE, Egwuata VE (1982) Female genital circumcision: management of urinary complications. Journal of Tropical Pediatrics, 28, 248–252

Almroth L, Elmusharaf S, El Hadi N et al. (2005) Primary infertility after genital mutilation in girlhood in Sudan: a case control study. The Lancet, 366, 385–391

Balk D (2000) To Marry and Bear Children? The Demographic Consequences of Infibulation in Sudan. Boulder, Co: Lynne Reinner Publisher Inc

Barstow DG (1999) Female genital mutilation: the penultimate gender abuse. Child Abuse and Neglect, 23(5), 501–510

Brady M (1999) Female genital mutilation: complications and risk of HIV transmission. AIDS Patient Care and STDs, 13(12), 709–716

Braddy CM, Files JA (2007) Female genital mutilation: cultural awareness and clinical considerations. Journal Midwifery Women's Health, 52, 158–163

De Silva S (1989) Obstetric sequelae of female circumcision. European Journal of Obstetrics and Gynecology and Reproductive Biology, 32, 233–240

Dirie MA, Lindmark G (1992) The risk of medical complications after female circumcision. East African Medical Journal, 69, 479–482

Dorkenoo E (1996) Combating female genital mutilation: an agenda for the next decade. World Health Statistics Quarterly, 49, 142–147

Eke N, Nkanginieme KE (2006) Female genital mutilation and obstetric outcome. The Lancet, 367, 1799–1800

Elmusharaf S, Elhadi N, Almroth L (2006) Reliability of self reported form of female genital mutilation and WHO classification: cross sectional study. British Medical Journal, 333, 124

Fourcroy JL (1983) Review of female circumcision. Urology, XX11(4), 458–461

Gerais AS, Bayoumi A (2001) Female Genital Mutilation (FGM) in the Sudan: A Community Based Study. University Press Khartoum

Gruenbaum E (2001) The Female Circumcision Controversy. Philadelphia: University of Pennsylvania Press

Hathout HM (1963) Some aspects of female circumcision. Journal of Obstetrics and Gynecology of the British Empire, 70, 505–507

Henrieka E, Dhar J (2003) Female genital mutilation in the Sudan: survey of the attitude of Khartoum University students towards this practice. Sexually Transmitted Infections, 79, 220–223

Hosken FP (1992) Genital and sexual mutilation of females. The Hosken Report. Third Review Edition. Women's International Network News (WINN), 18, 4

Jones SD, Ehiri JE, Anyanwu EC (2004) Female genital mutilation in developing countries: an agenda for public health response. European Journal of Obstetrics and Gynecology and Reproductive Biology, 116, 144–151

Kelly E, Hillard PJ (2005) Female genital mutilation. Current Opinion in Obstetrics and Gynecology, 17, 490–494

Kun KE (1997) Female genital mutilation: the potential for increased risk of HIV infection. International Journal of Gynecology and Obstetrics, 59(2), 153–155

Larson U, Okonofua FE (1999) Female circumcision and obstetric complications. International Journal of Gynecology and Obstetrics, 77(3), 255–265

Lawson JB (1967) Acquired gynatresia. In Lawson JB, Stewart DB (eds) Obstetrics and Gynecology in the Tropics and Developing Countries (pp. 543–545). London: Edward Arnold Ltd

Laycock HT (1950) Surgical aspects of female circumcision in Somali Land. The EAMJ, 445–450

Lightfoot-Klein H, Shaw E (1991) Special needs of ritually circumcised women patients. Journal of Obstetric, Gynecological, and Neonatal Nursing, 20, 102–107

Lockhat H (2004) Female Genital Mutilation: Treating the Tears. London: Middlesex University Press

Morris K (2006) Issues on female genital mutilation/cutting. The Lancet, 368(Sup 1), 564–567

Nour NM (2004) Female genital cutting: clinical and cultural guidelines. Obstetrical Gynecological Survey, 59, 272–279

Odoi AT (2005) Female genital mutilation. In Kwawukume EY, Emuveyan EE (eds) Comprehensive Gynecology in the Tropics (pp. 268–276). Accra, Ghana: Graphic Packaging Ltd

Ozumba BC (1992) Acquired gynatresia in eastern Nigeria. International Journal of Gynecology and Obstetrics, 37, 105–109

Population Reference Bureau (2001) Abandoning female genital mutilation: prevalence, attitudes, and efforts to end the practice. www.measurecommunication.org, cited 16 May 2008

Population Reference Bureau (2006) Abandoning Female Genital Mutilation/Cutting: An In-Depth Look at Promising Practices. Washington, DC: USAID

Rahman A, Toubia N (2000) Female Genital Mutilation: A Guide to Laws and Policies Worldwide. London: Zed

Royal College of Obstetricians and Gynecologists (RCOG) (2002) Female Genital Mutilation. RCOG Statement No.3

Rushwan H (1980) Ecological factors in pelvic inflammatory disease in Sudanese women. American Journal of Obstetrics and Gynecology, 138(7 pt 2), 877–879

Rushwan H (2000) Female genital mutilation (FGM) – management during pregnancy, childbirth and the postpartum period. International Journal of Gynecology and Obstetrics, 70(1), 99–104

Sanderson LP (1981) Against the Mutilation of Women. London: Ithaca Press

Shandall AA (1967) Circumcision and infibulation of females. Sudan Medical Journal, 178–212

Shell-Duncan B, Hernlund Y (eds) (2000) Female "Circumcision" in Africa: Culture, Controversy and Change. London: Lynne Rienner Publisher

Skaine R (2005) Female Genital Mutilation: Legal, Cultural and Medical Issues. Jefferson, NC: McFarland Publishers

Toubia N (1994) Female circumcision as public health issue. New England Journal of Medicine, 331, 712–716

Toubia NF, Sharief EH (2003) Female genital mutilation: have we made progress? International Journal of Gynecology and Obstetrics, 82, 251–261

UNICEF (2005a) Female Genital Mutilation/Cutting: A Statistical Exploration. http://www.unicef.org/publications/files/FGM-C_final_10 october.pdf, cited 25 December 2006

UNICEF (2005b) Changing a harmful social convention: female genital mutilation/cutting. http://www.unicef-icdc.org/publications/pdf/fgm-gb-2005, cited 22 October 2006

United Nations (2000) What is female genital mutilation? What actions are being taken to prevent it? United Nations Fact Sheet #3. New York: United Nations. http://www.un.org/geninfo/faq/factsheets/FS3.HTM, cited 21 May 2008

United Nations (2006) The impact of harmful traditional practices on the girl child. New York: United Nations. http://www.un.org/womenwatch/daw/egm/elim-disc-viol-girlchild/ExpertPapers/EP.4%20%20%20Raswork.pdf, cited 28 July 2008

United Nations (2008) Harmful traditional practices affecting the health of women and children. Fact Sheet # 23. http://www.unhchr.ch/html/menu6/2/fs23.htm, cited 16 May 2008

US Department of State (2001) Indonesia: Report on female genital mutilation (FGM) or female genital cutting (FGC). http://www.state.gov/g/wi/rls/rep/crfgm/10102.htm, cited 10 October 2008

Verzin JA (1975) Sequelae of female circumcision. Tropical Doctor, 163–169

WHO Study Group on Female Genital Mutilation and Obstetric Outcome (2006) Female genital mutilation and obstetric outcome: WHO collaborative prospective study in six African countries. The Lancet, 367, 1835–1841

World Health Organization (1995) Female genital mutilation. Report of a WHO Technical Working Group. WHO Document: WHO/FRH/WHD 96.10. Geneva: WHO

World Health Organization (1996) Female genital mutilation information pack. Gender and Women's Health Department. Geneva: WHO. http://www.who.int/docstore/frh-whd/fgm/infopack/english/fgm_infopack.htm, cited 12 December 2006

World Health Organization (1998) Female Genital Mutilation: An Overview. Geneva: WHO

World Health Organization (1999) Female genital mutilation – programmes to date: what works and what doesn't: a review. WHO Report No: WHO/CHS/WMH/99.5. Geneva: WHO, cited 9 June 2008

World Health Organization (2000a) A systematic review of the health complications of female genital mutilation including sequelae in childbirth. Geneva: WHO. http://www.who.int/reproductive-health/docs/systematic_review_health_complications_fgm.pdf, cited 9 June 2008

World Health Organization (2000b) Female Genital Mutilation: A Handbook for Frontline Workers. WHO Document: WHO/FCH/WMH/00.5. Geneva. World Health Organization

World Health Organization (2001) Female Genital Mutilation: Integrating the Prevention and the Management of Health Complications into the Curricula of Nursing and Midwifery. A student's manual. Geneva: WHO. www.mincava.umn.edu/categories/906, cited 9 June 2008

World Health Organization (2001a) Female Genital Mutilation: Integrating the Prevention and the Management of the Health Complications into the Curricula of Nursing and Midwifery, a Teacher's Guide. WHO Document: WHO/RHR/01.16. Geneva, World Health Organization

World Health Organization (2001b) Female Genital Mutilation: The Prevention and the Management of the Health Complications. Policy Guidelines for Nurses and Midwives. WHO Document: WHO/FCH/GWH/01.5; WHO/RHR/01.18. Department of Gender and Women's Health Department of Reproductive Health and Research Family and Community Health. Geneva: World Health Organization. https://www.who.int/reproductive-health/publications/rhr_01_18_fgm_policy_guidelines/fgm_policy_guidelines.pdf, cited 31 July 2008

World Health Organization (2006) Female Genital Mutilation – New Knowledge Spurs Optimism (Progress – Quarterly Brief of the UNDP/UNFPA/WHO/World Bank Special Programme of Research, Development and Research Training in Human Reproduction, Department of Reproductive Health and Research, #72). Geneva: WHO. http://www.who.int/reproductive-health/hrp/progress/72.pdf, cited 9 June 2008

World Health Organization (2008a) Eliminating Female Genital Mutilation: An Interagency Statement. Geneva: WHO. http://www.unifem.org/attachments/products/fgm_statement_2008_eng.pdf, cited 9 June 2008

World Health Organization (2008b) Female Genital Mutilation. http://www.who.int/topics/female_genital_mutilation/en/index.html, cited 29 May 2008

Worseley A (1938) Infibulation and female circumcision: a study of little-known custom. British Journal of Obstetrics and Gynecology, 45, 686–691

Chapter 11
Abortion and Postabortion Care

Andrzej Kulczycki

Learning Objectives After reading this chapter and answering the discussion questions that follow, you should be able to

- Critically analyze the history, incidence, and reasons for abortion from a global perspective.
- Identify and discuss differences in implementation of abortion laws and policies across different countries, and the public health implications with particular attention to unsafe abortion and abortion-related mortality and morbidity.
- Explain abortion techniques and safety and appraise the emerging trend toward earlier abortion in countries where abortion is safe and available.
- Discuss postabortion care – its evolution, current best practices, and examples.

Introduction

This chapter presents a global overview of abortion, examining its history and incidence, why women have abortions, and who has abortions. Abortion laws and policies, their implementation, and public health implications are discussed. Safe and unsafe abortion as well as abortion-related mortality and morbidity, conditions under which abortion occurs around the world and their health implications are presented. Also discussed are abortion techniques, safety and trend toward earlier abortion in countries

where abortion is safe and available. The chapter concludes with a discussion on postabortion care – its evolution, current best practices, and examples. We begin with some historical perspective.

Abortion has been with us since time immemorial. Spontaneous abortions, or miscarriages, occur in approximately 15% of clinically recognized pregnancies. Induced abortion, more commonly referred to as abortion, is the deliberate termination of pregnancy before viability (the point at which a fetus can survive independently outside the womb). Abortion is invariably a response to unwanted pregnancy and reflects a decision that may be due to a range of circumstances. Abortion may also have consequences for women's health if not performed under safe and hygienic conditions. Estimates suggest that approximately 68,000 deaths, or 13% of all maternal deaths, can be attributed to unsafe abortion. This is defined as the termination of an unwanted pregnancy either by persons lacking the necessary skills or in an environment lacking the minimal medical standards, or both (WHO 2003).

Due to the centrality of abortion in birth control and in women's lives, the contribution of unsafe abortion to maternal mortality and morbidity, the importance of efforts to reduce abortion and make it safer, and the immense passions associated with the topic, it is critical that we review why, how many, and under what conditions women around the world have abortions. It is also vital that we review efforts to reduce the incidence of abortion and to make it safer.

A. Kulczycki (✉)
University of Alabama at Birmingham, USA

J.E. Ehiri (ed.), *Maternal and Child Health*, DOI 10.1007/b106524_11,

Historical Perspective

Until the twentieth century, abortion was deemed unfit for public discussion in every country of the world. Women undergoing clandestine abortions were at high risk of being maimed and dying a lonely, gruesome death. This situation changed slowly with improvements in family planning, as abortion procedures became much safer, and as efforts to legalize abortion gained momentum. However, the topic remained largely off-limits in most countries and avoided at the international level until several high-profile UN conferences accorded greater attention to abortion. These included, in particular, the 1994 International Conference on Population and Development held in Cairo, and the 1995 Fourth World Conference on Women in Beijing. The Cairo conference was the first such intergovernmental meeting to deal with abortion as a public health issue, generating much acrimonious debate in the process (Kulczycki 1999).

Most countries criminalized abortion during the nineteenth century. Women's health, medical, legal, and religious leaders later took up the cause of legalizing abortion so as to reduce the toll of abortion-related mortality and morbidity. In the United States, for example, 201 deaths were officially attributed to abortion as late as 1965, 8 years before the procedure was legalized. This total accounted for 17 % of all reported maternal deaths that year, despite gains in the safety of abortion and adequacy of postabortion care over time. The true figure was undoubtedly higher because many deaths were ascribed to other causes so as to protect the name of women, their families, and those performing the abortions. Low-income women were disproportionately affected because they lacked the financial means to access safe abortion. Similarly today, poor women in countries where abortion is outlawed sometimes resort to self-induced abortion or, more often, seek dangerous, illegal abortion. Those with more resources typically manage to obtain a better quality procedure. They may also seek abortions in other jurisdictions, although this may result in a later-stage abortion and onward travel shortly afterward. This may prevent adequate rest and postabortion care if it is required, thereby increasing the risk of complications.

Historical and contemporary evidence demonstrates that outlawing abortion does not eliminate or lower its incidence. This is because it does not reduce unintended pregnancy, the underlying cause of abortion. Instead, outlawing abortion impacts the circumstances under which abortion occurs and is associated with adverse public health consequences for the woman, her family, and society. This is a major reason why many countries legalized abortion in the twentieth century.

Abortion Laws and Public Health Implications

Laws determine the official availability of abortion services. Nearly all Western democracies permit abortion under broad social and health grounds, enabling women to obtain a medically supervised and extremely safe abortion early in pregnancy. In contrast, Latin American, sub-Saharan African, and Arab countries have the most restrictive laws, generally allowing abortion only to save the life of a mother. South and South East Asian countries tend to restrict abortion, but India permitted abortion on broad grounds in 1971. Despite formal prohibitions on the procedure, Indonesia allows abortions to be performed in teaching hospitals as part of medical training and, along with Bangladesh, permits menstrual regulation before a pregnancy is confirmed. In East Asia, China and Vietnam have likewise allowed abortion under broad circumstances for several decades and have also promoted it as a means to reduce population growth.

On average, 6 in 10 women live in countries where early abortion is legally available to women on broad grounds, with 40% able to obtain the procedure on request, that is, without being required to specify a reason. One in four of the world's population reside in countries where abortion is allowed only to save a woman's life or is prohibited altogether; 10% of women have legal access to abortion only when deemed necessary to protect a woman's physical health or life, and 4% have access also if needed to protect a woman's mental health (United Nations 2002). Nevertheless, abortion is frequently performed in most countries that prohibit the procedure under almost all circumstances; about 41% of all procedures worldwide are illegal (WHO 2004). Those who live in extreme poverty are least likely to get a safe clandestine procedure performed by a physician under sanitary conditions. Those who are both poor and living in rural areas, without access to hospital care for the complications that may follow an abortion using crude procedures in unsanitary conditions, are at high risk of death.

England liberalized its abortion law in 1967, an action followed by many countries that had inherited English legal and parliamentary procedures. The US Supreme Court ruled in 1973 that restrictive state abortion laws were unconstitutional, thereby legalizing abortion throughout the country. As in other countries, decriminalization of abortion led to an initial increase in abortion rates that subsequently declined as contraceptive practice improved. The public health gains realized through reducing mortality and morbidity far exceed any demographic effect associated with a temporary reduction in the number of births. Evidence points to a strong correlation between less-restrictive abortion laws and policies, safer abortion, and lower maternal mortality. When Romania recriminalized abortion and banned contraceptives in 1966, maternal deaths soared, but after the procedure was legalized again in 1990, they fell sharply down from 159 to 83 deaths/100,000 live births within a year and continued to fall thereafter. This fall coincided with a rapid gain in contraceptive use as access to modern contraceptives improved. Hospital admissions for septic and incomplete abortion also fell sharply after South Africa legalized abortion in 1997.

Access to abortion is further conditioned by the actual implementation of laws and by societal and cultural views on sexuality and reproduction. In nearly all Latin American countries, abortion is only permitted in the event of a threat to a woman's life and is generally severely stigmatized, yet safe abortion services are readily accessible for those able to pay for them. In India, which closely followed the United Kingdom in allowing abortion on public health grounds, many women are driven to clandestine procedures, often performed by untrained persons in unhygienic conditions at sites other than registered government institutions. This is because women are not aware of the legal status of abortion and because services are insufficient to meet the demand. Service availability in rural areas remains largely limited to community health centers and rural hospitals, with few providers in primary health centers. Consequently, India has more abortion-related deaths than any other country. India's experience shows that legal abortion does not guarantee safety in an environment where broad access to services under sanitary conditions is impeded or where providers are not trained.

Abortion-Related Mortality and Morbidity

Each year, about 19 million women undergo unsafe abortions; 18.4 million of these women live in the economically less-developed countries and the rest live primarily in Eastern Europe (Table 11.1). One third of these women will suffer serious complications, but fewer than half will obtain the hospital treatment they need. About 68,000 deaths can be attributed to unsafe abortion, and still others to spontaneous abortion. If no new actions are taken, almost 100 million women alive today will experience the risk and trauma of an unsafe abortion during their lifetimes. Younger women are most affected, as two of every three unsafe abortions are experienced by 15–30-year-olds and one in seven, occur among women below age 20.

In parts of sub-Saharan Africa, perhaps one in three maternal deaths is due to abortion. African women experience the greatest risk of death from unsafe abortions, with a ratio of 1 in 150 compared to Asia's 1 in 250, Latin America's 1 in 800, and Northern countries' 1 in 3,700 (WHO 2004). Complications of spontaneous and induced abortion include sepsis, hemorrhage, toxic shock, damage to internal organs, and long-term conditions such as chronic pelvic pain and infertility. The consequences are especially serious for poor, young, and uneducated women. In many African countries, nonmarital adolescent pregnancies lead to expulsion from school, abandonment by the family, and sharply diminished life chances. Many such women will seek an abortion as a way out, but all too often lack the resources to obtain a safe abortion. In cultures where a woman's status still depends on her ability to give birth to many children, infertility arising from pregnancy termination may be devastating.

Morbidity from unsafe abortion is a huge public health problem. For decades, complications of illegal

Table 11.1 Global and regional estimates of incidence and mortality due to unsafe abortions

Region	Number of safe abortions (1,000s)	Unsafe abortions per 1,000 women aged 15–44	Number of deaths from unsafe abortions	Mortality from unsafe abortions per 100,000 live births	Percent of maternal deaths
World total	19,000	14	67,900	50	13
"More" developed countries	500	2	300	3	14
"Less" developed countries	18,400	16	67,500	60	13
Africa	42,000	24	29,800	100	12
Asia †	10,500	13	34,000	40	13
Europe	500	3	300	5	20
Latin America*	3,700	29	3,700	30	17
Oceana †	30	17	<100	20	7

†Excludes Australia, Japan, and New Zealand, although these countries are included in the total for developed countries
*Includes Caribbean states
Source: WHO (2004). Note that figures may not add to totals due to rounding

and unsafe abortion have been known to take up most maternity beds and obstetrics and gynecology budgets at the large urban hospitals of many developing countries. The cost of providing safe abortion services would be many times lower. Moreover, many women will not seek treatment, leading to lifelong suffering. Abortion-related mortality and morbidity are preventable. The glaring disparity between rich and poor countries in terms of abortion-related mortality and morbidity shows that it is the circumstances in which abortion takes place, including the presence or absence of legal and safe abortion care that determines the health consequences for women, rather than an abortion per se.

In more affluent countries that provide good access to safe abortion services, the procedure is far less likely than an injection of penicillin to cause death. Abortion is considerably safer than carrying a pregnancy to term (Cates et al. 2003). Although it is often asserted by those opposed to abortion that the procedure may be dangerous to other aspects of women's health, the body of accumulated evidence indicates that there is no link between abortion and breast cancer. There is no evidence to suggest a causal relationship between abortion and mental health problems. Any psychological impacts are likely associated with having an unwanted pregnancy to begin with or, if present, may be due to factors unrelated to either the pregnancy or abortion, such as being in an abusive relationship. This was acknowledged by former US

Surgeon General C. Everett Koop, a vocal opponent of abortion whose office spent 15 months reviewing all published studies on the topic (Kulczycki 1999). Evidence also indicates that abortion does not affect women's future fertility and birth outcomes, assuming it is performed safely.

Demography of Abortion

Estimates derived from a range of demographic techniques and pooled from an array of sources suggest that each year, approximately 46 million abortions occur worldwide (WHO 2004). Put another way, about one in four pregnancies end in abortion. While the incidence, distribution, and quality of abortions vary, there is no country in which abortion does not occur. The incidence of abortion is only known in detail for those countries in which abortion is legally permitted with few restrictions and the number of procedures is counted with a strong degree of completeness by an official government department. For many years, the lowest abortion rates in the world have been in the Netherlands, Belgium, and Scandinavia, now joined by Germany. These countries have some of the world's most liberal abortion laws, with services legal, free, and widely available; they also have a culture of contraceptive responsibility. In the United States, 1.3 million abortions occurred in 2002 and each year, 2 out of every 100 women aged 15–44 have an abortion. At the current rate, over one third of US women will have had an abortion by the time they reach age 45. These levels are higher than anywhere in Western Europe, Australia, or New Zealand, where contraceptive practice is more widespread and effective. The highest abortion rates in the world are found in many former Soviet Bloc republics. A 1999 survey documented that in Georgia, a woman would have about 3.7 abortions during her lifetime (Westoff 2005). A follow-up survey in 2005 indicated that the abortion rate had declined by 16%, but at 3.1 abortions per woman, it is still high even by regional standards.

The incidence of abortion is primarily a function of the incidence of unintended pregnancy rather than of the legal status of abortion. Unintended pregnancies are those not wanted at the time conception occurred, regardless of whether or not contraception was being used. Unintended pregnancy is a function of the level of sexual activity, the age at which women marry, desired family size, and contraceptive knowledge and use. It follows that abortion rates will be higher where desired family size and effective contraceptive use are low, regardless of the legal status of abortion, or cultural and religious sanctions against the practice. Thus, compared to Western Europe, abortion rates tend to be several times higher in Latin America and the Caribbean, in many sub-Saharan African countries, and in many Asian countries where contraceptive prevalence is low and abortion is heavily restricted. The US abortion rate is higher than that found in other Western nations because 49% of pregnancies are unintended, and about half of which are aborted.

A major cause of unintended pregnancy is lack of use or access to contraceptives. In the economically less-developed countries, over half of all sexually active women are at risk of an unintended pregnancy because they are using no contraceptive method at all, they are using a traditional method with high failure rates, or they are using a reversible method that demands regular resupply. However, even widespread modern contraceptive use will not entirely eliminate the need for recourse to abortion because no contraceptive works perfectly every time.

As fertility preferences fall, there is initially an increase in both contraceptive use and abortion. Evidence from a diverse set of countries shows that over time, abortion rates fall as levels of contraceptive use rise. In South Korea, average family size fell by over half between the 1960s and 1980s. Both contraceptive prevalence and abortion rates increased alongside the sharp decrease in desired family size. After some 20 years, the birth rate began to stabilize, the abortion rate plateaued, and contraceptive prevalence continued to rise (Marston and Cleland 2003). Russia has historically had one of the world's highest abortion rates, largely due to the poor accessibility and quality of the limited available contraceptive options, and the ready availability of abortion (legalized in 1955). Sexually active women tended to rely more on abortion rather than contraception to limit their family size. Many Russian women who wanted only two children had multiple abortions in their lifetimes, and as late as 1990, the abortion rate was well over 100 per 1,000 women of childbearing age. The situation finally changed in the early 1990s when the government began to promote contraceptive use. Family planning programs started to be subsidized, free contraceptives were distributed, and free market reforms opened the door to better quality, foreign-made modern contraceptives. As a result, modern contraceptive use experienced an 80% increase over 1988–1998, while the abortion rate fell by 53%.

Why Do Women Have Abortions?

Women have abortions for many reasons. Most women who terminate their pregnancies do so because doing otherwise would limit their ability to meet their current responsibilities and because they cannot afford the index child at that time. Even if it is dangerous or forbidden, many women will resort to abortion in order to protect their family from poverty or to conceal an illegitimate pregnancy where it is stigmatized. When asked for their reasons to have an abortion, 74% of recent US abortion patients cited concern for or responsibility to other individuals. Almost as many (73%) said they could not afford a baby then. In addition, 69% said that having a baby would interfere with their education, employment, or ability to care for dependents; almost half said they were having relationship problems or would have to raise the child as a single parent; and 38% did not wish to have another child because they had already completed their childbearing (Finer et al. 2005).

Characteristics of Women Who Obtain Abortions

Both unintended pregnancy and abortion rates are higher among some groups of women. These typically include women under age 30 (especially those aged 20–24), unmarried women, those in poverty, and those with more disadvantaged racial/ethnic minority status. In the United States, women in their 20s account for over half of abortions and almost two-thirds of all abortions are to never-married women. Women living below the federal poverty level are four times as likely to have an abortion as women living above 300% of the poverty level (44 vs. 10 per 1,000 women). US Hispanic and Asian women have slightly higher than average abortion rates, and Afro-American women are over twice as likely as women overall to have an abortion. Thus, 5% of Afro-American women have an abortion each year, compared to 3% of Hispanic women, 3% of Asian women, and 1% of Caucasian women. The abortion rate for Protestant women is slightly lower than for Catholic women (18 vs. 22 per 1,000), and for both groups it is lower than for those who do not identify with any religion (30 per 1,000).

It is often assumed that women who have abortions and women who have children are different, but in fact, they are the same women, at different points in their lives. In the United States, 6 in 10 women who have an abortion are already a parent (Jones et al. 2002) and over half of women who have an abortion intend to have children or more children in the future. These findings also indicate that most women who choose to have an abortion do so because they feel unable in their current circumstances to fulfill their parental responsibilities as they would like, or to provide the kind of

family support they believe their children deserve. With improved availability and new technologies for performing abortions, including medication abortion and vacuum aspiration with ultrasound, women are increasingly able to obtain an early-term abortion when it is safer and less traumatic. Within the United States, nine out of ten of all abortions are performed at or before 12 weeks' gestation, and three in five abortions occur at or before eight weeks' gestation. The proportion carried out at or before 6 weeks' gestation increased from 14% of all abortions in 1992 to 25% in 2001. Less than 1% of women who have had an abortion did so at, or after 21 weeks' gestation (Jones et al. 2002).

New Technologies and Earlier Abortion

Orthodox surgical methods of abortion include use of transcervical procedures such as vacuum aspiration, manual vacuum aspiration (MVA), and dilatation and curettage (D&C). Vacuum aspiration uses a plastic cannula or tube attached to either a hand-held vacuum syringe (MVA) or to an electric pump so as to evacuate the contents of the uterus. Although D&C is less safe, it remains widely used in developing countries. Medical methods involve the use of pharmacological drugs which are limited to nine weeks' gestation. Other technological improvements, including increased use of highly sensitive at-home urine pregnancy tests and the use of transvaginal ultrasonography, have also enabled a shift toward earlier abortions, which reduce the risk of complications.

Mifepristone remains limited to high-income countries where abortion is legal. It permits an alternative to surgical abortion in the first 9 weeks of pregnancy and is given under the supervision of a physician with the resulting abortion completed in the privacy of one's own home. Mifepristone, more commonly referred to as the abortion pill or by its earlier acronym, RU-486, was first approved in France in 1988 and then in other countries. A decade later, it accounted for over half of eligible early abortions in France, Scotland, and Sweden. With this new medication, a higher fraction of European women are now having abortions at or before 9 weeks than did so before the drug's introduction, which has not been associated with any increase in the overall abortion rate. In the United States, use of mifepristone has steadily increased since the drug's approval in 2000, but mostly at sites that also provide surgical abortion. Integration of the procedure into the health-care system has been slow.

Postabortion Care

Postabortion care (PAC) is a critical health-care service that can save women's lives in settings where abortion is performed unsafely. At minimum, PAC services should provide treatment for complications of spontaneous or induced abortion and strengthened family planning counseling and contraceptive method provision, both immediately after a procedure and in subsequent follow-up, to prevent unintended pregnancies that can lead to repeat abortions. Attempts to institute PAC services only gained momentum in the wake of the 1994 Cairo conference. International health organizations and donors then began providing technical and financial support for PAC programs. Several PAC models were introduced with links slowly developed between emergency abortion treatment services and comprehensive reproductive health care, focused primarily on clinical and related facility-based services from a health-care provider perspective. Attention was given to improving both technical competence in medical treatment of incomplete abortion and interpersonal communication with patients (Winkler et al. 1995). This also led to an increased stress on the holistic treatment of the patient as opposed to improving a single aspect of services, such as the use of MVA instruments.

Current best practices in PAC programming, like those in safe motherhood programming, show the importance of minimizing delays in receiving care. At the facility level, at least three types of services are needed. These include emergency treatment of postabortion complications, counseling on PAC treatment and family planning, including direct provision of contraceptives or referral, and referral for other reproductive health services. These might include, for example, STI/HIV prevention

education, screening, diagnosis, treatment, screening for sexual and/or domestic violence (with treatment as needed), and referral for medical, social, and economic services and support. Effective contraceptive methods should be initiated immediately postabortion or no later than 7 days, in order to prevent another unwanted pregnancy. Primary care facilities with limited health-care capacity can stabilize and refer clients with postabortion complications to hospitals for treatment, provide referrals for reproductive and other health services to other accessible facilities in providers' networks, and serve as a site for follow-up and provision of family planning counseling and methods to better space or prevent subsequent pregnancies.

International health organizations providing PAC assistance emphasize MVA as the preferred procedure for treating incomplete abortions. Although D&C is still widely used by hospitals in many countries for uterine evacuation, it requires general anesthesia and therefore a longer hospital stay, and is more costly. MVA is safer, less expensive, and can be performed effectively in low-resource settings. It can be provided using local anesthesia, enabling clients to safely leave the hospital within hours. Turkey and several Latin American countries have succeeded in institutionalizing the provision of the main elements of PAC (Billings and Benson 2005; Senlet et al. 2001). But in general, PAC programs have rarely been scaled up throughout the national health system and few postabortion care pilot projects have been expanded successfully. Numerous obstacles are frequently encountered in program implementation, typically due to political rather than technical reasons. In many countries, the political and cultural sensitivity of abortion makes even PAC programs vulnerable to political changes and charges, inadequate funding, and changes in hospital personnel. Since 2001, the U S government has instituted a "Global Gag Rule" that restricts non-governmental organizations (NGOs) in poor countries that receive USAID family planning funding from engaging in abortion-related activities, even with their own funds. This policy has prevented institutionalization of PAC services. Moreover, it has almost certainly increased the number of abortions through its disruption of family planning services.

Where emergency treatment for postabortion complications has been provided, it has traditionally been without family planning, counseling, and often contraceptive methods are not available on the OB/GYN ward where PAC services are provided. Integration between such services is often lacking because many family planning clinics in hospitals may be closed when women are discharged from the hospital after receiving treatment in a 24-h emergency setting. The development of integrated postabortion services within a family planning and reproductive health-care program has also been impeded in many countries by women's low socioeconomic status and normative restrictions on abortion. All these obstacles conspire to make the health-care concerns of women who need PAC care a low priority for governments and for many medical professionals. Additionally, legal and administrative constraints may force women to seek clandestine procedures from providers who cannot offer related reproductive health-care services.

The international health community has only recently begun to address some of the many sociocultural barriers that prevent women from seeking PAC services. For example, women may delay seeking care or not seek care at all if they are not the main family decision makers and cannot seek services autonomously, or if they do not recognize the urgency of a situation of postabortion complications. Facilities may also discriminate against PAC clients due to the stigma attached to abortion. Such barriers could be potentially reduced through working at the community level. An expanded and updated "Essential Elements of PAC" model has been proposed by family planning and reproductive health agencies, NGOs and donors (Post-abortion Care Consortium 2002). This adds the community and counseling as essential elements (Table 11.2).

Partnerships are increasingly emphasized with community members, community health workers, and formally trained service providers to improve and ensure the accessibility, acceptability, and use of quality PAC services. Under this model, counseling is not limited to family planning and contraceptive education and services. Rather, it should cover the full range of reproductive health, and other health and emotional needs, and concerns that arise for women in these circumstances. The revised PAC model has been extended in practice by the CATALYST Consortium of reproductive health and family planning agencies initiated by the US Agency for International Development (USAID). There are three core components to this promising initiative: (1) emergency treatment, (2) family planning counseling and provision, STI evaluation and treatment, and HIV counseling and/or referral for testing, and (3) community empowerment through community awareness and mobilization. Since 2003, CATALYST programs have been implemented and successfully scaled-up in Bolivia, Egypt and Peru (CATALYST

Table 11. 2 Essential elements of postabortion care

Community and service provider partnerships
- Prevent unwanted pregnancies and unsafe abortion
- Mobilize resources to help women receive appropriate and timely care for complications from abortion
- Ensure that health services reflect and meet community expectations and needs

Counseling
- Identify and respond to women's emotional and physical health needs and other concerns

Treatment
- Treat incomplete and unsafe abortions and potentially life-threatening complications

Contraceptive and family planning services
- Help women practice birth spacing or prevent an unwanted pregnancy

Reproductive and other health services
- Preferably provided on-site to ensure women's needs are met, or via referrals to other accessible facilities in providers' networks

Source: Postabortion Care Consortium (2002)

Consortium 2005). Several common elements have been identified:

(1) Provision of PAC training tailored to the type of facility in which the provider works and sensitizing providers to the situations of women who experience complications of abortion. For example, providers at primary care facilities were trained to recognize danger signs, stabilize, and refer clients to a higher level facility for emergency treatment. These providers were also trained to provide follow-up care, including family planning counseling and contraceptive methods to PAC clients.

(2) Community mobilization at all sites, whereby community participants (women, men, and adolescents) were provided with the tools and technical support needed to identify community problems and resources related to PAC, to develop and implement action plans, and to collaborate with local hospital authorities, in order to increase knowledge of, access to, and quality of PAC services. Community awareness sessions included, for example, disseminating information about safe behaviors for preventing unintended pregnancies, seeking immediate care in the event of complications of abortion and waiting at least 6 months before getting pregnant again. Community leaders and organizations were also engaged in this effort and communities involved in ongoing monitoring and evaluation.

(3) Creation and maintenance of a supportive policy environment at local, regional, and national levels, to facilitate integration of PAC services.

These steps have helped ensure political commitment and community empowerment, with transfer of responsibility to local communities and local governments. They are also facilitating program sustainability and scale-up. In Bolivia and Peru, community members additionally identified gender-based violence as an important cause of unintended pregnancy, miscarriage and induced abortion, underscoring the need to address another neglected community health problem. The CATALYST Consortium has also started to help local NGOs in Romania, Nepal, and Cambodia to identify community needs regarding PAC and to provide solutions that are socially and culturally adapted to their specific situations. The goal is to build awareness of PAC issues among communities and stakeholders and improve provider skills and PAC programming at all levels of facilities. By expanding from facility-based, clinical services to a more comprehensive public health model, PAC programs are increasingly providing prevention, treatment, counseling, and services to respond to women's reproductive health needs and concerns following an incomplete or unsafe abortion.

Conclusion

Abortion is an essential aspect of fertility regulation. Pregnancy is not always planned or welcomed, an awkward truth for some workers and researchers in the MCH field, as well as public health practitioners and policymakers. Some women conceive when they do not want to and pregnancy is not always trouble-free. Programs must address such problems. The role of improved contraceptive practice, particularly the use of more effective, long-acting methods, is critical to reducing the incidence of abortion. New technologies allow women to obtain earlier and safer, abortions. Laws and policies should reflect health concerns and access to safe abortion services. Laws and policies can be improved by decreasing the administrative obstacles to legal services (abortions performed under the indications allowed by a country's law) and by increasing the availability of legal services for safe abortion in public sector facilities.

Morbidity and mortality due to unsafe abortion continue to pose a serious global threat to women's health and lives. The costs of treating these complications are a major economic burden on limited health-care budgets, particularly in resource-poor settings. PAC programs are being implemented in a growing number of countries and increasingly recognize the need to build partnerships with communities. In addition to providing treatment for incomplete and unsafe abortion, such programs increasingly stress a continuum of postabortion care. Much more work is needed in this vital area to prevent unsafe abortion, reduce morbidity and mortality from incomplete and unsafe abortion, and improve the lives of women and their families.

Key Terms

Abortion	Fourth World Conference on	Miscarriage
Abortion-related mortality and	Women	Postabortion care
morbidity	Hemorrhage	Postabortion care consortium
Birth control	Illegal abortion	Pregnancy termination
CATALYST Consortium	Infertility	Safe motherhood
Chronic pelvic pain	International Conference on	Self-induced abortion
Contraceptive knowledge	Population and	Sepsis
Contraceptive responsibility	Development	Spontaneous abortion
Contraceptive use	Late-stage abortion	Toxic shock
Dilatation and curettage	Manual vacuum aspiration	Unintended pregnancy
(D&C)	(MVA)	Unsafe abortion
Family planning counseling	Maternal death	
Fetus	Mifepristone	

Questions for Discussion

1 Briefly summarize the reasons why women have abortion.
2 What factors account for the disparity in abortion-related morbidity and mortality between rich and poor countries?
3 Historical and contemporary evidence shows that outlawing abortion does not eliminate or reduce its incidence. Using specific country examples, discuss why this is the case.
4 Evidence shows that there is a strong correlation between less-restrictive abortion laws and policies, safer abortion, and low maternal mortality. However, experts say that for many less-developed countries, legalization of abortion may not guarantee safe abortion. Explain the rationale for this observation.
5 List the three elements of an effective postabortion care model. What factors hinder the implementation of effective postabortion services in less-developed countries?

References

Billings DL, Benson J (2005) Post-abortion care in Latin America: policy and service recommendations from a decade of operations research. Health Policy and Planning, 20(3): 158–166

CATALYST Consortium (2005) PAC Compilation Document. www.pathfind.org/site/DocServer/PAC_Compilation_Document.pdf?docID = 5585 Cited 2 August 2008

Cates W, Grimes DA, Schulz KF (2003) The public health impact of legal abortion: 30 years later. Perspectives on Sexual and Reproductive Health, 35(1): 25–28

Finer LB, Frohwirth LF, Dauphinee LA et al. (2005) Reasons U.S. women have abortions: quantitative and qualitative perspectives. Perspectives in Sexual and Reproductive Health, 37(3): 110–118

Jones RK, Darroch JE, Henshaw SK (2002) Patterns in the socioeconomic characteristics of women obtaining abortions in 2000–20001. Perspectives on Sexual and Reproductive Health, 34(5): 226–235

Kulczycki A (1999) The Abortion Debate in the World Arena. London: Macmillan and New York: Routledge

Marston C, Cleland J (2003) Relationships between contraception and abortion: a review of the evidence. International Family Planning Perspectives, 29(1): 6–13

Postabortion Care Consortium (2002) Essential elements of postabortion care: an expanded and updated model. Postabortion Care Consortium, PAC in Action, no. 2, special supplement. www.pac-consortium.org/site/PageServer? pagename = PAC_Model Cited 2 August 2008

Senlet P, Cagatay L, Ergin J et al. (2001) Bridging the gap: integrating family planning with abortion services in Turkey. International Family Planning Perspectives, 27(2): 90–95

United Nations (2002) Abortion Policies: A Global Review. Vols. 1–3. New York: United Nations

Westoff, C (2005) Recent Trends in Abortion and Contraception in 12 Countries. DHS Analytical Studies no. 8. Calverton, MD: ORC Macro

Winkler J, Oliveras E, McIntosh N (eds.) (1995) Postabortion Care: A Reference Manual for Improving Quality of Care. Baltimore, MD: Postabortion Care Consortium

World Health Organization (WHO) (2003) Safe Abortion: Technical and Policy Guidance for Health Systems. Geneva: World Health Organization

World Health Organization (WHO) (2004) Unsafe Abortion: Global and Regional Estimates of the Incidence of Unsafe Abortion and Associated Mortality in 2000, 4th ed. Geneva: World Health Organization

Part III
Specific Disease Concerns

Chapter 12
Malaria in Women and Children

Martin Meremikwu, Emmanuel Ezedinachi and John E. Ehiri

Learning Objectives After reading this chapter and answering the discussion questions that follow, you should be able to

- Explain the global burden of malaria, discuss its clinical manifestations, and appraise its health impact on women and children.
- Analyze the mechanisms and consequences of malaria and HIV co-infection and discuss current treatment, control and prevention strategies.
- Describe the challenges posed by vector resistance to insecticides, parasite resistance to antimalarials, climate change, wars/conflicts, and HIV/AIDS to malaria control and prevention efforts.
- Evaluate social, cultural, and economic limitations of community-based programs for malaria control and prevention.

Introduction

Malaria is caused by *Plasmodium*, a protozoan parasite transmitted through the bite of infected female anopheline mosquitoes. The four species of *Plasmodium* known to cause malaria in humans are *P. falciparum, P. malariae, P. ovale*, and *P. vivax*. *Plasmodium falciparum* is the most virulent of these species and is responsible for most cases of malaria infections and malaria deaths in sub-Saharan Africa. *Plasmodium vivax*, the second most common species of the malaria parasite, is more

prevalent in Asia and is rarely associated with acute complications of malaria or fatality. Box 12.1 presents definitions of some of the most commonly used terms in malaria epidemiology.

Figure 12.1 shows the global distribution of malaria transmission risk. Malaria transmission occurs in Africa, Asia, and the Americas, but sub-Saharan Africa bears over 80% of the global burden of malaria mortality (Ehiri et al. 2004). Malaria is still a major public health problem in parts of Southeast Asia with foci of high *P. falciparum* transmission and high incidence of multidrug resistance.

More than 40 species of *Anopheles* mosquitoes transmit malaria. *Anopheles gambiae*, which is the most efficient and resilient vector, is the predominant vector in most parts of tropical Africa, where it finds adequate rainfall, temperature, and humidity to support its breeding. Figure 12.2 provides an illustration of the life cycle of *Plasmodium* in the human and in the mosquito vector.

Spleen rates (percentage of the population with palpably enlarged spleen at any given time) and parasite rates (percentage of the population with malaria parasites in peripheral blood film at any given time) are traditionally used as malariometric indices to determine whether or not malaria is endemic in a given area. The entomologic inoculation rate (EIR) is believed to be a better measure of malaria transmission and risk of infection than spleen or parasite rates. However, it is more difficult to assess. EIR is the product of human biting rates (the number of mosquitoes biting a person over a given period of time) and the sporozoite rate (the proportion of vectors with sporozoites in the salivary glands) (Snow et al. 2004).

M. Meremikwu (✉)
Department of Pediatrics Institute for Tropical Disease Reasearch, University of Calabar, Calabar, Cross River State, Nigeria

Box 12.1 Definition of Terms

Anemia: A reduction in the number of circulating red blood cells or in the quantity of hemoglobin.

Anopheles: A genus of mosquito, some species of which can transmit human malaria.

Artemisinin: A drug used against malaria, derived from the Qinghao plant, *Artemisia annua* L.

Cerebral Malaria: A complication of *Plasmodium falciparum* malaria in which infected red blood cells obstruct blood circulation in the small blood vessels in the brain. When cerebral malaria is present, the disease is classified as severe malaria.

Chemoprophylaxis: Taking antimalarial drugs to prevent the disease.

Chloroquine: A drug used against malaria. A very safe and inexpensive drug, its value has been compromised by the emergence of chloroquine-resistant malaria parasites.

Drug Resistance: Drug resistance is the result of microbes changing in ways that reduce or eliminate the effectiveness of drugs, chemicals, or other agents to cure or prevent infections.

Endemic Malaria: Constant incidence over a period of many successive years in an area.

Epidemic: The occurrence of more cases of disease than expected in a given area or among a specific group of people over a particular period of time.

Erythrocyte: A red blood cell.

Erythrocytic Stage: A stage in the life cycle of the malaria parasite found in the red blood cells. Erythrocytic stage parasites cause the symptoms of malaria.

Gametocyte: The sexual stage of malaria parasites. Male gametocytes (microgametocytes) and female gametocytes (macrogametocytes) are inside red blood cells in the circulation. If they are ingested by a female *Anopheles* mosquito, they undergo sexual reproduction which starts the extrinsic (sporogonic) cycle of the parasite in the mosquito. Gametocytes of *Plasmodium falciparum* are typically banana- or crescent-shaped (from the latin falcis = sickle).

Hemoglobin: The red, oxygen-carrying protein found in red blood cells.

Hemolysis: Destruction of red blood cells. Malaria causes hemolysis when the parasites rupture the red blood cells in which they have grown.

Hyperreactive Malarial Splenomegaly (also called "tropical splenomegaly syndrome"): occurs infrequently and is attributed to an abnormal immune response to repeated malarial infections. The disease is marked by a very enlarged spleen and liver, anemia, and a susceptibility to other infections (such as skin or respiratory infections).

Hypoglycemia: Low blood glucose. Hypoglycemia can occur in malaria. In addition, treatment with quinine and quinidine stimulate insulin secretion, reducing blood glucose.

Immunity: Protection generated by the body's immune system, in response to previous malaria attacks, resulting in ability to control or lessen a malaria attack.

Leukocyte: White blood cell.

Lymphocyte: Leukocyte with a large round nucleus and usually a small cytoplasm. Specialized types of lymphocytes have enlarged cytoplasms and produce antibodies.

Merozoites: A daughter cell formed by asexual development in the life cycle of malaria parasites. Liver stage and blood stage malaria parasites develop into schizonts which contain many merozoites. When the schizonts are mature, they (and their host cells) rupture; the merozoites are released and infect red blood cells.

Monocyte: Leukocyte with a large, usually kidney-shaped nucleus. Within tissues, monocytes develop into macrophages which ingest bacteria, dead cells, and other debris.

Oocyst: A stage in the life cycle of malaria parasites, oocysts are rounded cysts located in the outer wall of the stomach of mosquitoes. Sporozoites develop inside the oocysts. When mature, the oocysts rupture and release the sporozoites, which then migrate into the mosquito's salivary glands, ready for injection into the human host.

Parasitemia: The presence of parasites in the blood. The term can also be used to express the quantity of parasites in the blood (e.g., 'a parasitemia of 2%").

Phagocyte: A type of white blood cell that can engulf and destroy foreign organisms, cells and particles.

Platelets: Small, irregularly-shaped bodies in the blood that contain granules. These cells are important components of the blood coagulation (clotting) system.

Presumptive Treatment: Treatment of clinically suspected cases without, or prior to, results from confirmatory laboratory tests.

Protozoan: Single-celled organism that can perform all necessary functions of metabolism and reproduction. Some protozoa are free-living, while others, including malaria parasites, parasitize other organisms for their nutrients and life cycle.

Residual insecticide spraying: Treatment of houses by spraying insecticides that have residual efficacy (i.e., that continue to affect mosquitoes for several months). Residual insecticide spraying aims to kills mosquitoes when they come to rest on the walls, usually after a blood meal.

Resistance: The ability of an organism to develop strains that are impervious to specific threats to their existence.

Schizogony: Asexual reproductive stage of malaria parasites. In red blood cells, schizogony entails development of a single trophozoite into numerous merozoites. A similar process happens in infected liver cells.

Schizont: A developmental form of the malaria parasite that contains many merozoites. Schizonts are seen in the liver-stage and blood-stage parasites.

Sequelae: Morbid conditions following as a consequence of a disease.

Severe Malaria: occurs when *P. falciparum* infections (often in persons who have no immunity to malaria or whose immunity has decreased) are complicated by serious organ failures or abnormalities in the patient's blood or metabolism, resulting in cerebral malaria, with abnormal behavior, impairment of consciousness, seizures, coma, or other neurologic abnormalities, severe anemia due to hemolysis (destruction of the red blood cells), hemoglobinuria (hemoglobin in the urine) due to hemolysis, pulmonary edema (fluid buildup in the lungs) or acute respiratory distress syndrome (ARDS), which may occur even after the parasite counts have decreased in response to treatment, abnormalities in blood coagulation and thrombocytopenia (decrease in blood platelets), cardiovascular collapse, shock, acute kidney failure, hyperparasitemia, where more than 5% of the red blood cells are infected by malaria parasites, metabolic acidosis (excessive acidity in the blood and tissue fluids), often in association with hypoglycemia (low blood glucose).

Splenomegaly: Enlargement of the spleen, found in some malaria patients. Splenomegaly can be used to measure malaria endemicity during surveys (e.g., in communities or in school children).

Sporozoite Rate: The proportion of female anopheline mosquitoes of a particular species that have sporozoites in their salivary glands (as seen by dissection), or that are positive in immunologic tests to detect sporozoite antigens.

Sporozoite: A stage in the life cycle of the malaria parasite. Sporozoites are produced in the mosquito and migrate to the mosquito's salivary glands. They can be inoculated into a human host when the mosquito takes a blood meal on the human. In the human, the sporozoites enter liver cells where they develop into the next stage of the malaria parasite life cycle (the liver stage or exo-erythrocytic stage).

Stable Malaria: A situation where the rate of malaria transmission is high without any marked fluctuation over years though seasonal fluctuations occur.

Strain: A genetic variant within a species.

Sulfadoxine–pyrimethamine: A drug used against malaria.

Trophozoite: A developmental form during the blood stage of malaria parasites. After merozoites have invaded the red blood cell, they develop into trophozoites (sometimes, early trophozoites are called "rings" or "ring stage parasites"); trophozoites develop into schizonts.

Uncomplicated Malaria: The classical, (but rarely observed) uncomplicated malaria attack that lasts 6–10 hours. It consists of a cold stage (sensation of cold, shivering), a hot stage (fever, headaches, vomiting, seizures in young children), and finally a sweating stage (sweats, return to normal temperature, tiredness).

The classical (but infrequently observed) uncomplicated malaria attacks occur every second day with the "tertian" parasites (*P. falciparum*, *P. vivax*, and *P. ovale*) and every third day with the "quartan" parasite (*P. malariae*). More commonly, the patient presents with a combination of symptoms that include fever, chills, sweats, headaches, nausea and vomiting, body aches, general malaise.

Unstable Malaria: A situation where the rate of malaria transmission changes from year to year.

Vaccine: A preparation that stimulates an immune response that can prevent an infection or create resistance to an infection.

Vector: An organism (e.g., *Anopheles* mosquitoes) that transmits an infectious agent (e.g. malaria parasites) from one host to the other (e.g., humans).

Source: Malaria Glossary – Centers for Disease Control and prevention
http://www.cdc.gov/malaria/glossary.htm

Malaria transmission can be perennial (occurring throughout the year), high, intense, and/or stable, low, unstable, and seasonal. High stable transmission of mostly *P. falciparum* associated with high incidence of severe illness and mortality among preschool children is the predominant pattern of malaria in most of sub-Saharan Africa. The average malaria incidence rates across several parts of Africa with high transmission are estimated at 1.4 per persons per year, 0.59 per persons per year, and 0.11 persons per year for age groups <5 years, 5–14 years, and ≥15 years, respectively (Snow et al. 2003). In low transmission areas, incidence rates of malaria are much lower, and differ only marginally between the young and older age groups. Malaria epidemics are more likely to occur in areas with seasonal and unstable transmission.

Burden of Malaria

Figure 12.3 illustrates the various pathways by which malaria contributes to poverty, under-development, malnutrition, and maternal and infant mortality. Some 300–500 million malaria episodes occur annually. Children under 5 years of age in sub-Saharan Africa and women who are pregnant for the first or second time bear the heaviest burden of malaria morbidity and mortality. An estimated 250 million episodes of clinical malaria occur in young sub-Saharan African children annually. About 1 million cases are cerebral malaria, 4 million cases are severe anemia, and approximately 1 million result in death. Estimates of malaria mortality show wide variation. A review of the literature on this subject shows that the number of deaths due to malaria in African children aged less than 5 years

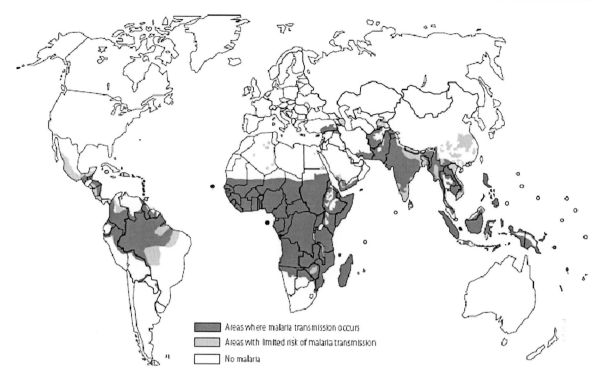

Fig. 12.1 Global distribution of malaria transmission risk, 2003. Source: WHO (2007)

could be between 625,000 and 1,824,000 annually (Breman et al. 2004).

About 250,000 of those that survive develop sequelae from neurological complications of *P. falciparum* malaria. Pregnant women are more vulnerable to adverse consequences of malaria than other adults. An estimated 10 million infections occur in pregnant women annually, resulting in 500,000 cases of severe maternal anemia and 500,000 low birth weight babies (Greenwood et al. 2005). In malaria-endemic countries of Africa, up to 40% of all outpatient clinic visits and between 20 and 50% of all hospital admissions are due to malaria (WHO 2003). Although the incidence of uncomplicated malaria is lower in adolescents aged 10–19 years than younger school aged and preschool children, the burden of malaria in this age group could be substantial in areas with high and stable transmission. A recent review of the epidemiology and pattern of malaria in adolescents estimates the clinical malaria rate in African adolescents aged 10–20

years to be 0.252 attacks per adolescent per year (Lalloo et al. 2006). Results of analyses based on rainfall and temperature data and geographic information system (GIS) population databases in areas with high and stable malaria transmission put the yearly estimate of the number of malaria attacks in children aged 0–4 years, 5–9 years, and 10–14 years at 81.3 million, 16.0 million, and 13.4 million, respectively.

Clinical Manifestation of Malaria

The clinical pattern and deleterious consequences of malaria infection vary, depending on the level of acquired malaria immunity of the individual and the pattern of malaria transmission in an area. In areas with high and stable malaria transmission, resident adults and older children acquire sufficient partial immunity to reduce the

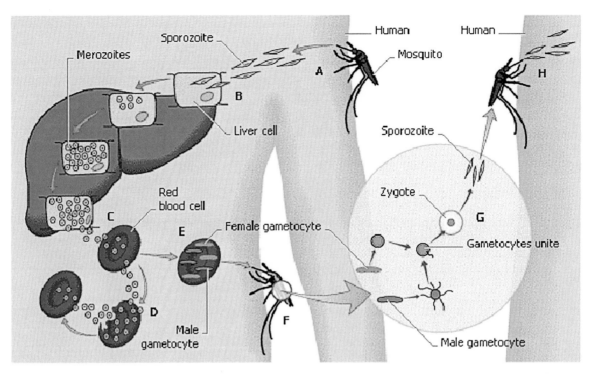

Fig. 12.2: Life cycle of *Plasmodium* parasite. Key: (**A**) Mosquito infected with the malaria parasite bites human, passing cells called sporozoites into the human's bloodstream. (**B**) Sporozoites travel to the liver. Each sporozoite undergoes asexual reproduction, in which its nucleus splits to form two new cells called merozoites. (**C**) Merozoites enter the bloodstream and infect red blood cells. (**D**) In red blood cells, merozoites grow and divide to produce more merozoites, eventually causing the red blood cells to rupture. Some of the newly released merozoites go on to infect other red blood cells. (**E**) Some merozoites develop into sex cells known as male and female gametocytes. (**F**) Another mosquito bites the infected human, ingesting the gametocytes. (**G**) In the mosquito's stomach, the gametocytes mature. Male and female gametocytes undergo sexual reproduction, uniting to form a zygote. The zygote multiplies to form sporozoites, which travel to the mosquito's salivary glands. (**H**) If this mosquito bites another human, the cycle begins again. Source: Microsoft Encarta (2008), http://encarta.msn.com/media_461541582_761566151_-1_1/life_cycle_of_the_malaria_parasite.html

Fig. 12.3 Pathways by which malaria contributes to morbidity, mortality, and under-development. Source: Adapted from Breman (2004)

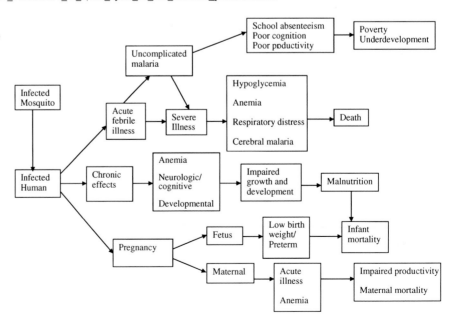

risk of severe and fatal malaria but younger children and pregnant women remain vulnerable to severe and complicated malaria. Malaria infection may be asymptomatic or symptomatic. The majority of malaria infections in areas where transmission is high and stable are asymptomatic. Even when malaria infection is asymptomatic, it is believed that the high prevalence of low parasitemic and asymptomatic malaria infections contribute to the high prevalence of mild and moderate childhood anemia. In these settings, young children who are less immune to the disease are more likely to have clinical malaria following infections.

The common symptoms of uncomplicated malaria are fever, poor appetite, aches, malaise, nausea, and vomiting. Uncomplicated malaria is the most common reason for which children and adults use the health service in sub-Saharan Africa. Uncomplicated malaria accounts for about 40 and 30% of outpatient attendance and hospital admissions, respectively. Malaria is also a leading cause of absenteeism and poor performance at work and school. Uncomplicated malaria is rarely fatal when treated promptly with effective antimalarial drugs. In preschool children, delayed treatment or failure to treat uncomplicated falciparum malaria could lead to rapid disease progression to severe and potentially fatal malaria within a period often less than 48 h from onset of illness. *Plasmodium falciparum* causes severe malaria through complex processes that involve immunological substances known as cytokines (John et al. 2000) leading to impaired perfusion and damage to tissues and organs. These pathological changes lead to clinical and laboratory features that are characteristic of severe and complicated malaria, namely cerebral malaria that is associated with impaired consciousness, repeated convulsions, severe malarial anemia, hypoglycemia, respiratory distress, and circulatory collapse. Children that die from malaria would have one or more of these signs. The risk of death is higher in patients with multiple signs (Schellenberg et al. 1999). Case fatality rate of complicated falciparum malaria is 10–50%. About 10–17% of those that survive cerebral malaria have residual neurological problems such as dyskinesia, cortical blindness, seizures, and learning disorders (Meremikwu et al.1997). Most of these disorders are resolved

within 6 months but about 2% persist for longer periods of time causing varying degrees of disability and impaired intellectual development (Murphy and Breman 2001).

Consequences of Malaria in Children and Adolescents

Anemia

Childhood anemia in low-income countries is caused by multiple factors including poor nutrition, malaria, intestinal parasites, HIV/AIDS, and inherited blood disorders (e.g., glucose-6-phosphate dehydrogenase (G-6-P-D) deficiency and sickle cell disease). In areas with high transmission, malaria is the leading etiological factor for anemia. The processes by which malaria causes anemia are not yet fully understood; however, malaria-related toxins and immunological factors are believed to cause increased hemolysis, increased splenic clearance of infected and uninfected red blood cells, and impaired production of red blood cells in the bone marrow (dyserythropoeisis). In areas of Africa with high malaria transmission, surveys have shown high prevalence rates of anemia (hemoglobin <11 g/dL) among infants and children under 5 years of age (as high as 50–80% in several areas). Most of these cases of anemia go unnoticed and untreated because they are mild and cause no symptoms. Although children with mild and chronic anemia do not feel distinct symptoms of illness, mild anemia is associated with chronic debility. It can cause such adverse effects as reduced activity and impaired cognition and learning. These chronic effects of malarial anemia in concert with malaria-related school absenteeism and neurological complications from cerebral malaria, adversely affect childhood development and education in sub-Saharan Africa (Mung'Ala-Odera et al. 2004).

Severe anemia (hemoglobin <5 g/dL) is a common acute complication of falciparum malaria. It is responsible for high case fatality and often follows massive hemolysis from a single episode of falciparum malaria. Repeated episodes or poorly treated episodes of uncomplicated malaria are fairly common pathways to severe anemia in infants and young children who are residents of areas with high and stable malaria transmission. In many communities in Africa where there are high levels of *P. falciparum resistance* to chloroquine and sulphadoxine–pyrimethamine, the continued use of failed drugs has resulted in an increase in the incidence of severe malarial anemia. Case fatality from severe malarial anemia varies from 1% in treated cases to over 30% when associated with other complications of falciparum malaria, especially respiratory distress and deep coma (John et al. 2000). Many more children with life-threatening severe malaria anemia do not have access to formal health care where adequate treatment and blood transfusion are possible. This indicates that overall case fatality from severe malarial anemia is likely to be much higher than reported. Blood transfusion for severe malaria-related anemia accounts for a remarkable proportion of new pediatric HIV infections in Africa (Crawley and Nahlen 2004).

Given the multifactorial nature of the etiology of childhood anemia, interventions to prevent or treat it should involve several approaches. For instance, mass de-worming of children and micronutrient supplementation programs are interventions that have the potential to reduce the burden of childhood anemia in developing countries (Briand et al. 2007). Insecticide-treated nets, chemoprophylaxis, and intermittent preventive treatment are malaria-specific interventions that have been shown to significantly reduce morbidity and mortality from malaria-related anemia (Briand et al. 2007). Malaria is a leading cause of hemolytic and vaso-occlusive crisis in African children and adolescents with sickle cell disease. Sickle cell disease is the most common inherited hematological disease among Africans. The prevalence of the sickle cell trait (heterozygous inheritance on an abnormal and a normal gene) can be as high as 25–40% in some parts of Africa with 1–3% affected by the disorder (inheritance of a pair of abnormal gene). A paradoxical relationship exists between the sickle cell gene and malaria. The sickle gene is believed to confer some measure of protection against malaria to those with the trait (one abnormal gene); however, it is a leading cause of morbidity and mortality among those with the disorder (two abnormal genes).

Malaria Nephropathy and Splenomegaly

Two other notable chronic effects of malaria in children and adolescents include malarial nephropathy and hyperactive malarial splenomegaly. Malarial nephropathy results from gradual damage of kidney cells by an antigen–antibody complex that is caused by previous malarial infection. There are no reliable data on the magnitude of renal morbidity which are caused by this malaria-induced pathology. However, it is believed that the problem is substantial. Hyperactive malarial splenomegaly (also called tropical splenomegaly syndrome) is another chronic, but less common presentation of malaria among children and adolescents in the tropics. This condition is characterized by an enlarged spleen, high levels of malarial immunoglobulin (IgM), sinusoidal lymphocyte infiltration, and resolution with prolonged antimalarial therapy.

Malaria in Pregnancy

Plasmodium falciparum and *P. vivax* are known to cause significant effects on maternal and child health during pregnancy. *Plasmodium falciparum* exerts the worst effects among all the species of malaria parasite. In sub-Saharan Africa, the transmission of *P. falciparum* is predominantly high and intense with high levels of morbidity and mortality among infants and pregnant women. The major consequences of malaria infection during pregnancy are clinical episodes of malaria, maternal anemia (hemoglobin concentration <11 g/dL), or severe anemia (hemoglobin concentration <8 g/dL), placental parasitemia, intrauterine growth retardation, preterm births, and low birth weight.

Table 12.1 shows the contribution of malaria to adverse maternal and child health outcomes. Malaria in pregnancy is estimated to account for up to 25% of cases of severe anemia, 10–20% of babies born with low birth weight, and 5–10% of neonatal and infant deaths are due to malaria-induced LBW (Greenwood et al. 2005). The effect of malaria in pregnancy is influenced by the level of malaria immunity acquired by the mother before pregnancy. This depends on the pattern and intensity of malaria transmission. The parasite species,

Table 12.1 Contribution of malaria to anemia, low birth weight, and infant deaths

Adverse health events	% of total
Maternal anemia	2–15
Low birth weight	8–14
Preterm birth	8–36
Intrauterine growth retardation	13–70
Infant death	3–8

Source: WHO-AFRO (2004)

the number of previous pregnancies, and the presence of human immunodeficiency virus (HIV) also remarkably impact malaria morbidity and mortality during pregnancy. In areas with high and stable malaria transmission, the prevalence and intensity of *P. falciparum* parasitemia are higher in pregnant women than in non-pregnant women. The majority of malaria infections in pregnant women living in high transmission areas are asymptomatic because of immunity acquired from repeated exposure to malaria before pregnancy. The adverse consequences of malaria during pregnancy in areas of high transmission are anemia, placental malaria, intrauterine growth retardation, and low birth weight. In areas of low or unstable transmission, acquired malaria immunity is low in all age groups. Pregnant women with malaria in this area are vulnerable to severe manifestation of the disease including cerebral malaria.

HIV and Malaria Co-infection

The evidence that malaria and HIV co-infection increases morbidity associated with both conditions has been confirmed by several studies (Snow et al. 2003). Impact of the complex interaction between malaria and HIV appears to be most profound in pregnancy and children. HIV infection in pregnancy is known to increase the risk of malaria infection (population attributable risk (PAR), 10–27%), maternal anemia (PAR, 12–15%), and low birth weight (PAR, 11–38%) (Steketee et al. 2001). The mechanism by which HIV infection alters malaria morbidity is not well understood. It is believed to be due to systemic and placental immunologic changes that are induced by HIV. In a Rwandan cohort study that included 228 HIV-positive and 229 HIV-

negative participants, the incidence of malaria was almost twice as high in the HIV-positive group (6.2 per 100 women-months) than in the HIV- negative group (3.5 per 100 women-months) (Ladner et al. 2002). A review of studies on malaria and HIV co-infection shows that HIV infection in pregnancy significantly increases the risk of peripheral and placental malaria parasitemia. Malaria in pregnant women infected by HIV is more likely to cause higher parasite densities, febrile illness, severe anemia, and low birth weight than malaria in those without HIV infection (Snow et al. 2003). In the absence of HIV infection, the deleterious effects of malaria in pregnancy, notably low birth weight and maternal anemia, were significantly worse in those pregnant for the first or second time than in those who have been pregnant for three or more times (Ter Kuile et al. 2004). With HIV co-infection, the pattern of malaria morbidity is similar across all categories of pregnant women (Ter Kuile et al. 2004).

A review of studies in areas of sub-Saharan Africa with high and stable malaria transmission shows that HIV-1 infection and clinically diagnosed AIDS increased the incidence of malaria 1.2-fold and 2-fold, respectively (Korenromp et al. 2005). In these high transmission areas, HIV-1 infection in children increased hospitalization for malaria and malaria case fatality 6-fold and 9.8-fold, respectively. At the same time in low transmission areas, the incidence of severe malaria and malaria case fatality increased 2.7-fold and 3.6-fold, respectively. The effect of HIV on malaria incidence is worse in HIV patients with lower CD4 counts. In adult patients living in high malaria transmission areas, HIV increased the malaria incidence 1.2-fold, 3-fold, and 5-fold when CD4 counts were ≥ 500, 200–499, and $<200/\mu L$, respectively (Korenromp et al. 2005).

The increase in morbidity and mortality associated with HIV and malaria co-infection, both of which are highly prevalent in most parts of sub-Saharan Africa, calls for more focused research in this area and for integration of service delivery. One way of achieving greater impact is the integration of malaria and HIV/AIDS control activities within maternal and child health programs. Achieving high coverage of insecticide-treated bed nets (ITNs) use and prompt access to treatment with artemisinin-based combination treatments (ACTs) would contribute to the reduction in the morbidity and mortality attributable to HIV co-infection with malaria in high transmission areas. In areas of low intensity and unstable transmission, widespread and effective indoor residual spraying combined with effective treatment using artemisinin-based combination therapy (ACT) is cost-effective and has been shown to significantly reduce malaria morbidity and mortality (Snow et al. 2003).

Strategies for Global Malaria Control

The following section provides a summary of the three-pronged approach to malaria control recommended by the World Health Organization's malaria control program (WHO 2005).

Vector Control

Indoor residual spraying, environmental management to eliminate mosquito breeding sites, and use of larvicides are known to be effective in reducing malaria when used in combination. Aerial and terrestrial spraying of insecticides is used in parts of South America and Asia to control malaria. This intervention strategy is cost intensive and low in effectiveness. It is therefore, not an appropriate control measure for sub-Saharan Africa given the complex terrains and weak economies of these malaria-endemic countries.

Prevention of Human–Vector Contact

Insecticide-treated bed nets (ITN) have been shown by studies in a variety of settings to be effective in reducing the incidence of clinical malaria by half and fatalities by about a third (Snow et al. 2003). Population coverage for ITN in most parts of Africa remains low (<20%). The low re-treatment rate at the expiration of the usual period of potency (6 months) was a major challenge, even in areas that achieved high ITN coverage. The development and widespread deployment of factory-treated nets with lifelong protective effects (LLINs) has eliminated the need to re-treat insecticide-treated nets. The persisting challenge is how to improve access to

ITNs by poor women and children who need to be protected from severe and fatal malaria. The Global Fund for Tuberculosis AIDS and Malaria is providing funding to countries in endemic low and middle-income countries to support this intervention. A systematic review of randomized controlled trials conducted in Africa showed that ITNs used in pregnancy compared to "no nets" significantly reduced the risk of placental malaria in all pregnancies (relative risk 0.79, 95% confidence interval 0.63–0.98). The review also showed that ITNs significantly reduced the risk of low birth weight (relative risk 0.77, 95% CI 0.61–0.98) and fetal loss in the first to fourth pregnancy (relative risk 0.67, 95% CI 0.47–0.97). However, this was not the case in women with more than four previous pregnancies (Gamble et al. 2006). In a large randomized controlled trial in communities with intense and perennial malaria transmission, ITN use significantly reduced the risk of severe malaria anemia, placental malaria, and low birth weight among those pregnant for the first to fourth time, but not in those pregnant for five or more times (Ter Kuile et al. 2003). The adherence to ITN use in pregnancy was shown to be significantly lower in adolescent and young women, who are most at risk for the deleterious consequences of malaria (Browne et al. 2001). This observation and the known risk of higher malaria morbidity associated with first pregnancy (involving mostly adolescent women) make it necessary to specially target this age group for intervention.

In summary, the limited risk assessments undertaken so far with regard to the safety of ITNs suggest that they are relatively safe. However, a cautionary note regarding the need to monitor the health effects of long-term exposure to insecticides in resource-poor settings has been presented by Ehiri et al. (2004). Although the use of mosquito nets is not new, mass use of ITNs as a population-based malaria control tool is a relatively new technology, and some uncertainty remains about the potential for problems as their use expands (Hirsch et al. 2002).

Treatment and Prevention with Drugs

Prompt treatment of malaria with efficacious and affordable antimalarials is a key component of the Global Malaria Control Strategy. The emergence and spread of malaria parasites (especially *P. falciparum*) resistant to the commonly used affordable antimalarials, like chloroquine (CQ) and sulphadoxine–pyrimethamine (SP), hampered malaria control in Africa and has deteriorated the malaria situation on the continent. The emergence of these multidrug-resistant malaria parasites led to the adoption of combination treatment options as the gold standards for treating malaria. The WHO (2006) recommends that the ideal drug combination should contain two drugs that are individually effective against the blood stages of the parasite and use completely different mechanisms to kill the parasite. Based on results from several well-conducted studies, the WHO recommended that combinations that contain artemisinin (a drug derived from the Chinese plant *A. annua L.*) or its derivatives and another structurally unrelated and more slowly acting drug provide the best therapeutic effects and are safe. This category of drug combinations is collectively known as artemisinin-based combination treatments (ACTs).

The advantages of artemisinin-based combination treatments (ACTs) have been outlined by the WHO to include the following (WHO 2006):

- Rapid substantial reduction of parasite biomass
- Rapid resolution of clinical symptoms
- Effective action against multidrug-resistant *P. falciparum*
- Reduction of gametocyte carriage, which may reduce malaria transmission
- No parasite resistance documented as yet with the use of artemisinin and its derivatives
- Few reported adverse clinical effects (note that pre-clinical data on artemisinin derivatives are limited)

Monotherapy with artemisinin derivatives requires multiple doses given for 7 days due to their characteristic short half-life. The other key advantage of artemisinin containing combination treatments (ACTs) is the shortened duration of treatment (3 days), with expected improvement in patient compliance to treatment. If the partner drug is effective, ACTs ensure prompt recovery and high cure rates. They are generally well tolerated. Replacing the older failing or failed monotherapies with effective drugs will reduce morbidity and mortality. The challenge, however, remains how to deliver

these drugs to the people that need them. Implementation of this policy would put significant cost burdens on national malaria control programs. However, the costs of failing to change, such as an increase in childhood deaths and high cost of hospitalization, make it a necessary and cost-effective program.

Affordability of ACTs is a major issue affecting their effective deployment in malaria control programs in sub-Saharan Africa. ACTs are generally too expensive for most people in low-income settings where malaria is endemic. While drugs such as chloroquine and sulphadoxine–pyrimethamine (SP), which were previously used for treating uncomplicated malaria, cost only a few US cents, the new ACTs cost about $2–$3.5 and even higher when not discounted. International efforts to address this issue championed by the Roll Back Malaria (RBM) partnership have yielded some positive results, especially through the Global Fund for Tuberculosis, AIDS and Malaria (Brundtland 2002). However, huge gaps still exist. Unfortunately access to prompt treatment with effective antimalarial drugs remains very low in many sub-Saharan countries, leading to the persistence of high malaria mortality rates. The reasons for poor access to treatment are mainly due to weak health systems that are poorly patronized by the populace and a lack of funds to procure and effectively deliver expensive artemisinin-based combination treatment (ACTs). ACTs are necessary since high levels of *P. falciparum* resistance have rendered chloroquine and sulphadoxine–pyrimethamine ineffective. These were the cheaper treatment options that have been used for several decades. Most children who become ill with malaria in these areas are usually treated at home with poor quality or inappropriately administered medicines that were purchased from local, often untrained drug vendors.

Antimalarial treatment policies, adopted by each country, depend on the epidemiology of the disease, including patterns of transmission, drug resistance, political environment, and economic context. The adoption of ACTs in sub-Saharan Africa was preceded by establishment of local evidence on the effectiveness of existing first- and second-line drugs which have demonstrated consistently high treatment failure rates due to parasite resistance (Snow et al. 2003). The WHO (2006) also

Box 12.2 Challenges of Community Delivery of Malaria Chemotherapy Through the Primary Healthcare System

Limitation of outreach capacity to geographically remote areas, and particularly to nomadic populations

  Inability to make efficient use of community resources (both human and material)

  Difficulty in achieving full community acceptance of chemotherapy

  Insufficient training of local health workers

  Lack of understanding of health problems and their solutions

  Potential ineffectiveness of the curative drug or drug dosage used, usually through the emergence of parasite resistance to the drug

  Undesirable side-effects of the drug

  Source: Jeffery (1984)

recommends that countries developing antimalarial treatment policies should strive to ensure that

- all populations at risk have access to prompt treatment with safe, good quality, effective, affordable, and acceptable antimalarial drugs and
- there is rational use of antimalarial drugs in order to prevent the emergence and spread of drug resistance induced by unduly high selection drug pressure on mutant malaria parasites.

Delivery of effective and safe antimalarial treatment to poor rural populations and those in difficult, hard-to-reach settings poses enormous challenges to malaria control programs in Africa. In many endemic countries, the formal health system is weak. Often the health system consists of a few ill-equipped health facilities run by inadequately trained and/or poorly motivated health personnel. The proportion of the people that access these services is so low that successful malaria treatment programs in Africa would be impossible without community-based delivery mechanisms including adequately trained and equipped informal community-based providers and caregivers who provide treatment and preventive services as close as possible to where people live and work. Delivering community health care such as malaria treatment services through primary healthcare centers has long been identified a big challenge by Jeffery (1984) as summarized in

Box 12.2. A careful appraisal of these factors in the context of the current situation of malaria control efforts in most endemic countries in sub-Saharan Africa shows situations that are as pertinent today as they were over two decades ago when they were highlighted by Jeffery (1984).

Home management of malaria (HMM), the strategy currently recommended by the WHO (Mendie et al. 2003) as an effective community delivery mechanism for antimalarial treatment, is likely to address some of the limitations highlighted in Box 12.2. The HMM strategy entails educating community health workers, volunteers, mothers, and caregivers to recognize symptoms of malaria and treat with appropriate antimalarial drugs (Mendie et al. 2003). Its goal is to ensure early recognition and prompt and appropriate response to malarial illness in under-5 children in the home and community by enabling health workers, mothers, and caregivers to recognize malarial illness early and take appropriate action. The WHO HMM strategy consists of four strategic components:

1. Ensure access to effective and good-quality antimalarial drugs (preferably pre-packed) at community level.

2. Ensure that community drug or service providers (e.g., patent medicine vendors, volunteer village health workers, community health extension workers) have necessary skills and knowledge to manage malaria.

3. Ensure an effective communication strategy to enable caregivers to recognize malarial illness early and take appropriate action.
4. Ensure good mechanisms for supervision, monitoring, and communication activities.

As shown in Chapter 27, integrated management of childhood illness (community IMCI) also addresses both preventive and curative aspects of malaria control by seeking to improve community and family practices.

Using Drugs to Prevent Malaria

Giving prophylactic antimalarial drugs to prevent malaria is a routine practice for non-immune persons visiting malaria-endemic areas. Malaria prophylaxis refers to daily or weekly administration of antimalarial drugs at a dose that is usually smaller than the therapeutic doses with a view to preventing clinical malaria. Intermittent preventive treatment (IPT) refers to full therapeutic doses of an antimalarial given at specified time points to presumptively cure asymptomatic malaria and prevent clinical malaria or such other adverse consequences as anemia or placental malaria. Usually, sulphadoxine–pyrimethamine (SP) is used for IPT as it requires a single dose and has a long half-life. The rationale is that intermittent treatment is likely to have fewer adverse events than prophylaxis because it is taken less often, and it is easier to deliver through clinics, reducing poor adherence with self-administration.

Chloroquine was the most widely used drug for malaria prophylaxis in pregnancy. The high prevalence of resistant strains, and the fact that most women adhered poorly to the weekly regimen required to achieve beneficial effects, rendered chloroquine chemoprophylaxis ineffective for malaria control in pregnancy. Meta-analysis included in a Cochrane systematic review of randomized controlled trials showed that IPT with sulphadoxine–pyrimethamine significantly reduced the risk of severe maternal anemia (relative risk 0.60, 95% CI 0.50–0.78; 2,243 participants), placental malaria (relative risk 0.35, 95% CI 0.27–0.47; 1,232 participants), and low birth weight (relative

risk 0.58, 95% CI 0.43–0.78; 1,399 participants) in women who were pregnant for the first or second time (Garner and Gülmezoglu 2006).

IPT with sulphadoxine–pyrimethamine (SP) along with consistent use of ITNS are currently recommended as cost-effective and evidence-based interventions to prevent the deleterious effects of malaria in pregnancy and to reduce the associated maternal and infant morbidity and mortality. Almost all the 35 countries in Africa with stable malaria transmission are already implementing intermittent preventive treatment in pregnancy (IPTp) with SP (Vallely et al. 2007). One of the key challenges with implementation of IPT is the high rate of parasite resistance to SP, and the lack of a safe and effective alternative to this antimalarial. In most parts of Africa SP failure exceeds 20% and surveillance data on the trends are lacking in most cases. The effectiveness of this intervention in areas with high SP failure rates is yet to be adequately studied. The suggestion that two and three doses of SP, respectively, should be used in areas with SP resistance <30 and 30–50% remains to be validated by robust research data. The continued use of IPT with SP in areas where SP resistance exceeds 50% also needs to be justified by research.

There is also the problem of how to handle malaria co-infection with HIV in areas with high prevalence of HIV. A third dose of SP for IPT has been recommended for areas with high HIV prevalence but there is a need to monitor impact on such outcomes as severe anemia and low birth weight, and to study possible drug interactions in those receiving anti-retroviral treatment. In malaria-endemic communities, use of antimalarial drugs for prophylaxis or intermittent preventive treatment (IPT) is recommended for only pregnant women and special vulnerable groups such as children with sickle cell disease. Several randomized controlled trials in malaria-endemic communities have shown consistently that malaria prophylaxis and intermittent preventive treatment of infants (IPTi) and young children are effective. A Cochrane systematic review and meta-analysis (Meremikwu et al. 2005) showed that receiving antimalarial drugs as prophylaxis or intermittent treatment reduced the incidence of clinical malaria episodes and severe anemia by about 50% in preschool children living in malaria-endemic communities. Two main reasons are commonly given for discouraging widespread use of malaria chemoprophylaxis in preschool children in endemic communities. The first reason is the concern that giving malaria prophylaxis to infants and young children living in malaria-endemic areas will delay or minimize their chances to acquire protective immunity and result in a rebound rise in the incidence of severe morbidity and mortality later in life.

The second reason is that poor compliance to weekly antimalarial drug prophylaxis could induce drug pressure and selection of mutant resistant strains of *P. falciparum*. Intermittent preventive treatment of infants (IPTi) with treatment doses of SP under direct observation at the time of routine immunization offers a better programmatic option, since it eliminates the problem of non-compliance and is expected to have little or no adverse effect or interfere with the child's ability to acquire malarial immunity. A major challenge to implementation of IPTi, among others, is the rising incidence of SP resistance which is the principal drug currently used for this intervention. There has also been a concern about the possible interaction between SP and the routine infant vaccines but this has not been supported by any strong evidence.

Malaria Vaccines

Timely and efficient deployment of efficacious vaccines is widely accepted as an effective child survival strategy. The development of a successful malaria vaccine especially against *P. falciparum* would contribute remarkably to reduction of the unacceptably high childhood death from malaria. Unfortunately decades of efforts at vaccine development have yet to meet this expected public health success. Developing vaccines against parasitic infections poses greater challenges than developing vaccines for virus and bacterial infections because of their more complex nature and larger genomes. The multiple stages of the malaria parasite and the different proteins they express pose additional challenges to the development of a potent malaria vaccine. An all-stage malaria vaccine capable of inhibiting growth or killing all of these different stages of malaria poses a complex challenge. Researchers involved in development of malaria vaccine devote their efforts to three key strategies that target the pre-erythrocytic and erythrocytic stages of the life cycle in humans (Fig. 12.2), and vaccines that induce antibodies in humans that can kill or prevent development of viable sexual forms ingested by the mosquito vectors. The pre-erythrocytic stage vaccines aim to prevent sporozoites (the stage of plasmodium that mosquitoes pass to humans) from invading and developing in the liver, while an asexual erythrocytic stage vaccine limits the invasion of erythrocytes or prevents their multiplication in the erythrocytes.

The complete mapping of the *P. falciparum* genome with a better understanding of the organism at sub-cellular and molecular levels coupled with recent advances in genomic and proteomic science has led to a remarkable increase in the number of candidate malaria vaccines. There is no time better than the present to scale up support for malaria vaccine research and development. The goal of most of the initial efforts of malaria vaccine development is complete prevention of the disease with the hope of eliminating malaria. The disappointing results of early malaria vaccine trials appear to have diminished this enthusiasm. Should efforts to develop a malaria vaccine capable of completely preventing clinical malaria fail, most public health experts and vaccine researchers advocate the goal of making malaria vaccines that ameliorate the severity of the disease and reduce the level of fatality. In Africa, where pregnant women and children bear the greatest burden of severe malaria, such a vaccine will be a significant addition to maternal and child health services and will help to reduce the burden of childhood disability attributable to cerebral malaria. The opportunities provided by better research tools and a better understanding of the *Plasmodium* and *Anopheles* genome make the prospects and possibilities of a malaria vaccine better today than ever before. Funding for malaria vaccine development and field trials has increased in recent years. However, it is still far short of the expected investment, given its huge potential for improving child survival and contributing to achievement of the millennium development goals (MDG).

Progress and Challenges of the Global Malaria Control Strategy

The inadequacies of health information systems and vital registration processes in most parts of sub-Saharan Africa make it difficult to obtain reliable records of malaria mortality. Facility-based records of deaths, when available, are not representative of the situation in the larger population given that the majority of sick children do not use health facilities and most deaths occur outside the formal health facilities. Most of the available mortality data from malaria-endemic areas are estimates and prospective mortality data from demographic surveillance systems validated by verbal autopsies (Snow et al. 2004). The inefficiency of health information systems and vital registration processes in sub-Saharan African countries makes it difficult to obtain sufficient and timely information to track the performance of malaria control programs. The malaria situation globally deteriorated in the past three decades. This resulted in increased malaria-related morbidity and mortality, especially in sub-Saharan Africa where emergence and spread of multidrug-resistant malaria parasites and breakdown of malaria control programs were the leading reasons, among others (Korenromp et al. 2003). Greenwood et al. (2005) have given an elaborate summary of the factors believed to

have contributed to the deterioration of the global malaria situation in Box 12.3.

While the discovery of additional malaria control measures such as a highly effective malaria vaccine should be expected to increase the gains of malaria control efforts, several appraisals and overviews of global malaria control efforts agree that the key reasons for the recent decline in the gains of malaria control efforts have not been the lack of effective malaria control measures. There is consensus that the four technical elements of the global malaria control strategy (Box 12.4) affirmed by the international ministerial conference held in Amsterdam under the auspices of the World Health Organization in 1992 have been essentially effective in the years preceding and succeeding the Amsterdam conference.

Careful study of malaria control scenarios (mostly in sub-Saharan Africa) that have failed, or achieved only minimal success with these same strategies, shows that these control programs lacked the pre-conditions for effectiveness of the global strategy (Box 12.5) as also outlined in the Amsterdam Ministerial Conference on Malaria.

When the RBM strategy was established in 1998, it was in response to these deficiencies. The RBM is a partnership between the WHO, other UN agencies, bilateral aid agencies, non-governmental organizations, and governments of

---

Box 12.3 Factors Contributing to Deterioration of the Malaria Situation

- Climate instability: drought and floods increased malaria transmission in different epidemiological circumstances
- Global warming may have led to increased malaria transmission especially in some highland areas
- Civil disturbances and unrest have resulted in the collapse of malaria control programs and refugee situations with attendant effects on malaria transmission across epidemiological areas and increased risk of epidemics
- Changes and increase in travel patterns within endemic areas and from non-endemic areas to endemic areas putting many non-immune people at risk
- HIV increases susceptibility to malaria and increases the burden on the health service
- Emergence and spread of drug resistant *P. falciparum* has been a key reason for deterioration of malaria situation in especially Africa and Southeast Asia
- Insecticide resistance: resistance to pyrethroids used for treated bed-nets has emerged in *Anopheles gambiae* (in West Africa) and *Anopheles funestus* (in southern Africa). High vector resistance to *Anopheles funestus* diminished the use of DDT for household spraying in southern Africa.

Source: Greenwood et al. (2005)

Box 12.4 Basic Technical Elements of the Malaria Control Strategy

- To provide early diagnosis and treatment
- To plan and implement selective, multiple and sustainable preventive measures: including vector control; personal protection (notably insecticide treated nets); and chemoprophylaxis/intermittent preventive treatment.
- To detect early, contain or prevent epidemics;
- To conduct focused research, and to regularly assess the country's malaria situation, including ecological, social and economic determinants of the disease.

Source: WHO (1992)

Box 12.5 Conditions for Effective Implementation of the Global Malaria Control Strategy

- Political Will: sustained political commitment from all levels and sectors of government
- Integration: malaria control should be an integral part of health systems, and be coordinated with relevant development programs in non-health sectors
- Community participation: communities should be full partners in malaria control activities
- Resource mobilization: adequate human and financial resources should be mobilized

Source: WHO (1992)

malaria-endemic countries. The RBM has a long-term goal of reducing malaria morbidity and mortality by at least half by 2010. RBM was not meant to be a new malaria control strategy but rather an organized global effort to facilitate the effective implementation of the global control strategy.

Conclusion

The evidence that large-scale and effective use of ITNs can reduce the incidence of malaria and malaria-related deaths is both strong and consistent (Lengeler 2000). Insecticide-treated mosquito nets (ITNs) can reduce all-cause childhood mortality by about a fifth; with about 6 lives saved for every 1,000 preschool children protected with ITN (Lengeler 2000). It is estimated that full ITN coverage in sub-Saharan Africa could prevent 370,000 child deaths per year (Lengeler 2000). Insecticide-treated nets are cost-effective, but endemic poverty and inadequate sensitization of people in malaria-endemic areas remain the major reasons for low use (Snow et al. 2003). The cost-effectiveness of ITNs (US $19–85 per disability-adjusted life year

(DALY)) is similar to most childhood vaccines (WHO 2003). When community coverage is high, ITNs not only protect those who sleep under them, but also those in the same dwelling (the home effect) and those living nearby (the community effect) (Snow et al. 2003).

The year 2005 marked the end of the target set by African Heads of State to achieve at least 60% access to prompt and effective treatment of malaria and 60% ITN coverage for under-5 children and pregnant women. However, most countries in sub-Saharan Africa fell far short of these targets. It was also in the same year that RBM set the landmark target of halving malaria mortality by 2010. Appraisal of malaria control efforts at the end of 2005 uniformly indicated that resources available for procurement of malaria control commodities (ACTs, ITN, and diagnostic kits) were grossly inadequate. The appraisal also showed that malaria control personnel at national and regional levels was inadequately equipped.

Donors and governments should develop effective mechanisms to monitor the access that children, adolescents, pregnant women, and children in difficult circumstances have to evidence-based treatment and preventive interventions for malaria. Donor funds specifically tagged to providing resources and infrastructure for effective management of severe and complicated malaria have been grossly inadequate. Supportive care for women and children with severe malaria is grossly impeded by weak health systems in malaria-endemic countries. Funds meant for providing adequate infrastructure and personnel for managing severe malaria should be tagged to bilateral and multilateral health system support grants.

Key Terms

Acquired malaria immunity	Impaired consciousness	*Plasmodium malariae*
Anemia	Infant mortality	*Plasmodium ovale*
Anopheles funestus	Insecticide-treated bed nets (ITNs)	*Plasmodium vivax*
Anopheles gambiense		Poor appetite
Artemisia annua	Integrated management of childhood illnesses (IMCI)	Population attributable risk (PAR)
Artemisinin-based combination therapy (ACT)	Intermittent preventive treatment (IPT)	Poverty
Artemisinin-based combination treatments (ACTs)	Intermittent preventive treatment of infants (IPTi)	Pregnancy
Blood transfusion		Preterm births
Case fatality rate	Intrauterine growth retardation (IUGR)	Relative risk
Cerebral malaria	Learning disorders	Repeated convulsions
Chloroquine	Lifelong protective effects (LLINs)	Residual spraying
Circulatory collapse		Respiratory distress
Cortical blindness	Low birth weight	Roll Back Malaria (RBM)
Cytokines	Malaise	Seizures
Dyserythropoeisis	Malaria-endemic countries	Severe anemia
Dyskinesia	Malaria vaccine	Severe malaria
Entomologic inoculation rate (EIR)	Malarial nephropathy	Sickle cell disease
Fetal loss	Malariometric indices	Sinusoidal lymphocyte infiltration
Fever	Maternal malaria	Splenomegaly
Global Malaria Control Strategy	Maternal mortality	Sporozoite
	Monotherapy	Sporozoite rate
Glucose-6-phosphate dehydrogenase (G6PD) deficiency	Mosquito	Stable malaria transmission
	Multidrug-resistant malaria parasites	Sulphadoxine–pyrimethamine (SP)
Hemoglobin	Nausea	Tropical splenomegaly syndrome
Hemolytic crisis	Parasite resistance	Uncomplicated malaria
Home management of malaria (HMM)	Parasitemia	Under-development
	Perennial malaria	Vaso-occlusive crisis
Hyperactive malarial splenomegaly	Placental malaria	Vector control
Hypoglycemia	*Plasmodium falciparum*	

Questions for Discussion

1 Globally, women, children, and adolescents in sub-Saharan Africa are known to bear the greatest burden of malaria morbidity and mortality. List any six factors most peculiar to the region that account for this high burden.

2 List five consequences of malaria infection in children and pregnant women.

3 An integrated approach is advocated as an efficient and cost-effective strategy for the management of malaria co-infection with HIV/AIDS. Briefly discuss what you understand by integrated management and describe how such an integrated approach might be operationalized in practice.

4 What are artemisinin-based combination treatments (ACTs) and what are the advantages of their use in the treatment of malaria?

5 What are the challenges of community delivery of malaria treatment through existing primary healthcare systems? Is home treatment of malaria a better option? Discuss the reasons for your position.

6 List six factors that contribute to the worsening of the global problem of malaria? How can these be addressed? What should be the role of Roll Back Malaria initiative in global malaria control?

References

Breman JG, Alilio MS, Mills A (2004) Conquering the intolerable burden of malaria: what's new, what's needed: summary. American Journal of Tropical Medical Hygiene, 71(Suppl 2), 1–15

Briand V, Cottrell G, Massougbodji A (2007) Intermittent preventive treatment for the prevention of malaria during pregnancy in high transmission areas. Malaria Journal, 6, 160

Browne EN, Maude GH, Binka FN (2001) The impact of insecticide-treated bednets on malaria and anemia in pregnancy in Kassena-Nankana district, Ghana: a randomized controlled trial. Tropical Medicine & International Health, 6, 667–676

Brundtland GH (2002) External evaluation of Roll Back Malaria. http://www.rbm.who.int/changeinitiative/externalevaluation.pdf, cited 21 May 2008

Crawley J, Nahlen B (2004) Prevention and treatment of malaria in young African children. Seminars in Pediatric Infectious Diseases, 15(3), 169–180

Ehiri JE, Anyanwu EC, Scarlett HP (2004) Mass use of insecticide-treated bednets in malaria endemic poor countries: public health concerns and remedies. Journal of Public Health Policy, 25(1), 9–22

Gamble C, Ekwaru JP, ter Kuile FO (2006) Insecticide-treated nets for preventing malaria in pregnancy. Cochrane Database of Systematic Reviews, Issue 2

Garner P, Gülmezoglu AM (2006) Drugs for preventing malaria in pregnant women. Cochrane Database of Systematic Reviews, Issue 4

Greenwood BM, Bojang K, Whitty CJM et al. (2005) Malaria. Lancet, 365: 1487–1498

Hirsch B, Gallegos C, Knausenberger W et al. (2002) Programmatic environmental assessment for insecticide-treated materials in USAID activities in sub-Saharan Africa. Agency for International Development (USAID), Office of Sustainable Development. http://www.afr-sd.org/documents/iee/docs/32AFR2_ITM_PEA.doc, cited 16 May 2008

Jeffery GM (1984) The role of chemotherapy in malaria control through primary healthcare: constraints and future prospects. Bulletin of World Health Organization, 62(Suppl.), 49–53

John CC, Sumba PO, Ouma JH (2000) Cytokine responses to Plasmodium falciparum liver-stage antigen 1 vary in rainy and dry seasons in highland Kenya. Infection and Immunity, 68(9), 5198–5204

Korenromp EL, Williams BG, Gouws E (2003) Measurement of trends in childhood malaria mortality in Africa: an assessment of progress toward targets based on verbal autopsy. Lancet Infectious Disease, 3, 349–358

Korenromp EL, Williams BG, de Vlas SJ (2005) Malaria attributable to the HIV-1 epidemic, sub-Saharan Africa. Emerging Infectious Diseases, 11(9), 1410–1419

Ladner JL, Leroy VR, Simonon A (2002) HIV infection, malaria, and pregnancy: a prospective cohort study in Kigali, Rwanda. American Journal of Tropical Medicine and Hygiene, 66(1), 56–60

Lalloo DG, Olukoya P, Olliaro P (2006) Malaria in adolescence: burden of disease, consequences, and opportunities for intervention. Lancet Infectious Disease, 6(12), 780–793

Lengeler C (2000) Insecticide-treated bednets and curtains for preventing malaria. Cochrane Database of Systematic Reviews, 2

Mendie K, Bosman A, Olumese P (2003) Effective delivery methods for malaria treatment. Reducing malaria's burden: evidence of effectiveness for decision makers. Technical Report Washington: Global Health Council, 39–45

Meremikwu MM, Asindi AA, Ezedinachi ENU (1997) The pattern of neurological sequelae of childhood cerebral malaria among survivors in Calabar, Nigeria. Central African Journal of Medicine, 43, 231–234

Meremikwu MM, Omari AAA, Garner P (2005) Chemoprophylaxis and intermittent treatment for preventing malaria in children. Cochrane Database of Systematic Reviews, Issue 4

Mung'Ala-Odera V, Snow RW, Newton CRJC (2004) The burden of the neuro-cognitive impairment associated with Plasmodium falciparum malaria in sub-Saharan Africa. American Journal of Tropical Medicine and Hygiene, 71(Suppl 2), 64–70

Murphy SC, Breman JG (2001) Gaps in childhood malaria burden in Africa: cerebral malaria, neurological sequelae, anemia, respiratory distress, hypoglycemia, and complications of pregnancy. American Journal of Tropical Medicine and Hygiene, 64(1, 2), S:57–67

Schellenberg D, Menendez C, Kahigwa E et al. (1999) African children with malaria in areas of intense Plasmodium falciparum transmission: features on admission to the hospital and risk factors for death. American Journal of Tropical Medicine and Hygiene, 61(3), 431–438

Snow RW, Craig MH, Newton CRJC (2003) The public health burden of Plasmodium falciparum malaria in Africa: deriving the numbers. Working Paper 11, Disease Control Priorities Project. In: The Disease Control Priorities Project (DCPP) Working Paper Series. Bethesda (Maryland): Fogarty International Center, National Institutes of Health

Snow RW, Korenromp EL, Gouws E (2004) Pediatric mortality in Africa: Plasmodium falciparum malaria as a cause or risk. American Journal of Tropical Medicine and Hygiene, 71(Suppl 2), 16–24

Steketee RW, Nahlen BL, Parise ME (2001) The burden of malaria in pregnancy in malaria-endemic areas. American Journal of Tropical Medicine and Hygiene, 64(1,2), S: 28–35

Ter Kuile FO, Terlouw DJ, Phillips-Howard PA et al. (2003) Reduction of malaria during pregnancy by permethrin-treated bed nets in an area of intense perennial malaria transmission in western Kenya. American Journal of Tropical Medicine and Hygiene, 68(Suppl 4), 50–60

Ter Kuile FO, Parise ME, Verhoeff FH et al. (2004) The burden of co-infection with human immunodeficiency virus type 1 and malaria in pregnant women in sub-Saharan Africa. American Journal of Tropical Medicine and Hygiene, 71(Suppl 2), 41–54

Vallely A, Vallely, L, Changalucha J et al. (2007) Intermittent preventive treatment for malaria in pregnancy in Africa: what's new, what's needed. Malaria Journal, 6:16

World Health Organization (1992) Ministerial Conference on Malaria. Amsterdam Netherlands 26–27 October. WHO CTD/MCM/92.3

World Health Organization (2003) Cost-effectiveness of social marketing of insecticide-treated nets for malaria control in the United Republic of Tanzania. Bulletin of the World Health Organization, 81(4), 269–276

World Health Organization (2004) A strategic framework for malaria prevention and control during pregnancy in the African Region. WHO Document: AFR/MAL/04/01. Brazzaville: World Health Organization Regional Office for Africa

World Health Organization (2005) World Malaria Report. Geneva: World Health Organization. http://www.rbm. who.int/wmr2005/html/map1.htm, cited 15 May 2008

World Health Organization (2006) Guidelines for the treatment of malaria. WHO/HTM/MAL/2006.1108. Geneva: World Health Organizagtion. Cited August 8, 2009

World Health Organization (2007) International travel and health: situation as of 1 January 2007. Geneva, World Health Organization. http://whqlibdoc.who.int/publications/2007/9789241580397, cited 21 May 2008

Chapter 13
The Global Burden of Childhood Diarrhea

Cynthia Boschi-Pinto, Claudio F. Lanata, and Robert E. Black

Learning Objectives After reading this chapter and answering the discussion questions that follow, you should be able to

- Define the different types of childhood diarrhea and distinguish their clinical manifestations.
- Describe the magnitude and unequal distribution of childhood diarrhea by age group and by different world regions.
- Analyze the relative contributions of different diarrhea pathogens, as well as environmental and socio-behavioral risk factors to the causation of childhood diarrhea.
- Appraise and prioritize the evidence base of various treatment and prevention options.

Introduction

Using data from the Child Health Epidemiology Reference Group (CHERG) of the Department of Child and Adolescent Health and Development, World Health Organization, this chapter provides a comprehensive overview of the current status of the global burden of childhood diarrhea, highlighting evidence of the relationship between diarrheal diseases and child health. To set the discussion in context, the chapter begins with a summary of the definition and description of clinical manifestations of childhood diarrhea. An exposition on the

global burden of childhood diarrheal morbidity and mortality is then provided by world regions and by age groups. The unequal distribution of diarrhea between rich and resource-poor countries is highlighted. The relative contributions of different diarrheal disease pathogens (enterotoxigenic *Escherichia coli*, *G. lamblia*, *Rotavirus*, *Campylobacter*, *Shigella*, *Cryptosporidium parvum*, *Entamoeba histolytica*, and *Vibrio cholerae*) as well as risk factors (access to clean water and sanitation, maternal education, poverty and undernutrition) are analyzed. The chapter appraises the evidence base of various treatment and prevention options, including promotion of exclusive breastfeeding, hand washing, vaccines, oral rehydration therapy (ORT), zinc supplementation, and improved access to basic care. It concludes with a call for prioritization of interventions to control diarrhea deaths in order to optimize the use of scarce resources. The need to monitor and evaluate progress toward reduction of global inequity in childhood diarrheal morbidity and mortality is also stressed.

Major changes are taking place worldwide in the area of child health as efforts are geared toward achievement of Millennium Development Goal (MDG) # 4 of reducing by two-thirds, between 2000 and 2015, under-5 mortality rates (Bryce et al. 2006; United Nations Development Programme 2003). This goal is, however, contingent on progress of other Millennium Development Goals (MDGs), particularly those related to eradication of extreme poverty and hunger and improvement of maternal health. Countries with the highest burden of neonatal and under-5 mortality are those with the highest burden of maternal mortality as well. The concept of

C. Boschi-Pinto (✉)
Department of Child and Adolescent Health and Development, World Health Organization, Geneva, Switzerland

continuum of care from mothers to neonates to infants and under-5s highlights the importance of jointly addressing maternal and child health. In the specific context of diarrheal disease for example, it is well known that children exclusively breastfed are about six times less likely to die of diarrhea than children who are not exclusively breastfed.

Definition and Clinical Manifestations

There is great variability in the definition of diarrhea in the literature. However, for most epidemiological studies, diarrhea is defined as a condition in which three or more liquid stools are passed within a 24-h period (Morris et al. 1994). Most diarrheal episodes terminate within a week (an episode is considered terminated if there are at least 2 days free of diarrhea); however, a few episodes may last longer and continue for 2 weeks or more. The World Health Organization (WHO 1988) defines persistent diarrhea as an episode that continues for at least 14 days. Dysentery is defined by the presence of blood in loose or liquid stools.

Diarrheal diseases may cause severe loss of water and electrolytes such as sodium, chloride, potassium, and bicarbonate. When there is inadequate replacement of liquid and electrolytes, children can become dehydrated. Although the early stages of dehydration present no signs or symptoms, as it advances, symptoms become pronounced and may progress to shock. If the child is not promptly rehydrated, death follows very rapidly. Case fatality rates in under-5s have been reported to be 0.2% in developing countries overall, ranging from 0.1 to 0.5%, and being highest in younger children (Institute of Medicine 1986). Dehydration can be prevented by giving the child more fluids than usual. Increased intake of fluids supplemented by oral rehydration salts together with continued feeding has proven to be a powerful intervention for the prevention of childhood deaths from diarrhea (Victora et al. 2000). Since the early 1980s, substantial efforts have been aimed at the reduction of diarrhea mortality. However, considerable morbidity and mortality attributable to diarrheal disease remain in less developed countries where poverty is the underlying factor.

Morbidity and Mortality Burden

Diarrhea is a very common disease among children in developing countries, with an estimated frequency of about 3 episodes per child per year. In addition, it is one of the major under-5 killers worldwide. The first estimates of diarrheal morbidity and mortality among children less than 5 years of age in developing countries were published in 1982, by Snyder and Merson. They followed two other methodologically comparable reviews by Bern et al. (1992) and Kosek et al. (2003). These studies have made available, important and continued sources of information and constitute together major evidence of the declining mortality trend from diarrheal diseases. Two decades ago, diarrhea was responsible for almost 5 million deaths among children under-5 (Snyder and Merson 1982). Estimates have shown a steady decline ever since: 3.3 million deaths in the 1990s (Bern et al. 1992) and 2.5 million in the year 2000 (Kosek et al. 2003). However, in spite of this decline, diarrhea is still the second leading cause of under-5 mortality globally.

As opposed to the decreasing mortality trend, the overall incidence of diarrhea has remained relatively stable over time. These three reviews have estimated a worldwide incidence of 2.2 episodes per child under-5 per year in the 1980s (Snyder and Merson 1982), 2.6 episodes per child under-5 per year in the 1990s (Bern et al. 1992), and 3.2 episodes per child under-5 per year in the year 2000 (Kosek et al. 2003).

The Child Health Epidemiology Reference Group (CHERG), coordinated by the Department of Child and Adolescent Health and Development of the World Health Organization (WHO), has recently commissioned a systematic literature review to identify articles published between 1990 and 2002 that reported diarrhea morbidity rates in children less than 5 years of age. Studies included in the review were community-based surveys carried out in low- and middle-income countries that reported frequent home visits. Studies of outbreaks and studies focused on HIV/AIDS patients were excluded from the review. Thirty-three papers were finally included in the analysis. Countries in which studies were carried out were grouped according to the six WHO regions of the world: Africa, Americas, Eastern Mediterranean, Europe, Southeast Asia, and Western Pacific regions.

The median incidence of diarrheal disease among under-5s in the studied countries was 3.5 episodes per child per year (Table 13.1), very similar to the 3.2 episodes per child under-5 per year estimated and reported by Kosek et al. (2003). Incidence rates were slightly higher in Africa, the Americas, and the Eastern Mediterranean region (5 episodes per child per year) than in Southeast Asia and the Western Pacific region (3 episodes per child per year). Rates were generally highest in children aged 6–23 months.

Information on the prevalence of diarrhea was obtained from the Demographic and Health Surveys

Table 13.1 Reported incidence (episodes per child per year) of diarrheal diseases among children less than 5 years of age and corresponding age-adjusted rates

Country/author(s)/year	0–5	6–11	12–23	24–35	36–47	48–59	Reported Incidence 0–4 years	Age-adjusted incidence 0–4 years
Guinea-Bissau (Mølbak et al. 1997)		13.0					10.2	10.2
Nigeria (Oni et al. 1991)	3.3	4.1	2.9	2.2				2.6
Kenya (Mirza et al. 1997)			3.5					3.1
Ghana (Morris et al. 1996)							2.5	2.5
Kenya (Thomas and Neumann 1992)			7.3					5.8
Zimbabwe (Root 2001)							2.0	2.0
Zimbabwe (Root 2001)							6.2	6.2
Age-adjusted median for (sub-Saharan) Africa								**5.0**
Brazil (Lima et al. 2000)			6.8				5.3	5.3
Brazil (Barreto et al. 1994)				7.1				7.7
Brazil (Linhares et al. 1996)		6.0						4.9
Chile (Ferreccio et al. 1991)		2.3	2.1	1.5	1.3	0.9	1.5	1.5
Honduras (Kaminsky 1991)		5.0	3.4	3.2	2.6	1.5	3.2	3.2
Mexico (Guerrero et al. 1998)		2.9						2.4
Guatemala (Cruz et al. 1992)			7.6					6.8
Peru (Yeager et al. 1991)	7.3	10.3	9.1	6.3				7.4

Table 13.1 (continued)

Country/author(s)/year	0–5	6–11	12–23	24–35	36–47	48–59	Reported Incidence 0–4 years	Age-adjusted incidence 0–4 years
Brazil (Schorling et al. 1990)	9.4	14.1	15.1	12.2	8.7	7.2	10.4	10.4
Brazil (Moore et al. 2000)		5.5	4.5	2.4				3.4
Mexico (Cravioto et al. 1990)		4.4	4.5					3.6
Argentina (Viboud et al. 1999)							0.8	0.8
Venezuela (Pérez-Schael et al. 1990)	2.4	1.8	1.7					1.8
Peru (Lanata et al. 1996)		8.3						6.8
Age-adjusted median for (Latin) America								**5.0**
Egypt (Naficy et al. 2000)	7.3	8.8	5.5	2.9				5.5
Pakistan (Chavasse et al. 1999)							7.1	7.1
Egypt (Abu-Elyazeed et al. 1999)		4.9	2.5	1.0				3.0
Pakistan (Van der Hoek et al. 2002)		5.8	5.2	5.1	2.1	1.6	3.9	3.9
Age-adjusted median for the Eastern Mediterranean region								**4.9**
Indonesia (Dibley et al. 1996)				0.8				0.9
Thailand (Punyaratabandhu et al. 1991)	2.0	2.4	1.2		0.4		0.9	0.9
Bangladesh (Baqui et al. 1993)	5.1	6.2	5.4	4.3	3.6	2.4	4.5	4.5
India (Gupta et al. 1996)	2.0	3.1	2.0	1.3	1.1			1.9
India (Lal 1994)		6.0	5.5	4.2				4.8
India (Rahmathullah et al. 1991)							5.6	5.6
Age-adjusted median for Southeast Asia								**3.1**
China (Chen et al. 1991)							2.3	2.3
Malaysia (Yap et al. 1992)							0.2	0.2
Papua New Guinea (Wyrsch et al. 1998)	2.7	5.4	5.1	2.8	1.5	1.2	3.0	3.0
Age-adjusted median for Western Pacific								**3.3**
Global median (25% and 75% IQI)	**3.3 (2.5–6.8)**	**5.5 (3.6–9.2)**	**4.5 (2.6–5.5)**	**3.0 (2.2–4.3)**	**2.1 (1.4–3.1)**	**1.6 (1.3–2.2)**	**3.6 (1.9–5.5)**	**3.5 (2.3–5.7)**

(DHS), which are nationally representative surveys that report on the occurrence of diarrheal disease episodes in the 2 weeks prior to the surveys. Data from these surveys were abstracted and analyzed to explore trends over time. Figure 13.1a suggests recent decrease in the prevalence of diarrheal disease in Africa, the Americas, and the Eastern Mediterranean region, while an increase is indicated in Southeast Asia and in the Western Pacific region. Nevertheless, these data should be interpreted with caution as they reflect information based on a 2-week period recall and do not take seasonality into account. Moreover, countries examined and averaged in region prevalence might not be the same in different periods of time. Other limitations are possible changes in questions and interviewers. Therefore, comparability over time cannot be directly inferred from these data and the interpretation of results is not straightforward. The distribution of diarrheal disease prevalence by age group was consistent over the years, showing a peak among children aged 6–11 months and declining thereafter (Fig. 13.1b).

Common sources of information for mortality level and cause of death are vital registration systems and nationally representative surveys. However, such data are scarce in less developed countries. Almost none of the countries that account for 98% of all under-5 deaths have vital registration systems to support accurate attribution of the causes of child deaths (Rudan et al. 2005). Nationally representative surveys such as DHS and the Multiple Indicators Cluster Surveys (MICS) do not usually collect or report causes of death. Therefore, the main currently available sources of data that allow the estimation of cause-specific mortality are special population epidemiological studies. The most important limitations of this type of studies are the lack of representativeness, possible site bias, and misclassification of causes of death. However, these remain the major or only source of cause-of-death information.

Geographic Distribution of Deaths Due to Diarrhea

Based on these latter data sources, it has been estimated that about 1.9 million children less than 5 years of age died from diarrheal diseases in the year 2004. The distribution of these deaths, however, is heavily unbalanced; the greatest mortality burden being in sub-Saharan Africa and in Southeast Asia, which account together for approximately 80% of all under-5 deaths due to diarrheal diseases. In contrast, the burden of diarrheal mortality in more developed regions has been reduced to very low levels: merely 1% in Europe and 3% in the region of the Americas (Boschi-Pinto et al. 2008). The estimated regional distribution of diarrheal deaths for the year 2004 is shown in Fig. 13.2.

Similarly, the distribution of diarrheal deaths between and within countries shows a wide variation. Some of the main reasons for this discrepancy are directly or indirectly linked to poverty. Poor access to water, sanitation and hygiene, poor housing, crowding and limited or no access to care constitutes some of the main risk factors for the development of diarrheal disease. Country- specific estimates have highlighted that low- and middle-income countries account for 99% of the global under-5 deaths caused by diarrheal diseases. The country-specific distribution of deaths due to diarrheal disease is shown in Fig. 13.3.

Strikingly, these estimates have also revealed that just 15 countries account for almost three-quarters of all under-5 diarrhea deaths worldwide (Boschi-Pinto et al. 2008). Eight out of these 15 countries are in sub-Saharan Africa and four are in Southeast Asia. This large variation on the distribution of diarrhea deaths is further witnessed within countries. In the Americas, Huicho et al. (2006) have shown that proportional mortality from diarrhea varied from 7% in the Peruvian coastal area to 9% in the Andean region to 11% in the jungle, in the period 1996–2000. A study carried out in southeast Brazil (Guimaraes et al. 2001) has shown a threefold difference (from 10.8 to 30.1%) in the proportions of infant deaths due to diarrhea between six districts under study. Even more appalling is the variation observed in Mexico (Mota 2000): an approximate 20-fold difference between the states of Chiapas (highest) and Sinaloa (lowest).

In India, a study carried out in six rural and three urban areas representing eight major national states showed that 88% of the infant deaths due to diarrhea occurred in rural areas while only 12% happened in urban sites (Tandon et al. 1987). Within districts in a rural area of Ethiopia, a sixfold difference in

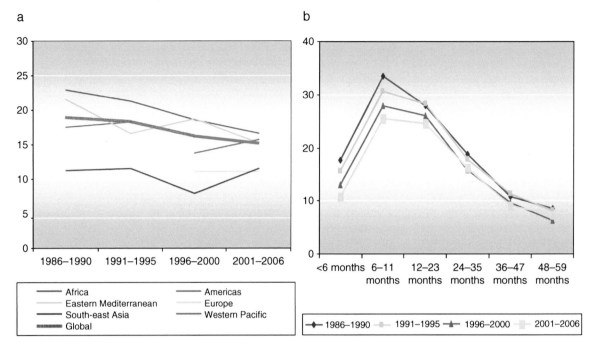

Fig. 13.1 (**a**) Global and regional trends in the prevalence of diarrheal diseases among children under-5 in the 2 weeks preceding DHS surveys by the WHO regions and time period. (**b**) Diarrhea prevalence among children under-5 in the 2 weeks preceding DHS surveys by age group and time period. Source: Macro International (2007)

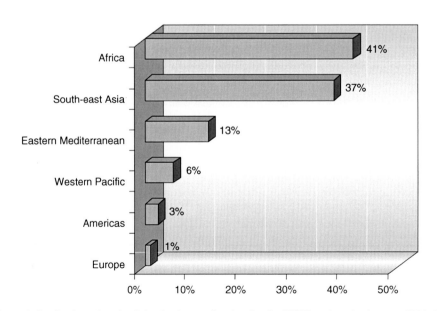

Fig. 13.2 Estimated distribution of under-5 deaths due to diarrhea by the WHO regions in the year 2004. Source: Boschi-Pinto et al. (2008)

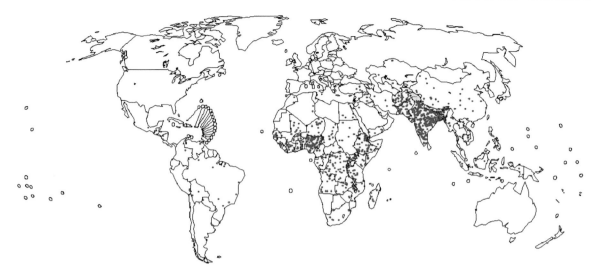

Fig. 13.3 Distribution of estimated number of deaths due to diarrheal disease among children under-5 in the year 2004 (1,000 deaths per dot). Source: Boschi-Pinto et al. (2008)

mortality rates was observed. Areas furthest away from the only health center in the district had the highest mortality burden (Shamebo et al. 1991).

Although DHS do not usually report causes of death, the 2004 survey carried out in Bangladesh (BDHS 2004) included this information. A fourfold variation in deaths due to diarrhea was revealed between the five divisions assessed (Fig. 13.4). Diarrhea proportional mortality ranged from 2.1% in Rajshahi division to 8.5% in Chittagong division.

Age Distribution of Deaths Due to Diarrhea

Diarrhea deaths are less frequent among neonates than among children 1–59 months of age, reaching its maximum burden between the first and the eleventh months of life, when breastfeeding tends to be terminated and infants are first exposed to adverse environmental factors such as contaminated water and food and lack of sanitation and of personal and

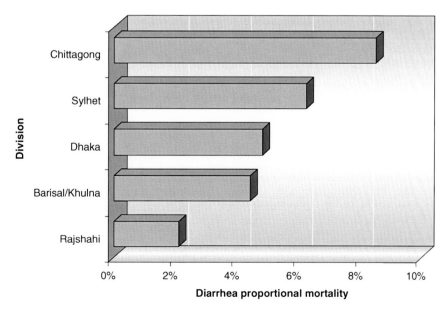

Fig. 13.4 Diarrhea proportional mortality among under-5s by Bangladeshi divisions. Source: Bangladesh DHS (2004)

domestic hygiene (Ehiri and Prowse 1999). The recent WHO estimates show that almost 95% of all under-5 deaths due to diarrhea occur after the first month of life (WHO 2005). Studies from different regions of the world, carried out at various periods of time, provide further evidence that diar-

children 4–5 years old. Hammer et al. (2006) have shown that, in a malaria holoendemic area of northwestern Burkina Faso, mortality attributed to acute gastrointestinal infection peaks among infants 6–11 months. Studies carried out in Asia (Baqui et al. 2001) have also shown that proportions are consis-

Table 13.2 Age distribution of diarrhea deaths among under-5s

References	Region	Period of study	Neonatal % (N)	1–11 months % (N)	<1 year % (N)	12–59 months %(N)	Total (0–59) diarrhea deaths (N)
Baqui et al. (1998)	Southeast Asia	1988–1993	8 (10)	45 (55)	53 (65)	47 (57)	122
Baqui et al. (2001)	Southeast Asia	1992–1996	6 (6)	57 (60)	63 (66)	37 (39)	105
Barros et al. (1987)	America	1982–1986	...	...	86 (25)	14 (4)	29
Bendib et al. (1993)	Africa	1985–1989	10 (27)	73(203)	83(230)	17 (46)	276
Campos et al. (1995)	America	1986	...	...	83 (35)	17 (7)	42
De Francisco et al. (1993)	Africa	1988–1989	10 (10)	37 (38)	47 (48)	53 (54)	102
Ekanem et al. (1994)	Africa	1991	0 (0)	24 (9)	24 (9)	76 (28)	37
Garrib et al. (2006)	Africa	2000–2002	0 (0)	43 (12)	43 (12)	57 (16)	28
Jinadu et al. (1991)	Africa	1987	...	...	59 (23)	41 (16)	39
Marsh et al. (1993)	Eastern Mediterranean	1988–1991	0 (0)	72 (13)	72 (13)	28 (5)	18
Stanton and Langsten (2000)	Eastern Mediterranean	1994–1996	12 (8)	38 (25)	50 (33)	50 (33)	66
Yassin (2000)	Eastern Mediterranean	1992–1996	10(8)	68 (53)	78 (61)	22 (17)	78
Median (25% and 75% IQI)	All	1990 (1987–1994)	**8% (0–10%)**	**45% (38–70%)**	**61% (47–83%)**	**39% (17–53%)**	**942 deaths**

rhea deaths are indeed less frequent among neonates (median = 8%; range: 0–12%) and highest among children 1–11 months (median = 45%; range: 24–73%). These studies are summarized in Table 13.2.

Studies that focused on slightly different age group breakdowns have shown similar patterns. In northern Nigeria (Bradley and Gilles 1984), deaths due to diarrhea had the following age pattern: 16% among neonates, 11% among children 1–5 and 6–11 months of age, 9% in children 1–2 and 2–3 years old, 6% among those 3–4 years old, and 8% among

tently lower among neonates (median 9%; range 3–15%) and are equal to or greater than 85% among children 1–11 months (median 91%; range 85–97%). Anand et al. (2000) reported that, in a rural area of a northern state in India, 12% of the 88 diarrhea deaths among infants that occurred in the period 1972–1974 were in the neonatal period, and 88% in the post-neonatal period. In this same area, in 1982–1984, 95% of diarrhea deaths happened after the 28th day of life and in 1992–1994 this proportion was equal to 97%. Similarly, studies from Bangladesh (Baqui et al. 2001) have shown that 85% of infant diarrhea deaths happened in the post-neonatal period in 1988–1993, increasing to 91% in 1992–1996.

Likewise, global diarrhea mortality rates are highest in the youngest (infants) than among children 1–4 years of age. Kosek et al. (2003) have reported a global median mortality rate more than twofold higher in infants (8.5 per 1,000 children per year) than in children 1–4 years (3.8 per 1,000 children per year) in the developing world.

Assessing "Trends" in Diarrhea Mortality

The decreasing trend in diarrhea mortality among children less than 5 years of age is largely documented. The first sources of evidence are the three reviews mentioned in the introduction of this chapter (Snyder and Merson 1982; Bern et al. 1992; Kosek et al. 2003). Regardless of the possible limitations inherent to these types of review and of the

lack of comparability with respect to some design issues, these studies constitute an important body of evidence of the burden of diarrheal diseases over time. Several other studies have also reported major reductions in diarrhea mortality rates as well as in the proportional mortality due to diarrhea over time (Table 13.3). Impressive decreases of 76 and 81% in mortality rates among infants and children 1–4 years of age, respectively, have been described by Miller et al. (1994) in Egypt during the 1980s. Guimaraes et al. (2001) also reported a decrease in proportional diarrhea mortality of more than 70% among Brazilian infants in the 1990s.

Further indication that, at least for some countries, diarrhea mortality has been declining over the years can be found in studies by Villa et al. (1999), Miller and Hirschhorn (1995), Victora et al. (2000), and Baltazar et al. (2002). These declining trends are reportedly owed to the progress in case management of diarrheal diseases.

Table 13.3 Decrease of diarrhea mortality over time among under-5s

References	Region	Period	Measure	Decrease (%)	Age group
Anand et al. (2000)	Southeast Asia	1983–1993	Proportional diarrhea mortality	31	1–11 months
Campos et al. (1995)	Americas	1986–1989	Number of diarrhea deaths	69	0–11 months
El-Rafie et al. (1990)	Eastern Mediterranean	1982–1987	Cause-specific mortality rate	58	0–11 months
El-Rafie et al. (1990)	Eastern Mediterranean	1982–1987	Cause-specific mortality rate	43	1–4 years
Guimaraes et al. (2001)	Americas	1980–1989	Proportional diarrhea mortality	58	0–11 months
Guimaraes et al. (2001)	Americas	1990–1998	Proportional diarrhea mortality	72	0–11 months
Gutierrez et al. (1996)	Americas	1984–1989	Proportional diarrhea mortality	28	0–59 months
Gutierrez et al. (1996)	Americas	1990–1993	Proportional diarrhea mortality	33	0–59 months
Huicho et al. (2006)	Americas	1996–2000	Proportional diarrhea mortality	82	0–59 months
Jaffar et al. 1997	Africa	1989–1993	Cause-specific mortality rate	64	0–11 months
Jaffar et al. (1997)	Africa	1989–1993	Cause-specific mortality rate	53	1–4 years
Miller et al. (1994)	Eastern Mediterranean	1980–1990	Cause-specific mortality rate	76	0–11 months
Miller et al. (1994)	Eastern Mediterranean	1980–1990	Cause-specific mortality rate	81	1–4 years
Mota-Hernández, (2000)	Americas	1990–1994	Cause-specific mortality rate	62	1–4 years
No authorship – report MoH, Mexico (1994)	Americas	1985–1993	Cause-specific mortality rate	69	0–59 months

Information on the proportion of deaths due to diarrheal disease was obtained from studies carried out between 1981 and 1998 in 25 countries from different regions of the world. These studies allowed the abstraction and plot of 69 data points that are shown in Fig. 13.5(a). Time period of the studies is distributed around an average mid-surveillance period 1985–1990. The plotting of the diarrhea proportional mortality obtained from these studies suggests a decreasing trend over time, possibly reflecting the secular downward trend in child mortality that has been accompanied by a decrease in the proportion of deaths due to diarrhea. As these studies were carried out in different sites and had different designs, the plot of the data points does not represent real-time trends. Yet, they provide some further indication of the decline in diarrhea proportional mortality over time. It is worth noting that the data used in these figures refer to studies that were mainly carried out in the late 1980s and early 1990s. This represents a more than 10-year lag time. Hence, this currently available data are unable to capture recent changes

due to interventions, coverage, or to new emerging diseases and competing causes of death.

Vital registration data on under-5 mortality rates (per 1,000 under-5 population) for 20 countries in Latin America from 1970 to 1990 have been published by Bern et al. (1992). Although these data represent real trends, they also have some severe limitations such as lack of comparability due to huge variability in the vital registration systems between countries (e.g., different coverage, underreporting rates, and miscoding of causes of death) and over time. Furthermore, where coverage is incomplete, the poorer population, with higher mortality rates and different patterns of causes of death, is likely to be underrepresented. Even within countries, these trends may be difficult to compare without a correction factor, as the systems and coverage tend to improve over time. Finally, these data also have the limitation of not capturing recent data and trends. Consequently, data presented in Fig. 13.5(a and b) should be interpreted with caution, especially if attempting to extrapolate them to recent years.

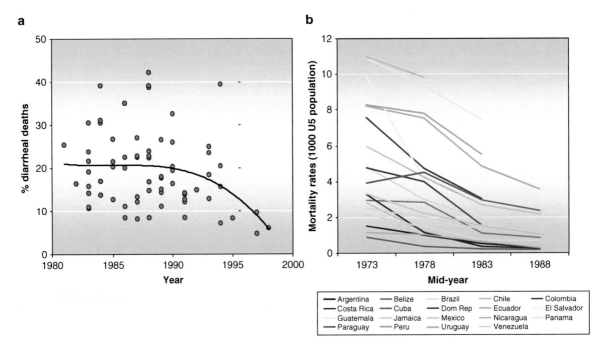

Fig. 13.5 (a) Proportion of deaths due to diarrhea among children under-5 by mid-year of study, 1981–1998. Source: Boschi-Pinto et al. (2008). (b) Diarrhea mortality rates (per 1,000 under-5 population) in some Latin American countries, 1970–1990. Source: Bern et al. (1992)

Etiology

Major pathogens involved in diarrheal diseases have been the focus of several community- and facility-based studies. Results from community-based studies are usually more representative of the overall occurrence of disease than facility-based studies, as their findings are independent of the severity of disease or care-seeking behavior. In community-based studies, enteropathogens have been generally identified and reported in about 50% of stool samples collected during episodes of diarrhea. In facility-based studies, this proportion was between 60 and 70%.

A recent review of studies published since 1990 showed that the enteropathogen most frequently isolated from stools in community-based studies was enterotoxigenic *E. coli*. This pathogen was identified in about 14% of samples collected during episodes of diarrhea. *Giardia lamblia*, enteropathogenic *E. coli*, and *Rotavirus* were identified as the next most commonly isolated pathogens, with reported prevalence between 8 and 10%. Other common enteropathogens included *Campylobacter, Shigella, C. parvum*, and *E. histolytica*.

In facility-based studies, rotavirus was the enteropathogen most frequently isolated, with a prevalence that varied between 18 and 25%. Bacterial pathogens such as enterotoxigenic *E. coli*, enteropathogenic *E. coli, Campylobacter*, and *Shigella* were also frequently identified. *Vibrio cholerae* is frequently isolated in some settings, and in more recent studies, *Norovirus* has been recognized as an important cause of severe diarrhea in both developed and developing countries.

Risk Factors

Some of the well-established determinants of diarrheal morbidity and mortality are socioeconomic status (Yeager et al. 1991), crowding, access to clean water and sanitation (Rahaman et al. 1985), and maternal education (Betrand and Walmus 1983). These main determinants of the development of diarrheal disease are intrinsically linked to poverty.

Place of residence within countries (rural or urban, districts, provinces, etc.), wealth, crowding, access to clean water and sanitation, and mother's education are all closely intertwined and denounce social inequalities that are reflected in the health status of the child. In some countries, disparities are also observed by sex of the child, girls being less likely to survive or to be taken to a health facility than boys (Larson et al. 2006). Diarrhea could well be considered as a "sentinel" disease in terms of inequities in general social welfare and in access to health care as it can be easily prevented and averted through affordable means.

Data from DHS surveys carried out in 41 countries between 2002 and 2007 have been analyzed, revealing a 34% increase in diarrhea prevalence in the 2 weeks before the survey among children of mothers with no education as compared to those children of mothers with secondary or higher level of education. Children living in rural settings had a 10% higher prevalence than children from urban areas.

The association of these risk factors and diarrheal mortality is exemplified in some studies. Gurgel et al. (1997) have shown that, in an urban setting in northeastern Brazil, higher diarrhea mortality rates were seen in districts with higher proportions of slums than in those with fewer slums ($p < 0.001$). Gutierrez et al. (1996) have shown a strong inverse correlation between under-5 mortality from diarrheal diseases and the proportion of literate women (Pearson correlation = 0.7958). In a metropolitan area of northeastern Brazil (Campos et al. 1995) and in rural districts of Sierra Leone (Amin 1996), higher proportions of diarrhea deaths were reported among children whose mothers had lower level of education than among those whose mothers had at least secondary school education. The DHS carried out in Bangladesh in 2004 has also examined the distribution of causes of death according to the level of mother's education. An increased 50% diarrhea mortality was observed among children whose mothers had lowest level of education.

The major route of transmission for diarrheal pathogens is the fecal–oral route. Consequently, both access to clean water and safe disposal of human feces are expected to reduce transmission of most pathogens. Poor sanitation, lack of access to clean water, and inadequate personal hygiene are responsible for an important proportion of childhood diarrhea. Therefore, hygiene and feces disposal practices at home are key determinant factors for reduction of the incidence of diarrheal disease. Contaminated water plays an important role in the transmission of some pathogens that cause diarrhea. Huttly et al. (1997) have shown that promotion of hand washing can reduce diarrhea incidence by an average of 33%. In a recent meta-analysis, Ejemot et al. (2008) found that interventions promoting hand washing resulted in a 29% reduction in diarrhea episodes in institutions in high-income countries (IRR 0.71, 95% CI 0.60–0.84; 7 trials) and a 31% reduction in such episodes in communities in low- or middle-income countries (IRR 0.69, 95% CI 0.55–0.87; 5 trials). However, effects on reduction of mortality have not been shown. Yet, another six observational studies did demonstrate a median reduction of 55% in all-cause child mortality associated with improved access to sanitation facilities (Esrey et al. 1985). Sanitation schemes such as latrines generally require proper education and active involvement of the community in order to be effective. The use of potties was identified as an important intervention to avoid fecal contamination of household's soil by toddlers (Yeager et al. 2002). Nevertheless, behavior change is complex, and significant resources are needed to tackle such interventions.

Synergy with Malnutrition

Diarrhea and undernutrition act synergistically in an implacable manner as frequent and prolonged episodes of diarrhea usually lead to malnutrition and malnutrition facilitates the progression of diarrhea toward death (Fontaine and Boschi-Pinto 2006). Strong evidence of such fatal synergy is provided by several studies worldwide. Community-based studies report an increased risk of mortality from diarrhea among children who had low weight for their age. In a study carried out in an urban setting of northeast Brazil, Gurgel et al. (1997) showed that diarrhea and malnutrition were recorded together in 26% of the 318 under-5 deaths caused by diarrhea. In rural India, Bhandari et al. (1992) have also demonstrated that severely malnourished children had a 24-fold higher diarrheal case fatality rate as compared to normally nourished children.

Moreover, the risk of dying from diarrheal disease has been shown to be proportional to the degree of malnutrition. A dose–response relationship was reported in studies from India (Bhandari et al. 1992), the Philippines (Yoon et al. 1997), and Sudan (Fawzi et al. 1997) and a review of six prospective studies (Pelletier et al. 1993) has demonstrated a consistent increase in mortality with poorer nutritional status. Caulfield et al. (2004) performed a combined analysis of data from 10 longitudinal community-based studies. The authors found that the relative risk of death from diarrhea was increased for children who were less than $-1z$ weight for age, and that the risk increased progressively with each z-score below the median. The authors further estimated that 61% of under-5 deaths attributable to diarrhea are associated with children being underweight.

Preventive and Treatment Interventions

Promotion of Exclusive Breastfeeding

Exclusive breastfeeding means no food or drink (not even water) other than breast milk is permitted, except for supplements of vitamins and minerals or necessary medicines. The WHO has established, based on sound evidence, that the optimal duration of exclusive breastfeeding is 6 months (WHO 2001). A meta-analysis of three studies carried out in developing countries shows that children under 6 months of age that are breastfed are six times less likely to die of diarrhea than infants who are not breastfed (WHO 2000). When exclusive breastfeeding is continued during diarrhea, it also diminishes the adverse impact of poor nutritional status. Estimates suggest that breastfeeding promotion could also decrease all-cause mortality in children under-5 by 13% (Jones et al. 2003).

Vaccines

One of the major complications of measles infection is diarrheal disease secondary to immunodeficiency. It has been estimated that high coverage of measles vaccines would prevent up to 3.8% of diarrheal episodes and 6–26% of under-5 deaths due to diarrhea (Feachem and Koblinsky 1983). Currently available vaccines against cholera are likely to be safe and offer reasonable protection for a limited period of time; however, they are rarely used in developing countries and only Vietnam has established routine cholera vaccination (Keusch et al. 2006). It has been estimated that rotavirus accounts for at least a yearly 475,000 deaths among under-5s (Parashar et al. 2003). In 1998, a live rotavirus vaccine was introduced in the United States (Glass et al. 1999), but it was withdrawn from the market due to the detection of an increased occurrence of intussusceptions among vaccinated children (CDC 1999). Two new vaccines have been recently introduced into the markets, which were proven to be safe and effective: an attenuated human rotavirus strain (Ruiz-Palacios et al. 2006) and a bovine-based tetravalent rotavirus vaccine (Vesikari et al. 2006). These vaccines are currently being used in several countries in the American region.

Oral Rehydration Therapy (ORT)

Case studies in countries such as Brazil (Victora et al. 1996), Egypt (Miller and Hirschhorn 1995), and Mexico (Gutierrez et al. 1996) have demonstrated an association between increased use of ORT and marked declines in mortality due to diarrhea. Oral rehydration therapy (ORT) was introduced in 1979, consisting of the oral administration of sodium, a carbohydrate, and water (Hirschhorn and Greenough 1991). It rapidly became the foundation for the control of diarrheal diseases, but scientific progress together with considerations on feasibility has led to a series of changes in the recommendations on the use of ORT for home treatment of diarrheal diseases. In the early 1980s, it was recommended that all diarrhea episodes should be treated with a solution of oral rehydration salts (ORS). With the recognition that access to ORS was limited and that more than two-thirds of diarrhea cases were not accompanied by dehydration, the focus thus shifted to the prevention of dehydration through recommended home fluids (RHFs). In 1988, continued feeding was added as one of the appropriate managements of diarrhea cases. Later, in 1990–1991, emphasis shifted to the amount of fluids given rather than the type of fluid. Finally, since 1993, more

importance has been given to increased fluids plus continued feeding (Victora et al. 2000).

A new ORS solution with lower salt and glucose content was launched by the WHO and UNICEF in May 2002. Some of the advantages of this new solution are reduced stool output and duration, less vomiting, and decreased need of intravenous fluids, thus improving acceptance by mothers and health workers.

Zinc Supplementation

A review of relevant clinical trials has indicated that zinc supplementation given during an episode of acute diarrhea reduces both duration and severity of the disease and could prevent about 300,000 child deaths each year (Black 2003). The WHO and UNICEF currently recommend that all children with acute diarrhea be given zinc for 10–14 days during and after diarrhea (WHO/UNICEF 2004). Zinc supplementation and the newly formulated ORS used in combination with promotion of exclusive breastfeeding, general nutritional support, and selective and appropriate use of antibiotics can further reduce the number of diarrheal deaths among children. Moreover, zinc supplements administered during 10–14 days have been shown to reduce the incidence of diarrhea in the following 2–3 months.

Access to, and Quality of, Care

Reductions in diarrheal mortality are known to be linked to increased utilization of health services. Figure 13.6 illustrates the differences in care seeking for diarrhea observed in 19 countries with available DHS data for the years 2005 and 2006. According to these data, the proportion of children with diarrhea in the 2 weeks preceding the survey that were reportedly taken to a health facility or provider showed a fivefold difference, varying from 14% in Rwanda to 70% in Uganda. In 17 of the 19 (89%) countries observed, appropriate care was sought in less than 50% of diarrheal cases and in 10 (53%) countries, less than 30% of the ill children were taken to either a health facility or provider.

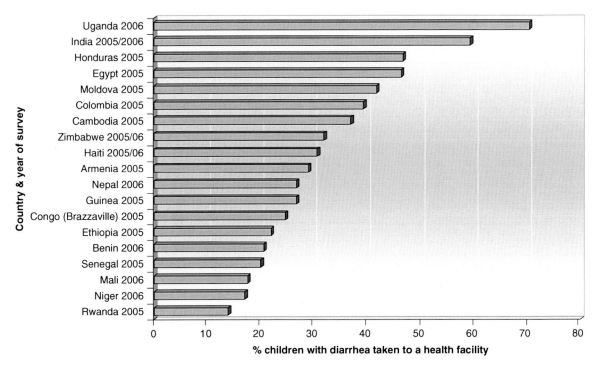

Fig. 13.6 Children under-5 with diarrhea symptoms who were taken to a health provider in some selected countries of the world 2005–2006. Source: DHS (2005–2006)

Some identified predictors of healthcare utilization by children with diarrheal disease include length of illness and maternal education. Children whose diarrhea last for 2 or more days are more likely to be taken to a health facility (Thind 2003) than those children whose diarrhea last for less than 2 days. Also, mothers with a higher level of education are more likely to take their children to a health facility during an episode of diarrhea than those with lower levels of education (Thind 2003). In an urban area of Guinea-Bissau, care-seeking behavior of mothers of deceased children in the post-neonatal period was investigated. Median time from the onset of symptoms to first consultation was 2 days for acute diarrhea and 14.5 days for chronic diarrhea cases. The health center was the place of first consultation for 56.5 and 66.7% of acute and chronic cases, respectively (Sodemann et al. 1997). In Bangladesh, the most common predictors for seeing a licensed provider, after adjustment for host and illness characteristics, were higher income, longer duration of illness,

and higher education of the mother. In rural settings, where access to licensed providers is much more restricted, the most important predictors were younger age of the child, longer duration of illness, and mother's education (Larson et al. 2006).

Overall, children who live in urban settings, children whose mothers have at least secondary school education, and those who are from households in the highest wealth quintile have a much higher likelihood of seeking treatment for diarrhea from a health professional or facility. Figure 13.7 illustrates the differences in care seeking according to the place of residence and level of mother's education in some selected countries. Considerable differences are also present in diarrhea case management according to the place of residence (urban–rural). Children with diarrhea living in urban areas are not only more likely to be taken to a health facility than children living in rural areas, but they are also more likely to be adequately treated with ORT and increased fluid intake.

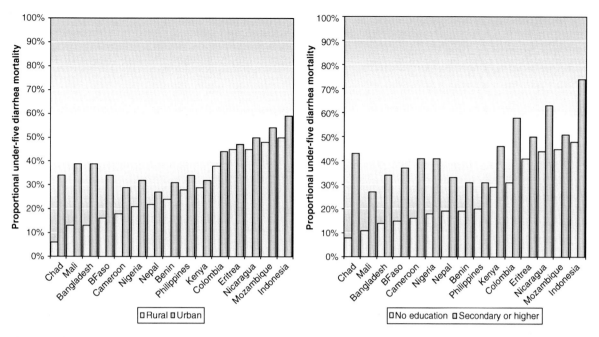

Fig. 13.7 Children under-5 with diarrhea symptoms taken to a health facility according to the place of residence (rural and urban) and level of mother's education. Source: DHS (2004)

Conclusions

Despite the decline in numbers and rates of diarrhea deaths worldwide over the past decades, diarrheal diseases remain the second leading single cause of death among children less than 5 years of age in the world. This burden is especially high in the African and Southeast Asia regions. Determinants of the disease and prevention measures are well established and case management is accessible, effective, and affordable.

Nevertheless, children from less privileged regions of the world suffer, on average, more than 3 episodes of diarrheal disease each year and almost 2 million under-5s continue to die every year as a consequence of diarrheal diseases. Careful planning and prioritization of interventions to control diarrhea deaths as well as monitoring and evaluating their progress in low-income areas are crucial to reduce under-5 diarrhea mortality toward the levels attained by more developed regions of the world.

Key Terms

Campylobacter	*Entamoeba histolytica*	Oral rehydration therapy
Case fatality rate	*Escherichia coli*	Persistent diarrhea
Cholera	Exclusive breastfeeding	Prospective studies
Cryptosporidium parvum	*Giardia lamblia*	*Rotavirus*
Dehydration	Maternal mortality	*Shigella*
Demography and Health Surveys (DHS)	Median incidence	Under-5 mortality
	Multiple Indicator Cluster Surveys (MICS)	*Vibrio cholerae*
Diarrhea episode		*z*-Score
Dysentery	Neonatal mortality	

Questions for Discussion

1. Estimates show a steady decline in childhood diarrheal mortality from 3.3 million deaths in the 1990s to less than 2 million currently. However, diarrhea remains the second leading cause of under-5 mortality globally, and although mortality has been decreasing, childhood diarrheal morbidity remains relatively stable. Why is this?

2. What factors explain the wide variations observed in the distribution of diarrheal deaths between and within countries? In a country such as India, for example, what factors would account for urban–rural differentials in childhood diarrhea mortality?

3. Diarrheal deaths are less frequent among neonates than among children 1–59 months of age. Why?

4. Explain the mechanisms for the synergistic relationship between childhood diarrhea and childhood malnutrition.

5. Various intervention strategies for reducing morbidity and mortality from childhood diarrhea have been evaluated, including promotion of exclusive breastfeeding, rotavirus vaccines, oral rehydration therapy, and zinc supplementation. Discuss the relative importance of each strategy based on available evidence.

References

Abu-Elyazeed R, Wierzba TF, Mourad AS et al. (1999) Epidemiology of Enterotoxigenic *Escherichia coli* Diarrhea in a Pediatric Cohort in a Periurban Area of Lower Egypt. Journal of Infectious Diseases, 179: 382–389.

Amin R (1996) Immunization coverage and child mortality in two rural districts of Sierra Leone. Social Science and Medicine, 42: 1599–1604.

Anand K, Kant S, Kumar G et al. (2000) "Development" is not essential to reduce infant mortality rate in India: experience from the Ballabgarh project. Journal Epidemiology and Community Health, 54: 247–253.

Baltazar JC, Nadera DP, Victora CG (2002) Evaluation of the national control of diarrhoeal disease programme in the Philippines, 1980–1993. Bulletin of World Health Organization, 80: 637–643.

Baqui AH, Black RE, Sack RB et al. (1993) Malnutrition, cell-mediated immune deficiency, and diarrhea: a community-based longitudinal study in rural Bangladeshi children. American Journal of Epidemiology, 137: 355–365.

Baqui AH, Black RE, Arifeen SE et al. (1998) Causes of childhood deaths in Bangladesh: results of a nationwide verbal autopsy study. Bulletin of the World Health Organization, 76: 161–171.

Baqui AH, Sabir AA, Begum N et al. (2001) Causes of childhood deaths in Bangladesh: an update. Acta Paediatrica, 90: 682–690.

Barreto ML, Santos LM, Assis AM et al. (1994) Effect of vitamin A supplementation on diarrhea and acute lower respiratory tract infections in young children in Brazil. Lancet, 344: 228–231.

Barros FC, Victora CG, Vaughan JP (1987) Causes of perinatal mortality in Pelotas, RS (Brazil). Use of a simplified classification. Revista de Saúde Pública, 21: 310–316.

Bangladesh Demography and Health Survey (DHS) (2004) Bangladesh: improving maternal and child health in the south-east Asia region http://unpan1.un.org/intradoc/groups/public/documents/APCITY/UNPAN022523.pdf Cited 2 August 2008.

Bendib A, Dekkar N, Lamdjadani N (1993) Factors associated with neonatal, infant and child mortality: Results of a national survey in Algeria. Archives of French Pediatrics, 50: 741–747.

Bern C, Martines J, de Zoysa I, Glass RI (1992) The magnitude of the global problem of diarrheal disease: a ten-year update. Bulletin of the World Health Organization, 70: 705–714.

Betrand WE, Walmus BF (1983) Maternal knowledge, attitudes and practice as predictors of diarrheal disease in young children. International Journal of Epidemiology, 12: 205–210.

Boschi-Pinto C, Velebit L, Shibuya K (2008) Estimating child mortality due to diarrhea in developing countries. Bulletin of the World Health Organization, 86: 710–717.

Bhandari N, Bhan MK, Sazawal S (1992) Mortality associated with acute watery diarrhea, dysentery and persistent diarrhea in rural north India. Acta Paediatrica Supplement 381: 3–6.

Black RE (2003) Zinc deficiency, infectious disease and mortality in the developing world. Journal of Nutrition, 133:1; 1485S–1489S.

Bradley AK, Gilles HM (1984) Malumfashi Endemic Diseases Research Project, XXI. Pointers to causes of death in the Malumfashi area, northern Nigeria. Annals of Tropical Medicine and Parasitology, 78: 265–271.

Bryce J, Terreri N, Victora CG et al. (2006) Countdown to 2015: tracking intervention coverage for child survival. Lancet, 368: 1067–1076.

Campos G, de J, Dos Reis Filho SA et al. (1995) Infant morbimortality due to acute diarrhea in a metropolitan area of northeastern Brazil, 1986–1989. Revista de Saúde Publica, 29: 132–139.

Caulfield LE, de Onis M, Blossner M et al. (2004) Undernutrition as an underlying cause of child deaths associated with diarrhea, pneumonia, malaria and measles. American Journal of Clinical Nutrition, 80: 193–198.

Centers for Disease Control and Prevention (1999) Intussusception among recipients of rotavirus vaccine. United States, 1998–1999. Morbidity and Mortality Weekly Report, 48: 577–581.

Chavasse DC, Shier RP, Murphy OA et al. (1999) Impact of fly control on childhood diarrhea in Pakistan: community-randomised trial. Lancet, 353: 22–25.

Chen KC, Lin CH, Qiao QX et al. (1991) The epidemiology of diarrheal diseases in southeastern China. Journal of Diarrheal Diseases Research, 9: 94–99.

Cravioto A, Reyes RE, Trujillo F et al. (1990) Risk of diarrhea during the first year of life associated with initial and subsequent colonization by specific enteropathogens. American Journal of Epidemiology, 131: 886–904.

Cruz JR, Bartlett AV, Mendez H et al. (1992) Epidemiology of persistent diarrhea among Guatemalan srural children. Acta Paediatrica Supplement, 381: 22–26.

De Francisco A, Hall AJ, Schellenberg JR et al. (1993) The pattern of infant and childhood mortality in Upper River Division, The Gambia. Annals of Tropical Pediatrics, 13: 345–352.

Dibley MJ, Sadjimin T, Kjolhede et al. (1996) Vitamin A supplementation fails to reduce incidence of acute respiratory illness and diarrhea in preschool-age Indonesian children. Journal of Nutrition, 126: 434–442.

Ehiri JE, Prowse JM (1999) Child health promotion in developing countries: the case for integration of environmental and social interventions? Health Policy and Planning 14: 1–10.

Ejemot RI, Ehiri JE, Meremikwu MM et al. (2008) Hand washing for preventing diarrhea. Cochrane Database of Systematic Reviews, Issue 1.

Ekanem EE, Asindii AA, Okoi OU (1994) Community-based surveillance of paediatric deaths in Cross River State, Nigeria. Tropical and Geographical Medicine, 46: 305–308.

El-Rafie M, Hassouna WA, Hirschhorn N et al. (1990) Effect of diarrheal disease control on infant and childhood mortality in Egypt. Report from the National Control of Diarrheal Diseases Project. Lancet, 335: 334–338.

Esrey SA, Feachem RG, Hughes JM (1985) Interventions for the control of diarrheal diseases among young children: improving water supplies and excreta disposal facilities. Bulletin of the World Health Organization, 63: 757–772.

Fawzi WW, Herrera MG, Spiegelman DL et al. (1997) A prospective study of malnutrition in relation to child mortality in the Sudan. American Journal of Clinical Nutrition, 65: 1062–1069.

Feachem RG, Koblinsky MA (1983) Interventions for the control of diarrheal diseases among young children: measles immunization. Bulletin of the World Health Organization, 61: 641–652.

Ferreccio C, Prado V, Ojeda A et al. (1991) Epidemiologic patterns of acute diarrhea and endemic shigella infections in children in a poor periurban setting in Santiago, Chile. American Journal of Epidemiology, 134: 614–627.

Fontaine O, Boschi-Pinto C (2006) Special Section: Diarrheal Diseases. Population Bulletin, 61: 10–13.

Garrib A, Jaffar S, Knight S et al. (2006) Rates and causes of child mortality in an area of high HIV prevalence in rural South Africa. Tropical Medicine and International Health, 11: 1841–1848.

Glass RI, Bresee JS, Parashar UD et al. (1999) First rotavirus vaccine licensed: is there really a need? Acta Paediatrica Supplement, 88: 2–8.

Guerrero ML, Noel JS, Mitchell DK et al. (1998) A prospective study of astrovirus diarrhea of infancy in Mexico City. Pediatric Infectious Disease Journal, 17: 723–727.

Guimaraes ZA, Costa MC, Paim JS et al. (2001) Decline and social inequalities of infant mortality caused by diarrhea. Revista da Sociedade Brasileira de Medicina Tropical, 34: 473–478.

Gupta DN, Sircar BK, Sengupta PG et al. (1996) Epidemiological and clinical profiles of acute invasive diarrhea with special reference to mucoid episodes: a rural community-based longitudinal study. Transactions of the Royal Society of Tropical Medicine and Hygiene, 90: 544–547.

Gurgel RQ, Andrade JM, Machado-Neto P et al. (1997) Diarrhea mortality in Aracaju, Brazil. Annals of Tropical Pediatrics, 17: 361–365.

Gutierrez G, Tapia-Conyer R, Guiscafré H et al. (1996) Impact of oral rehydration and selected public health interventions on reduction of mortality from childhood diarrheal diseases in Mexico. Bulletin of the World Health Organization, 74: 189–197.

Hammer GP, Some F, Muller O et al. (2006) Pattern of cause-specific childhood mortality in a malaria endemic area of Burkina Faso. Malaria Journal, 5: 47.

Mota HF (2000) Disminución de la mortalidad por diarrea en niños. Bol Med Hosp Infant Mex, 57: 32–40.

Hirschhorn N, Greenough WB (1991) Progress in oral rehydration therapy. Scientific American, 264: 50–56.

Huicho L, Trelles M, Gonzales F (2006) National and sub-national under-five mortality profiles in Peru: a basis for informed policy decisions. BMC Public Health, 6, 173.

Huttly SR, Morris SS, Pisani V (1997) Prevention of diarrhea in young children in developing countries. Bulletin of the World Health Organization, 75: 163–174.

Institute of Medicine (1986) Committee on Issues and Priorities for New Vaccine Development. New vaccine development: establishing priorities. Vol. II. Diseases of importance in developing countries. Washington, DC: National Academy Press.

Jaffar S, Leach A, Greenwood AM et al. (1997) Changes in the pattern of infant and childhood mortality in Upper River Division, The Gambia, from 1989 to 1993. Tropical Medical International Health, 2: 28–37.

Jinadu MK, Olusi SO, Agun JI et al. (1991) Childhood diarrhea in rural Nigeria. I. Studies on prevalence, mortality and socio-environmental factors. Journal of Diarrheal Diseases Research, 9: 323–327.

Jones G, Steketee RW, Black RE et al. (2003) Bellagio Child Survival Study Group. How many child deaths can we prevent this year? Lancet, 362: 65–71.

Kaminsky RG (1991) Parasitism and diarrhea in children from two rural communities and marginal barrio in Honduras. Transactions of the Royal Society of Tropical Medicine and Hygiene, 85: 70–73.

Keusch GT, Fontaine O, Bhargava A et al. (2006) Diarrheal diseases. In: Jamison DT, Breman JG, Measham AR, et al. eds. Diseases Control Priorities in Developing Countries (second edition). New York: Oxford University Press and the World Bank, pp. 371–388.

Kosek M, Bern C, Guerrant R (2003) The global burden of diarrheal disease as estimated from studies published between 1992 and 2000. Bulletin of the World Health Organization, 81: 197–204.

Lal S (1994) Surveillance of acute diarrheal diseases at village level for effective home management of diarrhea. Indian Journal of Public Health, 38: 65–68.

Lanata CF, Midthun K, Black RE et al. (1996) Safety, Immunogenicity, and protective efficacy of one and three doses of the Tetravalent Rhesus Rotavirus Vaccine in infants in Lima, Peru. Journal of Infectious Diseases, 174: 268–275.

Larson CP, Saha UR, Islam R et al. (2006) Childhood diarrhea management practices in Bangladesh: private sector dominance and continued inequities in care. International Journal of Epidemiology, 35: 1430–1439.

Lima AM, Moore SR, Barboza MS et al. (2000) Persistent diarrhea signals a critical period of increased diarrhea burdens and nutritional shortfalls: A prospective cohort study among children in northeastern Brazil. Journal of Infectious Diseases, 181: 1643–1651.

Linhares AC, Gabbay YB, Mascarenhas JD et al. (1996) Immunogenicity, safety and efficacy of tetravalent rhesus human reassortant rotavirus vaccine in Belem, Brazil. Bulletin of the World Health Organization, 74: 491–500.

Macro International (2006) India: DHS, 2005/2006 – Final Report (English). Calverton, MD: MEASURE DHS, Macro International Inc.http://www.measuredhs.com/pubs/pub_details.cfm?ID = 723 Cited 12 December 2008

Macro International (2007) Demography and Health Surveys, Global Childhood diarrhea 1986–2006. Calverton, MD: MEASURE DHS, Macro International Inc.

Marsh D, Majid N, Rasmussen Z et al. (1993) Cause-specific child mortality in a mountainous community in Pakistan by verbal autopsy. Journal Pakistan Medical Association, 43: 226–229.

Miller P, Hirschhorn N (1995) The effect of a national control of diarrheal diseases program on mortality: the case of Egypt. Social Science and Medicine, 40: S1–S30.

Miller P, Loza S, Terreri N et al. (1994) Diarrhea and mortality in Menoufia, Egypt. Journal of Diarrheal Diseases Research, 12: 173–181.

Mirza NM, Caulfield LE, Black RE et al. (1997) Risk factors for diarrheal duration. American Journal of Epidemiology, 146: 776–785.

Mølbak K, Jensen H, Ingholt L et al. (1997) Risk factors for diarrheal disease incidence in early childhood: a community cohort study from Guinea-Bissau. American Journal of Epidemiology, 146: 273–282.

Moore S, Lima AAM, Schorling JB et al. (2000) Changes over time in the epidemiology of diarrhea and malnutrition among children in an urban Brazilian shantytown, 1989 to 1996. International Journal of Infectious Diseases, 4: 179–186.

Morris SS, Cousens SN, Lanata CF, Kirkwood BR (1994) Diarrhea – defining the episode. International Journal of Epidemiology, 23: 617–623.

Morris SS, Cousens SN, Kirkwood BR et al. (1996) Is prevalence of diarrhea a better predictor of subsequent mortality and weight gain than diarrhea incidence? American Journal of Epidemiology, 144: 582–588.

Mota H (2000) Disminución de la mortalidad por diarrea en niños. Boletín Médico del Hospital Infantil de México, 57: 32–40.

Naficy AB, Rao MR, Holmes et al. (2000) Astrovirus diarrhea in Egyptian children. Journal of Infectious Diseases, 182: 685–690.

Oni GA, Schumann DA, Oke EA (1991) Diarrheal disease morbidity, risk factors and treatments in a low socioeconomic area of Ilorin, Kwara State, Nigeria. Journal of Diarrheal Diseases Research, 9: 250–257.

Parashar UD, Hummelman EG, Bresee JS et al. (2003) Global illness and deaths caused by rotavirus disease in children. Emerg Infect Dis, 9:565–572.

Pelletier DL, Frongillo EA Jr, Habicht JP (1993) Epidemiologic evidence for a potentiating effect of malnutrition on child mortality. American Journal of Public Health, 83: 1130–1133.

Pérez-Schael I, García D, Gonzáles M et al. (1990) Prospective study of diarrheal diseases in Venezuelan children to evaluate the efficacy of rhesus rotavirus vaccine. Journal of Medical Virology, 30: 219–229.

Punyaratabandhu P, Vathanophas K, Varavithya W et al. (1991) Childhood diarrhea in a low-income urban community in Bangkok: incidence, clinical features, and child caretaker's behaviors. Journal of Diarrheal Diseases Research, 9: 244–249.

Rahaman M, Rahaman MM, Wojtyniak B et al. (1985) Impact of environmental sanitation and crowding on infant mortality in rural Bangladesh. Lancet, 2, 28–31.

Rahmathullah L, Underwood BA, Thulasiraj RD et al. (1991) Diarrhea, respiratory infections, and growth are not affected by a weekly low-dose vitamin A supplement: a masked, controlled field trial in children in southern India. American Journal of Clinical Nutrition, 54, 568–577.

Root GP (2001) Sanitation, community environments, and childhood diarrhea in rural Zimbabwe. Journal of Health, Population and Nutrition, 19, 73–82.

Rudan I, Lawn J, Cousens S et al. (2005) Gaps in policy-relevant information on burden of disease in children: a systematic review. Lancet, 365: 2031–2040.

Ruiz-Palacios GM, Perez-Schael I, Velazquez FR et al. (2006) Safety and efficacy of an attenuated vaccine against severe rotavirus gastroenteritis. New England Journal of Medicine, 354: 11–22.

Schorling JB, Wanke CA, Schorling SK et al. (1990) A prospective study of persistent diarrhea among children in an urban Brazilian slum. American Journal of Epidemiology, 132: 144–156.

Shamebo D, Muhe L, Sandstrom A et al. (1991) The Butajira rural health project in Ethiopia: mortality pattern of the under fives. Journal of Tropical Pediatrics, 37: 254–261.

Snyder JD, Merson MH (1982) The magnitude of the global problem of acute diarrheal disease: a review of active surveillance data. Bulletin of the World Health Organization, 60: 605–613.

Sodemann M, Jakobsen MS, Mølbak K et al. (1997) High mortality despite good care-seeking behavior: a community study of childhood deaths in Guinea-Bissau. Bulletin of the World Health Organization, 75: 205–212.

Stanton B, Langsten R (2000) Morbidity and mortality among Egyptian neonates and infants: rates and associated factors. Annals of Tropical Medicine and Parasitology, 94: 817–829.

Tandon BN, Sahai A, Balaji LN et al. (1987) Morbidity pattern and cause specific mortality during infancy in ICDS projects. Journal of Tropical Pediatrics, 33, 190–193.

Thind A (2003) Diarrhea in the Dominican Republic: determinants of the utilization of children's health services. Journal of Tropical Pediatrics, 49: 93–98.

Thomas JC, Neumann CG (1992) Choosing an appropriate measure of diarrhea occurrence: examples from a community-based study in rural Kenya. International Journal of Epidemiology, 21: 589–593.

United Nations Development Programme (2003) Human Development Report: Millennium Development Goals: A Compact Among Nations to End Human Poverty. New York: Oxford University Press.

Van der Hoek W, Feenstra SG, Konradsen F (2002) Availability of irrigation water for domestic use in Pakistan: its impact on prevalence. Journal of Health, Population and Nutrition, 20: 77–84.

Vesikari T, Mason DO, Dennehy P et al. (2006) Safety and efficacy of a pentavalent human-bovine (WC3) reassortant rotavirus vaccine. New England Journal of Medicine, 354: 23–33.

Viboud GI, Jouve MJ, Binsztein N et al. (1999) Prospective cohort study of enterotoxigenic *Escherichia coli* infections in Argentinean children. Journal of Clinical Microbiology, 37: 2829–2833.

Victora CG, Olinto MT, Barros FC et al. (1996) Falling diarrhea mortality in Northeastern Brazil: did ORT play a role? Health Policy and Planning, 11: 132–141.

Victora CG, Bryce J, Fontaine O et al. (2000) Reducing deaths from diarrhea through oral rehydration therapy. Bulletin of the World Health Organization, 78: 1246–1255.

Villa S, Guiscafré H, Martínez H et al. (1999) Seasonal diarrheal mortality among Mexican children. Bulletin of the World Health Organization, 77: 375–380.

World Health Organization (WHO) (1988) Report of a WHO Meeting. Persistent diarrhea in children in developing countries. Geneva: World Health Organization. WHO/CDD/88.27 http://www.popline.org/docs/054768 Cited 2 August 2008.

World Health Organization (WHO) (2000) Collaborative Study Team on the Role of Breastfeeding on the Prevention of Infant Mortality. Effect of breastfeeding on infant and child mortality due to infectious diseases in less developed countries: a pooled analysis. Lancet, 355: 451–455.

World Health Organization (WHO) (2001) The optimal duration of exclusive breastfeeding. A systematic review. Geneva: WHO http://www.who.int/nutrition/publications/optimal_duration_of_exc_bfeeding_review_eng.pdf Cited 2 August 2008.

World Health Organization (WHO)/United Nations Children's Fund (UNICEF) (2004) Declaracion conjunta de la OMS y el UNICEF. Tratamiento clínico de la diarrea aguda. Geneva: World Health Organization. WHO/FCH/CAH/04.7 http://www.izincg.org/pdf/WHOUnicefdiarrheaStatementSPANISH.pdf?PHPSESSID=b44e4e7d8d0c278bf2278dc23c86754 Cited 2 August 2008.

World Health Organization (WHO) (2005) World Health Report 2005: Make every mother and child count. WHO: Geneva. http://www.who.int/whr/2005/whr2005_en.pdf Cited 2 August 2008.

Wyrsch M, Coakley K, Alexander N et al. (1998) Diarrhea morbidity in children in the Asaro Valley, Eastern Highlands Province, Papua New Guinea. Papua New Guinea Medical Journal, 41: 7–14.

Yap KL, Yasmin AM, Wong YH et al. (1992) A one year community-based study on the incidence of diarrhea and rotavirus infection in urban and suburban Malaysian children. Medical Journal of Malaysia, 47: 303–308.

Yassin KM (2000) Indices and sociodemographic determinants of childhood mortality in rural Upper Egypt. Social Science and Medicine, 51: 185–197.

Yeager BA, Lanata CF, Lazo F et al. (1991) Transmission factors and socioeconomic status as determinants of diarrheal incidence in Lima, Peru. Journal of Diarrheal Diseases Research, 9: 186–193.

Yeager BAC, Huttly SRA, Diaz J et al. (2002) An intervention for the promotion of hygienic feces disposal behaviors in a shanty town of Lima, Peru. Health Education Research, 17: 761–773.

Yoon PW, Black RE, Moulton LH et al. (1997) The effect of malnutrition on the risk of diarrheal and respiratory mortality in children <2 y of age in Cebu, Philippines. American Journal of Clinical Nutrition, 65: 1070–1077.

Chapter 14
Tuberculosis in Childhood and Pregnancy

Krishna Reddy, David Moore, and Robert Gilman

Learning Objectives After reading this chapter and answering the discussion questions that follow, you should be able to

- Present a concise overview of the global burden of TB among women and children, highlighting differences in trends in developed and less-developed countries.
- Identify risk factors for childhood TB and discuss the challenges of diagnosing and tracking TB in children.
- Describe the pathogenesis of TB and discuss the relationship between TB and HIV/AIDS.
- Appraise the global challenges posed by multi-drug-resistant TB.
- Critically assess options for treatment and prevention of TB among women and children, and discuss the associated challenges.

Childhood Tuberculosis: Introduction

The global prevalence of tuberculosis (TB) is greater now than ever before. The World Health Organization has declared TB a global emergency that is expected to account for over 30 million deaths in the next decade. It is estimated that between 2000 and 2020, almost 1 billion people will be newly infected with *Mycobacterium tuberculosis* and 200 million people will develop active disease. HIV infection has had a profound

impact on TB incidence, accounting for an estimated excess of 34% of new TB cases (Cantwell and Binkin 1997). Other factors contributing to the global resurgence of TB include poverty, overcrowding, increased travel and immigration, ineffective TB surveillance and control programs, emergence of multidrug-resistant TB, and non-completion of treatment regimens. TB control features among the health targets of the Millennium Development Goals (MDGs) of the United Nations because it is both primarily a disease of the poor and a cause of poverty for individuals, societies, and governments. Box 14.1 presents definitions of some of the most commonly used terms in TB epidemiology.

Of the estimated 8.3 million new TB cases diagnosed in 2000, approximately 11% were children (Nelson and Wells 2004), often diagnosed on the basis of exposure history and clinical signs and symptoms without microbiological confirmation. Most of these children are found in developing countries, where TB occurs at all ages; in industrialized countries, conversely, TB occurs primarily in older adults. Childhood TB is often overlooked in public health intervention planning. Many TB control programs do not consider the treatment of children to be of paramount importance because children tend to have lower bacillary loads and usually do not transmit TB. Nevertheless, childhood TB has important public health implications. TB in a child represents a sentinel event within a community, as childhood infection most often represents recent transmission from an infectious adult with pulmonary TB. In addition, the strains of *M. tuberculosis* that affect children are representative of the infectious strains currently being transmitted

K. Reddy (✉)
Internal Medicine, Massachusetts General Hospital, Boston, MA, USA

Box 14.1 Definition of Terms

Active TB: An illness in which TB bacteria are multiplying and attacking a part of the body, usually the lungs. The symptoms of active TB disease include weakness, weight loss (hence the name consumption or wasting), fever, no appetite, chills, and sweating at night and for TB of the lungs (pulmonary TB), severe cough, pain in the chest, and coughing up blood.

Anergy: The inability to react to a skin test because of a weakened immune system. This is often observed in HIV infection or other severe illnesses.

Antigen-specific anergy: This describes a lack of reaction by the body's defense mechanisms to foreign substances and consists of a direct induction of peripheral lymphocyte tolerance. An individual in a state of anergy often indicates that the immune system is unable to mount a normal immune response against a specific antigen.

Apgar scores: Simple and repeatable method to quickly and summarily assess the health of newborn children immediately after childbirth.

Bacille Calmette–Guérin (BCG): A vaccine for TB named after the French scientists who developed it, Calmette and Guérin. BCG is rarely used in the United States, but it is often given to infants and small children in other countries where TB is common.

BACTEC radiometric assay: Nonselective culture medium to be used as an adjunct to aerobic blood culture media for the recovery of mycobacteria, yeast, and fungi and is useful for rapid detection of microorganisms in clinical specimens.

Caseating granuloma: An organized collection of macrophages with central areas of necrosis that appears cheese-like and is peculiar to tuberculosis infection.

CD4 lymphocyte: A type of white blood cell which carries the CD4 cell surface receptor and helps the body fight infection through cell-mediated immunity.

Congenital TB: Congenital TB may occur as a result of maternal TB when it involves the genital tract or placenta. The signs and symptoms are nonspecific. Three possible modes of infection of the fetus have been proposed: Hematogenous infection via the umbilical vein, fetal aspiration of infected amniotic fluid, and fetal ingestion of infected amniotic fluid.

Contact tracing: The identification and diagnosis of persons who may have come into contact with an infected person. People who have been exposed to TB are screened for TB infection and disease.

Delayed hypersensitivity: Delayed hypersensitivity reactions are inflammatory reactions initiated by mononuclear leukocytes. The term delayed is used because it involves a secondary cellular response, which appears 48–72 h after antigen exposure.

Directly Observed Therapy Shortcourse (DOTS): A way of helping patients take their medicine for TB. If you get DOT, you will meet with a health-care worker every day or several times a week. You will meet at a place you both agree on. This can be the TB clinic, your home or work, or any other convenient location. You will take your medicine while the health-care worker watches.

Droplet nuclei: Very small droplets (1–5 μm in diameter) that may be expelled when a person who has infectious TB coughs or sneezes; they can remain suspended in the air for several hours, depending on the environment.

Ethambutol: A drug used to treat TB disease; it may cause vision problems. Ethambutol should not be given to children who are too young to be monitored for changes in their vision.

Extrapulmonary TB: Active TB disease in any part of the body other than the lungs (for example, the kidney, spine, brain, or lymph nodes).

False-negative reaction: A negative reaction to the tuberculin skin test in a person who has TB infection; it may be caused by anergy, recent infection (within the past 10 weeks), or very young age (younger than 6 months old).

False-positive reaction: A positive reaction to the tuberculin skin test in a person who does not have TB infection; it may be caused by infection with nontuberculous mycobacteria or by vaccination with BCG.

Ghon focus: A primary lesion of granulomatous inflammation caused by mycobacterium bacilli (tuberculosis) developed in the lung of a previously uninfected individual and only detectable by chest X-ray if it calcifies or grows substantially.

Ghon complex: A calcified focus of infection and an associated lymph node. These lesions are particularly common in children and can retain viable bacteria, so are sources of long-term infection and may be involved in reactivation of the disease in later life.

Hematogenous dissemination: Ability to spread by entering the blood directly by intravasating into venous capillaries.

Hepatotoxicity: Chemical-driven liver damage especially from drugs, especially antituberculosis drugs, e.g., rifampin and isoniazid. The liver plays a central role in transforming and clearing chemicals and is susceptible to the toxicity from these agents.

Induration: Swelling that can be felt around the site of injection after a Mantoux skin test is done; the reaction size is the diameter of the indurated area (excluding any redness), measured across the forearm.

Isoniazid: A medicine used to prevent active TB disease in people who have latent TB infection. INH is also one of the four medicines often used to treat active TB disease.

Latent TB: Persons with latent TB infection carry the organism that causes TB, but do not have TB disease, are asymptomatic, and are noninfectious. Such persons usually have a positive reaction to the tuberculin skin test.

Lowenstein-Jensen medium: A growth medium specially used for culture of *M. tuberculosis*. The media must be incubated for a significant length of time, usually 4 weeks, due to its slow doubling time compared with other bacteria (15–20 h).

Microscopic observation drug susceptibility (MODS): Culture method shown to be more sensitive, a faster and cheaper test than current culture-based tests for TB. It involves direct observation of *M. tuberculosis* and simultaneously yields drug resistance.

Miliary TB/Disseminated TB: A form of tuberculosis that is characterized by a wide dissemination into the human body and by the tiny size of the lesions (1–5 mm). Its name comes from a distinctive pattern seen on a chest X-ray of many tiny spots distributed throughout the lung fields.

Multidrug-resistant TB (MDR-TB): Active TB disease caused by bacteria resistant to two or more of the most important medicines: Isoniazid (INH) and Rifampin (RIF).

M. tuberculosis: Pathogenic bacterial species in the genus *Mycobacterium* and the causative agent of most cases of tuberculosis.

Natural history: The uninterrupted progression of a medical condition in an individual.

Perinatal TB: Tuberculosis can be acquired in the perinatal period. Infants may acquire tuberculosis (TB) by transplacental spread through the umbilical vein to the fetal liver, by aspiration or ingestion of infected amniotic fluid, or via airborne inoculation from close contacts (family members or nursery personnel).

Pleural effusions: Excess fluid between the two membranes that envelop the lungs called the pleural space.

Primary TB: Occurs when a person first becomes infected. This is when the body forms tubercles on the lungs to contain the bacteria. There are rarely any symptoms with primary TB.

Pulmonary TB: Active TB disease that occurs in the lungs, usually producing a cough that lasts 3 weeks or longer. Most active TB disease is pulmonary.

Pyrazinamide: A drug used to treat TB disease, usually during the initial phase of treatment; this should not be given to pregnant women.

Reactivation TB: Postprimary TB resulting either from the reactivation of a latent primary infection or, less commonly, from the repeat infection of a previously sensitized host.

Rifampin: A drug used to treat TB disease, also used for preventive therapy in people with a positive skin test reaction who have been exposed to isoniazid-resistant TB. Rifampin has several possible side effects (for example, hepatitis, turning body fluids orange, and drug interactions).

Sensitivity: Measures the proportion of actual positives which are correctly identified as such (i.e., the%age of sick people who are identified as having the condition).

Smear-negative: Sputum smear test which involves staining of three sputum samples for acid-fast bacilli, and negative acid-fast bacilli smear results (three) from sputum is considered smear-negative.

Smear-positive: For a smear to be positive, there must be at least 5,000–10,000 acid-fast bacilli per milliliter of sputum.

Specificity: Measures the proportion of negatives which are correctly identified (i.e., the%age of well people who are identified as not having the condition).

Sputum induction: Indicated on patients with suspect tuberculosis who are unable to cough and produce an adequate sputum sample. Involves making a patient breath 3% hypertonic solution via a jet nebulizer for approximately 30 min, then the patient is instructed to induce a deep cough from their chest and not to expectorate saliva or postnasal drip but a specimen from their chest.

Stegen–Toledo Criteria: This is based on signs and symptoms, such as persistent cough, abnormal findings of chest radiography, and contact with a patient with active tuberculosis for diagnosis of pediatric tuberculosis. Patients are classified into four categories: for unlikely tuberculosis, the score was 0–2; for suspected tuberculosis, 3–4; for probable tuberculosis, 5–6; and for highly probable tuberculosis, ≥ 7.

String test: Involves swallowing a string to obtain a sample from the upper part of the small intestine. The sample is then tested to detect the presence of intestinal parasites or acid-fast bacilli. The string test is rarely used in the United States.

TB meningitis: Infection of the meninges – the system of membranes which envelops the central nervous system. Fever and headache are the cardinal features.

Teratogenic: Able to disturb the growth and development of an embryo or fetus.

Tubercle bacilli: Another name for *M. tuberculosis* organisms, which cause TB disease

Tuberculin: A protein extracted from *M. tuberculosis* that is used in a skin test to determine if a person has been exposed to tuberculosis. The tuberculin preparation in most common use today is purified protein derivative (PPD) tuberculin. PPD is injected (or multiple punctured) into the skin. The PPD tuberculin test done by intradermal injection is also known as the Mantoux test.

Tuberculin skin test (TST)/Mantoux test: A test that is often used to detect latent TB infection. A liquid called tuberculin is injected under the skin on the lower part of your arm. If a reaction is seen at and around the site of injection, the test is positive (you probably have latent TB infection).

Source: U.S. Department of Health and Human Services (2007)

in the community as a whole. Thus, identification of childhood TB is important for assessing overall TB control in a population. Furthermore, infected children represent the pool from which a significant proportion of future cases of adult TB will arise.

The biggest obstacle to attaining accurate epidemiologic data of TB in children – and to prevention and control of the disease in this population – is diagnosis. Unlike adults, in whom bacteriologic confirmation is the mainstay of diagnosis, children are found to be positive on culture or smear in only 20–30% of treated TB cases. Adequate diagnostic specimens are difficult to obtain in children because children rarely produce sufficient sputum and, even when they do, their specimens usually contain very low concentrations of mycobacteria. Compounding the diagnostic dilemma are the limitations of most existing diagnostic tests: the more sensitive tests (automated mycobacterial culture tools such as MBBacT and BACTEC) are very expensive, while traditional, less expensive tests (such as Lowenstein-Jensen culture) are slow and have poor sensitivity. Thus, because of limited resources and personnel in endemic areas, limited efforts are made to bacteriologically confirm a diagnosis of TB in a child. Consequently, many children with TB are never diagnosed or registered as cases of TB. On the other hand, a proportion of children treated for TB may not actually have the disease; clinical scoring systems used for diagnosis in the absence of bacteriologic confirmation suffer from poor specificity.

The increasing burden of TB and HIV in children around the world perpetuates a cycle of malnutrition and poverty. The paucity of accurate epidemiological data combined with the substantial TB-associated morbidity and mortality among children in high-burden settings underscore the need for a more precise and thorough picture of TB in this population.

Surveillance and Global Burden

Limitations of Existing Data

The global burden of tuberculosis in children is unclear. Accurate statistics are limited due to the difficulty of diagnosing TB in children, the lack of commonly used standard case definitions, the inadequate surveillance systems in developing countries, and the dearth of importance given to childhood TB by TB control programs (Shingadia and Novelli 2003). There are very few epidemiologic studies of TB in children, and many of the available studies were conducted in areas with relatively low incidences of TB, or in hospital-based populations, who may not be representative of the general pediatric population. Furthermore, differences in methodology and case definitions complicate any potential comparisons between countries. In studies published to date, case definitions of childhood TB are rarely based on bacteriology, but instead on a variable combination of contact history, clinical symptoms, chest radiography, and tuberculin skin testing. Analyses of these algorithms have demonstrated poor sensitivity (Hesseling et al. 2002).

Another limitation of surveillance data in some places is the delay in reporting TB cases to local and national control programs. A study of tuberculous meningitis in South African children revealed that only 56% of cases had been registered (Berman et al. 1992). This is particularly notable because meningitis is the most lethal form of TB and therefore among the most likely to be reported, in theory. In 1991, the International Union Against Tuberculosis and Lung Disease (IUATLD) declared that reliable statistics regarding the incidence of childhood TB can be obtained only in developed countries (Hershfield 1991). Thus, there is a need for more accurate identification of the burden of TB in the pediatric population in developing countries where the burden of disease is the greatest.

Global Trends

In spite of the drawbacks of existing data, some conclusions can be drawn with regard to global trends in childhood TB. In developing countries, TB in children constitutes 15–40% of the total number of TB cases (Mwinga 2005). In developed countries, the proportion tends to be less than 5%. During the 1990s, adult TB case numbers increased in every region of the world except Western Europe; it is likely that childhood TB also increased in these regions. The trend in TB rates varies across countries. Among industrialized countries, some have witnessed a sustained decline in the incidence of childhood TB, while others have experienced a slowing in the rate of decline or even a reversal. Many developing countries, meanwhile, have observed increases in incidence. For example, almost all African countries have reported an increase in notification rates, and some have seen their rates more than quadruple compared to those in the 1970s (Mwaba et al. 2003). Though pediatric TB appears to be increasing in many parts of the world, the increase may reflect a reporting bias, in that areas with little change or a decrease may be less likely to publish these results.

The United States has had a well-established system of TB surveillance since 1953. After years of declining overall TB case rates, the United States saw an increase in the TB case rate from 1984 to 1992, coinciding with the HIV epidemic (Nelson and Wells 2004). During this period, the number of childhood TB cases rose by 40%. The trend was later reversed largely through public health interventions. Incidence rates in children in the United States have been declining since 1992. In England and Wales, the TB rate decreased from 7/100,000 in 1978 to 3.2/100,000 in 2003 (Chintu and Mwaba 2005). In developed countries, TB rates tend to be higher among foreign-born children. In the United States, childhood TB case rates are substantially higher among ethnic and racial minorities and the foreign-born than among Caucasians (Starke 1999).

Most developing countries have seen an increase in published case rates of childhood TB. In Botswana, reported case rates in children ages 9 and under increased from 199/100,000 in 1996 to 229/100,000 in 2000 (Nelson and Wells 2004). In Tanzania, TB surveillance among children under age 15 revealed that case rates increased from 38/100,000 in 1996 to 45/100,000 in 2000 (Nelson and Wells 2004). Smear-positive cases accounted for only 8% of all TB reported in children in Tanzania. A recent autopsy study of children dying of respiratory disease in Zambia found evidence of TB in 20% of cases, in many of which TB was diagnosed only postmortem (Chintu et al. 2002). The rates of adult and childhood TB in South Africa are among the highest in the world: a prospective, clinic-based study in South Africa found the incidence of TB among the adult population (≥ 13 years of age) to be 845/100,000/year, while the incidence in the child (<13 years of age) population was 441/100,000/year (Marais et al. 2006b).

In Latvia, TB case rates in children increased from 7.5/100,000 in 1991 to 38.9/100,000 in 2000 (Nelson and Wells 2004). In Russia, childhood TB case rates increased from 7.5/100,000 in 1989 to 18.6/100,000 in 2001 (Nelson and Wells 2004). Meanwhile, in Peru, case rates of childhood TB actually decreased from 61/100,000 in 1994 to 43/100,000 in 2000; cases of TB meningitis in children under age 5 decreased from 3.4/100,000 in 1992

to 0.8/100,000 in 2000 (Nelson and Wells 2004). These changes paralleling a decline in adult TB case rates attributed to an effective DOTS program in the country. A bacille–Calmette–Guérin (BCG) vaccine campaign may have contributed to the decrease in TB meningitis.

Risk Factors

Factors contributing to the risk of becoming infected with *M. tuberculosis* and developing active TB disease can be divided into those that increase transmission and those that increase susceptibility. Marais et al. (2005) summarized many of these factors (Box 14.2). The risk of developing TB and the clinical manifestations of the disease in childhood vary by age. Studies of the natural history of childhood TB (conducted before 1950, prior to the advent of chemotherapy) revealed that age at the time of infection is the most important determinant of risk of progression from *M. tuberculosis* infection to active disease in immunocompetent children (Marais et al. 2004). Largely because their immune defenses are relatively immature, young children

---

Box 14.2 Risk Factors for Transmission of M. tuberculosis and Development of Tuberculosis

Community Level: Transmission	Individual Level: Susceptibility
Number of infectious cases	Immune compromise
Duration of infectiousness	Malnutrition
Delayed diagnosis	Substance abuse
Delayed treatment	HIV
Ineffective treatment	Age
Exposure	Genetic susceptibility
Duration	Immune stimulation
Proximity	Immunization
Mycobacterial load	Environmental mycobacteria
Crowding	Local defenses
	Poverty

Source: Marais et al. (2005)

carry the greatest burden of disease among the pediatric population, being the most likely to develop active disease after infection with *M. tuberculosis* and the most likely to have significant signs or symptoms of TB (Vallejo et al. 1994) and extrapulmonary and severe disseminated disease. The lowest age-specific rates of TB in most populations are usually found in children between the ages of 5 and 14, sometimes called the "favored age."

It is not clear why children of these ages are apparently protected, to a degree, from developing TB, though it suggests an effect of the maturing immune system. The gender ratio for childhood TB is about 1:1, whereas in adults the disease is found more commonly in men.

Pathogenesis

Infection Versus Disease

Traditionally, a distinction has been made between "infection" and "disease" with respect to tuberculosis (Box 14.3). When a person with transmissible TB disease coughs or sneezes, microorganisms are expelled in droplets into the air and can be inhaled by another person. After this initial exposure, some children will become infected with *M. tuberculosis*. This is marked by conversion of the tuberculin skin test (TST). A positive reaction to the TST represents delayed-type hypersensitivity – the individual mounts an immune response to the tuberculin antigen after (presumably) having been exposed previously to the antigen in *M. tuberculosis*. A person with a positive TST and no signs or symptoms of active disease is said to be latently "infected" with *M. tuberculosis*. The annual risk of infection (ARI) has been reported to be 1–2% in many endemic regions and up to 5% in some (Cauthen et al. 2002).

Following *M. tuberculosis* infection in HIV-negative adults, the lifetime risk of developing active TB is about 5–10%; the lifetime risk is considered to be higher when infected with *M. tuberculosis* as a child. In HIV-infected adults, the risk of progression to active disease is approximately 10% per year. Active "disease" occurs when clinical manifestations of tuberculosis become

Box 14.3 Latent Infection Versus Disease

Latent Infection

- *M. tuberculosis* spreads to lung of new host from person with infectious tuberculosis
- Contained by host immunologic response
- Most commonly detected by tuberculin skin test; interferon blood assay is newer technique
- New host is not infectious
- May or may not require treatment
- Treatment is generally with isoniazid alone

Disease

- Referred to as "tuberculosis"
- Mycobacteria are no longer contained by immune cells
- Some cases are infectious (depends on location and mycobacterial load; rare in children)
- Diagnosed by detection of mycobacteria in patient specimens (gold standard) and/or combination of radiographic findings, clinical history and exam, and contact tracing
- Lungs are most common site, but can affect many other sites
- Treatment requires multiple drugs

apparent, either by clinical signs and symptoms or by chest radiograph. The term "tuberculosis," or TB, is generally used to refer to those who have active disease and not to those with infection only. The distinction between infection and disease is made partly because disease requires treatment (with three or more drugs) while treatment for infection (with a single drug) may or may not be indicated. The risk of a child becoming infected with *M. tuberculosis* depends on contact and environmental factors. The risk of a child developing TB disease following infection is affected by host immunologic and genetic characteristics.

Early Pathogenesis

Initial infection in the lung results in a Ghon focus and regional lymphadenitis. This primary complex may not be obvious on a chest radiograph. In most children, the complex resolves spontaneously. Some children, especially infants, may develop progressive lymphadenopathy. Alternatively, in progressive primary tuberculosis, the primary parenchymal infiltrate can progress to a caseating lesion. This lesion may rupture into the pleural or pericardial spaces leading to effusions. Erosion of caseating lesions into pulmonary vessels can result in hematogenous dissemination to the lung or to distant anatomic sites. The most common manifestation of this is miliary tuberculosis, which usually affects infants and young children. Older children and adolescents tend to develop adult-type reactivation disease. Cavitating disease becomes a more common manifestation of tuberculosis in children over 10 years of age, and these children pose a transmission risk similar to that of adults.

Transmissibility

In order for tuberculosis to be transmissible, the disease must spread into the bronchial tree, generally via progressive liquefaction and caseation followed by cavity formation. In the majority of children with tuberculosis, the disease remains in the lymph nodes and does not extend to the bronchus. When disease does spread in children, it often occurs via the blood. Therefore, TB in children is rarely transmissible and rarely positive on sputum smear. Another reason for the low infectiousness of children with TB is the paucibacillary nature of childhood TB. Cavitation, which is fairly common in adults and rare in young children, represents a breeding ground for *M. tuberculosis*. Estimates of the number of tubercle bacilli found in TB lesions are 10^7–10^9 in cavities, and 10^2–10^5 in solid caseous areas (Moulding 1999); nevertheless, acid-fast bacilli are usually difficult to find in histological sections. Since most children, especially those with lymph node disease, have relatively small amounts of caseation and cavitation and low bacillary numbers, tubercle bacilli are relatively difficult to detect in their specimens.

Pulmonary TB can be "smear-positive" or "smear-negative" cases, depending on whether the organism is detected on acid-fast bacillus smears of sputum specimens. Whether a patient has smear-positive or smear-negative disease depends on the person's load of mycobacterial bacilli as well as the availability of a diagnostic sample from the diseased lung segment. The source cases with the greatest likelihood of transmitting *M. tuberculosis* to others are those with sputum smear-positive pulmonary disease. However, those with sputum smear-negative pulmonary TB have also been shown to contribute to transmission; one study showed that 17% of *M. tuberculosis* transmission was attributed to smear-negative, culture-positive adults (Behr et al. 1999). Those with only extrapulmonary TB are rarely infectious.

Nutrition and Tuberculosis

Malnutrition may play an important role in the progression of tuberculosis in children by altering immune function. Malnourished children have been found to have diminished CD4 lymphocyte activation capacity and cytokine production (Rodriguez et al. 2005). The type of malnutrition may also be important. A study in Uganda found a significantly lower CD4 lymphocyte count in children with nonedematous malnutrition as compared to those with edematous malnutrition (Bachou et al. 2006). The TST also appears to be affected by malnutrition. A negative TST correlated strongly with malnutrition in Peruvian children presenting with a presumptive diagnosis of pulmonary TB (Salazar et al. 2001). In a study of randomly selected Peruvian adults, protein-deficient patients had antigen-specific anergy to tuberculin but not to candida or tetanus antigens (Pelly et al. 2005).

Clinical Presentation

The presentation and clinical features of TB in children differ from those in adults. Children infected with *M. tuberculosis* develop active disease very rapidly, even in a matter of weeks. Studies of the natural history of TB indicate that over 95% of children who develop active TB do so within 12 months after initial infection

(Marais et al. 2006b). In adults, there is a much greater incidence of TB caused by reactivation of dormant organisms. There is usually a period of years to decades between infection and reactivation-type disease. Thus, the clinical distinction between primary infection and disease is less clear in children than it is in adults, and the approach to diagnosis and prevention differs between children and adults.

Symptoms of childhood TB may differ between developing and developed regions. A study of Peruvian children revealed that the typical symptoms of pulmonary TB in this population was similar to those in adults (Salazar et al. 2001). In developed countries, children usually have minimal or no symptoms at the time of presentation with TB. Case ascertainment strategies may partly account for the difference.

Of those who are symptomatic, the most common manifestations are chronic cough, fever, and weight loss, or failure to gain weight. Over half of children with TB initially have minimal symptoms and require chest radiograph to confirm the diagnosis. However, in many children with presumed TB, chest radiograph shows no abnormalities.

Spectrum of Disease

Childhood TB is often reported as a single disease entity despite the fact that it includes a wide spectrum of pathology with important prognostic implications. A prospective, clinic-based study in South Africa (Marais et al. 2006c) reported the manifestations of childhood TB: of 439 children treated for TB during the study period, 85 (19.4%) were later classified as not having TB (due to lack of bacteriologic or histologic confirmation of TB and lack of radiographic and extrapulmonary signs of TB); 307 (69.9%) were classified as having intrathoracic TB only; 72 (16.4%) had extrathoracic TB only, including central nervous system, abdominal, osteoarticular, and skin disease; and 25 (5.7%) had both intra- and extrathoracic TB. Twenty-six children (5.9%) were diagnosed with disseminated (miliary) TB or tuberculous meningitis. Young children (<3 years of age) and HIV-infected children – whose immune systems are immature and compromised, respectively – were prone to developing disease manifestations indicative of poor organism containment, such as miliary disease.

Diagnosis

The accurate diagnosis of pediatric tuberculosis is a major challenge. Misdiagnosis of childhood pulmonary TB has multiple origins, including the nonspecificity of signs and symptoms, low bacillary load, inherent limitations of current diagnostic assays, and techniques used to obtain samples (Eamranond and Jaramillo 2001) (Box 14.4 and Table 14.1). The mainstay of diagnosis in adults – bacteriologic confirmation – is of limited use in children because their disease spreads much less frequently to the bronchus and, therefore, tubercle bacilli will not appear in sputum samples. Early diagnosis depends on early symptomatic presentation and sensitive diagnostic tools. Factors such as limited access to health care (which, in turn, is affected by poverty and discrimination) contribute to delays in diagnosis. Delays in diagnosis increase the morbidity and mortality of childhood TB for the patient and increase the duration of infectivity of those patients who are infectious, thereby adding to the public health problem.

Box 14.4 Challenges of TB Diagnosis in Children

- Sputum specimens difficult to acquire
- Low mycobacterial counts → false-negative smear stains and cultures
- Inherent limitations of diagnostic assays
- Nonspecific clinical signs and symptoms
- Nonspecific radiographic findings
- Barriers to access to health care
- Relatively limited importance in national TB control programs

Table 14.1 Advantages and disadvantages of various methods for diagnosis of tuberculosis

Diagnostic method	Advantages	Disadvantages
Smear microscopy	Rapid, low tech	Very low sensitivity
Lowenstein-Jensen culture	Definitive diagnosis	Low sensitivity, very slow, requires biosafety area
Automated mycobacterial culture	Definitive diagnosis, reasonable sensitivity	Very costly and requires biosafety area
MODS culture	Definitive diagnosis, good sensitivity, fast and simultaneous drug sensitivity testing	Requires biosafety area
PPD	Good for screening, can aid in diagnosis	Does not distinguish between infection and disease, false positives and false negatives occur, less useful in endemic regions
PCR	Rapid	Poor sensitivity, costly, requires qualified lab personnel, false positives due to contamination
Chest radiograph	Aids in detection of lung pathologies	Not available in some areas; low sensitivity and specificity
Thorax CT	Enhanced visualization of small lesions	Costly, requires scanner

Source: Eamranond and Jaramillo (2001)

Differences in Diagnostic Approaches in Developing and Developed Regions

In developed countries, diagnosis of childhood TB is generally based on tuberculin skin testing, chest radiograph, history of exposure to an adult with infectious TB, and culture of gastric washings, naso-pharyngeal aspirate, or induced sputum. In developing countries (especially in rural areas), diagnosis is more complicated due to lack of radiological machines, microscopes, and tuberculin skin testing, as well as a greater risk of specimen contamination during transport (Eamranond and Jaramillo 2001). Because many childhood TB cases in developed countries are detected by population-based tuberculin skin testing or by contact tracing, many children are asymptomatic at the time of diagnosis. In developing regions, in contrast, most childhood TB is diagnosed by evaluation of children with symptomatic disease.

Limitations of Clinical Diagnosis

Nonspecific clinical signs and symptoms complicate the diagnosis of childhood TB. The diagnosis is sometimes confused with that of other pulmonary diseases, such as pneumonia and asthma. Studies attempting to identify signs and symptoms to be applied to the diagnosis of pulmonary TB have shown poor sensitivity and specificity. A critical review found that various clinical scoring systems are limited by a lack of standard symptom definitions and adequate validation (Hesseling et al. 2002). Another study examined WHO criteria – assessing the combination of (1) recent weight loss or failure to gain weight adequately, (2) cough or wheezing for >2 weeks, and (3) recent household contact with an adult case of pulmonary TB – and demonstrated a positive predictive value of only 63% as compared to culture-confirmed TB or probable TB (as demonstrated by chest radiograph or tuberculin skin test reaction greater than 15 mm) (Houwert et al. 1998). Among children in Lima, Peru, the triad of cough lasting ≥2 weeks, fever, and TST ≥10 mm had a positive predictive value of 73% and sensitivity of 44% for culture-positive pulmonary disease (Salazar et al. 2001). Marais et al. (2006b) reported that in a prospective, community-based study of symptom-based diagnosis of childhood tuberculosis in South Africa, the combination of cough of 2 weeks duration, failure to thrive during the previous 3 months, and fatigue had a sensitivity of 62.6%, specificity of 89.8%, and positive predictive value of 83.6% for confirmed or probable TB in HIV-uninfected children ≥3 years of age. These criteria were less accurate in HIV-infected children and children under 3 years of age.

Clinical scoring systems such as the Stegen–Toledo criteria (Toledo and Stegen 1979) (Box 14.5) incorporate factors such as positive culture, TB granuloma, positive TST, and clinical suspicion for the diagnosis of TB. These scoring systems may be useful when there is a positive culture or TB granuloma, as these are given the most weight in the scoring system. However, these are not the situations when diagnosis is in doubt. A more typical scenario is a child with negative or pending culture data and inconclusive radiograph – in this situation the Stegen–Toledo scoring system is less useful in diagnosing TB.

Tuberculin Skin Test (TST)

In endemic areas, a positive TST reaction is the most commonly used sign of *M. tuberculosis* infection. In very young children, a positive TST represents recent infection by definition, and, because of the high risk of progression to active disease in young children, is often a trigger for initiation of preventive chemotherapy. However, TST usefulness is limited by false-positive and false-negative results (Box 14.6). In endemic areas, a positive TST is common in randomly selected healthy children, thereby limiting the test's ability to diagnose active disease. The risk of exposure and infection increases with age as the child is exposed to more tubercle bacilli in the community. In a shantytown on the outskirts of Lima, Peru, rates of positive purified protein derivative (PPD) skin test reactions were 12% in the 0–1-year-old age group, 18% in the 2–4-year-old group, 24% in the 5–14-year-old group, 60% in the 15–24-year-old group, and 68% in the ≥25-year-old group (Getchell et al. 1992). In industrialized countries, conversely, less than 5% of children may be positive.

Once exposed and infected, tuberculin reactivity becomes apparent in 3–6 weeks in most children, but very young children may take up to 3 months to develop a positive tuberculin skin test, due to their immature immune systems. The TST is negative in up to 10% of children with culture proven TB and up to 40% of those with TB meningitis (Walls and Shingadia 2004); this low negative predictive value limits the usefulness of TST as a diagnostic rule-out tool.

Effect of BCG Vaccination on TST

In areas with a high BCG vaccine coverage, which includes most TB endemic regions, there is debate regarding the utility of TST. BCG vaccination can complicate the interpretation of a subsequent tuberculin skin test, namely by causing false-positive reactions. Our data from a peri-urban shantytown in Lima, Peru with high rates of TB and BCG vaccination indicate that people with two or more BCG scars have significantly larger TST reactions, even after adjusting for potential risk factors (Saito et al. 2004). A study in Brazil of children ages 7–14 found that the proportion of PPD reactions $\geq$10 mm was 14.2% in those with no BCG scar, 21.3% in those with 1 scar, and 45.0% in those with 2 scars (Bierrenbach et al. 2003). On the other hand, in a prospective cohort study of BCG-vaccinated newborns in Lima, at 6 months of age only 3 of 68 vaccinated infants had a TST greater than 10 mm, and all 3 had household contact with a known case of active TB (Santiago et al. 2003). A study of TST in children ages 3–60 months in Botswana, also an area with a high rate of BCG vaccination, found that 79% had 0-mm induration, 7% had a reaction 10 mm or greater, and 2% had a reaction 15 mm or greater (Lockman et al. 1999). Together, these results suggest that the age at time of TST and the lapse between BCG and TST may influence the relative utility of TST in areas of high BCG coverage.

Microbiological Diagnosis

The gold standard for diagnosing adult TB, bacteriologic confirmation, is of limited use in children for reasons previously described. In many endemic and resource-poor areas, sputum smear microscopy is the only diagnostic test available for TB. The Directly Observed Therapy Shortcourse (DOTS) strategy for global TB control targets sputum smear-positive cases. This poses a problem for control of TB in children. Even when specimens are obtained, smear microscopy is positive in less than 10–15% of children with suspected TB (Zar et al. 2005). The yield is higher in older children and in children with adult-type, cavitating disease. Culture

yields are also low – reportedly less than 30–40% in children with suspected TB (Zar et al. 2005), though it is difficult to define cases in the absence of a microbiological gold standard. A prospective study in Peru (Oberhelman et al. 2006) found that of 165 children with clinically suspected TB, only 15 (9%) had a confirmed positive culture for TB in a clinical specimen (stool, nasopharyngeal aspirate, or gastric aspirate). Of the 59 children with "highly probable" TB (Stegen–Toledo score of 7 or higher), 10 (16.9%) had a positive culture. A more recent study of bacteriologic yield in South African children for whom there was radiographic suspicion of intrathoracic TB and who received antituberculosis treatment revealed that 122 (62.2%) of the 196 subjects from whom specimens were collected had bacteriologic confirmation by culture or sputum smear (Marais et al. 2006a). Children with uncomplicated lymph node disease comprised the largest proportion (47.9%) of the group and had the lowest bacteriologic yield (34.7%). It is important to emphasize that this study included only children with radiographic evidence of TB, and that for many children, multiple, nonroutine specimens (such as gastric aspirates, nasopharyngeal aspirates, induced sputum, and pleural fluid aspirates) were assessed. Of the total cohort of 307 children, 68.7% were tested for HIV and 8.1% were found to be HIV-positive.

Lowenstein-Jensen medium is the most commonly used medium for culturing *M. tuberculosis* in resource-poor areas, but its clinical utility is limited by lengthy incubation periods – up to 7–10 weeks in some cases. The BACTEC radiometric assay improves the yield of positive cultures from clinical specimens and has a shorter incubation time for detection (9–14 days). However, it is not commonly used in resource-poor settings because of the very high costs of the instruments.

There is an urgent need for a more sensitive and rapid method of diagnosing TB in children. A new technique that has potential in this realm is the microscopic observation drug susceptibility assay (MODS). This is an inexpensive method for detection of *M. tuberculosis* (and thus definitive diagnosis of active disease) based on culturing the organism in a liquid medium (Moore et al. 2004). The assay also offers the benefit of simultaneous isoniazid and rifampicin susceptibility testing. Studies in adults (Moore et al. 2006) and children (Oberhelman et al. 2006) in Peru have found MODS to be more sensitive and more rapid than the traditional Lowenstein-Jensen culture method in isolating *M. tuberculosis* from sputum (in adults) and from nasopharyngeal aspirates, gastric aspirates, and stool (in children). In the pediatric population, mean time to isolation of *M. tuberculosis* was 11 days for MODS and 26 days for Lowenstein-Jensen ($p<0.001$) (Oberhelman et al. 2006).

Specimen Acquisition

Further complicating diagnosis is the difficulty in obtaining bacteriologic specimens. Children under 8 years of age rarely produce adequate sputum and tend to swallow it when they do. Other options for obtaining specimens include sputum induction or retrieval of swallowed sputum from the stomach by gastric aspiration. The yield of *M. tuberculosis* from three consecutive morning gastric aspirates from children with TB has been reported as 28–65% (Zar et al. 2005). This procedure is limited by contamination with nontuberculous acid-fast organisms from the mouth, need for an overnight fast, collection of multiple specimens, discomfort for the child and health-care personnel, and, in many cases, hospital admission. Nasopharyngeal aspiration yields results comparable to gastric aspiration, but the former offers the benefits of being minimally invasive and not requiring hospitalization or fasting (Franchi et al. 1998). However, nasopharyngeal aspiration has yet to be widely used because it provokes coughing and is not well tolerated by some children.

Sputum induction was demonstrated to be well tolerated in children, and it provides good diagnostic yield (Zar et al. 2005). A novel application of an old technique for specimen acquisition from the stomach is the string test, in which a capsule containing a coiled string is swallowed and maintained in situ for 4 h prior to removal through the mouth via the other end of the string. The string can then be examined by culture. This procedure was well tolerated by children as young as 4 years of age in a TB study (Chow et al. 2006) and as young as 1 year of age in a more recent study of detection of *Helicobacter pylori* (personal communication). In another study, the string test was found to be more effective than induced sputum for diagnosing TB in HIV-positive adults (Vargas et al. 2005), who, like children, tend to have difficulty in producing a sputum specimen for TB diagnosis.

Contact Tracing

The most efficient method of finding children newly infected with *M. tuberculosis* is by contact tracing of adults with transmissible pulmonary TB. Many children with radiographic signs of TB have no physical findings and are discovered only via contact tracing. WHO guidelines advise active screening of all children under 5 years of age in household contact with an adult with sputum smear-positive TB disease. Contacts can be screened for TB by physical exam, TST, and chest radiography. Contact tracing and screening, while theoretically of great use, are not widely employed in resource-poor settings as these would place an excessive burden on the health-care system for relatively small gains in public health and detection of active cases. The large number of adult cases and the limited availability of screening tests like TST and chest radiography limit the use of contact tracing in children. In these settings, it is recommended that scarce resources for contact screening and tracing be focused on those children with the highest risk of progressing from initial infection to active disease, namely children <3 years of age and immunocompromised children.

Extrapulmonary TB

Tuberculosis most commonly affects the lungs (pulmonary TB), but it can also affect sites outside of the lungs. As a proportion of total tuberculosis cases, extrapulmonary tuberculosis is more common in children than in adults. Of reported cases of TB in children under 15 years of age in the United

States between 1985 and 1994, 22% were extrapulmonary only; the proportion was 25% in children under 4 years of age (Ussery et al. 1996). In comparison, the rate among the general US population between 1991 and 1994 was 16%, as reported by the Centers for Disease Control.

Children under age 6 can develop central nervous system and disseminated TB in less than 3 months after infection. Thus, severe extrapulmonary forms of TB can manifest before the TST becomes reactive. The rapid progression and propensity for extrapulmonary spread place children at risk for the most severe clinical outcomes of TB. In a study of Peruvian children presenting with presumptive pulmonary TB, concurrent extrapulmonary TB was noted in 21 (16%) of 135 children; those with positive culture who were found to have extrapulmonary TB were significantly younger than those without signs or symptoms of extrapulmonary disease (Salazar et al. 2001). Because presumptive pulmonary TB was a criterion for entry, it is likely that the proportion of extrapulmonary cases among total TB cases (not just the proportion of pulmonary cases that have an extrapulmonary component) is actually higher.

Superficial lymphadenitis is the most common form of extrapulmonary TB; bones, joints, and skin can also be affected. The most serious forms of extrapulmonary TB in children are tuberculous meningitis and disseminated (miliary) disease; the latter occurs after hematogenous spread to distant organs. Eighty of TB meningitis cases occur in children 4 years of age and younger. A study of TB in England and Wales found that about 4% of children with TB had central nervous system (CNS) disease (Kumar et al. 1997). The overall mortality of CNS TB has been reported to be 13%, with about half of survivors developing permanent neurological sequelae.

HIV

Trends in TB-HIV Co-infection

HIV has had a profound impact on the global burden of TB, with average annual TB case rates since

---

> **Box 14.7 Impact of HIV on Childhood Tuberculosis**
>
> - HIV in adults → TB in adults → TB in children
> - Further limits utility of tuberculin skin test
> - Diagnosis of TB can be confused with that of other HIV-related illnesses
> - Increases mortality rate from TB
> - Increases TB relapse rate

1985 increasing twice as fast in countries with high HIV seropositivity rates as compared to those with low or intermediate HIV rates (Cantwell and Binkin 1997). HIV has brought the problems of a "telescoping down" of the time to development of active disease (Daley et al. 1992), an increase in the TB reactivation risk of coinfected individuals, and a rapid spread of drug-resistant disease (Shafer et al. 1995) (Box 14.7). Adults with HIV are at greatly elevated risk for both primary and reactivation TB, as well as for recurrent episodes due to exogenous reinfection. Among patients with HIV, concomitant TB doubles the risk of death, independent of the CD4 count (Whalen et al. 1995).

In many developing countries, childhood TB has increased along with the emergence of the HIV pandemic in adults and in children. In a study of 45 HIV-infected children admitted to the infectious diseases ward of a hospital in Lima, Peru, it was found that 8 (17%) had evidence of TB either by positive culture or by PCR (Ramirez-Cardich et al. 2006). Some studies of childhood TB have shown a concordance between increasing case rates of childhood TB and increasing rates of HIV-infected adults in the community (Starke 1999). In countries with high HIV infection rates, there is an increasing number of children with dual HIV and TB infection (Mukadi et al. 1997). One study from Zambia found that the prevalence of HIV-1 in children with TB increased from 24% on 1989 to 68% in 1992 (Luo et al. 1994). A more recent pediatric autopsy study also found high rates of coinfection at autopsy (Chintu et al. 2002). However, although there is some evidence that TB rates are higher in HIV-infected children than in the general pediatric population, the evidence is not as strong as that for adults. In fact, many studies worldwide have failed to find an increased rate of TB in HIV-infected children as compared to HIV-negative children, though this may reflect difficulties in case ascertainment. Moreover, the increased tendency for extrapulmonary TB in HIV-infected patients is more pronounced for adults than for children. Even when examining the HIV pandemic only in adults, HIV's effects on childhood tuberculosis can be appreciated. High rates of HIV infection in adults are associated with high rates of adult TB. Infectious adults can transmit TB to children, thereby increasing rates of latent infection and TB disease among children.

Mortality from TB-HIV Coinfection

Children with HIV have a greater risk of death from TB and have higher TB relapse rates than children without HIV. The mortality rate from TB was found to be up to six times greater in Ethiopian children who were HIV-seropositive as compared to those who were HIV-seronegative (Palme et al. 2001). A study from Cote d'Ivoire showed that during a 6-month treatment period for TB, mortality rates among HIV-positive children with CD4 under 10 and HIV-negative children were 50% and 4%, respectively (Mukadi et al. 1997).

Additional Diagnostic Challenges

In children infected with HIV, TB diagnosis poses challenges additional to those described earlier. First, bacteriologic confirmation, as in children not infected with HIV, is difficult to obtain. Second, the presentation of HIV disease itself may be quite similar to that of TB in the absence of HIV coinfection. In both, common presentations include malnutrition, fever, night sweats, weight loss, failure to thrive, and cough. The clinical presentation of TB in HIV-infected children with relatively preserved immunocompetence can be very similar to that in children without HIV. However, with increasing levels of immunosuppression in children with HIV,

the risks of mycobacteremia and extrapulmonary TB increase. Third, chest radiographic findings may also be very similar among TB and non-TB HIV-related disease. Our data indicate that, among hospitalized children with HIV in Peru, radiographic changes were similar among TB-positive and TB-negative patients (Ramirez-Cardich et al. 2006). Furthermore, many other HIV-associated pulmonary diseases, such as *Pneumocystis carinii* pneumonia and lymphocytic interstitial pneumonitis, mimic TB in terms of signs, symptoms, and findings on chest radiography. Chronic HIV-related signs and symptoms and the rapid progression of TB seen in this population limit the utility of symptom-based diagnosis and chest radiography.

Other obstacles to early diagnosis are the difficulty in obtaining specimens suitable for diagnosis and the limited utility of TST in this population. Studies have found TST to be less useful in children with HIV (Palme et al. 2001), most likely because of anergy. The sensitivity of TST has been reported as 50% or less in HIV-infected children with bacteriologically confirmed TB, even with an induration size cutoff of 5 mm.

Multidrug-Resistant Tuberculosis (MDR-TB)

Drug resistance impairs response to standard treatment, resulting in increased mortality (Park et al. 1996). Drug resistance initially arises in patients who do not adhere to anti-TB treatment; others can later become infected with these resistant strains. Therefore, a reduction in drug-resistant and multidrug-resistant (MDR, defined as resistance to isoniazid and rifampicin) tuberculosis depends on the proper allocation of public health resources to ensure that patients complete their appropriate treatment regimen. Children rarely contribute to the emergence of drug-resistant tuberculosis because of the paucibacillary nature of their disease. They can, however, be infected by drug-resistant strains originating from adult patients with high bacillary loads.

Because of the previously mentioned difficulties in securing a microbiologic diagnosis in children, drug-resistant TB is difficult to confirm. Consequently, there is limited data in the literature about MDR-TB in children. Usually, the diagnosis will be made based on confirmation of drug resistance in the index (usually adult) case. Other times diagnosis is made only after the child fails first-line treatment. In general, the types of strains encountered in children will reflect those found in the community; resistance patterns in children have been found to be similar to those of adults from the same areas. A study of TB culture-positive children conducted in South Africa between 1994 and 1998 found that 5.6% were resistant to isoniazid and 1% was multidrug resistant (Schaaf et al. 2000). These results were similar to surveillance data from adults during the same period: 3.9% isoniazid resistance and 1.1% multidrug resistance.

HIV and MDR-TB

The HIV pandemic appears to be contributing to the spread of MDR-TB. In a recent hospital-based study of consecutive adults with laboratory-proven tuberculosis in Lima, Peru (Kawai et al. 2006), 31 (43%) of 72 patients with HIV had MDR-TB, whereas 20 of 215 (9%) of non-HIV-infected patients had MDR-TB. In Peru, MDR-TB is associated with previous TB treatment, previous isoniazid preventive therapy, hospitalizations, and care in centers for people with HIV, all of which link HIV to MDR-TB (Kawai et al. 2006). Though there is limited information on MDR-TB in children infected with HIV, it can be appreciated that children can contract drug-resistant *M. tuberculosis* from adults.

Vaccination

The Bacille Calmette–Guérin (BCG) vaccine is the world's most widely used vaccine. However, in contrast to the decrease in caseloads seen with increased vaccine coverage against other diseases like polio and measles, there has been an increase in TB rates despite high BCG coverage. BCG plays a narrow role in the prevention of TB. Neonatal BCG

Box 14.8 BCG Vaccination

- Effective in preventing tuberculous meningitis and miliary tuberculosis
- Globally, no clear efficacy in preventing pulmonary (transmissible) TB
  - Utility depends on geographic region – appears to be less effective closer to the equator
- Effect may wane over time
- No proven benefit of repeat vaccination
- May complicate interpretation of tuberculin skin test

---

vaccination protects primarily against disseminated forms of TB during early childhood (Box 14.8). On% a worldwide basis, BCG does not clearly provide protection against pulmonary TB; there is great variation in the literature regarding the efficacy of the vaccine. Reported protection from pulmonary TB ranges from 0% in South India to 77% in the UK Medical Research Council trial (Hart and Sutherland 1977). A meta-analysis across different populations, study designs, and forms of TB found that BCG's protection (in terms of relative risk or odds ratio) against all forms of TB was approximately 0.52 when approximated from case–control studies, while its protection against tuberculous meningitis and disseminated infection in children was 0.64 and 0.78, respectively (Colditz et al. 1994).

A study in Malawi reported that BCG did not protect against pulmonary TB but did protect against leprosy (Ponnighaus et al. 1992); the latter finding has been corroborated in other studies. A large study in India found that BCG offered no overall protection against adult-type TB and a low level of overall protection (27%; 95% CI = –8 to 20) in children (Datta et al. 1999). A meta-analysis revealed that study sites at a greater distance from the equator were associated with a higher efficacy of BCG vaccine (Wilson et al. 1995). Geographic differences in exposure to environmental mycobacteria may explain, in part, the variation in BCG efficacy across different populations (Black et al. 2002). Other possible contributing factors include the use of different BCG preparations, genetic susceptibility, nutrition levels, and other socioeconomic variables. The long-term efficacy of BCG is not clear. A study in American Indians and Alaska natives found that BCG reduced TB incidence by 52% and that the efficacy persisted for 50–60 years (Aronson et al. 2004). In contrast, a review of 10 randomized trials of BCG showed that efficacy waned over time – an annual decrease of 5–14% in the rate ratio of TB in unvaccinated versus vaccinated individuals (Sterne et al. 1998). The WHO recommends BCG vaccination at birth except to babies with symptomatic HIV infection, though symptomatic HIV infection at birth is not common. However, in many TB-endemic areas, BCG is recommended for all infants as early as possible. A review of BCG administration to infants with asymptomatic HIV infection found that the benefits outweigh the risks of complications (O'Brien et al. 1995). There is no proven benefit of repeat vaccination.

Preventive Chemotherapy

Preventive chemotherapy is recommended for some children latently infected (as determined by TST) with *M. tuberculosis*. Because the TST is not adequately sensitive to exclude infection with *M. tuberculosis*, preventive chemotherapy is also recommended for those in household contact with known cases of infectious tuberculosis. A study in the United States demonstrated the benefit of 12 months of isoniazid therapy in reducing complications from progression of *M. tuberculosis* infection (Comstock et al. 1974). Preventive chemotherapy with isoniazid for 6–9 months has been shown to reduce the risk of TB in infected children by at least two-thirds. However, poor adherence limits the effectiveness of this regimen. Hepatotoxicity from isoniazid preventive therapy is extremely rare among children; a prospective cohort study in the United States found that none of 1,468 patients under age 15 who received isoniazid prophylaxis developed hepatotoxicity (Nolan et al. 1999).

Preventive Chemotherapy in Children with HIV

Because HIV-infected children coinfected with *M. tuberculosis* are thought to be at high risk of progression to active tuberculosis, preventive chemotherapy is recommended in this group, as well as in HIV-infected children recently exposed to an adult with infectious TB. However, in the literature, there is very limited data on the efficacy of preventive chemotherapy in HIV-infected children. In HIV-infected adults with positive TSTs, isoniazid prophylaxis for 6 months reduced TB risk by about 70%, according to one study (Halsey et al. 1998).

Treatment

Treatment of children with tuberculosis follows the same principles as treatment of adults. Treatment of drug-susceptible TB, reviewed elsewhere (Enarson et al. 2005), generally consists of a 2-month intensive phase of 3–4 drugs (often isoniazid, rifampicin, pyrazinamide, and streptomycin and/or ethambutol) and a 4–6 month continuation phase (often isoniazid and rifampicin). Tuberculosis is entirely curable if an appropriate medication regimen is followed. Treatment failure and the emergence of drug-resistant strains of *M. tuberculosis* can arise when treatment regimens are not completed, such as when a patient stops taking the medicines as soon as his/her symptoms improve. The Directly Observed Therapy Shortcourse (DOTS) strategy is promoted by the World Health Organization to increase the likelihood that treatment will be completed. However, DOTS is not always carried out, particularly in resource-poor settings. MDR-TB, when detected, is treated with second-line drugs, which are more costly and more toxic than first-line drugs.

Conclusions

Despite the availability of effective treatment, childhood tuberculosis continues to be a major problem in many parts of the world, and in fact is increasing in incidence in some regions (Box 14.9). Accurate epidemiologic data are limited because of the difficulties in

Box 14.9 Childhood Tuberculosis – Conclusion

- Childhood TB is increasing in many parts of the world
- Global pandemic of HIV is contributing to resurgence of childhood TB
- Accurate epidemiologic data is limited
- Differences in presentation and methods of diagnosis in developed versus developing regions
- Difficult to establish diagnosis

  - Clinical signs and symptoms are nonspecific
  - Clinical scoring scales are usually not useful
  - Diagnostic specimens are difficult to obtain from children
  - Microbiologic assays used in endemic regions have poor sensitivity for diagnosis of childhood TB as children have relatively low bacillus loads

- BCG vaccine reduces risk of the most severe forms of TB but is not clearly effective in reducing risk of pulmonary (infectious) TB
- High rate of latent infection and malnutrition in endemic regions confounds interpretation of tuberculin skin test
- Emergence of drug-resistant strains complicates treatment

establishing standard case definitions, obtaining bacteriologic confirmation, and ensuring proper surveillance at local, regional, and national levels. Key differences exist between developed and developing regions in terms of presentation and diagnosis of TB.

It is important to note that particular schemes for prevention and diagnosis may be more appropriate for some regions as opposed to others. In developed countries, detection of latent infection (and thus prevention of active disease) is accomplished through tuberculin skin testing. This is more difficult to carry out in endemic regions because of the high background level of positive tuberculin skin tests and the high prevalence of BCG vaccination, malnutrition, and HIV infection, which complicate the interpretation of skin test results.

BCG vaccination, while effective in reducing the risk of severe manifestations like miliary disease and tuberculous meningitis, is not clearly effective in reducing the risk of pulmonary TB. The global HIV pandemic is contributing to the resurgence of TB among children. While there is no definitive evidence that HIV increases the risk of developing TB among children, this relationship is more clearly defined in adults, who can then spread TB to children. HIV has been shown to increase mortality and relapse rates from TB among children. The challenges to diagnosis of childhood TB include the nonspecific signs and symptoms, the difficulties in obtaining specimens from children, and the low sensitivity of bacteriologic assays carried out in endemic regions. The emergence of drug-resistant strains of TB underscores the need for more effective methods of establishing microbiologic diagnosis and assessing drug sensitivity.

Maternal and Congenital Tuberculosis: Introduction

Women face a growing burden of tuberculosis. Epidemiologic studies have demonstrated that women have a higher rate of progression from infection to active disease than men and a higher case-fatality rate (Holmes et al. 1998). Several factors may contribute to the apparent lower frequency of tuberculosis in women (Box 14.10). Some studies have suggested differences in the immune responses of women and men. An alternative explanation is that there is no biological difference, but care-seeking behaviors are gender dependent. In particular, women may be more affected than men by physical, geographic, and economic barriers to accessing health-care services. In many societies, women take on multiple occupations – namely, taking care of the family and home and doing agricultural and other types of work outside the home. Thus, many women lack the time and resources necessary to seek care and to adhere to TB treatment regimens, including directly observed therapy (DOT), as suggested by a randomized control trial of DOT (Zwarenstein et al. 1998).

Stigma may also play a role in TB burden in women. Although both men and women may face stigma associated with TB, women – particularly

> ### Box 14.10 Tuberculosis in Pregnancy – Conclusion
>
> - The increase in HIV and TB among women of childbearing age has led to an increase in TB in pregnant women
> - Pregnancy does not appear to increase the risk of developing TB
> - Symptoms of TB may be confused with common manifestations of pregnancy
> - Fetal and maternal outcomes depend on location of disease, point of disease progression and pregnancy at which diagnosis is made, and adherence to treatment
> - Isoniazid, rifampicin, and ethambutol are considered safe to use during pregnancy
> - Congenital TB is rare
> - Diagnosis is generally made in the context of a recent maternal history of TB

those who are coinfected with HIV – may be more susceptible in many societies. With respect to tuberculosis and pregnancy, much of the literature is outdated and difficult to interpret in the context of current management practices. Nevertheless, some conclusions may be drawn using existing data. Because of the increase in the proportion of persons with TB who are women of childbearing age, there has been an increase in the number of women with TB who become pregnant. The greatest burden of TB for women is during their childbearing years (ages 15–49). However, there is no clear increase in the risk of developing TB during pregnancy. Because pregnancy may be one of the few times when some women have contact with the health-care system, it is an opportune time to screen for TB for high-risk individuals and/or persons living in endemic areas. This also implies that enhanced case ascertainment may affect the reported case rates of TB in the population of pregnant women as compared to other populations.

Effect of Pregnancy on Tuberculosis

Tuberculosis in pregnant women has been a controversial topic since the days of Hippocrates, who believed that pregnancy has a beneficial effect on TB. Some thought that the enlarging uterus, via increases in abdominal and thoracic pressures, helped to close pulmonary cavities and that the hormonal alterations of pregnancy improved the course of the disease. In the mid-1800s, an opposing view emerged. A review of 24 patients reported that pregnancy worsened the course of TB (Grisolle 1850). Some suggested that woman with pulmonary TB should not marry, if married should not conceive, if pregnant should terminate, and if delivered should not breast-feed (Tripathy and Tripathy 2003). A study published by Hedvall in 1953 challenged this notion. Two hundred and fifty women (370 pregnancies) with TB were followed throughout pregnancy – before the arrival of antituberculosis drugs – 9% of the subjects improved, 7% worsened, and 84% remained unchanged during pregnancy. During the first postpartum year, 9% improved, 15% worsened, and 76% remained stable. None of the women died during pregnancy, and none of the infants developed congenital TB. The findings of this study are often cited as the natural history of TB in pregnancy. There is no clear evidence of an altered risk of becoming infected with *M. tuberculosis*, progressing to active disease, or reactivating latent infection during pregnancy. Still, there were some concerns about the risk of progression of TB during the postpartum period, though over time this has been rejected by most studies. There is no evidence that pregnancy increases the risk of TB among women with HIV. A case–control study of HIV-positive and HIV-negative pregnant women in the Dominican Republic found that pregnancy did not increase the risk of developing active TB in either group (Espinal et al. 1996).

Presentation and Diagnosis

The presentation of TB in pregnant women is generally similar to that in nonpregnant women. However, one study found that pregnant patients with TB were significantly more likely to be asymptomatic than their nonpregnant counterparts and were significantly more likely to present with unilateral, non-cavitary, smear-negative disease (Carter and Mates 1994). Up to 20% of pregnant women with TB have been found to be asymptomatic (Good et al. 1981). Again, because pregnant women are more likely to seek health care than their nonpregnant counterparts, more cases of TB may be detected incidentally.

Diagnosis may be delayed by the nonspecific nature of early symptoms and the high background frequency of malaise and fatigue in pregnancy (Doveren and Block 1998). Llewelyn et al. (2000) found a median lapse of 7 weeks between onset of symptoms and diagnosis of TB in 13 pregnant women. Further complicating diagnosis is the fact that pregnant women are more likely to postpone having chest radiography (Doveren and Block 1998); this makes investigation of smear-negative TB, in particular, more difficult. Despite its limitations, TST can still be used as an indicator of latent infection as pregnant women are not at higher risk of cutaneous anergy than their nonpregnant counterparts (Jackson and Murtha 2001).

Treatment of Latent Infection in Pregnancy

Preventive chemotherapy with isoniazid is recommended for some pregnant women with latent infection with *M. tuberculosis*, as determined by TST. Threshold induration size of TST is generally similar to that among the general population. Initial reports suggested an increased risk of isoniazid-induced hepatitis in pregnant women, but more recent analyses have suggested that this was an artifact due to overreporting (Ormerod 2001). Nevertheless, preventive chemotherapy for latent infection is usually postponed until after delivery.

Treatment of Active Disease in Pregnancy

Before the arrival of antituberculosis drugs, advanced TB caused substantial mortality for both mother and child. One study found a 30–40% mortality rate in patients with advanced TB (Schaefer et al. 1975). With regard to treatment of active TB in pregnancy, the primary concern is the risk of teratogenicity. Some first-line drugs (isoniazid, rifampicin, and ethambutol) are considered to be safe in

pregnancy. Little is known about pyrazinamide's effects on the fetus; thus it is generally avoided. Streptomycin is known to be teratogenic with about one in six fetuses developing palsies of the vestibulocochlear nerve or deafness.

The use of isoniazid, rifampicin, ethambutol, and pyrazinamide has been considered compatible with breast-feeding (Brost and Newman 1997). There have been no reports of adverse events among infants of nursing mothers receiving these drugs. MDR-TB is difficult to treat in pregnant women because some of the medicines that would be used in the treatment have adverse or unknown effects on the fetus (Tripathy and Tripathy 2003). Cases of MDR-TB in pregnancy should be managed on an individualized basis.

Perinatal and Maternal Outcomes

Disparate perinatal and maternal outcomes from TB in pregnancy have been described. One study noted increased abortion rates, high levels of pre-eclampsia, and increased levels of difficult labor requiring intervention in women with TB (Bjerkedal et al. 1975). Other studies have noted overall good fetal outcomes (Schaefer et al. 1975). Recent studies have demonstrated that fetal and maternal outcomes depend on the location of disease (pulmonary or extrapulmonary), the point (early or late) in the pathophysiologic course at which diagnosis is made, the point of pregnancy at which the diagnosis is made (with cases with late diagnosis having worse fetal outcomes (Figueroa-Damian and Arredondo-Garcia 1998)), and adherence to treatment. A study in Mexico found that pregnant women with TB who began antituberculosis treatment during the first trimester had perinatal morbidity outcomes similar to those in women without TB, while those who started treatment later in pregnancy had significantly higher obstetrical morbidity and neonatal mortality (Figueroa-Damian and Arredondo-Garcia 1998). After a follow-up study of 215 pregnant women with active pulmonary TB, de March (1975) came to the conclusion that neither pregnancy, birth, nor lactation predisposed women for any risk of relapse of pulmonary TB when it is adequately treated.

These studies indicate the need for early diagnosis and treatment of TB in pregnant women. TB is not a medical indication for abortion, as good maternal and fetal outcomes can be obtained, particularly if diagnosed and treated early.

Congenital and Perinatal Tuberculosis

Congenital tuberculosis has been defined as TB lesions in an infant plus one of the following: (1) lesions in the first week of life, (2) primary hepatic complex or caseating granuloma, (3) documented TB infection of placenta or endometrium, (4) exclusion of postnatal transmission by separation of the infant from the mother and other potential sources of infection (Cantwell et al. 1994). These criteria have become increasingly difficult to follow in current practice. Congenital TB is rare, especially if the mother has been treated appropriately during pregnancy. It occurs almost exclusively when the placenta is actively infected; thus, pulmonary TB in the mother poses little risk of congenital TB. Congenital TB may be suspected if aggressive broad spectrum antibiotics are ineffective and tests for other congenital infections are negative. If the mother is known to have TB, and if she has been diagnosed recently, the suspicion is further raised (Ormerod 2001). TST is not useful for detection in infants since it is always negative initially and can take several months to become positive. Thus, diagnosis relies on clinical suspicion and contact investigation – a maternal history of TB exposure is important in diagnosis – and demonstration of acid-fast bacilli in tissue or fluids; gastric aspirates are recommended. Mortality rates from congenital TB approaching 50% have been described (Nemir and O'Hare 1985).

Perinatal TB, acquired after birth, can occur via airborne infection from the mother, adult caregiver, or another infectious adult contact (nurses, healthcare workers) (Burk et al. 1978). Transmission of *M. tuberculosis* in breast milk has not been reported, although theoretically it could occur if the mother has a tuberculous breast abscess. If the mother has active TB, expressed breast milk can be used to feed the infant until the mother is deemed noninfectious, at which point direct breast-feeding can commence (Jones 2001).

HIV

A resurgence of TB among pregnant women in New York in the early 1990s was linked to HIV coinfection (Margono et al. 1994). More recently, in endemic communities, cases of active TB are increasing among pregnant women; this increase appears to be associated with the HIV epidemic as opposed to pregnancy itself. In endemic communities, HIV testing is generally recommended only for high-risk women diagnosed with active TB, as HIV testing of all TST-positive women would not be economically feasible.

Extrapulmonary Tuberculosis

In endemic areas, extrapulmonary TB is becoming more prevalent among pregnant women; this is partly associated with the HIV pandemic. There is some evidence that extrapulmonary TB represents a relatively high proportion of total TB cases among pregnant women (Kothari et al. 2006). TB at extrapulmonary sites can adversely affect the outcome of pregnancy. A study in India of pregnancy outcomes in women with TB found significantly higher frequencies of hospitalization during pregnancy, fetal growth retardation, and low Apgar scores in women with extrapulmonary TB (other than TB lymphadenitis) as compared to uninfected women (Jana et al. 1999). Tuberculous lymphadenitis had no effect on perinatal outcome.

Conclusion

Because of the increase in incidence of HIV and TB among women of childbearing age, there has been an increase in the incidence of TB in pregnant women (Box 14.9). However, the data on TB in pregnancy are limited. Pregnancy does not appear to increase the risk of developing TB. Diagnosis of TB in pregnant women may be delayed by nonspecific symptoms, which can be confused with common manifestations of pregnancy. Fetal and maternal outcomes depend on the location of disease, the points of disease progression and pregnancy at which diagnosis is made, and adherence to treatment. Isoniazid, rifampicin, and ethambutol are considered safe for use during pregnancy.

Congenital TB is rare. Diagnosis relies on clinical suspicion, especially with a recent history of maternal TB.

Key Terms

Acid-fast bacilli (AFB)	Extrapulmonary TB	Superficial lymphadenitis
Active TB	Extrathoracic TB	TB granuloma
Anergy	Fetal growth retardation	TB meningitis
Annual risk of infection (ARI)	Ghon focus	Teratogenic
Antigen-specific anergy	Hematogenous dissemination	Tubercle bacilli
Apgar scores	Hepatotoxicity	Tuberculin skin test (TST)
Bacille Calmette-Guérin (BCG)	Induration	Perinatal tuberculosis
BACTEC radiometric assay	Intrathoracic TB	Presumptive diagnosis
Caseating granuloma	Isoniazid	Primary TB
Caseating lesion	Latent TB	Progressive lymphadenopathy
Cavitating disease	Lowenstein-Jensen medium	Progressive primary TB
CD4 lymphocyte	Microscopic observation drug susceptibility (MODS)	Pulmonary TB
Chest radiograph		Purified protein derivative (PPD)
Congenital TB	Miliary TB	
Contact tracing	Multidrug-resistant TB (MDR-TB)	Pyrizinamide
Delayed hypersensitivity		Reactivation TB
Directly Observed Therapy Shortcourse (DOTS)	Mycobacterial load	Regional lymphadenitis
	Natural history	Rifampicin
Droplets	Specificity	Sensitivity
Effusions	Sputum induction	Smear-negative
Ethambutol	Stegen–Toledo criteria	Smear-positive
Exogenous reinfection	String test	

Questions for Discussion

1. List any five factors that contribute to the global resurgence of TB.
2. Discuss any three reasons why diagnosis, monitoring, and treatment of TB in children have implications for community control of TB.
3. List five challenges that are usually encountered in diagnosing TB in children using currently available methods. In a 1,000 word narrative, discuss any three of these.
4. The Director of Child Health Services in a rural health department in a TB-endemic less-developed country in sub-Saharan Africa is planning to embark on mass TST and BCG vaccination campaign for infants and young children as a means of controlling TB. As the regional MCH program director, what advice would you give him/her regarding evidence of the effectiveness of this intervention?

References

Aronson NE, Santosham M, Comstock GW et al. (2004) Long-term efficacy of BCG vaccine in American Indians and Alaska Natives: A 60-year follow-up study. Journal of the American Medical Association, 291(17), 2086–2091

Bachou H, Tylleskar T, Downing R et al. (2006) Severe malnutrition with and without HIV-1 infection in hospitalized children in Kampala, Uganda: differences in clinical features, haematological findings and CD4+ cell counts. Nutrition Journal, 5, 27

Behr MA, Warren S, Salamon H et al. (1999) Transmission of *Mycobacterium tuberculosis* from patients smear-negative for acid-fast bacilli. Lancet, 353(9151), 444–449

Berman S, Kibel MA, Fourie PB et al. (1992) Childhood tuberculosis and tuberculous meningitis: high incidence rates in the Western Cape of South Africa. Tuberculosis and Lung Disease, 73(6), 349–355

Bierrenbach AL, Cunha S, Barreto M et al. (2003) Tuberculin reactivity in a population of schoolchildren with high BCG vaccination coverage. Revista Panama de Salud Publica, 13(5), 285–293

Bjerkedal T, Bahna SL, Lehmann EH (1975) Course and outcome of pregnancy in women with pulmonary tuberculosis. Scandinavian Journal of Respiratory Diseases, 56(5), 245–250

Black GF, Weir RE, Floyd S et al. (2002) BCG-induced increase in interferon-gamma response to mycobacterial antigens and efficacy of BCG vaccination in Malawi and the UK: two randomized controlled studies. Lancet, 359(9315), 1393–1401

Brost BC, Newman RB (1997) The maternal and fetal effects of tuberculosis therapy. Obstetrics and Gynecology Clinics of North America, 24(3), 659–673

Burk JR, Bahar D, Wolf FS et al. (1978) Nursery exposure of 528 newborns to a nurse with pulmonary tuberculosis. Southern Medical Journal, 71(1), 7–10

Cantwell MF, Binkin NJ (1997) Impact of HIV on tuberculosis in sub-Saharan Africa: a regional perspective. International Journal of Tuberculosis and Lung Disease, 1(3), 205–214

Cantwell MF, Shehab Z, Costello A et al. (1994) Brief report: congenital tuberculosis. New England Journal of Medicine, 330(15), 1051–1054

Carter EJ, Mates S (1994) Tuberculosis during pregnancy. The Rhode Island experience, 1987 to 1991. Chest, 106(5), 1466–1470

Cauthen GM, Pio A, ten Dam HG (2002) Annual risk of tuberculous infection. 1988. Bulletin of the World Health Organization, 80(6), 503–511; discussion 501–502

Chintu C, Mudenda V, Lucas S et al. (2002) Lung diseases at necropsy in African children dying from respiratory illnesses: a descriptive necropsy study. Lancet, 360(9338), 985–990

Chintu C, Mwaba P (2005) Tuberculosis in children with human immunodeficiency virus infection. International Journal of Tuberculosis and Lung Disease, 9(5), 477–484

Chow F, Espiritu N, Gilman RH et al. (2006) La cuerda dulce – a tolerability and acceptability study of a novel approach to specimen collection for diagnosis of pediatric pulmonary tuberculosis. BMC Infectious Diseases, 6, 67

Colditz GA, Brewer TF, Berkey CS et al. (1994) Efficacy of BCG vaccine in the prevention of tuberculosis. Meta-analysis of the published literature. Journal of the American Medical Association, 271(9), 698–702

Comstock GW, Livesay VT, Woolpert SF (1974) The prognosis of a positive tuberculin reaction in childhood and adolescence. American Journal of Epidemiology, 99(2), 131–138

Daley CL, Small PM, Schecter GF et al. (1992) An outbreak of tuberculosis with accelerated progression among persons infected with the human immunodeficiency virus. An analysis using restriction-fragment-length polymorphisms. New England Journal of Medicine, 326(4), 231–235

Datta M, Vallishayee RS, Diwakara AM (1999) Fifteen year follow up of trial of BCG vaccines in south India for tuberculosis prevention. Tuberculosis Research Centre (ICMR), Chennai. Indian Journal of Medical Research, 110, 56–69

de March AP (1975) Tuberculosis and pregnancy. Five- to ten-year review of 215 patients in their fertile age. Chest, 68(6), 800–804

Doveren RF, Block R (1998) Tuberculosis and pregnancy–a provincial study (1990–1996). Netherlands Journal of Medicine, 52(3), 100–106

Eamranond P, Jaramillo E (2001) Tuberculosis in children: reassessing the need for improved diagnosis in global control strategies. International Journal of Tuberculosis and Lung Disease, 5(7), 594–603

Enarson PM, Enarson DA, Gie R (2005) Management of tuberculosis in children in low-income countries. International Journal of Tuberculosis and Lung Disease, 9(12), 1299–1304

Espinal MA, Reingold AL, Lavandera M (1996) Effect of pregnancy on the risk of developing active tuberculosis. Journal of Infectious Diseases, 173(2), 488–491

Figueroa-Damian R, Arredondo-Garcia JL (1998) Pregnancy and tuberculosis: influence of treatment on perinatal outcome. American Journal of Perinatology, 15(5), 303–306

Franchi LM, Cama RI, Gilman RH et al. (1998) Detection of *Mycobacterium tuberculosis* in nasopharyngeal aspirate samples in children. Lancet, 352(9141), 1681–1682

Getchell WS, Davis C, Gilman J et al. (1992) Basic epidemiology of tuberculosis in Peru: a prevalence study of tuberculin sensitivity in a Pueblo joven. American Journal of Tropical Medicine and Hygiene, 47(6), 721–729

Good JT Jr., Iseman MD, Davidson PT et al. (1981) Tuberculosis in association with pregnancy. American Journal of Obstetrics and Gynecology, 140(5), 492–498

Grisolle A (1850) De l'influence que la grossesse et laphthisie pulmonaire exercant reciproquement l'unesur l'autre. Archives of General Medicine, 22:41

Halsey NA, Chaisson RE, Matts JP et al. (1998) Randomized trial of isoniazid versus rifampicin and pyrazinamide for prevention of tuberculosis in HIV-1 infection. Lancet, 351(9105), 786–792

Hart PD, Sutherland I (1977) BCG and vole bacillus vaccines in the prevention of tuberculosis in adolescence and early adult life. British Medical Journal, 2(6082), 293–295

Hedvall E (1953) Pregnancy and tuberculosis. Acta Medica Scandinavica Supplement, 286, 1–101

Hershfield E (1991) Tuberculosis in children: guidelines for diagnosis, prevention and management (a statement of the scientific committees of the IUATLD). Bulletin of the International Union Against Tuberculosis and Lung Disease, 66, 61–67

Hesseling AC, Schaaf H, Gie R et al. (2002) A critical review of diagnostic approaches used in the diagnosis of childhood tuberculosis. International Journal of Tuberculosis and Lung Disease, 6(12), 1038–1045

Holmes CB, Hausler H, Nunn P (1998) A review of sex differences in the epidemiology of tuberculosis. International Journal of Tuberculosis and Lung Disease, 2(2), 96–104

Houwert KA, Borggreven P, Schaaf et al. (1998) Prospective evaluation of World Health Organization criteria to assist diagnosis of tuberculosis in children. European Respiratory Journal, 11(5), 1116–1120

Jackson TD, Murtha AP (2001) Anergy during pregnancy. American Journal of Obstetrics and Gynecology, 184(6), 1090–1092

Jana N, Vasishta K, Saha S et al. (1999) Obstetrical outcomes among women with extrapulmonary tuberculosis. New England Journal of Medicine, 341(9), 645–649

Jones CA (2001) Maternal transmission of infectious pathogens in breast milk. Journal of Pediatric Child Health, 37(6), 576–582

Kawai V, Soto G, Gilman R et al. (2006) Tuberculosis mortality, drug resistance, and infectiousness in patients with and without HIV infection in Peru. American Journal of Tropical Medicine and Hygiene, 75(6), 1027–1033

Kothari A, Mahadevan N, Girling J (2006) Tuberculosis and pregnancy – results of a study in a high prevalence area in London. European Journal of Obstetrics and Gynecologic Reproductive Biology, 126(1), 48–55

Kumar D, Watson JM, Charlette A et al. (1997) Tuberculosis in England and Wales in 1993: results of a national survey. Thorax, 52(12), 1060–1067

Llewelyn M, Cropley I, Wilkinson RJ et al. (2000) Tuberculosis diagnosed during pregnancy: a prospective study from London. Thorax, 55(2), 129–132

Lockman S, Tappero JW, Kenyon TA et al. (1999) Tuberculin reactivity in a pediatric population with high BCG vaccination coverage. International Journal of Tuberculosis and Lung Disease, 3(1), 23–30

Luo C, Chintu C, Bhat G et al. (1994) Human immunodeficiency virus type-1 infection in Zambian children with tuberculosis: changing seroprevalence and evaluation of a thioacetazone-free regimen. Tuberculosis and Lung Disease, 75(2), 110–115

Marais BJ, Gie RP, Schaaf HS et al. (2004) The natural history of childhood intra-thoracic tuberculosis: a critical review of literature from the pre-chemotherapy era. International Journal of Tuberculosis and Lung Disease, 8(4), 392–402

Marais BJ, Gie RP, Schaaf HS et al. (2006a) The spectrum of disease in children treated for tuberculosis in a highly endemic area. International Journal of Tuberculosis and Lung Disease, 10(7), 732–738

Marais BJ, Hesseling AC, Gie RP et al. (2006b) The bacteriologic yield in children with intrathoracic tuberculosis. Clinical Infectious Diseases, 42(8), e69–e71

Marais BJ, Hesseling AC, Gie RP et al. (2006c) The burden of childhood tuberculosis and the accuracy of community-based surveillance data. International Journal of Tuberculosis and Lung Disease, 10(3), 259–263

Marais BJ, Obihara C, Warren RM et al. (2005) The burden of childhood tuberculosis: a public health perspective. International Journal of Tuberculosis and Lung Disease, 9(12), 1305–1313

Margono F, Mroueh J, Garely A et al. (1994) Resurgence of active tuberculosis among pregnant women. Obstetrics and Gynecology, 83(6), 911–914

Moore DA, Mendoza D, Gilman R et al. (2004) Microscopic observation drug susceptibility assay, a rapid, reliable diagnostic test for multidrug-resistant tuberculosis suitable for use in resource-poor settings. Journal of Clinical Microbiology, 42(10), 4432–4437

Moore DA, Evans CA, Gilman RH et al. (2006) Microscopic-observation drug-susceptibility assay for the diagnosis of TB. New England Journal of Medicine, 355(15), 1539–1550

Moulding T (1999) Pathogenesis, pathophysiology, and immunology: clinical orientations. In: D Schlossberg (ed.), Tuberculosis and Non-Tuberculous Mycobacterial Infections. Philadelphia: W.B. Saunders, pp. 48–56

Mukadi YD, Wiktor S, Coulibaly I et al. (1997) Impact of HIV infection on the development, clinical presentation, and outcome of tuberculosis among children in Abidjan, Cote d'Ivoire. Aids, 11(9), 1151–1158

Mwaba P, Maboshe M, Chintu C et al. (2003) The relentless spread of tuberculosis in Zambia – trends over the past 37 years (1964–2000). South African Medical Journal, 93(2), 149–152

Mwinga A (2005) Challenges and hope for the diagnosis of tuberculosis in infants and young children. Lancet, 365(9454), 97–98

Nelson LJ, Wells CD (2004) Global epidemiology of childhood tuberculosis. International Journal of Tuberculosis and Lung Disease, 8(5), 636–647

Nemir RL, O'Hare D (1985) Congenital tuberculosis. Review and diagnostic guidelines. American Journal of the Disabled Child, 139(3), 284–287

Nolan CM, Goldberg SV, Buskin SE (1999) Hepatotoxicity associated with isoniazid preventive therapy: a 7-year survey from a public health tuberculosis clinic. Journal of the American Medical Association, 281(11), 1014–1018

Oberhelman RA, Soto-Castellares G, Caviedes L et al. (2006). Improved recovery of *Mycobacterium tuberculosis* from children using the microscopic observation drug susceptibility method. Pediatrics, 118(1), e100–e106

O'Brien KL, Ruff AJ, Louis MA et al. (1995) Bacillus Calmette–Guérin complications in children born to HIV-1-infected women with a review of the literature. Pediatrics, 95(3), 414–418

Ormerod P (2001) Tuberculosis in pregnancy and the puerperium. Thorax, 56(6), 494–499

Palme IB, Gudetta B, Degefu H et al. (2001) Risk factors for human immunodeficiency virus infection in Ethiopian children with tuberculosis. Pediatric Infectious Disease Journal, 20(11), 1066–1072

Park MM, Davis AL, Schluger NW et al. (1996) Outcome of MDR-TB patients, 1983–1993. Prolonged survival with appropriate therapy. American Journal of Respiratory and Critical Care Medicine, 153(1), 317–324

Pelly TF, Santillan CF, Gilman RH et al. (2005) Tuberculosis skin testing, anergy and protein malnutrition in Peru. International Journal of Tuberculosis and Lung Disease, 9(9), 977–984

Ponnighaus JM, Fine PE, Sterne JA et al. (1992) Efficacy of BCG vaccine against leprosy and tuberculosis in northern Malawi. Lancet, 339(8794), 636–639

Ramirez-Cardich ME, Kawai V, Oberhelman RA et al. (2006) Clinical correlates of tuberculosis co-infection in HIV-infected children hospitalized in Peru. International Journal of Infectious Disease, 10(4), 278–281

Rodriguez L, Gonzales C, Flores L et al. (2005) Assessment by flow cytometry of cytokine production in malnourished children. Clinical and Diagnostic Laboratory Immunology, 12(4), 502–507

Saito M, Bautista CT, Gilman RH et al. (2004) The value of counting BCG scars for interpretation of tuberculin skin tests in a tuberculosis hyperendemic shantytown, Peru. International Journal of Tuberculosis and Lung Disease, 8(7), 842–847

Salazar GE, Schmitz T, Cama R et al. (2001) Pulmonary tuberculosis in children in a developing country. Pediatrics, 108(2), 448–453

Santiago EM, Lawson E, Gillenwater K et al. (2003) A prospective study of bacillus Calmette–Guérin scar formation and tuberculin skin test reactivity in infants in Lima, Peru. Pediatrics, 112(4), e298

Schaaf HS, Gie RP, Beyers N et al. (2000) Primary drug-resistant tuberculosis in children. International Journal of Tuberculosis and Lung Disease, 4(12), 1149–1155

Schaefer G, Zervoudakis IA, Fuchs FF et al. (1975) Pregnancy and pulmonary tuberculosis. Obstetrics and Gynecology, 46(6), 706–715

Shafer RW, Small PM, Larkin C et al. (1995) Temporal trends and transmission patterns during the emergence of multidrug-resistant tuberculosis in New York City: a molecular epidemiologic assessment. Journal of Infectious Diseases, 171(1), 170–176

Shingadia D, Novelli V (2003) Diagnosis and treatment of tuberculosis in children. Lancet Infectious Diseases, 3(10), 624–632

Starke JR (1999) Tuberculosis in infants and children. In: D Schlossberg (ed.), Tuberculosis and Nontuberculous Mycobacterial Infections (Fourth Edition). Philadelphia: W.B. Saunders, pp. 303–324

Sterne JA, Rodrigues LC, Guedes IN (1998) Does the efficacy of BCG decline with time since vaccination? International Journal of Tuberculosis and Lung Disease, 2(3), 200–207

Toledo A, Stegen G (1979) Criterios de diagnóstico en tuberculosis infantil (Diagnostic criteria for pediatric tuberculosis). Revista Mexicana de Pediatría, 46, 239–243

Tripathy SN, Tripathy SN (2003) Tuberculosis and pregnancy. International Journal of Gynaecology and Obstetrics, 80(3), 247–253

U.S. Department of Health and Human Services (2007) *Glossary of Terms Related to TB*. Atlanta, Georgia: Centers for Disease Control and Prevention. http://www.cdc.gov/tb/faqs/qa_glossary.htm Cited August 9, 2009

Ussery XT, Valway SE, McKenna M et al. (1996) Epidemiology of tuberculosis among children in the United States: 1985 to 1994. Pediatric Infectious Disease Journal, 15(8), 697–704

Vallejo JG, Ong LT, Starke JR (1994) Clinical features, diagnosis, and treatment of tuberculosis in infants. Pediatrics, 94(1), 1–7

Vargas D, Garcia L, Gilman RH et al. (2005) Diagnosis of sputum-scarce HIV-associated pulmonary tuberculosis in Lima, Peru. Lancet, 365(9454), 150–152

Walls T, Shingadia D (2004) Global epidemiology of pediatric tuberculosis. Journal of Infection, 48(1), 13–22

Whalen C, Horsburgh CR, Hom D et al. (1995) Accelerated course of human immunodeficiency virus infection after tuberculosis. American Journal of Respiratory Critical Care Medicine, 151(1), 129–135

Wilson ME, Fineberg HV, Colditz GA (1995) Geographic latitude and the efficacy of bacillus Calmette–Guérin vaccine. Clinical Infectious Diseases, 20(4), 982–991

Zar HJ, Hanslo D, Apolles P et al. (2005) Induced sputum versus gastric lavage for microbiological confirmation of pulmonary tuberculosis in infants and young children: a prospective study. Lancet, 365(9454), 130–134

Zwarenstein M, Schoeman JH, Vundule C (1998) Randomized controlled trial of self-supervised and directly observed treatment of tuberculosis. Lancet, 352(9137), 1340–1343

Chapter 15
Impact of HIV on the Health of Women, Children, and Families in Less Developed Countries

Hoosen M. Coovadia and Nigel C. Rollins

Learning Objectives After reading this chapter and answering the discussion questions that follow, you should be able to

- Present a brief description of the global prevalence of HIV/AIDS among women, children, and adolescents.
- Summarize the impact of HIV/AIDS on the family and community, including the challenges posed by the increasing scale of AIDS orphans globally.
- Discuss factors that increase women's vulnerability to HIV/AIDS.
- Evaluate strategies for the prevention and comprehensive management of women, adolescents, and children at risk of HIV/AIDS.

Introduction

This chapter presents an overview of the global burden of HIV/AIDS with a focus on women and children. It begins with a discussion of the prevalence of the disease among women, highlighting the factors that increase women's vulnerability to HIV/AIDS, including biological factors (the greater anatomical, physiological, and pathological features that increase the likelihood of women more than men being infected in sexual intercourse), social factors (e.g., stigma, discrimination, and sexual violence), political factors (e.g., compromised political rights and repressive legislation), economic factors

(e.g., poverty), cultural factors (e.g., subordinate position of women, emphasis on male-directed and controlled prevention methods), and access to care (especially limited for women in rural areas). The chapter progresses to discuss strategies for prevention of HIV among women and emphasizes the need for improved antenatal care services with effective counseling on options for prevention of mother-to-child transmission, cervical barrier methods of prevention (e.g., diaphragms, female condoms, microbicides, and HIV vaccine), and detection and treatment of sexually transmitted infections, especially those due to herpes virus 2. With regard to HIV/AIDS among children, the chapter provides an overview of the global burden of the disease and its impact on this population group. A discussion of strategies for comprehensive management of children at risk for HIV/AIDS is provided. The chapter concludes with an examination of the impact of HIV/AIDS on the family and community, highlighting the challenge posed by the increasing scale of AIDS orphans globally. It is recommended that prevention programs targeted at women and children should aim at creating social, political, economic, and cultural environments that empower women, challenge stigma and discrimination against women, and aggressively combat poverty, gender, and racial inequalities.

HIV/AIDS is one of the worst pandemics to have ever afflicted humankind. More than 22 million people have already died from the disease since it was first recognized in the United States in 1981. It is one of the major killers of human beings, together with tuberculosis and malaria. Human history has been punctuated by major pandemics, times without number, that swept across countries and through populations. Some of the better known

H.M. Coovadia (✉)
Nelson R. Mandela School of Medicine, University of Natal, South Africa

J.E. Ehiri (ed.), *Maternal and Child Health*, DOI 10.1007/b106524_15,
© Springer Science+Business Media, LLC 2009

diseases are plague (the "Black Death") which devastated Europe in the fourth and fifteenth centuries, smallpox, tuberculosis, syphilis, and influenza which threatens the world once again. By the end of 2005 there were about 38.6 million persons (range = 33.4–46.0 million) who were estimated to be infected with HIV globally. The total number of people living with HIV/AIDS had gone up during the previous 2 years in all regions of the world, except the Caribbean. An estimated 4.1 million people became newly infected with HIV and 2.8 million lost their lives to AIDS. Globally, the number of persons becoming newly infected every year peaked in the late 1990s and stabilized thereafter. However, in some countries, the incidence of HIV continues to increase. Sub-Saharan Africa, which contains 10% of the global population, is the hardest hit with about 24.5 million, which is roughly two-thirds of the global burden (UNAIDS 2007). The epidemic is quite diverse throughout the continent with most countries following the worldwide trend, while in some countries, the epidemic continues to increase. With an estimated 5.5 million (4.9 million–6.1 million) people living with HIV (UNAIDS 2006), South Africa is the country with the largest number of infections in the world. The country's Department of Health estimates that 18.3% of adults (15–49 years) were living with HIV in 2006 (Department of Health, South Africa 2007). More than half (55%) of all South Africans infected with HIV reside in the KwaZulu-Natal and Gauteng provinces (Dorrington et al. 2006). Staggering increases in HIV during the past decade have been quite dramatic in some African countries: this is illustrated by the rapid escalation of HIV in South Africa where the antenatal clinic prevalence has gone up from <1% in 1990 to 20% in the year 2000. A corresponding rise in adult mortality has paralleled this increase (UNAIDS 2007). However, in recent years, there has been stabilization or a promising decline in prevalence in Uganda, Kenya, Tanzania, Rwanda, Zambia, Zimbabwe, Burkina Faso, and Ghana (UNAIDS 2007). In South Africa, the latest HIV data collected at antenatal clinics suggest that HIV infection levels might be leveling off, with HIV prevalence in pregnant women at 30% in 2005 and 29% in 2006 (Department of Health, South Africa 2007).

A key characteristic of this epidemic is that it often affects the most disadvantaged and poorest communities worldwide, groups who are at the margins of society, or sections of the population subordinated to those who hold political, economic, and social power. These include women and men in developing countries, women in all societies, gay men, intravenous drug users, alcohol abusers, and children. This chapter is about two of these groups, women and children in developing countries. We discuss aspects of the disease in these groups with which we are most familiar through our professional and personal lives.

Mothers

HIV in Women: Prevalence

Of the roughly 40 million persons who are HIV infected and who remain alive, 17.5 million (16.2–19.3) are women of child-bearing age (UNAIDS 2005). There was an increase of a million more HIV-infected women in 2005 compared to 2003 (UNAIDS 2005). There were similar increases in numbers of HIV-infected women (about 2 million) in south and Southeast Asia (UNAIDS 2005). About 70% of all women (i.e., 13.5 million) who are HIV infected are in sub-Saharan Africa. Globally, about 46% of all those who are HIV infected are women (15–49 years old), and in the Caribbean, North Africa, and the Middle East it is roughly 50%; in sub-Saharan Africa it is 57%. It is the young (15–24 years old) who are most vulnerable. In sub-Saharan Africa, adolescent women are three to six times more likely to become HIV infected than their male peers, and in southern Africa, this proportion is up to 75%. Therefore, there is a very large pool of women who could potentially give birth to children who would be either HIV infected themselves or be exposed to the virus in the womb and during childbirth every year. Some hundreds of thousands of children could also become HIV infected due to breastfeeding. In southern Africa, the overall HIV prevalence at antenatal clinics is about 20%; in Botswana, Swaziland, and Kwa-Zulu/Natal in South Africa, the figures range from 30 to 40% (Department of Health, South Africa 2007).

Vulnerability of Women to HIV

HIV adversely affects every dimension of women's sexual and reproductive health: pregnancy, childbirth, use of contraceptives, infant feeding choices, exposure to and treatment of sexually transmitted diseases, and vulnerability to sexual violence. HIV worsens some reproductive health diseases, increases the severity of others, decreases fertility, and affects sexual health. The reasons for the disproportionate burdens of HIV among women are multiple and not always clearly understood (Collazos et al. 2007). The key reasons accounting for the vulnerability of women to HIV are a combination of biological and social factors (Box 15.1). Biological factors relate to the greater anatomical, physiological, and pathological features which increase the likelihood of women more than men to be infected in sexual intercourse. Social factors are determined by the exposure of women to risky contextual factors, sexual customs, and practices. The primary route of HIV transmission in Africa, accounting for 85% of all

---

Box 15.1 Factors that Increase Women's Vulnerability to HIV

- Biological factors: HIV risk two to four times higher for women than men
- Social factors: coercive sex, especially young women
- Political factors: compromised political rights; regressive legislation
- Economic factors: poverty and food insecurity disproportionately affect more women than men
- Cultural factors: subordinate position of women; use of condoms
- Access to health services: often restricted, especially rural women
- Reproductive health services: antenatal and other services often unavailable, inaccessible, and inadequate; family planning often limited to technical services without provision of comprehensive sexual health services or options for prevention of mother-to-child transmission and infant feeding

---

infections, is through heterosexual contact (African Union 2006), while across Asia, infection occurs mostly through intravenous drug use and commercial sex workers (UNAIDS 2005).

There are a number of social, political, and cultural reasons for the increased vulnerability of women to HIV. Younger women, in particular, are culturally and socially unable to negotiate safer sex, including the use of condoms, with their male partners; they are often subjected to coercion in sexual relations, and their rising expectation of modern life encourages them into sexual liaisons with older men (transactional or barter sex) who may have more resources but also higher HIV prevalence. Women, especially at younger ages and in rural areas, are less well informed about HIV transmission than young males. Education can make a difference in gaining knowledge on HIV/AIDS and may reduce acquisition of HIV – but knowledge does not assure choice and autonomy. Women are often subjected to physical and sexual violence, and although this occurs in most regions of the world, it is especially damaging to the health of women in regions where HIV is prevalent (Zablotska et al. 2007). There is considerable overlap between HIV, sexually transmitted diseases, and violence (Karamagi et al. 2006). It is known that women with HIV are more likely to have experienced sexual and physical violence than women without HIV. Women have learned that disclosure of their HIV status may entail serious problems and cannot be lightly undertaken. In some settings, more in Africa than in the developed world, in excess of 20% of women disclosing their HIV status to partners have met with negative responses, including violence. Frequently, violence against women and children occurs within families or within the circle of acquaintances and friends of the family. Coercive sex and rape are often antecedents of HIV infection in some African countries. It has been estimated that 2 million girls (5–15 years of age) are coerced into the sex trade every year, and that a third to half of married women in some regions are subjected to physical abuse by their partners. Women who suffered food insecurity and hunger more frequently agreed to sex without condoms, intergenerational sex, and multiple partners (Weiser et al. 2007). Persistent and residual cultural practices, such as female genital mutilation (FGM) (see Chapter 10), may predispose women to sexually transmitted diseases, including HIV; 130 million women in the world are said to be living with the effects of this destructive practice. Partner infidelity often places women at risk of being the passive victims of sexually transmitted diseases. Marriage and their own fidelity are insufficient to protect women against acquiring HIV. In southern Africa (Harare, Durban, Soweto) 66% of women had one lifetime partner and 79% had abstained from sex until marriage at 17 years. Yet 40% of young women were HIV infected (Chen et al. 2007). In India, most females have been HIV infected by their husbands who had contracted the infection from sex workers (UNAIDS 2005). In Colombia, 72% of women who were HIV positive at antenatal clinics were in stable relationships (UNAIDS 2005).

Shame, stigma, and discrimination hinder women with HIV or at risk for HIV from protecting themselves or seeking assistance and support (Ehiri et al. 2005). Social and cultural taboos on sexuality aggravate the position. These factors prevent women from making autonomous decisions for their personal and family health and benefit, including preventing them from accessing health and other services which may offer counseling, prophylaxis, treatment, and care. Poverty and lack of education and economic opportunities ensure that women stay in a subordinate position in society.

Political rights may be compromised: in some developing countries legislation bars women from entering into independent contracts, denies them the right to inherit land and property, and binds them to regressive laws on marriage, divorce, and child custody (Krishnan et al. 2008). Conflicts, famines, wars (see Chapter 7), internal and external migrations, and foreign occupation affect women more than they do men, exposing them to sexual exploitation and risks, and multiple health, social, and financial difficulties (Parker et al. 2000). Trafficking of young women, often into commercial sex work, and criminalization of sex workers add to the structural conditions that increase the risk of HIV infection.

In addition, there are biological factors determining vulnerability to HIV which are more prominent in women than men. The risk of becoming HIV infected during unprotected sexual intercourse is two to four times higher for women than men. Sexually transmitted infections are more common in women; these infections may compromise the integrity of the vaginal mucosa, rendering women more vulnerable to HIV transmission. Young women in particular have immature cervices and less vaginal secretions; these make them prone to vaginal lacerations during sex. Sexually transmitted infections in women's HIV-infected partners may increase the viral load in these partners and raise their propensity to transmit HIV sexually. There are more than 340 million cases of curable sexually transmitted infections every year, with women having greater vulnerability than men (UNAIDS 2006). The high prevalence of vaginal infections among women in Africa [bacterial vaginosis (30–60%); vulvovaginal candidosis (10–13%); trichomonas vaginalis (7–23%)] predisposes them to HIV transmission (Chen et al. 2007). Despite the high risk that these infections pose for the spread of HIV, health services for prevention and treatment are poorly cocoordinated, and coverage is low (UNAIDS 2006). Women are said to progress to severe HIV disease at lower viral loads and higher CD4 counts than men (Umeh and Currier 2005; Gilad et al. 2003; Napravnik et al. 2002; Suligoi 1997). Although this requires better evidence; ovulatory hormones may play a role in this effect. The implications of these virological and immunological characteristics are that initiation of antiretroviral therapy for women should be at lower viral loads.

HIV/AIDS Among Adolescents

Although the burden of HIV/AIDS among adolescents has been discussed in Chapter 24 (Adolescent Health), it is germane to mention here that youth aged 15–25 years are at high risk for infection and represent the population group with the largest number of infected persons. Over 10 million HIV infections worldwide are among youth aged 15–24 years, which represent almost 7,000 infections per day (United Nations 2001). Over half of all new infections occur among adolescents (UNAIDS 2003; Senderowitz 1997). In Africa and the Caribbean, the epidemic disproportionately affects young women, with infection rates for young women two to three times higher than for young men.

Targeting adolescents is regarded as a feasible means of halting the spread of infections, for they have not yet established deep-rooted behavioral patterns and may therefore, be more amenable to prevention interventions in comparison to older people (Cowan 2002; Aggleton and Rivers 1998). This promising aspect of working with adolescents, however, also requires that programs be carefully designed and attuned to the particular characteristics of, and culture inherent among, adolescents (Population Council 2000). To be effective, interventions must take account of the basic truths of adolescent behavior: exploration, experimentation, and rebellion, which can often lead to early initiation of sex, multiple sex partners, and lack of condom use (Magnussen et al. 2004). Attitudes of invincibility also seriously alter the adolescents' perception of HIV/AIDS/STD risks (Magnussen et al. 2004). In addition, social forces combine with these behaviors to form in the adolescent, ingrained negative messages that subsume positive, healthy behaviors and attitudes. For example, poverty, the shift from rural to urbanized cultures, the exploitative economic power of "sugar daddies" (Silberschmidt and Rasch 2001), delayed marriage, and pervasive gender inequality block access to condoms and information, and place adolescents in precarious, high-risk situations (Magnussen et al. 2004). Thus, interventions predicated on the idea that there are equal rights in a sexual relationship may be counterproductive in many cultures (Stanton et al. 1998).

Magnussen et al. (2004) conducted a review of the effectiveness of interventions to prevent HIV/AIDS among adolescents using data from the literature. Only studies that included a control group, and which involved pre- and post-intervention assessments were included. Outcomes assessed included changes in safe sex practices (abstinence, condom use, limitation of sexual partners, avoidance of casual sex), knowledge about HIV/AIDS transmission and prevention methods, perception of HIV/AIDS/STD risks, self-efficacy with regard to condom negotiation and refusal of sex, uptake of voluntary counseling and testing (VCT), and reduction in incidence of HIV/AIDS/STDs. Studies were assessed in terms of intervention format (e.g., education, role-play, video), duration, and setting (school or community based). Reported improvements in outcome measures in intervention versus control groups were assessed. Sixteen studies met the inclusion criteria;

thirteen of these were conducted in Africa and three in Latin America. Twelve of the sixteen studies were school based and four were community based. It was found that the interventions reviewed were not resoundingly successful in achieving their goals of increasing knowledge of HIV/AIDS, altering attitudes, improving negotiation and communication skills, or in influencing positive behavior evidenced through consistent condom use, abstinence, or reducing the number of partners (Magnussen et al. 2004).

ABC (abstinence, be faithful, use condoms) is promoted as the foundation of prevention messages but is often not applicable or practiced by groups at risk, and oversimplifies the determinants of infection and opportunities for prevention. For example, women in Africa often do not live under fair and just social conditions or have sufficient economic power to negotiate condom use or the right to refuse sex. Therefore, other interventions are required. The subordinate position of women in many affected societies mandates the development of women-controlled prevention measures. These include the use of female condoms and detection and treatment of sexually transmitted infections, especially those due to herpes virus 2. Promising, but as yet unproven interventions, which may be especially useful to women include cervical barriers such as diaphragms, microbicides, and HIV vaccines. Male circumcision may prove to be effective; it has been demonstrated to reduce HIV transmission to males in a controlled trial in South Africa (Flynn et al. 2007; Muller et al. 2003), but what is urgently needed is evidence that male circumcision will reduce HIV transmission to females. The use of antiretrovirals (ARVs) (for prevention, post-exposure prophylaxis, and for treatment in the form of highly active antiretroviral therapy [HAART]) may not be sufficient on its own to prevent HIV transmission; ARVs will have to be combined with reduction of risky sexual behavior.

HIV in Women: Health Services Provision

Health service inadequacies and subjective factors are the key reasons for avoidable deaths in women. Lack of healthcare facilities, personnel and transport, and delays in providing treatment are the major administrative avoidable factors; personal beliefs, such as fatalism and non-caring attitudes, are also responsible. Of those who need HAART, less than 10% in Africa and less than 15% in Asia have access to it. However, due to new scale-up initiatives through United Nations agencies ("3×5" and Universal Access Programmes), up to 350,000 deaths were averted in 2005 (WHO/ UNAIDS 2003). Prevention interventions are available to less than 20% of those at risk of acquiring HIV in developing countries. Women-directed prevention services are often more deficient than those for both sexes. For example, antiretroviral therapy increased from 7% of those who required it in developing countries in 2003 to 20% in 2005, prevention services to reduce mother-to-child transmission of HIV expanded from 7.6 to 9.0%, and antiretroviral prophylaxis for prevention of mother-to-child transmission (PMTCT) went up from 3.3 to 9.2% during the same period (WHO/ UNAIDS 2005). While PMTCT coverage further increased to 34% in 2007 (UNAIDS 2007), this is still grossly inadequate and represents a failure of commitment and prioritization by governments, UN agencies, and civil society itself. There are, however, some successes: prevention activities are reducing HIV prevalence among young women (and men) in Uganda (Green et al. 2006), among sex workers and their clients in Thailand, Cambodia, Senegal, and India, and among intravenous drug users in Brazil (Piot et al. 2001).

The coverage of antenatal clinic services is often patchy in sub-Saharan Africa. About 40–50% of the poorest pregnant women lack access to antenatal clinic services and to a professional healthcare provider. The coverage for effective neonatal care is even worse. Counseling at such health facilities on options for prevention of transmission of HIV to the infant is critical. These are of considerable value for HIV-infected women as the risks of a premature birth and of low birth weight infants are not negligible. HIV-infected women fare worse than uninfected women: they are more likely to experience more adverse pregnancy outcomes, complications, and mortality. They are more often anemic, have pregnancy-induced high blood pressure, lower weight, and more infections of the urinary tract. They also experience greater frequency of syphilis, vaginal discharge, and increased severity of complications such as tuberculosis, malaria, miscarriages, and stillbirths. They are more likely to die from cervical cancer secondary to undiagnosed human papilloma virus (HPV) infection, and especially so when living in rural areas. Malnutrition may also supervene. Yet, HIV-related symptoms are rarely documented in antenatal notes presumably because health workers rarely ask the necessary questions. In countries with the highest infant deaths, there are also unacceptable maternal deaths. In South Africa, HIV-related maternal deaths increased steadily from 14.5% in 1998 to 20.1% in 2002–2004; HIV accounted for more than 50% of non-obstetric maternal mortality. The most common reasons for these maternal deaths are an absence of practical guidelines for midwives' antenatal assessments and for management of pregnancies in HIV-positive women (McIntyre 2003).

Voluntary counseling and HIV testing (VCT) centers are often inadequately provided. VCT centers are a gateway to a very large number of other public services such as welfare, health, support organizations, advice on safe and satisfying sexual lives, and referral to abuse centers. Counseling may also strengthen women's resolve to deal with violence, adhere to treatment schedules, and make appropriate decisions on infant feeding. In order to avoid dealing with HIV/AIDS as a special disease, and thereby exacerbating stigma and discrimination, many African countries are beginning to treat HIV/AIDS as a routine problem, and providing advice and tests as is done for other common disorders.

Psychosocial support is essential for HIV-infected women and is often neglected in developing countries. Counseling and testing for HIV is in itself insufficient to provide the depth of psychological support required to deal with anxiety, distress, fear, denial, guilt, etc. Specially trained individuals who are very often either unavailable or unaffordable are needed to provide individual, couple, family, group, and community counseling on HIV/AIDS.

Family planning services can play a supportive role during the HIV epidemic, as both HIV and reproductive health disorders are rooted in poverty, gender discrimination, and social marginalization. In Africa, the coverage is often restricted and integration with reproductive health and other services is uncommon. This diminishes potential synergies in disease prevention and control. These services can provide HIV prevention messages (condom use, abstinence, fidelity) and manage sexually transmitted diseases. Family planning centers can improve prevention of mother-to-child transmission programs by promoting interventions that decrease incidence of HIV in women of child-bearing age (primary prevention), and which prevent unintended pregnancies. Fifty percent of unintended pregnancies globally are terminated annually, 19 million unsafely (see Chapter 11). Therefore, access to safe and legal abortion is essential. The complicated interactions between antiretrovirals and hormonal contraceptives may also be addressed at these facilities.

HIV in Women and Pregnant Women: Impact

In the most seriously affected countries in southern Africa, AIDS has become the main cause of maternal death in all age groups. Measurements of the burden of disease in South Africa confirm that AIDS is a major cause of death among all women (with the 25- to 29-year age group being at most risk) and that these women have a higher mortality than men (47% versus 33%). Diarrhea, tuberculosis, and lower respiratory tract infection are the other important causes of years-of-life lost.

Children

Epidemiology

Nearly all HIV-positive children in developing countries became HIV infected through transmission of the disease from their mothers during pregnancy, through delivery, and postnatally from breastfeeding. The highest transmissions occur during delivery and from breastfeeding. HIV-infected children and HIV-uninfected children born to HIV-infected women (who are also considered to be vulnerable to many adverse medical and social problems) are the face of the AIDS epidemic which is often ignored. They often remain invisible to policy makers, program implementers, and service providers. About 2.3 million children under the age of 15

years are living with HIV worldwide, of whom 2.0 million are in sub-Saharan Africa. Many of them have no access to specific care and treatment, and they survive or die depending on their chances of joining the queue for general child health prevention and treatment services.

Impact of HIV on Children

HIV is a lethal disease in adults and children. Whereas clinical features and deterioration in many adults become prominent only 9–10 years after infection, the decline in health is much more rapid in children. The mortality from childhood HIV, in the absence of treatment and care, is very high, with a quarter to a third dying before 1 year of age, and the majority before their fifth birthday. It is estimated that children constitute 14% of the total HIV infections worldwide, but they account for 18% of all deaths due to AIDS. In 2005, about 570,000 children died from HIV/AIDS. Sickness and death are often due to the HIV disease process itself, as it erodes and destroys vital tissues and organs. More often, morbidity and mortality in children are due to a relentless destruction of the immune system which opens the floodgates to multiple infections and cancers. It follows that the types of infections that supervene are those that are latent and common in the environment. In Africa, the overwhelming causes of ill health and of death are pneumonias (often due to pneumocystis and bacteria), diarrhea, sepsis, malnutrition, and tuberculosis. In endemic areas, malaria is also important. These diseases are generally indistinguishable from those in the general population of children, except that they are more frequent and the clinical manifestations are more severe than in HIV-uninfected children. Even in countries where HIV prevalence is high, the proportion of children with HIV/AIDS is fairly small – in South Africa it is less than 10% of all children. It follows that thousands of children die of common diseases without any indication of their underlying HIV status. In the most severely affected countries, under 5 deaths attributable to HIV/AIDS vary considerably from across the regions, reaching roughly 45% in Botswana. In Africa as a whole,

AIDS was responsible for 2% of under 5-year mortality in 1990; this had risen to 6.5% in 2003 (Newell et al. 2004a; Zaba et al. 2004). Globally, however, it has been estimated that a fraction of under 5-year mortality is caused by HIV/AIDS, and that prevention activities relevant for HIV in children could prevent 150,000 of the 11 million child deaths from the common diseases that occur annually (Coovadia and Schaller 2008).

The latter part of the last century had witnessed the creation and global spread of a number of health programs aimed at preventing major diseases and reducing mortality in children. The benefits were gratifying and resulted in improving survival and falling mortality rates. In sub-Saharan Africa, many of these gains are being reversed by the impact of the AIDS epidemic. Infant mortality rates in this region have increased by more than 19%; in South Africa, where the under 5 mortality had fallen to 55 per 1,000 births by 1994, it has now risen to about 87 per 1,000 births (Coovadia and Schaller 2008). The global community has formulated ideas on further progress in global health by establishing the Millennium Development Goals: the figures given above for maternal mortality and the rates for child mortality reduce the prospects of success in meeting these goals by 2015. In industrialized countries, HIV infection in infants and children is a rapidly diminishing problem (McIntyre and Gray 2002); mortality rates for HIV-infected children and adolescents have decreased from 5% in 1996 to currently less than 1% (Volmink et al. 2006).

Prevention of Mother-to-Child Transmission (PMTCT) of HIV

Box 15.2 presents a summary of strategies for comprehensive management of children at risk of HIV. Striking reductions in perinatal transmission (during late pregnancy and delivery) of HIV and longer child survival within research cohorts have been achieved by comprehensive prevention of mother-to-child transmission (pMTCT) programs. The use of antiretrovirals in pMTCT programs has been critical for their success. However postnatal transmission (through breastfeeding) remains unresolved; in 2003 an estimated 300,000 infants of a

Box 15.2 Comprehensive Management of Children at Risk of HIV

- Prevention of HIV infection in women of child-bearing age
- Family planning for HIV-infected women
- Options for termination of pregnancy in HIV-infected women
- Prevention of mother-to-child transmission of HIV
- Diagnosis of HIV infection in infants and children
- Care of HIV-uninfected children born to HIV-infected women
- Clinical staging of HIV infection
- Clinical management of HIV-infected children
- Antiretroviral therapy
- Chronic care of HIV-infected children
- Terminal care of HIV-infected children
- Counseling and psychosocial support
- Nutritional care
- Family support
- Referral to welfare and social services

total of 700,000 newly infected by HIV had been infected through breastfeeding (WHO 2004a).

A number of earlier trials in Africa and Thailand, using drugs and combination antiretrovirals (ARVs) appropriate for developing regions, found that in non-breastfeeding women, zidovudine (AZT) can reduce transmission by between 50 and 70%, while in women who breastfeed this reduction varies between 63% at 6 weeks and 23% at 24 months (WHO 2004b). The reduced efficacy at 24 months is due to continued transmission of HIV through breast milk. Even when the mother is not able to get to a clinic to give birth and receive the appropriate ARVs, postpartum nevirapine (NVP) to the infant can reduce MTCT significantly, to 20.9% at 6–8 weeks, while NVP + AZT reduces transmission to 15.3% (WHO 2004b). When combined with elective caesarean section and avoidance of all breastfeeding, these interventions have reduced the risk of HIV transmission to infants to approximately 1% (WHO 2008).

Total avoidance of breastfeeding by an HIV-positive mother is patently very effective in preventing transmission of the virus to the child through this route. However, this option is not feasible for the majority of women in developing regions, mainly due to stigma of HIV associated with avoidance of breastfeeding, costs of formula, difficulties in hygienic preparation of artificial milks, lack of refrigeration and electricity, and unsafe or erratic water and formula supplies. Most importantly, the dangers of formula feeding – morbidity and deaths due to diarrhea and pneumonia, which are the result of contamination by polluted water and addition of unhygienic foods – often outweigh the risks of HIV transmission (Coutsoudis et al. 1999; Coovadia et al. 2007). Mixed breastfeeding (breast milk and other foods/liquids), which is the most common type of breastfeeding universally, increases the risk of HIV transmission (Magoni et al. 2005). Solids are recommended for infants only in the weaning period. Six months of exclusive breastfeeding (EBF), where the infant is fed breast milk only, with no other foods or liquids, is optimal for child growth and development. Solids given too early in infancy have been consistently shown to have deleterious effects on child health and increase HIV transmission (Magoni et al. 2005). However, in better resourced areas these differences have not been detected, which reinforce the UNAIDS guidelines on replacement feeding in HIV-infected women, viz. "where replacement feeding is acceptable, feasible, affordable, sustainable and safe, avoidance of all breastfeeding is recommended, otherwise exclusive breastfeeding is recommended for the first few months" (WHO/UNICEF/UNAIDS 2004). In developing countries, EBF for the first 6 months is very often more appropriate, as this is affordable, may lead to lower HIV transmission than mixed feeding, and improve infant survival (Coovadia et al. 2007; Magoni et al. 2005; Coutsoudis et al. 1999).

Community-based interventions to support EBF within HIV-infected and uninfected populations, have been successful in changing behavior from mixed to exclusive breastfeeding (Bland et al. 2008; Orne-Gliemann et al. 2006; Bhandari et al. 2003; Haider et al. 2000; Rodriguez-Garcia et al. 1990). Even in high prevalence HIV countries, breastfeeding could prevent 13% of under-5 deaths; while in low HIV prevalence countries, about 15% of under-5 deaths could be averted (WHO 2004a).

As the majority of HIV-positive children acquire the virus from their mothers, it makes sense that, in addition to the use of antiretrovirals during the perinatal period, most pediatric infections can be averted by preventing maternal HIV infection in the first place or by preventing of unwanted pregnancies by HIV-positive women. Indeed, a recent study undertaken in eight African countries showed that reducing the HIV prevalence of women by as little as 1.5% or decreasing the number of unwanted pregnancies in HIV-positive women by only 16% yielded a reduction in MTCT equivalent to that achieved using single-dose nevirapine (sdNVP), given to the mother during labor and to the infant directly after birth (Sweat et al. 2004).

The addition of short courses of ARVs to sdNVP in both breastfed and formula fed infants greatly decreases the risk of HIV infection in the infant, and the World Health Organization (2006) recommends that AZT + sdNVP be given to otherwise healthy HIV-infected women to prevent MTCT. Over 24 months, average MTCT of HIV without ARVs is between 30 and 45%, with combination ARVs these figures drop to between 2 and 3% in non-breast-feeding babies and around 5% in breastfeeding populations (WHO 2004a).

Access to Treatment

Box 15.3 summarizes the impact of AIDS on children. Less than 5% of HIV-positive children

---

Box 15.3 Impact of AIDS on Children

- Loss of family and identity;
- Depression;
- Reduced well-being;
- Increased malnutrition, starvation;
- Failure to immunize or provide health care;
- Decline in health status;
- Increased demands on labor;
- Loss of schooling/educational opportunities;
- Loss of inheritance;
- Forced migration;
- Homelessness, vagrancy, crime;
- Increased street living;
- Exposure to HIV infection.

who require AIDS treatment have access to it. A recent study from the United States suggests that appropriate treatment for HIV/AIDS in children may reduce pneumocystis pneumonia 14-fold, bacteremia 10-fold, and bacterial pneumonia 5-fold (Klugman 2007; Fisher et al. 2001). More than 90% of HIV-infected children are in Africa and they have the least access to the services they require. Expensive drugs, lack of trained personnel, inadequate health facilities such as hospitals and clinics, and budgetary constraints were believed to be extreme barriers to implementation of combination antiretrovirals for children and adults in developing countries. Experience has proven that these barriers are surmountable.

Families

Impact on the Family

HIV/AIDS wreaks havoc on many aspects of social and economic life, especially on the family (Box 15.4). The consequences of parental death on children can be extensive. Globally, there are about 15.0 million AIDS orphans, of whom 12.3 million are in sub-Saharan Africa, and most of the latter (8.5 million) are in east and southern Africa. By 2010 it is estimated that sub-Saharan Africa will have 18.4 million AIDS orphans (UNAIDS/UNICEF/USAID 2002). Welfare services and child care support from the state to households ravaged by the disease is paltry. In Botswana 34.3% of households that require support for orphans receive it, in Kenya the figure is 10.3%, and in Ethiopia 3.6% (UNAIDS/UNICEF/USAID 2002). It is tragic that the catastrophic effects of apartheid on infant and child development and on the fulfillment of their potential are being repeated by the HIV/AIDS epidemic in South Africa.

Family life, at the very center of nurturing and caring activities for the tender young, remains under threat as it has been throughout modern times in South Africa. There has been an unremitting erosion of the integrity of African family life

---

Box 15.4 Potential Impact of AIDS on Family and the Community

Relationships

- Intra-family conflict;
- Rejection of family member;
- Stigmatization, discrimination and isolation;
- Death of member, grief;
- Increased number of multi-generational households lacking middle generation;
- Change in family composition and in adult and child roles.

Resources

- Impoverishment;
- Loss of labor;
- Loss of income for medical care and education;
- Forced migration;
- Time and money spent for funerals.

Resilience

- Demoralization;
- Stress;
- Inability to parent and care for children;
- Dissolution;
- Long-term pathologies (increased depressive behavior in children).

*Community stresses**

- Reduced labor;
- Increased poverty;
- Inability to maintain infrastructure;
- Loss of skilled labor, including health workers, teachers and agricultural extension workers;
- Loss of agricultural inputs and labor;
- Reduced access to healthcare;
- Elevated morbidity and mortality;
- Psychological stress and breakdown;
- Inability to marshal resources for community-wide funding schemes or insurance.

*Source: Besley (2006)

---

for more than 150 years. Colonial depredations, migrations, urbanization, and industrialization shaped the evolution of early African family structure; apartheid twisted the shape and form of the extended family. AIDS now looms large to wreak further damage and leave behind a trail of thousands of orphans and vulnerable children. This disastrous epidemic will cast a dark shadow well into the future of these countries, unless extraordinary measures are taken to control the disease and mitigate its effects on family life.

The impact of AIDS on families is well known. In a recent 40-country study in Africa (UNAIDS 2006), 16.5% of households with children, mostly female headed households, were caring for orphans and more than 90% of orphans who had lost both parents were being cared for by extended families. Both the insidious progression of the silent undetected infection, and the relentless march of the overt disease, eats away steadily at the fabric of the nuclear or extended family. All that finally exists is the frayed and torn remnants of a family structure, with children insecurely bound to desperate and frail grandmothers, and lives punctured by frequent and recurring illnesses. The financial and personal burdens become overwhelming as there is loss of productive capacity of parents, decrease in incomes, and an increase in health costs, poverty, starvation, and destitution. Orphaned children (both HIV uninfected and HIV infected) and other children in the household suffer greatly from malnutrition, infectious diseases, homelessness, depression, fear, guilt, shame, and death. Children of HIV-infected mothers with advanced AIDS are 3.5 times more likely to die irrespective of their own HIV status, when the mother dies the children are more than 4 times at risk of death (Newell et al. 2004b, Zaba et al. 2005). Children are often forced to assume headship of the family and home; there is little for shelter, food, education, hygiene, and personal needs, less for comfort and enjoyment, and nothing but emptiness tinged with fear for the times ahead. Poverty increases the exposure to child abuse and sexual coercion. Already about 25,000 children are sexually abused annually in South Africa (Lauren 2004). HIV/AIDS accounts for some of these 25,000 and likely many more are too far removed from social concern to comprise even a statistic. The figures are stupefying: more than half of all South African men do not live with their

children for sustained periods. Indeed, a World Bank study (Subbarao and Coury 2004) showed that only about 4 out of 10 children in South Africa whose mothers had died lived with their fathers; this compares with 9 out of 10 in Malawi and Zambia. Dr. Mamphela Ramphele, who was head of the University of Cape Town and worked at the World Bank, observes that even when men are there, they "die" as husbands and parents because of alcohol, drugs, and other social ills (Ramphele 2005). In a study by Professor Linda Richter of the University of KwaZulu/Natal and her colleagues (Richter et al. 2005) a majority of the men expressed deep guilt, both personally and socially, for the ills experienced by women and children. The burden of care for children, orphaned or affected by HIV/AIDS, in South Africa is borne largely by women, especially young women who are themselves desperately vulnerable to HIV.

Conclusion

It is sobering to remember that in the face of such an unprecedented global catastrophe, the breadth and diversity of the issues which have to be learned from experience and experiment remain enormous. The scientific challenges that still have to be confronted and overcome, the national and international policies and programs that remain unattended to and are yet to be implemented are huge. We have dealt with a small and specific area only. A comprehensive response to the vulnerability of women to HIV, and the afflictions and distress caused to them by the infection, is a central pillar in the strategy to confront and control this epidemic. A credible program for women would include the following: scaling-up VCT, prevention, treatment, and care (including psychosocial support); establishing child- and women-friendly, equitable, effective, and efficient health services; preserving and protecting breastfeeding during the HIV epidemic and implementing appropriate infant; feeding policies; and including men in HIV policies. The following basic interventions could avert substantial numbers of maternal deaths: policies and training on implementing appropriate

guidelines on management of HIV-positive pregnant women, and improved access to comprehensive essential obstetric care and to safe abortion
services (Box 15.5). Programs directed at women
should aim at creating social, political, economic,
and cultural environments which empower
women; counteract stigma and discrimination
against women; and aggressively combat poverty,
and racial and gender inequalities.

**Box 15.5 Prevention of HIV Infections
in Women**

- Interventions proven to work: condoms for
  men and women; promotion of safe sexual
  behaviors (delayed sexual debut, reduction in
  number of casual sexual partners)
- Potential, but unproven interventions:
  male circumcision; combination antiretrovirals; chemoprophylaxis of herpes sim-
  plex virus-2 and treatment of HSV-2 infections; treatment of non-pathogenic vaginal
  infections; pre-exposure prophylaxis;
  microbicides, diaphragms; penile hygiene;
  HIV vaccines.

Key interventions for children include scaling
up of prevention services to reduce MTCT as
described in this text, strengthening HIV-specific
treatment programs, and improving general child
health treatment, prevention, and care services,
and improving the care of orphans and vulnerable
children (Box 15.6). It is imperative that implementing authorities in Africa expand their
pMTCT services using ARV regimens best suited
for their social and economic conditions, integrate
HIV services into general child health services,
provide sound programs on infant feeding, and
monitor and evaluate all of these. It is now clear
that combination antiretroviral treatment
(HAART) is feasible, affordable, safe, and effective among children in developing countries.

The current problem is one of scale – the
small proportion treated of the large numbers
in need demands urgent expansion of treatment
programs in Africa. The key limitations that

Box 15.6 Care for AIDS Orphans

- Provide access to shelter, food, education,
  healthcare.
- Facilitate care and other grants from state
  welfare services.
- Socio-economic improvements to house-
  hold (e.g., household income).
- Combat stigma and discrimination.
- Prevent exploitation and abuse.
- Protect inheritance.

---

have to be overcome include shortage of trained
health personnel, a dearth of adequately
equipped and functioning health facilities, and
equitable and efficient health systems. The
family is the quintessential unit in a just and
benevolent society; it can be the foundation for
reconstructing communities ravaged by AIDS
and for preventing the spread of the infection
by HIV. Accordingly, the integrity and functioning of families in HIV-endemic regions should be
promoted, protected, and supported. Belsey
(2006) suggests the following child-related strategies for affected families: strengthen capacity of
families to protect and care for children;
improve capacity of children and young people
to meet their own needs; strengthen community
responses and create an enabling social environment; and ensure appropriate legislation and services in government. A comprehensive account
of policies, programs, and services to strengthen
families and communities within HIV-endemic
regions has been documented by Dairo and
Aglobitse (2004).

Finally, it bears repeating that the fundamental
success of many health promotion measures and
the effects of health interventions for children
depend on the environment in which they are
born and in which they grow, develop, and mature.
Reversing poverty and improving the social, economic, and political position of African people are
essential to addressing these contextual factors
for children, as indeed they are for African societies as a whole.

Key Terms

Abstinence, be faithful, use condoms (ABC) Antiretrovirals (ARVs) CD4 count Commercial sex work Condom use Endemic Exclusive breastfeeding (EBF) Female genital mutilation (FGM) Gender inequality Heterosexual contact	Highly active antiretroviral therapy (HAART) HIV/AIDS Human papilloma virus (HPV) Mother-to-child transmission (MTCT) Nevirapine (NVP) Pandemic Pneumocystis carinii pneumonia	Prevention of mother-to-child transmission (PMTCT) Safe sex practices Single-dose nevirapine (sdNVP) Transactional sex Viral load Voluntary counseling and testing (VCT) Zidovudine (AZT)

Questions for Discussion

1. In an essay of about 1,000 words, discuss factors that increase women's vulnerability to HIV/AIDS.
2. What factors limit the potential of ABC (abstinence, be faithful, use condoms) programs to reduce the incidence of HIV/AIDS among women in less developed countries?
3. Discuss the current state of knowledge and recommendations regarding the prevention of mother-to-child transmission of HIV using antiretroviral drugs.
4. Describe the current state of knowledge and international recommendations regarding breastfeeding and prevention of mother-to-child transmission of HIV/AIDS.
5. Summarize the impact of HIV/AIDS on

   a. children's health and well-being
   b. the family
   c. the community

References

African Union (AU) (2006) Update on HIV/AIDS control in Africa. Special Summit of the African Union on HIV/AIDS, Tuberculosis and Malaria (ATM), 2–4 May, 2006, Abuja, Nigeria, http://www.africa-union.org/root/au/conferences/past/2006/may/summit/doc/en/SP_ExCL_ATM3I_-HIV_UPDATE.pdf, cited 11 August 2008

Aggleton P, Rivers K (1998) Interventions for adolescents. In: Gibney L, DiClemente RJ, Vermund SH (Eds.) Preventing HIV in Developing Countries: Biomedical and Behavioral Approaches. New York: Plenum Press, pp. 231–255

Belsey MA (2006) AIDS and the Family: Policy Options for a Crisis in Family Capital. Department of Economic and Social Affairs. New York: United Nations, 126 pp

Bhandari N, Bahl R, Mazumdar S et al. (2003) Effect of community-based promotion of exclusive breastfeeding on diarrheal illness and growth: a cluster randomised controlled trial. Lancet, 361(9367), 1418–1423

Bland RM, Little KE, Coovadia HM et al. (2008) Intervention to promote exclusive breast-feeding for the first 6 months of life in a high HIV prevalence area. AIDS, 22(7), 883–891

Chen L, Jha P, Stirling B et al. (2007) Sexual risk factors for HIV infection in early and advanced HIV epidemics in sub-Saharan Africa: systematic overview of 68 epidemiological studies. PLoS, 2(10), e1001, http://www.pubmedcentral.nih.gov/picrender.fcgi?artid=1994584andblobtype=pdf, cited 11 August 2008

Collazos JA, Asensi VB, Carton JAB et al. (2007) Sex differences in the clinical, immunological and virological parameters of HIV-infected patients treated with HAART. AIDS, 21(7), 835–843

Coovadia HM, Rollins NC, Bland RM et al. (2007) Mother-to-child transmission of HIV-1 infection during exclusive breastfeeding in the first 6 months of life: an intervention cohort study. Lancet, 369(9567), 1107–1116

Coovadia HM, Schaller JG (2008) HIV/AIDS in children: a disaster in the making. Lancet, 372 (9635), 271–273

Coutsoudis A, Pillay K, Spooner E et al. (1999) Influence of infant-feeding patterns on early mother-to-child transmission of HIV-1 in Durban, South Africa: a prospective cohort study. Lancet, 354 (9177), 471–476

Cowan FM (2002) Adolescent reproductive health interventions. AIDS, 78:315–318

Dairo AE, Aglobitse DM (2004) Strengthening Families and Communities for HIV/AIDS Prevention and Care:

Community Partnership Approach. Abstract presented at XV International AIDS Conference Bangkok, Thailand 11–16 July

Department of Health South Africa (2007) National HIV and Syphilis Antenatal Prevalence Survey, South Africa 2006. Pretoria, South Africa: Department of Health, http://www.doh.gov.za/docs/reports/2007/hiv/part1.pdf, cited 11 August 2008

Dorrington RE, Johnson L, Bradshaw D et al. (2006) The Demographic Impact of HIV/AIDS in South Africa: National and Provincial Indicators for 2006. Cape Town, Centre for Actuarial Research, South African Medical Research Council and Actuarial Society of South Africa, http://www.mrc.ac.za/bod/Demographi-cImpactHIVIndicators.pdf, cited 11 August 2008

Ehiri JE, Anyanwu E, Jolly P (2005) AIDS-related stigma in sub-Saharan Africa: its contexts and potential intervention strategies. AIDS and Public Policy Journal 20(1/2), 25–39

Fisher RG, Nageswaran S, Valentine ME et al. (2001) Successful prophylaxis against Pneumocystis carinii pneumonia in HIV-infected children using smaller than recommended dosages of trimethoprim–sulfamethoxazole. AIDS Patient Care STDS, 15(5), 263–269

Flynn P, Havens P, Brady M et al. (2007) Male circumcision for prevention of HIV and other sexually transmitted diseases. Pediatrics, 119 (4), 821–822

Gilad J, Walfisch A, Borer A et al. (2003) Gender differences and sex-specific manifestations associated with human immunodeficiency virus infection in women. Eur J Obstet Gynecol Reprod Biol, 109:199–205

Green EC, Halperin DT, Nantulya V et al. (2006) Uganda's HIV prevention success: the role of sexual behavior change and the national response. AIDS and Behavior, 10 (4), 335–346

Haider R, Ashworth A, Kabir I et al. (2000) Effect of community-based peer counselors on exclusive breastfeeding practices in Dhaka, Bangladesh: a randomized controlled trial. Lancet, 356 (9242), 1643–1647

Joint United Nations Program on HIV/AIDS (UNAIDS)/ United Nations Children's Fund (UNICEF)/United States Agency for International Development (USAID) (2002) Children on the Brink, 2002. A Joint Report on Orphan Estimates and Program Strategies, http://data.unaids.org/Topics/Young-People/childrenonthebrink_en.pdf, cited 12 August 2008

Joint United Nations Program on HIV/AIDS (UNAIDS) (2003) AIDS Epidemic Update 2003. Geneva: Joint United Nations Program on HIV/AIDS (UNAIDS)

Joint United Nations Programme on HIV/AIDS (UNAIDS) (2005) AIDS Epidemic Update 2004. Geneva: Joint United Nations Programme on HIV/AIDS (UNAIDS), http://www.unaids.org/bangkok2004/GAR2004_pdf/UNAIDS-GlobalReport2004_en.pdf, cited 12 August 2008

Joint United Nations Programme on HIV/AIDS (UNAIDS) (2006) Report on the Global AIDS Epidemic, 2006. Geneva: Joint United Nations Programme on HIV/AIDS (UNAIDS), http://data.unaids.org/pub/GlobalReport/2006/2006_GR-ExecutiveSummary_en.pdf, cited 11 August 2008

Joint United Nations Programme on HIV/AIDS (UNAIDS) (2006) AIDS Epidemic Update 2005.

Geneva: Joint United Nations Programme on HIV/AIDS (UNAIDS), http://www.unaids.org/epi/2005/doc/EPIupdate2005_pdf_en/epi-update2005_en.pdf, cited 11 August 2008

Joint United Nations Programme on HIV/AIDS (UNAIDS) (2007) AIDS Epidemic Update 2007. Geneva: Joint United Nations Programme on HIV/AIDS (UNAIDS), http://data.unaids.org/pub/EPISlides/2007/2007_epiupdate_en.pdf, cited 11 August 2008

Karamagi CA, Tumwine JK, Tylleskar T et al. (2006) Intimate partner violence against women in eastern Uganda: implications for HIV prevention. BMC Public Health, 20(6), 284

Klugman K (2007) Recent discoveries in prevention of pneumococcal disease. Abstract Presented at the 17th European Congress of Clinical Microbiology and Infectious Diseases. ICC, Munich, Germany, 31 Mar–04 Apr 2007. European Society of Clinical Microbiology and Infectious Diseases, http://www.blackwellpublishing.com/eccmid17/abstract.asp?id = 55996, cited 24 November, 2008

Krishnan S, Dunbar MS, Minnis AM et al. (2008) Poverty, gender inequities, and women's risk of human immunodeficiency virus/AIDS. Ann N Y Acad Sci, 1136:101–110

Lauren W (2004) Sexual abuse of young children in Southern Africa. J Child and Adolescent Mental Health, 16(2), 127–129

Magoni M, Bassani L, Okong P et al. (2005) Mode of infant feeding and HIV infection in children in a program for prevention of mother-to-child transmission in Uganda. AIDS, 19(4), 433–437

Magnussen L, Ehiri JE, Ejere HOD et al. (2004). Interventions to prevent HIV/AIDS among adolescents in less developed countries: are they effective? International Journal of Adolescent Medicine and Health, 16(4), 303–323

McIntyre J (2003) Mothers infected with HIV: reducing maternal death and disability during pregnancy. British Medical Bulletin, 67, 127–135

McIntyre J, Gray G (2002) What can we do to reduce mother to child transmission of HIV? BMJ, 324(7331), 218–221

Muller M, Volmink J, Deeks J et al. (2003) Male circumcision for prevention of heterosexual acquisition of HIV in men. Cochrane Database Systematic Reviews, Issue 3

Napravnik S, Poole C, Thomas JC et al. (2002) Gender difference in HIV RNA levels: a meta-analysis of published studies. J Acquir Immune Defic Syndr, 31, 11–19

Newel ML, Brahmbhatt H, Ghys PD (2004a) Child mortality and HIV infection in Africa: a review. AIDS, 18(Suppl 2), S27–S34

Newell ML, Coovadia H, Cortina-Borja M et al. (2004b) Mortality of infected and uninfected infants born to HIV-infected mothers in Africa: a pooled analysis. Lancet, 364(9441), 1236–1243

Orne-Gliemann J, Mukotekwa T, Miller A et al. (2006) Community-based assessment of infant feeding practices within a programme for prevention of mother-to-child HIV transmission in rural Zimbabwe. Public Health Nutr, 9(5), 563–569

Parker RG, Easton D, Klein CH (2000) Structural barriers and facilitators in HIV prevention: a review of international research. AIDS, 14(Suppl 1), S22–S32

Piot P, Coll Seck AM (2001) International response to the HIV/AIDS epidemic: planning for success. Bulletin of the World Health Organization, 79, 1106–1112

Population Council (2000) FOCUS on Young Adults: End of Project Report. Advancing Young Adult Reproduction. New York: Population Council

Ramphele M (2005) Steering by the stars: Migrancy, family dissolution and fatherhood.2005 quoted in: The Fatherhood Project Final Report submitted to Ford Foundation. www.hsrc.ac.za/RPP-Fatherhood-1.phtml, cited 28 November 2008

Richter L, Dawes A, Higson-Smith C (2005) Sexual Abuse of Young Children in Southern Africa. Pretoria: HSRC Press

Rodriguez-Garcia R, Aumack KJ, Ramos A (1990) A community-based approach to the promotion of breastfeeding in Mexico. J Obstet Gynecol Neonatal Nurs, 19(5), 431–438

Senderowitz J (1997) Young people and STDs/HIV/AIDS: Part II: Programs to address the problem. FOCUS/Pathfinder International.

Silberschmidt M, Rasch V (2001) Adolescent girls, illegal abortions and "sugar-daddies" in Dar es Salaam: vulnerable victims and active social agents. Social Science and Medicine, 52(12), 1815–1826

Subbarao K, Coury D (2004) Reaching out to Africa's orphans: a framework for public action. Africa Region Human Development Working Paper Series. Washington, DC: World Bank, Africa Region, http://siteresources.worldbank.org/INTHIVAIDS/Resources/375798-1103037153392/ReachingOuttoAfricasOrphans. pdf, cited 12 August 2008

Stanton BF, Li X, Kahihuata J (1998) Increased protected sex and abstinence among Namibian youth following a HIV risk-reduction intervention: a randomized, longitudinal study. AIDS, 12:2473–2480

Suligoi B (1997) The natural history of human immunodeficiency virus infection among women as compared with men. Sex Transm Dis, 24, 77–83

Sweat MD, O'Reilly KR, Schmid GP (2004) Cost-effectiveness of nevirapine to prevent mother-to-child HIV transmission in eight African countries. AIDS, 18(12), 1661–1671

Umeh OC, Currier JS (2005) Sex Differences in HIV: natural history, pharmacokinetics, and drug toxicity. Curr Infect Dis Rep, 7, 73–78

United Nations (2001) Special Session on HIV/AIDS. Fact Sheet: Preventing HIV/AIDS Among Young People. New York: United Nations, June

Volmink J, Siegfried NL, van der Merwe L et al. (2006) Antiretrovirals for reducing the risk of mother-to-child transmission of HIV infection. Cochrane Database of Systematic Reviews 2006, Issue 4

Weiser SD, Leiter K, Bangsberg DR et al. (2007) Food Insufficiency Is Associated with High-Risk Sexual Behavior among Women in Botswana and Swaziland. PLoS Med, 4(10), e260

World Health Organization (WHO) (2008) WHO Expert Consultation on New and emerging evidence on the use of antiretroviral drugs for the prevention of mother-to-child transmission of HIV Geneva, 17–19 November 2008, http://www.who.int/hiv/topics/mtct/mtct_conclusions_consult. pdf, cited 26 February 2009

World Health Organization (WHO)/United National Fund for Population Activities (UNFPA) (2006) Sexual and reproductive health of women living with HIV/AIDS. Guidelines on care, treatment and support for women living with HIV/AIDS and their children in resource-constrained settings. Geneva/New York: WHO/UNICEF

World Health Organization (WHO)/Joint United Nations Program on HIV/AIDS (UNAIDS) (2003) Treating 3 million by 2005: making it happen – the WHO strategy. The WHO and UNAIDS Global Initiative to provide antiretroviral therapy to 3 million people with HIV/AIDS in developing countries by the end of 2005. Geneva: World Health Organization (WHO)/Joint United Nations Program on HIV/AIDS (UNAIDS), http://www.who.int/3by5/publications/documents/en/3by5StrategyMakingItHappen.pdf, cited 11 August 2008

World Health Organization (WHO) (2004a) Antiretroviral drugs for treating pregnant women and preventing HIV infection in infants. Guidelines on care, treatment and support for women living with HIV/AIDS and their children in resource-constrained settings. Geneva: World Health Organization, http://www.who.int/hiv/pub/mtct/en/arvdrugsguidelines.pdf, cited 12 August 2008

World Health Organization (WHO) (2004b) HIV transmission through breastfeeding: a review of available evidence. Geneva: World Health Organization, http://www.unfpa.org/upload/lib_pub_file/276_filename_HIV_PREV_BF_GUIDE_ENG.pdf, cited 12 August 2008

World Health Organization (WHO)/United Nations Children's Fund (UNICEF)/Joint United Nations Programme on HIV/AIDS (UNAIDS) (2004) HIV and infant feeding: guidelines for decision- makers. Geneva: World Health Organization, http://whqlibdoc.who.int/hq/2003/9241591226.pdf, cited 12 August 2008

World Health Organization (WHO)/Joint United Nations Program on HIV/AIDS (UNAIDS) (2005) Estimated percent of people on antiretroviral therapy among those in need: situation as of June 2005. Geneva: World Health Organization (WHO)/Joint United Nations Program on HIV/AIDS (UNAIDS). http://www.who.int/hiv/facts/cov0605map/en/index.html, cited 11 August 2008

World Health Organization (WHO) (2006) Antiretroviral drugs for treating pregnant women and preventing HIV infection in infants in resource-limited settings towards universal access: recommendations for a public health approach. 2006 version. Geneva: World Health Organization, http://www.who.int/hiv/pub/guidelines/WHOPMTCT.pdf, cited 13 August 2008

Zaba BA, Whiteside AB, Boerma JT et al. (2004) Demographic and socioeconomic impact of AIDS: taking stock of the empirical evidence. AIDS, 18(Suppl 2), S1–S7

Zaba B, Whitworth J, Marston M et al. (2005) HIV and mortality of mothers and children: evidence from cohort studies in Uganda, Tanzania, and Malawi. Epidemiology, 16(3), 275–280

Zablotska IB, Gray RH, Koenig MA et al. (2007) Alcohol use, intimate partner violence, sexual coercion and HIV among women aged 15–24 in Rakai, Uganda. AIDS and Behavior (Epub ahead of print)

Chapter 16
Malnutrition and Maternal and Child Health

Olaf Müller and Albrecht Jahn

Learning Objectives After reading this chapter and answering the questions that follow, you should be able to

- Identify the various manifestations of undernutrition (hunger, undernourishment, stunting, wasting, underweight, protein-energy malnutrition, and micronutrient deficiency) and describe their management and control.
- Identify the global magnitude of obesity among women and children.
- Identify and discuss the various biological, environmental, sociocultural, and behavioral factors that underlie malnutrition (overnutrition and undernutrition) among women and children.
- Appraise the evidence base of interventions to prevent malnutrition among women and children and assess the feasibility of achieving the Millennium Development Goal target of reducing by half of 1990 figures, the proportion of people who suffer from hunger.

Introduction

Malnutrition represents an imbalance between the nutrients the body needs and the nutrients it receives. It, therefore, includes undernutrition (inadequate intake of calories and/or nutrients) and overnutrition (consumption of too many calories or too much of any specific nutrient – protein, fat, vitamin, mineral, or other dietary supplement).

O. Müller (✉)
Department of Tropical Hygiene and Public Health, Medical Faculty, Ruprecht-Karls-University of Heidelberg, Germany

Box 16.1 presents a glossary of terms that were frequently in this chapter. The nutritional status of women and children is particularly important because of its far-reaching effects on overall population health and economic development. As an example (Blössner and de Onis 2005), a malnourished mother is likely to give birth to a low-birth-weight (LBW) baby who is susceptible to disease and premature death. This undermines the economic development of the family and society and continues the cycle of poverty and malnutrition (Fig. 16.1).

Maternal and child undernutrition remains a globally dominant public health challenge, and is a particular problem in the impoverished communities of developing countries (Caulfield et al. 2006). Southern Asia and sub-Saharan Africa (SSA) are the geographic regions with the highest prevalence of malnutrition from undernutrition. Diets in these populations are frequently deficient in macronutrients (protein, carbohydrate, and fat) and/or micronutrients (electrolytes, minerals, and vitamins) which can lead to protein-energy malnutrition (PEM) and specific micronutrient deficiencies (MND), respectively. Industrialized countries and urbanized areas of developing countries have the highest prevalences of malnutrition in the form of overweight or obesity, since energy-dense foods that lack micronutrients are common and inexpensive.

PEM and MND significantly overlap, and the lack of one micronutrient is typically associated with other MNDs. PEM occurs in an estimated 1 billion people worldwide and MNDs affect at least 2 billion people. The most important MNDs are deficiencies in iron, iodine, vitamin A, and zinc. The prevalence of vitamin C, D, and B deficiency has

Box 16.1 Definition of Terms

Hunger: the body's way of signaling that it is running short of food and needs to eat something. Malnutrition can lead to hunger and may be present in individuals who are normal or overweight because of micronutrient deficiencies ("hidden hunger").

Malnutrition: a state in which the physical function of an individual is impaired to the point where he or she can no longer maintain natural bodily capacities such as growth, pregnancy, lactation, learning, physical work, disease resistance, and/or recovery from disease. The term covers a range of problems from being dangerously thin (see *underweight*) or too short for one's age (see *stunting*) to being deficient in vitamins and minerals (see *micronutrient deficiency*) or being too fat (see *obesity*). Malnutrition is measured not by the quantity of food consumed but by age and physical measurements of the body, such as weight and/or height.

Undernourishment: describes the status of people whose food intake does not include enough calories (energy) and micronutrients (essential vitamins, minerals, and electrolytes) to meet minimum physiological needs. The term is a measure of a country's ability to gain access to food and is normally derived from Food Balance Sheets prepared by the UN Food and Agriculture Organization (FAO).

Stunting: reflects shortness-for-age; an indicator of chronic malnutrition and calculated by comparing the height-for-age of a child with a reference population of well-nourished and healthy children.

Wasting: reflects a recent and severe process that has led to substantial weight loss, usually associated with starvation and/or disease; calculated by comparing weight-for-height of a child with a reference population of well-nourished and healthy children; often used to assess the severity of emergencies because it is strongly related to mortality.

Underweight: measured by comparing the weight-for-age of a child with a reference population of well-nourished and healthy children.

Protein-energy malnutrition: occurs when food intake does not include enough calories from macronutrients (protein, carbohydrate, and fat).

Micronutrient deficiency: occurs when food intake does not include the right type or amount of micronutrients.

Overweight/Obesity: measured by comparing weight-for-height by age, or body mass index (BMI) for age (WHO 2008a), reflects over-consumption of some macronutrients (protein, carbohydrate, or fat).

declined greatly in recent decades (Müller and Krawinkel 2005). The prevalence of overweight and obesity is increasing across the world (Wang and Lobstein 2006). In particular, countries undergoing transition to developed economies are beginning to see a rise in the prevalence of overweight and obesity (Wang and Lobstein 2006). These countries will bear a double burden of disease from malnutrition – both under- and overnutrition.

The high prevalence of infectious diseases is a major determinant for the burden of malnutrition from undernutrition in developing countries (Rice et al. 2000). By interfering with the immunological capacity to defend against infectious diseases, malnutrition is a major underlying cause of morbidity and mortality (Fig. 16.2). Malnutrition remains the most important risk factor for the burden of diseases globally (Lopez et al. 2006). It is the direct cause of about 300,000 deaths per year and is indirectly responsible for about half of the roughly 11 million deaths per year in young children (Lopez et al. 2006). Malnutrition also contributes significantly to the roughly half a million women who die during pregnancy or childbirth annually (Freedman et al. 2005). The risk for morbidity and mortality is directly correlated with the degree of malnutrition. However, most of the morbidity and mortality burden is associated with low to moderate malnutrition, which has important implications for control strategies (Caulfield et al. 2006).

Fig. 16.1 The cycle of poverty and malnutrition. Source: Bhagwati et al. (2004)

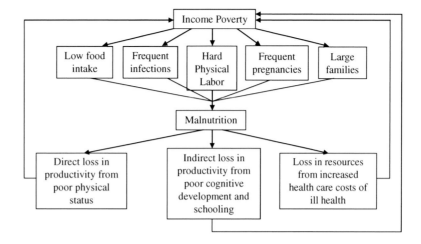

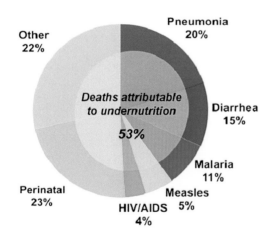

Fig. 16.2 Leading causes of death in children under 5 years in developing countries and the contribution of undernutrition. Source: World Health Report (WHO 2003); Caulfield et al. (2004)

The disability-adjusted life years (DALY) lost attributed to diseases in under five children, in addition to maternal and perinatal conditions, nutrition deficiencies, and endocrine disorders, amount to 42% of the global disease burden (Mason et al. 2006). Thus, programs covering aspects of women and children's health and nutrition address a substantial proportion of global health problems. The interaction of health and nutrition is evident in the experiences of a number of large-scale community-based programs in Asia. From these projects, it was concluded that health interventions are less effective when nutrition is

not addressed concurrently. Both better health and better nutrition are required for child survival and development (Mason et al. 2006).

While infectious diseases are a main contributor to the burden of undernutrition in developing countries, chronic diseases associated with overnutrition are also on the rise. The United Nations has estimated that by 2015, non-communicable diseases associated with overnutrition will surpass undernutrition as the leading causes of death in low-income countries (Tanumihardjo et al. 2007). Developing countries will be faced with the challenge of managing and controlling both infectious and chronic diseases simultaneously.

Poverty is the main underlying cause of undernutrition (Fig. 16.3). Women of reproductive age and children are the populations most affected by malnutrition due to biological and socioeconomic factors. Malnutrition further exacerbates poverty through increased costs of health services, reduced working capacities, impaired school performances, and probable long-term effects on the prevalence and severity of chronic diseases during adulthood (Caulfield et al. 2006). Poverty in low-income countries is less likely to be associated with obesity, as it is mainly the wealthy individuals in these countries that have access to refined foods and live sedentary lifestyles. However, obesity in high-income countries is highest in impoverished populations because of economic factors that favor high energy intake and low micronutrient intake (Tanumihardjo et al. 2007).

The degree and distribution of PEM and MND in a given population depends on a number of direct

Fig. 16.3 Determinants of malnutrition. Source: Müller and Krawinkel (2005)

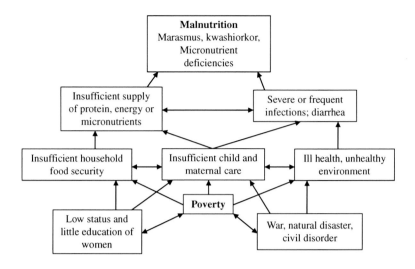

and indirect factors. Direct factors include breast-feeding habits and types and amounts of foods eaten by an individual. Indirect factors are extremely broad and include the political and economic situation, the level of education and sanitation, season and climate conditions, food production capacity, cultural and religious food customs, the prevalence of infectious diseases, existing nutrition programs, and the availability and quality of health services (Müller and Krawinkel 2005). Similarly, the prevalence of overweight and obesity in a population depends on various individual and environmental factors, such as diet, exercise, and the role of the built environment in supporting healthy behaviors.

The following sections provide an overview of the global burden of disease related to malnutrition among women of reproductive age and children with particular reference to protein-energy malnutrition, micronutrient deficiency, and obesity. For each of these, we examine the magnitude of the problem globally, determinants, management and control.

Protein-Energy Malnutrition

Burden of Disease

Worldwide, an estimated 852 million people were undernourished in 2000–2002, with the great majority (815 million) living in developing countries; roughly 150 million of this burden is in children under 5 years

of age (Müller and Krawinkel 2005). The absolute number of cases has not changed much over the last decade. However, while there were major reductions in the number of PEM cases in China during this period, this reduction was balanced by a corresponding increase in the rest of the developing world (Müller and Krawinkel 2005).

In children, PEM is defined by comparing age- and sex-specific weights and heights with the corresponding weights and heights of a healthy reference population (Fig. 16.4). The resulting z-scores are the difference between the weight or height and the corresponding median value in the reference population, divided by the standard deviation of the

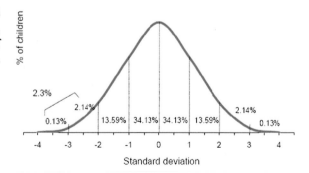

Fig. 16.4 Normal distribution of child growth for the NCHS/WHO reference population.[a] Source: Blössner and de Onis (2005)

[a]The distribution of child growth is shown as a function of standard deviation (SD) range. Child prevalences are shown as percentages between the SD ranges.

reference population (Caulfield et al. 2006). A weight below two standard deviations of normal weight for age is defined as underweight, a height below two standard deviations of normal height for age is defined as stunting, and a weight below two standard deviations of normal weight for height is defined as wasting. While wasting indicates recent weight loss, stunting is usually the product of chronic weight loss and the term underweight encompasses both stunting and wasting. Globally, information on prevalence of underweight is much more available than on stunting and wasting. However, there is good correlation between stunting and underweight.

Of all children under the age of 5 years in developing countries, about 31% are underweight, 38% are stunted, and 9% are wasted, with the highest prevalences in Asia and sub-Saharan Africa (Müller and Krawinkel 2005) (Table 16.1). However, malnutrition is not mainly a problem of politically unstable areas and it is not mainly associated with acute disaster. More often it is a silent emergency in otherwise stable communities (Gross and Webb 2006). In areas of such silent emergencies, there are major differences in the degree of malnutrition and associated childhood mortality even between neighboring villages (Müller and Becher 2006).

Besides an insufficient supply of macronutrients, severe and chronic infectious diseases constitute the major cause for PEM development. Figure 16.5 illustrates the relationship between malnutrition and infection.

In particular, diarrhea, but also, other bacterial (e.g., pneumonia, septicemia), viral (e.g., measles), and parasitic (e.g., malaria, helminth infections), diseases are responsible. Decreased food intake resulting from anorexia, impaired nutrient absorption, increased metabolic requirements, and associated nutrient losses are the directly underlying mechanisms (Müller and Krawinkel 2005).

In children, PEM usually manifests between 6 months and 2 years of age and is associated with early weaning, inappropriate introduction of complementary food, low-protein diet, and severe or frequent infection. Complementary feeding is the process of introducing other foods and liquids into the diet when breast milk alone is no longer sufficient (Caulfield et al. 2006). Major problems with complementary feeding are as follows: complementary food is introduced too early or too late (ideal timing is around 6 months of age); foods are served too infrequently, in insufficient amounts, or their consistency or energy density is inappropriate; the micronutrient content of foods is inadequate or other factors in the diet impair the absorption of

Table 16.1 Prevalence of PEM in under 5-year-old children in 1995 for UN regions

	Stunting (%)	Underweight (%)	Wasting (%)
Africa	39	28	8
Asia	41	35	10
Latin America and Caribbean	18	10	3
Oceania	31	23	5

Source: FAO (2004)

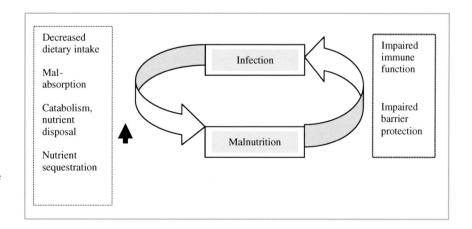

Fig. 16.5 Interdependence of infection and nutrition. Source: Adapted from Brown (2003)

foods; and microbial contamination occurs (Caulfield et al. 2006).

Severe malnutrition consists of wasting and/or edema and is prevalent almost exclusively in children. Marasmus, one of the three principal types of protein-energy malnutrition, is severe wasting, marasmic kwashiorkor is severe wasting in the presence of edema, and kwashiorkor is edema (Müller and Krawinkel 2005). The word "kwashiorkor" originates from the Ga language in Ghana and implies the "disease that the young child developed when displaced from his mother by another child or pregnancy." Early marasmus occurs in infancy and is frequently associated with contaminated bottle feeding (leading to illness) in urban areas (Müller and Krawinkel 2005).

In women of reproductive age, PEM is defined as a body mass index (BMI) below 18.5–20, according to different sources. In SSA a BMI below 18.5 can be found in 10–20% of women, with higher rates during acute famine; an even higher prevalence is observed in some South Asian countries, such as Bangladesh, with up to 40% of women being affected (Begum and Sen 2005). Assessing the consequences of maternal malnutrition is complicated, as the resulting ill health affects the mothers as well as their children. Mothers are directly affected by a higher risk of maternal death and morbidity due to maternal depletion, anemia, increased susceptibility

to infections, and mechanical delivery complications in cases of stunting.

The best documented and studied adverse outcome of maternal malnutrition is intrauterine growth retardation, resulting in low birthweight and ultimately in increased perinatal and neonatal mortality rates. According to a recent WHO report, women with a BMI below 20 have a 1.8 higher risk of low birthweight. Using the example of Nepal, it was estimated that 12.3% of all neonatal deaths are attributable to maternal malnutrition (Blössner and de Onis 2005). Low-birthweight rates are consequently regarded as the best proxy for maternal malnutrition in international health statistics. The overall pattern is similar to childhood malnutrition with the highest rates observed in Asia, followed by Africa (Table 16.2).

The negative health effects of maternal malnutrition in children continue after birth as intrauterine growth retardation contributes to stunting, which predisposes girls to delivery complications later in life, and finally affects the next generation (Fig. 16.6).

Furthermore, there is ample evidence that a number of chronic diseases in adulthood such as diabetes and hypertension are triggered by "fetal malnutrition" through fetal programming (Caulfield et al. 2006). Maternal and child malnutrition often go hand in hand, as they share many of the

Table 16.2 Percentage and number of low-birthweight infants by UN regions in 2000

	Percentage of low-birthweight infants	Number of low-birthweight infants (1,000s)	Number of live births (1,000s)
World	**15.5**	**20,629**	**132,882**
Asia	**18.3**	**14,195**	**77,490**
- Eastern	5.9	1,203	20,537
- South-central	27.1	10,819	39,937
- Southeastern	11.6	1,360	11,743
- Western	15.4	813	5,273
Africa	**14.3**	**4,320**	**30,305**
Oceania	**10.5**	**27**	**255**
Latin America and Caribbean	**10.0**	**1,171**	**11,671**
North America	**7.7**	**343**	**4,479**
Europe	**6.4**	**460**	**7,185**

Source: UNICEF and WHO (2004)

Fig. 16.6 Malnutrition throughout the life cycle. Source: ACC/SCN (2006)

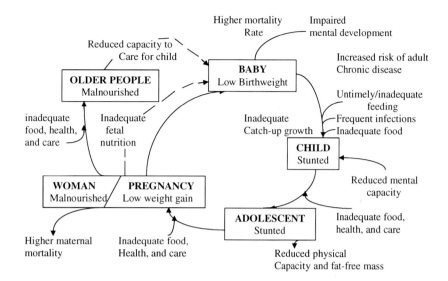

same socioeconomic risk factors such as poverty and illiteracy (Müller and Krawinkel 2005). This is well illustrated in a study in Bangladesh (Begum and Sen 2005), where maternal as well as child malnutrition was closely linked to the poverty level (Table 16.3).

and sodium intake in the first phase when emergency measures take care of the risk of hypoglycemia, hypothermia, and dehydration. Oral, enteral, and parenteral volume load needs to be checked carefully in order to avoid the imminent heart failure. Finally, it is recommended to always treat the severely mal-

Table 16.3 Mother's and child's nutritional status by household poverty level in Bangladesh

Mother's average BMI				Percentage of malnourished children(< 2SD)		
Poverty level	BMI	Below 18.5	Below 16	Underweight	Wasted	Stunted
Extreme poor	18.7	52.9	9.1	59.2	12.8	54.8
Moderate poor	19.1	45.9	5.9	49.8	10.6	46.7
Middle non-poor	20.0	35.3	4.5	40.9	10.0	39.5
Top non-poor	21.0	27.6	2.4	34.8	7.8	28.9

Source: Begum and Sen (2005)

Management and Control

Compared to marasmus, kwashiorkor and marasmic kwashiorkor consistently have a much higher case fatality rate. The high mortality indicates the need for a systematic approach to the severely malnourished patient. In addition to an appropriate diet, a complex management scheme is mandatory to reduce mortality (Müller and Krawinkel 2005). Essential steps are the reduction of volume, protein,

nourished child with an effective broad-acting antibiotic – even when that child does not manifest the symptoms of an infection (Müller and Krawinkel 2005). Management strategies for severe PEM have been changed in recent years to community-based therapeutic care which has substantially increased coverage and reduced mortality (Collins et al. 2006).

While previous efforts to combat PEM were to a large degree focused on identifying and treating severely malnourished patients, recent efforts emphasize prevention through combined nutritional and disease interventions (Caulfield et al. 2006). Preventive interventions to improve dietary intake range from income generation to nutritional education, to food prize subsidies and food supplementation (Müller and Krawinkel 2005). To address infectious diseases as a cause of PEM, promotion of breastfeeding, improved water supply and sanitation, and hygiene education as well as functioning health services are all of major importance (Caulfield et al. 2006).

With regard to breastfeeding, a consensus has been reached that 6 months is the recommended duration of exclusive breastfeeding and that the decision about the total duration of breastfeeding should be left to the mother (Caulfield et al. 2006). Promotion of exclusive breastfeeding is particularly effective through lay support and it has been estimated that such programs would reduce under-five mortality by 13% (Caulfield et al. 2006).

Community-based programs targeted at improving complementary feeding have mostly achieved good coverage and it has been estimated that they have the potential to reduce under-five mortality by 6% in developing countries (Mason et al. 2006). Usually interventions require a combination of community-based and facility-based activities, with sufficient support from regional and/or central levels. For comprehensive nutrition programs in poor countries it has been estimated that an amount of US $5–10 per child would be the minimum and US $10–20 would be advisable for reducing underweight prevalence by around 1–2% per year (Mason et al. 2006). As both coverage and intensity are the main determinants for effectiveness, underfunded programs often fail to achieve targets. With regard to staff requirements, an effective staff-to-population ratio appears to be 1:500 for full-time employed community workers and 1:10 or 1:20 for part-time volunteer community workers. For its successful program, Thailand trained 600,000 volunteer village workers (1% of the population) who operated at about 1:20 for part-time work with similar supervision ratios (Mason et al. 2006). Motivation is key to success, with supportive supervision, status considerations, and small financial or in-kind remunerations all having a role.

Except in very poor populations, supplementary feeding is not considered cost-effective (Mason et al. 2006). However, child survival programs have used supplemental food as an incentive to participate in other interventions. Such an approach has been used for example in the Integrated Child Development Service Program of India. It has been estimated that such programs have the potential to reduce PEM by 2.0–2.5% per year (Caulfield et al. 2006). However, few programs have used a comprehensive approach toward optimizing feeding practices, and proper evaluation of such interventions is lacking.

High immunization coverage and early and correct management of infectious diseases play a major role in the prevention and treatment of PEM (Caulfield et al. 2006). In children of poor communities, treatment of helminth infections three times per year had a positive effect on child growth and development (Nemer et al. 2001). PEM and diarrhea regularly interact in a vicious cycle, but control of diarrhea depends not only on the medical sector. Hand-washing interventions can reduce the risk of diarrhea by about 45% and are considered cost-effective (Caulfield et al. 2006).

Growth monitoring has been regarded as a potentially important instrument in child health clinics. However, there is often a lack of appropriate follow-up action, which may explain why a review by Garner et al. (2000) found no evidence of its effects on child health. It is recognized that messages for correct nutrition are largely universal and that growth monitoring is not the only model for service delivery (Caulfield et al. 2006). In its multifaceted horizontal approach, the WHO-supported Integrated Management of Childhood Illness (IMCI) initiative also addresses malnutrition (Chapter 27). This intervention has recently been shown to be effective (Müller and Krawinkel 2005).

Unlike in child health, most current Safe Motherhood programs do not include components which specifically target maternal PEM. However, there is a range of relevant activities implemented as part of antenatal care programs, the most important being the promotion of adequate and balanced diet through health education in antenatal classes. These include information about the specific nutritional requirements during pregnancy and lactation and options to cover these using locally available and acceptable types of food. Harmful traditional restrictions to pregnant women's diets – if existing and relevant – may also be addressed in a culturally acceptable way, where these may play a major role. Weight monitoring during pregnancy will identify women with inadequate weight gain (< 1 kg/month in the second and third trimesters) who should be counseled and followed up on an individual basis as part of antenatal care. The presumptive treatment of malaria and helminth infections, recommended as a routine intervention in antenatal care in endemic countries by WHO, contributes to improving the nutritional status of pregnant women even if this is not the primary objective of these interventions. Direct food supplementation is not considered an effective approach because its cost-effectiveness is questionable, it would not reach women preconceptionally or in early pregnancy, and it would pose logistical problems (Huffman et al. 2001). However, it may have to be considered in situations of acute natural or man-made disaster, e.g., in refugee communities. Given the obvious link between PEMs, poverty, and female education, long-term strategies to reduce maternal malnutrition will have to focus on broader issues (Table 16.3).

Micronutrient Deficiencies

Burden of Disease

Micronutrient deficiencies (MNDs) that are of particular global concern are iron, folic acid, iodine, vitamin A, and zinc. Iron is an essential part of hemoglobin, myoglobin, and different enzymes. Its deficiency mainly leads to anemia but may also have a number of other adverse effects (Caulfield et al. 2006). About 1 billion people suffer globally from iron deficiency anemia, mainly young children and pregnant women in developing countries. Iron deficiency is usually caused by a low intake due to poor diet, chronic iron loss due to parasitic infections (e.g., hookworm, schistosomiasis, whipworm), or elevated iron needs (e.g., during pregnancy and early childhood) (Zimmermann and Hurrell 2007). Diet is the most important determinant, with bioavailability (the extent to which the nutrients can be used by the body) being considered as important as iron content. Iron exists in plant foods, but it is more plentiful and bioavailable in meat.

Iron deficiency affects around 50% of all pregnancies worldwide, with a wide regional variation. In Africa, prevalence ranges from 2% in a local survey in Egypt to 73% in Wad Medani, Sudan; national data for Mozambique indicate a prevalence of 48%. In Asia, estimates range from 5% in Tehran, Iran, to 94% in low socioeconomic-level pregnant women in Coimbatore, India. South American data range from 4% in Santiago, Chile, to 65% in Lima, Peru (González-Cossío 2006). According to the World Health Report 2002, about one-fifth of perinatal mortality and one-tenth of maternal mortality in developing countries are attributable to iron deficiency. Correspondingly, there is a high prevalence of anemia in pregnancy (hemoglobin below 11 g/dL) in these countries, with a reported prevalence of 35–75%. At least half of all anemia cases in pregnancy have been attributed to iron deficiency (Walraven 2006).

Folic acid deficiency is also associated with anemia. Folic acid is critically important for fetal development as it is an essential cofactor in the nucleotide biosynthesis. Its deficiency constitutes a well-established risk factor for neural tube defects and potentially other malformations; periconceptual folic acid supplementation reduces the prevalence of neural tube defects by 70% (Fikree and Fariyal 2006).

The term iodine deficiency disorders (IDD) has replaced the terms endemic goiter and cretinism. IDD occurs mainly in inland areas far from the sea and is highly prevalent in many developing countries. Pregnant women and young children are the main risk groups. Lack of iodine leads to reduced production of thyroid hormone and stimulation of thyroid-stimulating hormone (TSH) production. It is estimated that globally about 740 million people are iodine deficient, up to 300 million have goiter, and 20 million are brain damaged due to the effects of maternal iodine deficiency on fetal development (Müller and Krawinkel 2005). Iodine deficiency is considered a public health problem if goiter is detected in more than 5% of the school-aged population (Caulfield et al. 2006).

Vitamin A deficiency disorders (VADD) are again mainly a problem in children and pregnant women. It is estimated that 250 million children are affected by vitamin A deficiency worldwide, mainly in developing countries (Caulfield et al. 2006).

VADDs are associated with significantly increased morbidity and mortality in children and pregnant women. Vitamin A deficiency contributes to anemia development and is essential for eye and immune system functioning. VADD are the most common causes of blindness in children, leading to xerophthalmia in 3 million and consequent blindness in 300,000 preschool children each year. While diarrhea morbidity and mortality has clearly been shown to be associated with vitamin A deficiency, the evidence for associations with acute lower-respiratory-tract infections (ARI) and malaria is much weaker (Müller and Krawinkel 2005).

The global burden of zinc deficiency has only recently become fully recognized (Caulfield et al. 2006). Zinc deficiency is frequent in developing countries, affecting up to 2 billion people. Zinc deficiency interferes with a number of biological functions such as gene expression, protein synthesis, skeletal growth, gonad development, appetite, and immunity. Zinc deficiency has consequently been demonstrated to be a major determinant for diarrhea and pneumonia, but there is conflicting evidence regarding its role in malaria and growth retardation (Müller and Krawinkel 2005). It has furthermore been associated with complications in pregnancy and childbirth, lower birthweight, and increased infectious disease morbidity and mortality. Meat is a good source of zinc, while fiber and phytates inhibit the absorption. Thus, populations living on plant-based diets are at a high risk for deficiency.

Management and Control

The provision of micronutrients through food with a high content of absorbable micronutrients is considered the best way for preventing micronutrient deficiencies. In communities where an adequate intake of micronutrients is not possible, specific preventive and curative micronutrient interventions are needed (Müller and Krawinkel 2005). There is a growing consensus on the importance of multiple micronutrient interventions in populations with a high prevalence of malnutrition (Müller and Krawinkel 2005). A special kind of intervention is the provision of "sprinkles" and fat-based spreads (like

peanut butter), which contain multiple micronutrients to be mixed with food. A principle limitation of all these interventions except dietary diversification is the orientation on single nutrients, leaving plant ingredients (e.g., phytosterols and fiber) outside the scope despite their role for the prevention of cancer and cardiovascular diseases.

Micronutrient supplementation is usually provided through the existing health services and with priority to vulnerable populations such as pregnant women and children (Müller and Krawinkel 2005). While some micronutrients have to be taken daily or weekly (e.g., iron and zinc), others can be stored in the body and have only to be given in intervals of months to years (e.g., vitamin A and iodine). However, delivery, compliance, and potential toxicity need to be considered. For iron deficiency in childhood, iron-fortified weaning foods and low-dose iron supplements are advocated by WHO and UNICEF (Caulfield et al. 2006; Zimmermann and Hurrell 2007). Iron supplementation is associated with significantly reduced anemia incidence rates and reversal of developmental delays in preschool children of poor countries. However, despite the recommendations of iron supplementation for pregnant women and young children being in place for decades, progress in anemia control has been slow. The main reasons for this are lack of political commitment and problems with prolonged adherence to daily supplementation. Moreover, there remains a controversial discussion on the risk–benefit ratio of providing iron supplementation to young children living in malaria endemic regions (Sazawal et al. 2006).

Increasing zinc intake is a complex task (Caulfield et al. 2006). Possible interventions are supplementation, fortification, and dietary diversification. Currently, the WHO recommends zinc only for the treatment of diarrhea and severe malnutrition. However, there is strong evidence that zinc supplementation is highly effective in the prevention of diarrhea and pneumonia. Practicable models for zinc supplementation programs still have to be developed.

Vitamin A supplementation can be curative or preventive. It has been shown to reduce blindness and infectious disease morbidity and mortality, and this intervention is now widely implemented (Caulfield et al. 2006). Supplementation has been associated with a 20–30% reduction in all-cause mortality in young children. Vitamin A capsules providing 200,000 international units have at least 90% prophylactic efficacy for 4–6 months against xerophthalmia. High-dose oral supplementation is recommended every 4–6 months for children under 5 years in areas of vitamin A deficiency. Vitamin A supplements are frequently delivered through immunization programs, but the safety and efficacy of supplementation during pregnancy and early infancy continues to be discussed controversially. Vitamin A deficiency has also been addressed through food fortification programs in South America and Southeast Asia.

Micronutrient fortification is generally considered superior to supplementation in the long term, as costs are lower and compliance is better. However, most experience with food fortification comes from developed countries, with salt and sugar being the usual carriers (Caulfield et al. 2006). Until today, only iodine fortification is globally successful. From 1990 through 1998, the number of countries with salt iodization programs has increased from 46 to 93, and more than two-thirds of people living in the 130 IDD-affected countries have access to iodized salt. In Latin America, there is some experience with iron fortification of wheat flour, but fortification of sugar with vitamin A failed due to high costs and potential toxicity (Caulfield et al. 2006; Zimmermann and Hurrell 2007). Fortification approaches are generally limited to populations with access to and availability of the fortified products. However, in regions of severe iodine deficiency, high-dose iodine supplementation is also successfully used.

Diet-based strategies are probably the most promising approach for a sustainable control of MND (Müller and Krawinkel 2005). Increasing dietary diversification through consumption of a broad variety of foods, preferably accessed through home gardens and small livestock production, has been shown to be effective. Households should be informed and supported to increase production of dark-green leafy vegetables, yellow and orange fruits, poultry, eggs, fish, and milk. A possible future strategy to prevent MND is the *breeding* of micronutrient-rich crops employing either a conventional breeding technique or a genetic modification of existing crops (Müller and Krawinkel 2005).

However, the achieved concentrations of micronutrients in these crops are very low. For vitamin A, it is unknown whether or not ß-carotin from the "golden rice" is bioavailable and how much rice needs to be consumed to cover the needs; for iron the concentrations in bioengineered rice are not higher than in natural varieties, e.g., basmati or jasmine rice.

Micronutrient supplementation for pregnant and lactating women is part of almost all antenatal care programs, including the supplementation of iron and folic acid, which is recommended by WHO. Beyond that, various combinations of micronutrients have been suggested for routine supplementation during pregnancy by agencies such as UNICEF and national authorities. These combinations usually include iron, folate, iodine, zinc, calcium, magnesium, other minerals and a range of vitamins (Huffman et al. 2001). While many of these components may be beneficial, evidence from randomized trials currently only support the supplementation of iron, folate, and iodine, according to the evidence compiled in WHO's reproductive health library (version 10). In HIV-infected mothers a multivitamin combination substantially improved perinatal outcomes and maternal T-cell counts (Fawzi et al. 1998).Given the late attendance in antenatal care – most women present themselves in the second or third trimester – and logistical problems in ensuring a constant supply in many developing countries, the potential benefit of micronutrient supplementation is often lost. Thus, micronutrient supplementation through antenatal care is not the magic bullet that it may seem. Finally, it is no substitute for population-based interventions to improve the nutritional status at the population level and to improve women's health throughout the life cycle.

Underlying Factors Contributing to Protein-Energy Malnutrition and Micronutrient Deficiencies

Complicating the ability to procure appropriate nutrition are interactions between underlying factors associated with micronutrient deficiencies and malnutrition. Contributing factors to micronutrient deficiencies and malnutrition can be grouped into three categories: individual factors, community/ sociocultural factors, and physical environmental factors (Fig. 16.7). Individual factors are characteristics that are intrinsic to a person, including age, gender, and health status. For example, having a diarrheal infection decreases the body's ability to absorb nutrients (Bhutta et al. 2008). Community or sociocultural environmental factors include community practices, customs, and attitudes that affect nutrition and feeding patterns. Physical environmental factors involve overarching influences that are beyond the community and individual levels and affect the availability of diverse food sources that are safe and healthy. Both community environment and physical environment comprise the overarching group of environmental factors. Individual factors often interact with environmental factors through behavior to impact nutrition. For example, a child's age and gender can determine what they eat. This is based on food customs and parental education in their community.

Social Cognitive Theory (SCT) holds that personal and environmental factors as well as attributes of behavior affect a person's behavior (Glanz et al. 2002). This theory has been determined to be an appropriate model for food behaviors (Parraga 1990). According to this theory, self-efficacy is central to behavior change. This theory focuses on the interaction of personal factors, environmental factors, and behavior. In regard to risk factors for malnutrition, personal factors include individual factors and some sociocultural factors. The environment includes community and surroundings, as well as some sociocultural factors, influencing availability of safe and healthy food. In this way, issues such as the self-efficacy of individuals and a community that supports proper nutrition can play an important role in countering malnutrition. Public

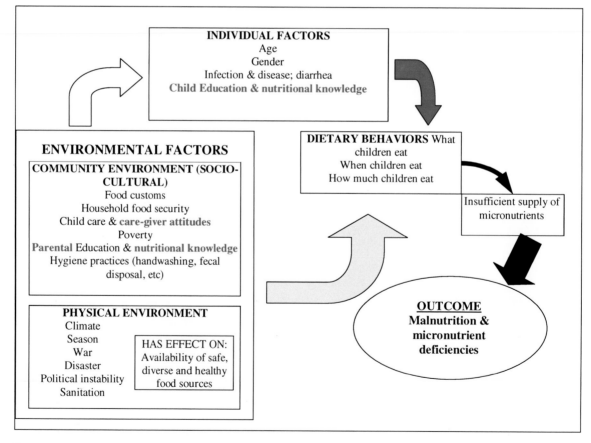

Fig. 16.7 Underlying factors contributing to malnutrition and micronutrient deficiencies. Source: Adapted from Mueller and Krawinkel (2005); Based on SCT conceptual model (Glanz et al. 2002).

health programming aimed at improving maternal and child health through nutrition can use innovative behavioral approaches in addition to providing nutrition and healthcare, such as appropriate education, identifying environmental barriers, and understanding nutritional practices on individual, family, and societal levels.

Obesity

Burden of Disease

The term malnourishment has traditionally meant undernutrition. However, malnutrition should also be used to refer to overnutrition (Tanumihardjo et al. 2007). While overweight and obesity are often thought of as problems of developed nations, recent studies have found the prevalence of childhood overweight and obesity to be increasing across the world (Wang and Lobstein 2006). These increases are particularly pronounced for developed countries and urbanized populations, but the economic development and urbanization of developing countries are correlated with overweight increases in these regions as well (Wang and Lobstein 2006). Both under- and overnutrition can result from inadequate food supply and other conditions of poverty. Therefore, countries undergoing economic transition may experience problems with both under- and overnutrition concurrently (Tanumihardjo et al. 2007). Both conditions of malnutrition cannot be considered separately from issues of food insecurity, disparities in socioeconomic status within and between countries, unequal global trade arrangements, and the global occurrence of cultural, social, and epidemiological transitions (Darnton-Hill and Coyne 1997; Anonymous 2008).

Comparing data across countries is often difficult because of differing measurements and definitions of overweight and obesity. Also, criteria for classification vary. The global prevalence of overnutrition is increasing, with few exceptions. Wang and Lobstein (2006) found that this increase occurs at the fastest rate in developed countries and urbanized areas, but also occurs in transitional and low-income countries.

From the 1970s to the 1990s the prevalence of obesity has doubled or tripled in countries in North America and South America, Europe, Australia, and Japan. These areas have the highest levels of overweight and obesity in the world, and Southeast Asia and sub-Saharan Africa have the lowest overall prevalence, which is also reflected by respective levels in children (Fig. 16.8). Countries currently experiencing economic growth (Brazil, Chile, Mexico, and Egypt) have overweight prevalences nearing industrialized countries. It is estimated that by 2010, 46% of school-age children in the Americas will be overweight, along with 41% in the eastern Mediterranean region, 38% in Europe, 27% in the west Pacific, and 22% in Southeast Asia (Wang and Lobstein 2006). Sufficient data for Africa were unavailable for prevalence projection. There is a shortage of data on the prevalence of overweight in lower-income countries, particularly those with large underweight populations. The global prevalence of overweight in developing countries was thought to be 3.3% (although some countries were much higher) in 1995 (de Onis and Blössner 2000). Out of 34 countries, trends suggest that prevalence was decreasing in 8, stable in 14, and increasing in 16. The highest prevalences were in the Middle East, North Africa, and Latin America.

Transitioning developing countries are beginning to bear a double burden of disease from malnutrition – both under- and overnutrition (Fig. 16.8). A study of Pakistani school children found that over a decade there was only a slight non-significant decrease in underweight children, but an increase in overweight children from 3.0 to 5.7% (Jafar et al. 2008). In a comparative study of wasting and obesity among preschool children in 94 countries that used weight-for-height distribution, it was found that for developing countries levels of wasting are generally higher than those of overweight (de Onis and Blössner 2000). In Africa and Asia they may be 2.5–3.5 times higher. The overall prevalence of overweight in developing countries was found to be 3.3%, compared with the overall prevalence of wasting of 9.4%. Levels of wasting and overweight varied by country, with wasting ranging from 0 to 23.3% and overweight from 1 to 14.4%. Forty-five percent of developing countries had more overweight than wasting, 48% had more wasting than overweight, and three countries (Uzbekistan, Kiribati, and Algeria) had similarly high levels of overweight and wasting. However, while 45

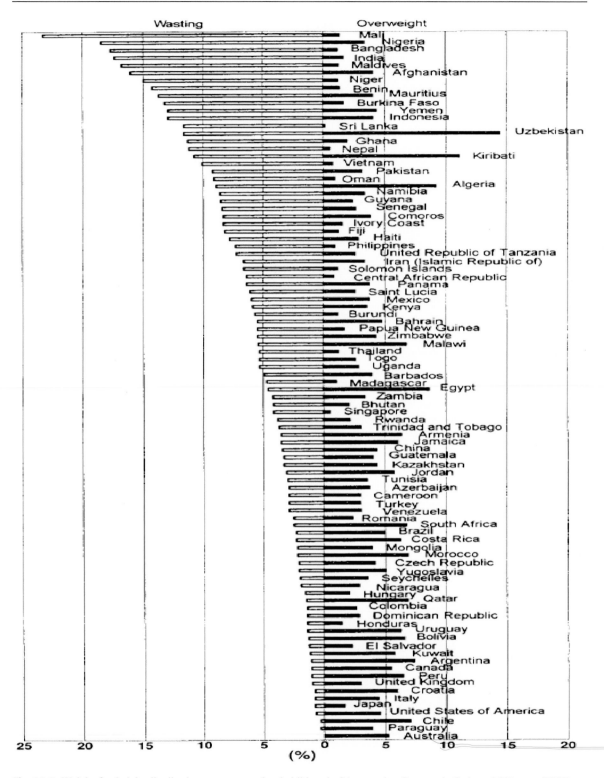

Fig. 16.8 Weight-for-height distribution among preschool children in 94 countries. Source: de Onis and Blössner (2000)

countries have wasting >5%, and 18 have wasting > 10%, only 21 countries have overweight > 5%, and merely 2 have overweight > 10%. This suggests that wasting is still a much more significant health concern than overweight for most developing countries, despite recent increases in the prevalence of overweight.

The double burden is evident in the occurrence of under- and overnutrition within the same household. Garrett and Ruel (2005) investigated the prevalence of a stunted child and overweight mother in the same household. In low- and middle-income countries, this prevalence is generally below 10%. It occurs most frequently in Latin America, followed by Africa and then Asia (less than 5%). Overweight mothers are common in many developing countries. In Latin America, country rates of overweight among mothers ranged from approximately 30–50%, except in Haiti (12%). In Africa, the range was from 4% in Madagascar to 55% in Egypt. Former Soviet Union countries had rates of ~15%, significantly more than the 4% in Bangladesh and 2% in Nepal. The prevalence of overweight is greater in urban areas than rural areas (except in Kazakhstan). Child stunting is common even in countries with a high prevalence of overweight mothers, although the prevalence of stunting is more common in rural rather than urban areas. The prevalence of households with a stunted child and overweight mother exceeds 10% in Bolivia, Guatemala, Peru, and Egypt. High prevalence occurs when there are both high overweight and high stunting levels. This prevalence is generally greatest in rural areas.

The divide between urban and rural populations is also evident. One in 8 children in urban China was overweight in 1997, and this is projected to be 1/5 in 2010, compared with a projected rural rate of only 1/14 (Wang and Lobstein 2006). However, Mendez et al. (2005) examined the association of adult female overweight with urban/rural distribution and level of income in 36 developing countries (Fig. 16.9).

They found that while increasing country income and urbanization was associated with a higher prevalence of overweight in general, it also narrowed the gap between urban and rural overweight. Among women of low socioeconomic status in higher-income developing countries, overweight remained high for both urban (51%) and rural (38%) women. Lower and middle-income countries are undergoing transition from under- to overnutrition, and having the burden of both. In countries with high prevalence of low birthweight there is a greater risk of stunting and, in turn, later availability of food may lead to an increase in body weight but not height proportionately (Wang and Lobstein 2006). Countries with stunting >50% may have many children at risk for this and subsequent chronic diseases (Wang and Lobstein 2006). This could also explain the occurrence of overweight mothers with stunted children, as the mothers themselves may have been stunted as children leading to a greater risk for obesity (Garrett and Ruel 2005).

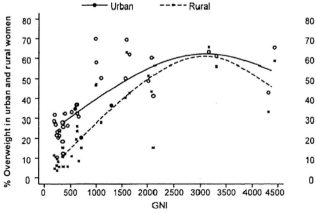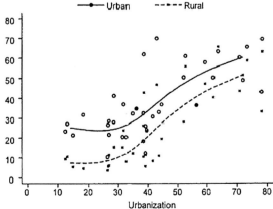

Fig. 16.9 Prevalence of overweight (BMI ≥ 25) in women aged 20–49 in 36 developing countries by gross national income (GNI) and level of urbanization. Source: Mendez et al. (2005)

Risk for overweight also depends on the economic state of a country and on the socioeconomic status of an individual within that country. In general, risk for overweight increases as a country's economy improves. Reversal in economic development can lead to a decline in overweight (Russia, Poland, Cuba), and recovery can lead to a rapid increase in obesity (Croatia and East Germany) (Wang and Lobstein 2006; Franco et al. 2008). Within countries, overweight is more prevalent in socially disadvantaged individuals in high-income countries, while advantaged individuals are more at risk in low-income countries (Friel et al. 2007).

Wealthy individuals in poor countries are those who can afford energy-dense, nutritious foods. They are also able to lead more sedentary lives. These are two contributors to overweight. In rich countries, risk to the poor may be explained by healthier foods being more expensive than less healthy foods, with all economic factors favoring high energy intake and low micronutrient intake, characteristics that lead to weight gain and obesity (Tanumihardjo et al. 2007). Low-income groups are also affected by constraints on their ability to travel to buy food, lack of healthy options in their immediate vicinity, and constraints on leading an active life (Friel et al. 2007).

Tanumihardjo et al. (2007) found that across the world, living in poverty is a better predictor of overweight and obesity than race or ethnicity. The relationship between obesity and poverty is shown in Fig. 16.10. In the United States for example, adult obesity is most prevalent in citizens of African origin, with nearly 50% of black women having a BMI greater than 30. However, the prevalence of obesity correlates with the prevalence of poverty among race/ethnicities, such that race/ethnicities with the greatest poverty levels also have the highest levels of obesity.

They also found that obesity is associated with a lack of family resources and food insufficiency. Food insecurity is the lack of access to safe and healthy food at a level sufficient for well-being. Food insecurity may lead to overweight when the limited foods available have sufficient or excess energy density, but fail to meet the body's micronutrient requirements (potentially leaving the consumer still hungry). These types of food are often cheaper than fruits, vegetables, and whole grains. Households classified as having food insecurity actually have the highest BMI and prevalence of obesity.

A person's physical environment affects his or her ability to maintain a healthy weight. Friel et al. (2007) found that inequities that lead to food insecurity are likely to correlate with lower access to material and psychosocial support for healthy behaviors and constraints on work availability and flexibility. Community design influences an individual's ability to walk to get to places, have spaces for recreation, and have the convenience of reliance on cars. Sedentary work, disinclination to active transport, and easy access to high-energy food all underlie risk for overweight. Friel et al. (2007) also found that globally, there is an increasing prevalence of refined foods, high-saturated fat foods, and reductions in energy expenditure. Increased trade between countries and changes in the food industry has saturated the market with foods that are cheap, high-energy, and low in nutrients. Bulk purchases, convenient food, and oversized proportions are becoming readily available, and advertising often focuses on increasing the desirability of unhealthy food. These findings are complemented by Garrett and Ruel (2005) who found that increases in economic development and urbanization lead to the consumption of processed foods with more sugar, salt, and fat, and increasingly sedentary jobs and use of labor-saving technologies.

Obesity increases risk for a number of chronic diseases, including diabetes and heart disease (Garrett and Ruel 2005). In the United States, obesity is the

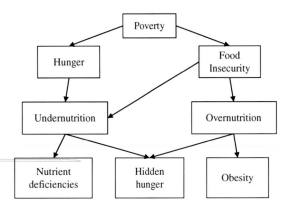

Fig. 16.10 Obesity and poverty. Source: Tanumihardjo et al. (2007)

second leading cause of death after smoking, with its direct and indirect costs amounting to US $117 billion in 2000 (Wang and Lobstein 2006). While clinically significant morbidity rates related to obesity are rare in children, childhood obesity has been shown to confer risks for long-term morbidity and mortality, including high blood pressure, diabetes, respiratory disease, orthopedic problems, and psychosocial disorders (de Onis and Blössner 2000; Yoon et al. 2006). Persistence into adulthood is a concern. Increasing prevalence rates of overweight and obesity worldwide suggest that the burden of chronic disease is going to increase, even in adolescence and early adulthood (Wang and Lobstein 2006).

Management and Control

Available reviews of interventions for overweight and obesity focus on individual behavioral factors such as diet and exercise. They are located primarily in industrialized countries and target adult populations. Therefore, they have limited generalizability to pediatric populations and for prevention purposes. These studies are additionally affected by high attrition rates (many around 40%) that limit

the certainty of conclusions. Efforts to manage and control the growing obesity epidemic need to address its multiple determinants (Fig. 16.11). These include an individual's environment and health behaviors.

Special attention has been given to children and adolescents, as overweight and obesity at younger ages may persist throughout life and confer greater risks for morbidity and mortality. While physical risk from obesity at young ages is rare, social isolation and its effects on psychosocial development are of concern (de Onis and Blössner 2000). Additionally, persistence of childhood overweight and/or obesity into adulthood is common, with a half to a third of overweight adolescents becoming overweight adults (Wang and Lobstein 2006). Stunted children are particularly at risk for weight gain disproportionate to height increases, and early catch-up growth interventions are necessary in order to prevent this (Wang and Lobstein 2006). In general, eating and activity habits formed in childhood may carry to adulthood, and parents should be encouraged to model good eating habits for their children (de Onis and Blössner 2000). There is also evidence that breastfed infants self-regulate their energy intake better than formula-fed infants. This suggests that breastfeeding may be a protective factor against overweight (de Onis and

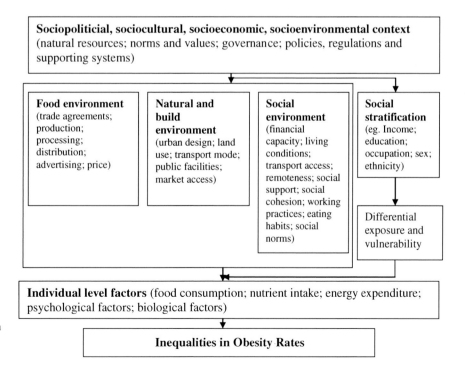

Fig. 16.11 Conceptual framework of the social determinants of inequities in obesity. Source: Friel et al. (2007)

Blössner 2000). Reducing the promotion of energy-dense food to children is a potential strategy (Wang and Lobstein 2006).

Prevention efforts involving diet and exercise interventions targeting children were found in meta-analysis to be ineffective at preventing weight gain, despite improvements in diet, increased exercise, and increased knowledge of healthy behaviors (Summerbell et al. 2005). The authors suggest that the lack of effect may be due to failure of the studies to take into account the complexity of the problem and the diversity of its determinants.

Friel et al. (2007) found environmental factors that affect health behaviors to be present at the local, national, and global levels. Local influences are those that directly influence an individual's nutritional intake and energy expenditure. Strategies for increasing healthy food intake include urban planning for access to nutritious food and local community food initiatives. Strategies for increasing energy expenditure focus on physical education in schools and other methods of encouraging active transport. The opportunity for exercise and reduction of car transport are important factors. In Brazil, the Agita Sao Paulo physical activity program (Matsudo et al. 2003) increased physical activity in the general population using a multi-strategy approach. This approach included building, widening, and removing obstacles from paths, building exercise tracks with shade and water available, maintaining green areas, and creating bicycle storage close to public transport stations, schools, and workplaces, and encouraging mass active transport through implementing private and public incentive policies.

At the national level, support and reinforcement of local initiatives is essential. For example, Norway reversed its shift toward high-fat, energy-dense diets by using food subsidies, price manipulation, retail regulations, clear nutrition labeling, and public education (Norwegian Nutrition Society 2004). Mauritius was also successful with a strategy including price policies, agricultural policies, and widespread educational activities (United Nations 1997). Coherence is necessary for inter-sector action at the national and international levels. For example, *Healthy Food For All*, in Ireland (EPHA 2008), is a multi-agency, equality-oriented program that focuses on access, affordability, and availability of food.

Internationally, trade is an important issue related to the prevalence of overweight. There is a need for trade agreements that allow most people to benefit, and regulation of global food marketing to prevent exploitation of vulnerable societies and populations. The World Health Organization (WHO 2008b) has created a global strategy for diet, physical activity, and health that focuses on national food and agricultural policies. Their aim is the development of multisectoral policies that promote public health in general, physical activity, and educational information.

Targeting the population at all levels is essential. Direct approaches such as changing an individual's behavior, through personal skills and enhancement of the local environment have limited sustainability and transferability. Additionally, uptake is generally higher for groups with greater social status. This serves to potentially increase the disparity between socioeconomic levels. Successful actions should address national and international support for the equitable distribution of nutritious food and local environments that lend themselves to healthy behaviors.

Given the increasing co-occurrence of under- and overnutrition in the same countries and households, new strategies will have to be developed to address both conditions simultaneously. Most programs that address food insecurity do not address obesity (Tanumihardjo et al. 2007). Garrett and Ruel (2005) found that successful strategies from Brazil, China, and Finland included community involvement and ownership, capacity-building for community organizations, evidence-based information and counseling, inclusion of the food industry in labeling and regulation, and support for physical exercise. Quality needs to be emphasized over quantity, as well as the importance of child care and feeding, not just household access to food.

Conclusion

A review of interventions that show evidence of effectiveness in addressing maternal and child undernutrition was recently published by the Maternal and Child Undernutrition Study Group (Bhutta et al. 2008). According to the group, potentially viable interventions include promotion of breastfeeding, promotion of complementary feeding, micronutrient interventions, and general supportive strategies to improve family and community nutrition. They also suggest a reduction of disease burden through promotion of hand-washing practices and strategies to reduce the burden of malaria in pregnancy (Table 16.4).

Only multiple and synergistic interventions embedded in true multisectoral programs will have sustainable impact on the reduction of malnutrition. This is because malnutrition has many causes and synergistic relationships with diarrhea, reduced immunity, and disease (Bhutta et al. 2008). These need to include large-scale agricultural and micronutrient interventions, provision of safe drinking water and sanitation, education and support on better diets, special attention to vulnerable groups such as pregnant women and young children, and quality health services. Nutrition education focusing on locally available protein- and micronutrient-rich plants should be considered as a particularly effective and sustainable intervention. In the long run, however, only a sufficient consideration of contextual factors such as women's status and education, social inclusion, community organization,

literacy, and political commitment will have a sustainable effect on health and nutrition leading to overall development and improvement of living standards (Ehiri and Prowse 1999).

Sub-Saharan Africa (SSA) is considered to be trapped in poverty with decreasing food production per capita and consequently increasing hunger and poverty (Sanchez and Swaminathan 2005). Community-based health and nutrition programs have been more successful in developing countries outside SSA. Reasons may have to do with lack of community participation, lack of infrastructure and staff, insufficient emancipation from former colonial or existing neo-colonial repressive conditions, unrestricted donor influences, and lack of political commitment (Mason et al. 2006). The first Millennium Development Goal is to eradicate extreme poverty and hunger by 2015. The two targets associated with this goal are (i) to reduce by half of 1990 figures, the proportion of people living on less than a dollar a day, and (ii) to reduce by half of 1990 figures, the proportion of people who suffer from hunger (The United Nations Millennium Project 2005). Prospects for achieving these targets vary by region as they are influenced by the range of

Table 16.4 Interventions that affect maternal and child undernutrition

Sufficient evidence for implementation in all 36 countries	Evidence for implementation in specific, situational contexts
Maternal and birth outcomes	
Iron folate supplementation	Maternal supplements of balanced energy and protein
Maternal supplements of multiple micronutrients	Maternal iodine supplements
Maternal iodine through iodization of salt	Maternal de-worming in pregnancy
Maternal calcium supplementation	Intermittent preventive treatment for malaria
Interventions to reduce tobacco consumption or indoor air pollution	Insecticide-treated bednets
Newborn babies	
Promotion of breastfeeding (individual and group counseling)	Neonatal vitamin A supplementation
	Delayed cord clamping
Infants and children	
Promotion of breastfeeding (individual and group counseling)	Conditional cash transfer programs (with nutritional education)
Behavior change communication for improved complementary feeding	De-worming
Zinc supplementation	Iron fortification and supplementation programs
Zinc in management of diarrhea	Insecticide-treated bednets
Universal salt iodization	
Hand-washing or hygiene interventions	
Treatment of severe acute malnutrition	

Source: Bhutta et al. (2008)

social, economic, and political factors already referenced in this chapter. Estimates by de Onis et al. (2004) project that the prevalence of childhood underweight will increase by 9% in sub-Saharan Africa. In eastern Africa, it is projected to increase by 25%. Only northern Africa is likely to reach the Millennium Development Goal target for hunger reduction with a forecasted reduction in the prevalence of childhood underweight from 9.5% in 1990 to 4.2% in 2015 (de Onis et al. 2004). Figure 16.12 presents the 2015 projections of the prevalence of underweight children for the African sub-regions compared with the Millennium Development Goal for those sub-regions. The prevalence of underweight is projected to be reduced from 35.1 to 18.5% in Asia between 1990 and 2015. Eastern Asia shows the largest improvement with a projected decline of 84% during the same time period.

Southeastern and South Central Asia were forecasted to experience substantial improvements, with reductions in the prevalence of underweight of 49 and 42%, respectively (de Onis et al. 2004). Nevertheless, both sub-regions will have high levels of childhood underweight in 2015. Western Asia was estimated to be the Asian sub-region with the lowest reduction in the prevalence of childhood underweight (29%). An 8.7% decrease is projected for Latin America and all of its regions are projected to experience decreasing trends with changes of −72% for the Caribbean, −54% for Central America, and −65% for South America (de Onis et al. 2004).

According to the United Nation's MDG progress report in 2006 (United Nations 2006), chronic hunger – measured by the proportion of people lacking the food needed to meet their daily needs – has declined in the developing world. But progress overall is not fast enough to reduce the number of people who go hungry, which increased between 1995–1997 and 2001–2003. An estimated 824 million people in the developing world were affected by chronic hunger in 2003 (United Nations 2006). The worst affected regions – sub-Saharan Africa and southern Asia – have made progress in recent years although advances have not kept pace with those of the early 1990s. Beyond that, increases in food prices and other adverse macroeconomic developments threaten to reverse the downward trend and have already resulted in an estimated additional 50 million people going hungry in 2007 (FAO 2008; Anonymous 2008).

It is germane to note that progress toward achievement of the other seven MDGs would directly or indirectly contribute to major reductions of undernutrition in developing countries (Sachs and McArthur 2005). Discouraging as the above statistics are, a review by the UN Millennium Project (2005) concludes that hunger can be halved by 2015 and even eradicated with deliberate and timely implementation of seven recommended interventions (Box 16.2).

The main challenge of the MDGs is the financing and the implementation of effective interventions at scale. Although the GAVI Alliance and the Global Fund for AIDS, Tuberculosis and Malaria (GFATM) have added significant funds to health programs in poor countries, funding is still below the required levels. Also, sustainability is an issue and additional financing instruments are only able

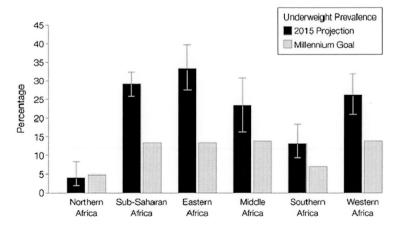

Fig. 16.12 Projections of Underweight Prevalence in African sub-regions in 2015 compared with the Millennium Development Goal. Source: de Onis et al. (2004)

Box 16.2 Recommendations for Halving Hunger by 2015

1. *Move from political commitment to action*

   - Advocate political action to meet intergovernmental agreements to end hunger
   - Strengthen the contributions of donor countries and national governments to activities that combat hunger
   - Improve public awareness of hunger issues and strengthen advocacy organizations
   - Strengthen developing country organizations that deal with poverty reduction and hunger
   - Strengthen accurate data collection, monitoring, and evaluation

2. *Reform policies and create an enabling environment*

   - Promote an integrated policy approach to hunger reduction
   - Restore budgetary priority to the agricultural and rural sectors
   - Build developing country capacity to achieve the hunger goal
   - Link nutritional and agricultural interventions
   - Increase poor people's access to land and other productive resources
   - Empower women and girls
   - Strengthen agricultural and nutrition research
   - Remove internal and regional barriers to agricultural trade
   - Increase the effectiveness of donor agencies' hunger-related programming
   - Create vibrant partnerships to ensure effective policy implementation

3. *Increase the agricultural productivity of food-insecure farmers*

   - Improve soil health
   - Improve and expand small-scale water management
   - Improve access to better seeds and other planting materials
   - Diversify on-farm enterprises with high-value products
   - Establish effective agricultural extension services

4. *Improve nutrition for the chronically hungry and vulnerable*

   - Promote mother and infant nutrition
   - Reduce malnutrition among children under five years of age
   - Reduce malnutrition among school-age children and adolescents
   - Reduce vitamin and mineral deficiencies
   - Reduce the prevalence of infectious diseases that contribute to malnutrition

5. *Reduce vulnerability of the acutely hungry through productive safety nets*

   - Build and strengthen national and local early warning systems
   - Build and strengthen national and local capacity to respond to emergencies
   - Invest in productive safety nets to protect the poorest from short-term shocks and to reduce long-term food insecurity

6. *Increase incomes and make markets work for the poor*

   - Invest in and maintain market-related infrastructure
   - Develop networks of small rural input traders
   - Improve access to financial services for the poor and food-insecure
   - Provide and enforce a sound legal and regulatory framework
   - Strengthen the bargaining power of the rural and urban poor in labor markets

- Ensure access to market information for the poor
- Promote and strengthen community and farmer associations
- Promote alternative sources of employment and income

7. *Restore and conserve the natural resources essential for food security*

- Help communities and households restore or enhance natural resources
- Secure local ownership, access, and management rights to forests, fisheries, and rangelands
- Develop natural resource-based "green enterprises"
- Pay poor rural communities for environmental services.

Source: The UN Millennium Project (2005)

to cover some aspects of maternal, neonatal, and child health (Costello and Osrin 2005).

According to recent estimates, the total donor cost of supporting the global MDG financing gap is around US $100 billion per year which is equivalent to the annual costs of the United States for the war in Iraq or roughly one-tenth of the global military budget. This amount equals 0.5% of total donor gross national product (GNP), well within the long-standing 0.7% commitment for development aid (Sachs and McArthur 2005). As shown in Table 16.4 (Bhutta et al. 2008), effective interventions for addressing undernutrition among women and children are already known and the underlying determinants of undernutrition, poverty, poor

education, disease burden, and lack of women's empowerment have been widely discussed in the literature (Ehiri and Prowse 1999).

Practical action is urgently needed to optimize the benefits of these known interventions. To ensure progress in the reduction of undernutrition and its associated consequences in less developed countries, it is time the plethora of evidence on effective interventions were translated into large-scale population-based programs. With increased funding by international health and development agencies, these interventions should be backed with adequate community and political support and participation. Only then can there be visible and sustained improvement in global maternal and child malnutrition.

Key Terms

Malnutrition	Overweight	Growth monitoring
Undernutrition	Obesity	Safe Motherhood
Hunger	Sedentary lifestyle	Xerophthalmia
Underweight	Anorexia	Protein-energy malnutrition
Stunting	Marasmus	Micronutrient deficiency
Wasting	Disability-adjusted life years	Complementary foods
Low birthweight	Millennium Development	Complementary feeding
Poverty	Goals	Exclusive breastfeeding
Fetal malnutrition	Food supplementation	Body mass index (BMI)
Micronutrient fortification	Food insecurity	
Undernourishment	Kwashiorkor	

Questions for Discussion

1. What are the consequences of maternal undernutrition?
2. Discuss the various approaches for the management and control of protein-energy malnutrition and micronutrient deficiencies, identifying evidence of effectiveness of each approach.
3. Community-based health and nutrition programs have not been as effective in sub-Saharan Africa as they have been in other developing countries. Why?
4. In 2005, the United Nations Millennium Project proposed seven recommendations for halving world hunger by 2015 (Box 16.2). How attainable are these recommendations? Using one developing country as a specific example, what are the potential barriers against implementation of these recommendations?
5. In their review of the effectiveness of interventions for addressing maternal and child undernutrition, the Maternal and Child Undernutrition Study Group (Bhutta et al. 2008) concluded that only multiple and synergistic interventions embedded in true multisectoral programs will have sustainable impact. With appropriate and specific examples, discuss what they mean by this.

References

Administrative Committee on Coordination/Sub-committee on Nutrition (ACC/SCN) (2006) Nutrition through the life cycle. In: Fourth Report of the World nutrition situation. Administrative Committee on Coordination/Sub-committee on Nutrition – (ACC/SCN) the UN system's forum for nutrition, http://www.unsystem.org/scn/archives/rwns04/index.htm, cited 5 August 2008

Anonymous (2008) Finding long-term solutions to the world food crisis. Lancet 371, 1389

Begum S, Sen B (2005) Maternal health, child well-being and intergenerationally transmitted chronic poverty: does women's agency matter? Institute for Development Policy and Management, University of Manchester, Working Paper No. 8

Bhagwati J, Fogel R, Frey B et al. (2004) Ranking the opportunities. In: B Lomberg (ed.) Global Crises, Global Solutions. Cambridge University Press, Cambridge

Bhutta ZA, Ahmed T, Black RE et al. (2008) What works? Interventions for maternal and child undernutrition and survival. Lancet 371(9610), 417–440

Blössner M and de Onis M (2005) Malnutrition: quantifying the health impact at national and local levels. WHO Environmental Burden of Disease Series, No. 12. Geneva: World Health Organization

Brown KH (2003) Diarrhea and malnutrition. Journal of Nutrition 133(1), 328S–332S

Caulfield LE, de Onis M, Blössner M et al. (2004) Undernutrition as an underlying cause of child deaths associated with diarrhea, pneumonia, malaria, and measles. American Journal of Clinical Nutrition 80, 193–198

Caulfield LE, Richard SA, Rivera JA et al. (2006) Stunting, wasting and micronutrient deficiency disorders. In: Jamison et al. (eds.) Disease Control Priorities in Developing Countries. Oxford University Press and the World Bank

Collins S, Dent N, Binns P et al. (2006) Management of severe acute malnutrition in children. Lancet 368, 1992–2000

Costello A, Osrin D (2005) Viewpoint: the case for a new Global Fund for maternal, neonatal, and child survival. Lancet 366, 603–605

Darnton-Hill I, Coyne ET (1997) Feast and famine: socio-economic disparities in global nutrition and health. Public Health Nutrition l(1), 23–31

de Onis M, Blössner M (2000) Prevalence and trends of overweight among preschool children in developing countries. American Journal of Clinical Nutrition 72, 1032–1039

de Onis M, Blössner M, Borghi E et al. (2004) Estimates of global prevalence of childhood underweight in 1990 and 2015. JAMA 291(21), 2600–2606

Ehiri JE, Prowse JM (1999) Child health promotion in developing countries: the case for integration of environmental and social interventions? Health Policy and Planning 14(1), 1–10

European Public Health Alliance (EPHA) (2008) Healthy Food for All Initative – Ireland, http://www.epha.org/a/2523, cited 5 August 2008

Fawzi WW, Msamanga GI, Spiegelman D et al. (1998) Randomized trial of effects of vitamin supplements on pregnancy outcomes and T cell counts in HIV-1-infected women in Tanzania. Lancet 351, 1477–1482

Fikree H, Fariyal F (2006) Routine folate supplementation in pregnancy: RHL commentary. The WHO Reproductive Health Library, No. 9, Update Software Ltd, Oxford

Food and Agricultural Organization of the United Nations (FAO) (2004) Undernourishment around the world. In: The state of the food insecurity in the world, 2004. Rome: Food and Agricultural organization (FAO)

Food and Agricultural Organization of the United Nations (FAO) (2008) About 50 million more hungry people in 2007: Hunger on the rise due to soaring food prices, http://www.fao.org/newsroom/en/news/2008/1000866/index.html, cited 20 August 2008

Franco M, Ordunez P, Caballero B et al. (2008) Obesity reduction and its possible consequences: what can we learn from Cuba's Special Period? Canadian Medical Association Journal 178, 1032–1334

Freedman LP, Waldman RJ, de Pinho H et al. (2005). Transforming health systems to improve the lives of women and children. Lancet 365, 997–1000

Friel S, Chopra M, Satcher D (2007) Unequal weight: equity oriented policy responses to the global obesity epidemic. British Medical Journal 335, 1241–1243

Garner P, Panpanich R, Logan S (2000) Is routine growth monitoring effective? A systematic review of trials. Archives of Disease in Childhood 82(3), 197–201

Garrett J, Ruel MT (2005) The coexistence of child undernutrition and maternal overweight: prevalence, hypotheses, and programme and policy implications. Maternal and Child Nutrition 1, 185–196

Glanz K, Rimer BK, Lewis FM (2002) Health behavior and health education: theory, research and practice. San Fransisco: Wiley and Sons

González-Cossío T (2006) Routine iron supplementation during pregnancy: RHL commentary. The WHO Reproductive Health Library, No. 9, Update Software Ltd, Oxford

Gross R, Webb P (2006) Wasting time for wasted children: severe child undernutrition must be resolved in non-emergency settings. Lancet 367, 1209–1211

Huffman SL, Zehner ER, Harvey P et al. (2001) Essential health sector actions to improve Maternal Nutrition in Africa. Regional Centre for Quality of Healthcare, Makerere University and LINKAGES, Kampala

Jafar T, Qadri Z, Islam M et al. (2008) Rise in childhood obesity with persistently high rates of under-nutrition among urban school aged Indo-Asian children. Archives of Disease in Childhood 93(5), 373–378

Lopez AD, Mathers CD, Ezzati M et al. (2006) Global and regional burden of disease and risk factors, 2001: systematic analysis of population health data. Lancet 367, 1747–1757

Mason JB, Sanders D, Musgrove P et al. (2006) Community health and nutrition programs. In: Jamison et al. (eds.) Disease Control Priorities in Developing Countries. Oxford University Press and the World Bank

Matsudo SM, Matsudo VR, Araujo TL et al. (2003) The Agita São Paulo Program as a model for using physical activity to promote health. Revista Panamericana de Salud Pública, 14(4)

Mendez MA, Monteiro CA, Popkin BM (2005) Overweight exceeds underweight among women in most developing countries. American Journal of Clinical Nutrition 81, 714–721

Müller O, Becher H (2006) Malnutrition and child mortality in developing countries. Lancet 367, 1978

Müller O, Krawinkel M (2005) Review: Malnutrition and health in developing countries. Canadian Medical Association Journal 173, 279–286

Nemer L, Gelband H, Jha P, Duncan T (2001) The evidence base for interventions to reduce malnutrition in children under five and school-age children in low and middle-income countries. CMH Working Paper Series. Commission on Macroeconomics and Health. Geneva: WHO

Norwegian Nutrition Society (2004) 8th Nordic Nutrition Conference: Public Health Nutrition, http://www.nse-info.no/nordic/Nordic.pdf, cited 5 August 2008

Parraga IM (1990) Determinants of food consumption. Journal of American Dietetic Association 90, 661–663

Rice AL, Sacco L, Hyder A et al. (2000) Malnutrition as an underlying cause of childhood deaths associated with infectious diseases in developing countries. Bulletin of the World Health Organization 78, 1207–1221

Sachs JD, McArthur JW (2005) The Millennium Project: a plan for meeting the Millennium Development Goals. Lancet 365, 347–353

Sanchez PA, Swaminathan MS (2005) Hunger in Africa: the link between unhealthy people and unhealthy soils. Lancet 365, 442–444

Sazawal S, Black RE, Ramsan M et al. (2006) Effects of routine prophylactic supplementation with iron and folic acid on admission to hospital and mortality in preschool children in a high malaria transmission setting: community-based, randomized, placebo-controlled trial. Lancet 367, 133–143

Summerbell CD, Waters E, Edmunds LD et al. (2005) Interventions for preventing obesity in children. Cochrane Database of Systematic Reviews, Issue 3

Tanumihardjo SA, Anderson C, Kaufer-Horwitz M et al. (2007) Poverty, obesity, and malnutrition: An international perspective recognizing the paradox. Journal of the American Dietetic Association 107, 1966–1972

United Nations Children's Fund (UNICEF) (2004) Low birthweight: country, regional and global estimates. United Nations Children's Fund/World Health Organization. Geneva/New York: WHO/UNICEF

United Nations Millennium Project (2005) Halving hunger: it can be done. New York: United Nations Development Program (UNDP). Task Force on Hunger, http://www.unmillenniumproject.org/documents/HTF-SumVers_FINAL.pdf, cited 5 August 2008

United Nations (1997) Republic of Mauritius, http://www.un.org/esa/earthsummit/morit-cp.htm, cited 5 August 2008

United Nations (2006) The Millennium Development Goal Report 2006. New York: United Nations Development Program (UNDP), http://mdgs.un.org/unsd/mdg/Resources/Static/Products/Progress2006/MDGReport2006.pdf, cited 5 August 2008

Walraven G (2006) Treatments for iron-deficiency anemia in pregnancy: RHL commentary. The WHO Reproductive Health Library, No. 10, Update Software Ltd, Oxford

Wang Y, Lobstein T (2006) Worldwide trends in childhood overweight and obesity. International Journal of Pediatric Obesity 1, 11–25

World Health Organization (WHO) (2003) World Health Report – Shaping the Future. Geneva: World Health Organization, http://www.usaid.gov/our_work/global_health/nut/echareas/malnutrition_chart.html, cited 5 August 2008

World Health Organization (WHO) (2004) Inheriting the World. The Atlas of Children's Health and the Environment. Geneva: World Health Organization

World Health Organization (WHO) (2008a) Child Growth Standards, http://www.who.int/childgrowth/standards/bmi_for_age/en/index.html, cited 5 August 2008

World Health Organization (WHO) (2008b) Diet and Physical Activity: A Public Health Priority, http://www.who.int/dietphysicalactivity/en/, cited 5 August 2008

Yoon KH, Lee JH, Kim WK et al. (2006) Epidemic obesity and type 2 diabetes in Asia. Lancet 368, 1681–1688

Zimmermann MB, Hurrell RF (2007) Nutritional iron deficiency. Lancet 370, 511–520

Chapter 17
The Global Burden of Obstetric Fistulas

L. Lewis Wall

Learning Objectives After reading this chapter and answering the discussion questions that follow, you should be able to

- Discuss the global burden of obstetric fistula.
- Analyze the biomedical and sociocultural causes of obstetric fistula, using the Worldwide Fistula Fund's pathways to the development of obstetric fistula.
- Appraise prevention strategies for obstetric fistulas as they relate to the provision of timely obstetric services, health systems development, and cultural changes.

Introduction

This chapter presents an overview of the global burden of obstetric fistula. Using the Worldwide Fistula Fund's pathways to the development of obstetric fistula, the biomedical and sociocultural causes of the condition are analyzed, including the role of obstructed labor, women's low status in society, malnutrition, illiteracy, limitation in access to emergency obstetric services, early marriage, and traditional harmful practices. The consequences (medical and social) of obstetric fistula as well as treatment options and challenges are discussed. The chapter concludes with an appraisal of short- and long-term prevention strategies as they relate to the provision of appropriate and timely obstetric services, health systems development, and cultural changes that institutionalize gender equity from birth through the life course.

An obstetric fistula is an abnormal opening between a woman's bladder and her vagina (sometimes between her rectum and vagina, or involving other structures) that develops as a result of obstetric injury, most commonly from prolonged obstructed labor (Fig. 17.1). Although this condition was common in the United States and Europe 150 years ago, advances in obstetric care have eliminated obstetric fistula from the collective memory of industrialized societies. However, it remains a pressing and much-neglected issue for women in impoverished, non-industrialized countries, perhaps afflicting as many at 3.5 million women in Africa and Asia alone (Wall et al. 2005). To set this chapter in proper context, operational definitions of a number of technical terms that are used frequently are presented in Box 17.1.

Because obstetric fistulas will not heal on their own (they require surgical repair) women who develop this condition face a future of severe stigmatization due to the constant incontinence of urine (and perhaps feces) that dominates their lives. Yet most women who develop a fistula are young when this injury occurs, sometimes only 12 or 13 years old (Holme et al. 2007; Wall 2006a; Wall et al. 2004; Onolemhemhen and Ekwempu 1999).

Obstructed Labor and Its Consequences

Humans have the most complicated obstetrical mechanics of any primate species. This is due to the uniquely problematic combination of the upright, bipedal human posture and the large size of the human fetus. The upright human posture imposes certain mechanical constraints on human pelvic

L.L. Wall (✉)
Department of Obstetrics and Gynecology, Washington University School of Medicine, St. Louis, Missouri, USA

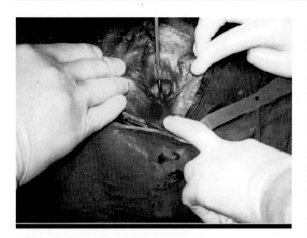

Fig. 17.1 Vesicovaginal fistula with probe. In the above figure, a metal probe has been inserted through the woman's urethra and the end of the probe can clearly be seen in her bladder, due to a large fistula where the bladder base should be. Source: Wall (2006a)

anatomy that are not present in other animal species that do not habitually walk upright on two legs. The pelvis of our closest biological relative (the chimpanzee, *Pan troglodytes*), for example, is configured as a simple cylinder, with the pelvic inlet, the mid-pelvis, and the pelvic outlet all aligned with one another along a single axis with an elongated anterior–posterior plane. As a result, birth for a chimpanzee fetus is a "straight shot" through the pelvis, a simple downward drop from the pelvic brim through an unconstricted mid-pelvis and out through a capacious pelvic outlet that opens posteriorly. This anatomical configuration means that parturition for the chimpanzee is a rapid process that proceeds relatively unhindered.

The human situation is much more complicated. Human birth requires the fetus to traverse a pelvis in which not only the inlet, the mid-pelvis, and the outlet have different dimensions but also the planes of those dimensions are not aligned along a single axis. As a result, the human fetus must constantly change its configuration as it proceeds through the birth canal utilizing a complicated, seven-step mechanism involving engagement, descent, flexion, internal rotation, extension, external rotation, and expulsion in the normal process of labor (Smellie 1752). If there is disproportion between the size of the head and the maternal pelvis, if there is a fetal malpresentation (such as a transverse lie), or if there are bony or soft-tissue

Box 17.1 Definition of Terms

- A fistula is an abnormal communication or passageway between two body cavities or organs that are not normally connected (Wall 2006a).
- An obstetric fistula is a fistula that develops during childbirth, most commonly from prolonged obstructed labor (Wall 2006a).
- Obstructed labor occurs when the descent of the fetus through the birth canal is arrested and no further progress can be made in spite of strong uterine contractions. This can be overcome only by operative intervention. Obstructed labor causes fistulas through pressure necrosis: the fetal head pushed against the mother's pelvic bones crushes the soft tissues trapped between these two bony plates, shutting off their blood supply and resulting in the death of these tissues (Arrowsmith et al. 1996).
- A vesicovaginal fistula is a fistula that develops between a woman's bladder and her vagina, resulting in continuous loss of urine (Wall 2006a).
- A rectovaginal fistula is a fistula that develops between a woman's rectum and her vagina, resulting in continuous loss of bowel contents (Wall 2006a).

abnormalities present, labor may become arrested. Obstructed labor occurs when the fetus cannot descend any further through the maternal pelvis, in spite of strong uterine contractions. When this occurs, the resulting "obstetric dilemma" can be overcome only by surgical intervention. In industrialized countries this usually means the performance of a prompt cesarean delivery. In impoverished, non-industrialized countries with a poor medical infrastructure, this usually means either a long delay before appropriate obstetrical care is received or simply no care at all. Under these circumstances, obstetric catastrophes are common.

When obstructed labor is allowed to continue unrelieved, the fetal head (or other presenting part, in cases of non-vertex presentations) is wedged ever more tightly into the mother's pelvis as the force of the uterine contractions continues unabated. As the head has reached an immoveable bony obstacle, further its descent becomes impossible (Fig. 17.2).

The soft tissues of the mother's pelvis – her bladder, urethra, vagina, cervix, and rectum – become compressed between these two bony plates and sustain a serious crush injury. Eventually the pressure exerted by this process cuts off the blood supply to these tissues and they die. In well over 90% of cases, the fetus also dies from asphyxiation (Dolea and AbouZahr 2003). In a day or two the dead fetus slowly macerates, decaying enough so that its tissues soften and it can change its conformation in its mother's pelvis, eventually sliding out of her vagina

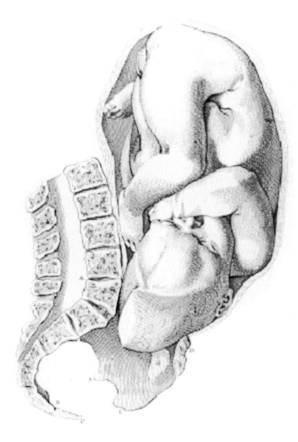

Fig. 17.2 Obstructed labor. It is an 18th-century obstetrical engraving showing obstructed labor. The distance between the pubic symphysis and the sacrum is too narrow to allow passage of the fetal skull, the descent of which has been arrested at this point. Note the pronounced overlapping of the fetal parietal bones as a result of this process. Source: Smellie (1752)

as a tragic stillbirth. If the mother survives this ordeal (which may last as long as 5 or more days) – and many women do not survive – she is often left with a constellation of crippling injuries called the obstructed labor injury complex (Table 17.1).

The most common injury from obstructed labor is a vesicovaginal fistula, a hole between a woman's bladder and her vagina (Fig. 17.1). In this situation the tissues of the vesicovaginal septum which normally separate these two organs have been destroyed by pressure necrosis and have sloughed off. The woman with this unfortunate condition loses all urinary control: the urine simply runs out of her bladder, into her vagina, across her perineum, and down her legs, 24 hours a day. Not only is this physically uncomfortable (for the urine irritates the skin and forms encrustations on her vulva) but also the resultant odor and social embarrassment lead to further stigmatization, ostracism, depression, and social withdrawal. If the woman is unfortunate enough to have sustained a rectovaginal fistula as well, her situation is even worse due to the constant commingling of urine and feces to which she is subjected (Wall 2006a).

The location and nature of the fistula that develops in obstructed labor is determined by the point at which labor becomes obstructed, the amount of pressure applied to the surrounding tissues, the duration of that compression, and the nature of the tissues thus compressed. In addition to the fistula itself, many women develop profound vaginal scarring with widespread destruction of neighboring tissues that makes subsequent surgical reconstruction difficult (Wall et al. 2005).

Epidemiology of Obstetric Fistulas

Obstetric fistulas no longer exist in the industrialized world because pregnant women have universal access to emergency obstetric services, but fistulas remain tragically common in impoverished, non-industrialized countries. Current estimates (which are the result of educated guesswork rather than detailed epidemiological studies) suggest that there are as many as 3.5 million women in underdeveloped countries with an unrepaired vesicovaginal or

Table 17.1 Spectrum of injuries seen in the obstructed labor injury complex

Acute obstetric injury
  Hemorrhage, especially postpartum hemorrhage from
    uterine atony
  Intrauterine infection and/or systemic sepsis
  Deep venous thrombosis
  Massive vulvar edema
  Pathological uterine retraction ring (Bandl's ring)
  Uterine rupture

Urologic injury
  Vesicovaginal fistula
  Urethrovaginal fistula
  Ureterovaginal fistula
  Complex combinations of fistulas (vesicocervical,
    vesicouterine, etc.)
  Urethral damage, including complete loss of the urethra
  Urinary stress incontinence
  Secondary hydroureteronephrosis and chronic
    pyelonephritis
  Renal failure

Gynecologic injury
  Amenorrhea
  Vagina scarring and stenosis, often with loss of coital
    function
  Cervical damage, including complete loss of the cervix
  Secondary pelvic inflammatory disease
  Secondary infertility

Gastrointestinal injury
  Rectovaginal fistula
  Acquired rectal atresia
  Anal sphincter injury with resulting anal incontinence

Musculoskeletal injury
  Osteitis pubis and related injuries to the pelvic bones
  Diffuse trauma to the pelvic floor

Neurological injury
  Foot drop (injury to the lumbosacral nerve plexus and/or
    common peroneal nerve)
  Neuropathic bladder dysfunction

Dermatological injury
  Chronic excoriation of the skin from maceration by urine
    and feces

Fetal/neonatal injury
  Approximately 95% perinatal case fatality rate
  Neonatal sepsis
  Neonatal birth asphyxia
  Neonatal birth injury, including scalp necrosis, nerve
    palsies, and intracranial hemorrhage.

Psychosocial injury
  Social isolation
  Divorce
  Worsening poverty
  Malnutrition
  Depression, sometimes leading to suicide

Source: Arrowsmith et al. (1996)

rectovaginal fistula, with tens (if not hundreds) of thousands of new cases developing each year (Wall and Arrowsmith 2007). Since obstetric fistulas are not generally fatal by themselves, the number of women suffering from this condition continues to grow.

Because obstetric fistulas are a form of severe obstetric morbidity, their prevalence tends to track maternal mortality statistics. The vast majority of maternal deaths (99% each year) occur in the impoverished parts of Africa, south Asia, and similar parts of the world (Mathers and Loncar 2006). Most maternal deaths (especially in the developing world) are due to a handful of consistent (and persistently deadly) causes: hemorrhage, infection, hypertensive disorders of pregnancy, complications of unsafe abortion, and obstructed labor. In most cases of maternal death, multiple factors contribute to the final outcome, but in those parts of the world where obstructed labor is common and maternal mortality is high, obstetric fistulas will be a prevalent problem. Case series from developing countries suggest that around 2% of women who develop prolonged obstructed labor will develop a fistula (Dumont et al. 2001). The World Health Organization's Global Burden of Disease Study (Dolea and AbouZahr 2003) suggests that there were 6.5 million cases of obstructed labor in the least developed regions of the world each year. If 2% of these women develop an obstetric fistula, then there would be 130,000 new fistula cases each year in these countries.

Social Causes of Fistula Formation

Obstetric fistulas are caused by the interaction of biological factors (obstructed labor) and the social environment in which those biological factors are found (Fig. 17.3). The principal cause of obstructed labor is cephalopelvic disproportion. The factors that lead to cephalopelvic disproportion are both biological and social. Proper nutrition in childhood is critical if young women are to reach reproductive age in a state of overall good health (Konje and Oladipo 2000) but equally important is the age at which marriage takes place and when entry into reproductive life begins.

Fig. 17.3 Pathways to development of obstetric fistula. Source: Wall (2005)

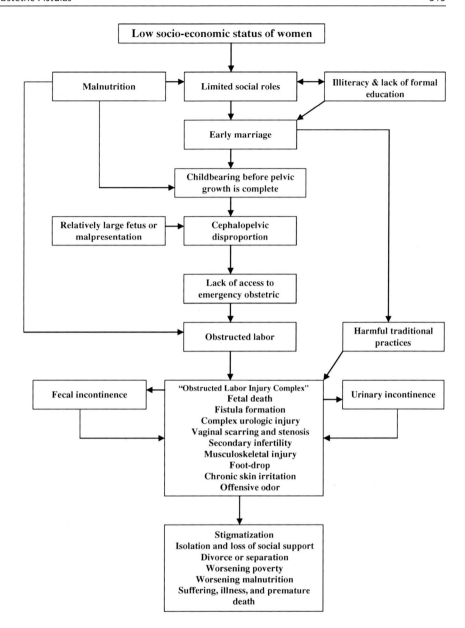

Because females reach the point of reproductive potential before they attain full growth in pelvic capacity, obstructed labor is more common in populations where girls marry soon after menarche and begin to have children in their early teens, while they are still children themselves (Moerman 1982). Societies in which this pattern is replicated tend to be societies in which even adult women (much less young teenage girls) have low social status, poor economic prospects, limited social roles, and poor access to education. Often women who have grown

up in these societies have faced nutritional discrimination as children, further hindering their pelvic growth. Lack of education has consistently emerged in studies as a marker for obstetric morbidity and mortality, probably because poorly educated women are less likely to gain access to the healthcare system when obstetric complications arise.

Once labor becomes obstructed, prompt intervention is necessary if the cascade of complications that can result from this process (Obstructed Labor Injury Complex) is to be avoided. Most often this requires prompt delivery by cesarean section, but access to effective obstetric surgery is often limited and delayed, with tragic consequences. It must be emphasized that an obstetric fistula can occur in *any* pregnancy – even among women who have successfully given birth previously – if labor becomes obstructed and prompt access to emergency obstetric care is not available. Thaddeus and Maine (1994) have investigated the causes of delay affecting obstetric emergencies in which the pregnant women subsequently die. Their discussion can equally be applied to obstetric fistula formation because the fundamental assumption underlying their work applies in both cases: in order to avoid a catastrophic outcome when an obstetric emergency arises (hemorrhage, sepsis, hypertensive crisis, obstructed labor) women must receive prompt access to competent emergency care. When care is delayed, the outcome is often poor. What causes delay in the treatment of obstructed labor? Thaddeus and Maine (1994) describe three principal causes of delay in scenarios that result in maternal death: (1) delay in deciding to seek care; (2) delay in arriving at a suitable health-care facility; and (3) delay in receiving appropriate care at that facility.

In many poor countries, childbirth is regarded as a natural phenomenon that should take place outside of the hospital/clinic setting. Most births in sub-Saharan Africa take place at home, generally in the presence of family members or a traditional birth attendant, whose specific duties and responsibilities will vary greatly among different cultures. When an obstetric complication such as prolonged labor arises, the immediate questions that need to be asked are: Is this a problem? What is causing it? What should be done about it? The assumptions from which one starts in trying to answer these questions have a direct impact on what happens subsequently. For example, in many parts of Africa trouble in childbirth is often attributed to some kind of moral failure on the part of the laboring woman. Difficult labor is frequently seen as retribution from God or the ancestors for adultery or some other moral lapse, rather than being the product of faulty obstetrical mechanics. In such cases the efforts of the birth attendants may well be directed toward getting the woman to confess "what she has done" rather than to seek medical attention. The decision to seek care for an obstetric problem involves economic costs, both the costs of transportation and the "opportunity costs" (lost wages, lost time working in the fields, etc.) that may be incurred. Often, particularly in cases of prolonged labor, the easiest decision is just to "wait and see what happens" in the hope that the woman will eventually deliver the baby by herself and that everything will come out all right in the end. Once labor has lasted over 24 hours, this is particularly dangerous. In many parts of Africa (particularly in northern Nigeria) women are normally expected to stay secluded within the family compound and are not normally allowed to travel without male accompaniment or permission. If the appropriate male authority figure is not present during obstructed labor, delays may be encountered before permission can be secured to take the woman to a health-care facility. Once the decision has been made that some kind of intervention is appropriate, the intervention that is chosen may still not lead to appropriate treatment. In many parts of southern Nigeria, for example, charismatic "spiritual churches" run maternity homes where the primary services provided are prayer and religious rituals rather than advanced obstetric care. Whatever the moral or spiritual value that such services may have, they are not effective in relieving the mechanical obstacle to delivery in obstructed labor. This only leads to further delay. In some cases the therapy chosen may actually be directly harmful to the laboring woman. For example, some recipes used by traditional healers in treating women in prolonged labor in parts of Africa do appear to have oxytocic properties that enhance uterine contractility and result in more forceful contractions. While this might be useful in labors in which progress is slow due to uterine inertia, giving such medications to a woman who is in obstructed labor will only accelerate the likelihood of a catastrophic outcome by increasing the pressure of the fetal head on the entrapped tissues.

In other cases traditional therapy itself may lead directly to the formation of a fistula. Among the Hausa people of northern Nigeria obstructed labor is often attributed to a condition known locally as *gishiri* ("salt") (Wall 2002). When *gishiri* is present, it is said that a film or web has grown over the vaginal outlet, hindering birth. The traditional treatment for this diagnosis is to consult with a traditional barber surgeon, who takes a knife or other sharp instrument and makes a series of random cuts in the vagina. In theory this removes the obstructing "web," but in reality it is far more likely to cause bleeding, infection, and direct injury to the urethra, bladder, vagina, and/or rectum than to open the vaginal outlet in any significant way to speed delivery.

After the decision has been made to seek care at a clinical facility, the task of arranging transportation begins. Depending on where the laboring woman is located, it may be difficult even to get to a serviceable road, particularly during the rainy season. She may have to walk for miles while in labor just to get to a location where road transportation might be available. If she is unable to walk due to her condition, she may have to be carried on a litter by family members or balanced on the handlebars of a bicycle while the rider tries to navigate down a footpath through the bush. Even if transportation is available, the owner or the driver of the vehicle may not wish to carry a pregnant woman in difficult labor for fear of soiling the vehicle, losing business from other passengers, incurring the wrath of angry ancestral or other spirits, or being held liable should she have an obstetric mishap while en route to the hospital. The state of roads in many parts of Africa is appalling, the vehicles not much better, and mechanical failures, accidents, and unpredictable delays are commonplace. It is also not unheard-of, for vulnerable people to face extortion from the purveyors of transportation in their time of need (Wall 2006a).

Once the woman in obstructed labor has reached the hospital, her dilemma is not yet over. Many women with obstetric complications make heroic efforts to get medical care only to find that it is not available at the facility they have reached and they must set out again on another journey to a different place in order to get help. Many African hospitals – particularly in rural areas – do not have anyone on staff that can perform a cesarean delivery (Elkins and Wall 1996). And even if such capabilities exist (at, for example, a major university teaching hospital in the capital city), the facility may be so overwhelmed with emergency cases that the suffering patient has to wait in line among the other obstetric emergencies that are stacked up waiting for the only available operating theater to become free. Patients who arrive at a hospital needing an emergency

cesarean section may still have to go to the market to find intravenous fluids, sterile gloves, antibiotics, and other necessary surgical supplies, which they themselves must bring to the hospital before an operation can begin. In many cases, "payment in advance" may be demanded before an operation can start, and sadly, there are many documented cases in which hospital personnel have demanded bribes before they would provide life-saving obstetrical services to vulnerable, suffering women in labor (Wall 2006a).

In most parts of sub-Saharan Africa, the maternal health-care system is broken and few people are trying to fix it. This has led some authors to conclude that the much heralded "Safe Motherhood" initiative launched in the 1980s has become "an orphan initiative." Correcting this problem is an urgent international public health issue (Weil and Fernandez 1999).

Treatment

A woman who presents to hospital immediately after surviving obstructed labor needs prompt supportive care with intravenous fluids, antibiotics, and placement of an indwelling urinary bladder to decompress the bladder and allow it to rest. The process of obstructed labor usually compresses the bladder neck and urethra so tightly that the woman may not have been able to urinate for several days. In these cases, her bladder generally will be distended, atonic, and often bleeding from the trauma it has sustained. Prompt decompression and relief of the overdistension is necessary both to provide patient comfort and to prevent further damage to the bladder. If a fistula is already present, immediately instituting prolonged catheter drainage will prevent further injury and may even allow the fistula to heal spontaneously over the course of several weeks. Sometimes prolonged bladder drainage is successful even with relatively large fistulas if it is instituted immediately after the injury is apparent. If the fistula is long standing, prolonged bladder drainage is unlikely to be curative, and surgical intervention will probably be needed.

It is not the purpose of this chapter to describe the surgical repair of obstetric fistulas in detail, for their manifestations vary widely, as do the specific surgical techniques needed to deal with specific types of injury. Some fistulas are simple and their repair is straightforward. Other fistulas are extremely complicated, accompanied by multiple other pelvic injuries, and may require extensive pelvic reconstructive surgery to repair the damage. Some fistulas are totally inoperable. The first consistently successful surgical operations to repair vesicovaginal fistulas were performed in the late 1840s by American surgeon J. Marion Sims, who initially developed his technique by operating on a small group of African-American slave women with fistulas who had been given to him by their owners for the purpose of attempting to cure them (Wall 2006b). He housed them in a small hospital he constructed behind his home in Montgomery, Alabama, for this purpose. Desperate for cure, stigmatized by their injuries, and ostracized even within their own slave society, these women eventually became Sims' surgical assistants, helping him operate on one another in turn until he was finally successful in closing their fistulas. This process of therapeutic surgical experimentation lasted nearly 4 years during which time one slave woman, Anarcha, underwent 30 operations before she was cured (Wall 2006b).

Although there have been many advances in surgical technology and many changes in surgical technique, the basic principles involved in vesicovaginal fistula repair have not changed much in the last 75 years. Fistula repair involves surgical separation of the tissue planes of the overlying vagina from the underlying bladder, wide mobilization of those tissues so that the hole in the bladder can be closed (originally with permanent sutures that had to be removed after several days, now with absorbable suture material). The bladder repair must be watertight and this should be confirmed at the time of surgery. Ideally, the bladder should be closed in two layers for greater strength, although this may not be possible in all circumstances. In many cases, particularly when the fistula is large or when it is surrounded by dense scar tissue, it is often desirable to bring a fresh blood supply into the surgical site by mobilizing a vascular pedicle of uninjured tissue from another nearby location (such as the bulbocavernosus fat pad underlying one of the vulvar labia) and suturing this in place over the bladder repair

(Wall 2005). After this is done, the vaginal incision is closed separately. The bladder should be drained with an indwelling urinary catheter for a prolonged period of time (usually 10–14 days) so that it does not become distended with urine, create pressure on the suture line, and result in breakdown of the repair and a recurrence of the fistula (Wall 2005).

Fistula surgery can usually be done under spinal anesthesia, at low cost, using standard surgical instruments and sutures. It rarely requires access to "high technology" to be successful. Physicians with basic surgical skills can learn to repair straightforward, uncomplicated fistulas in short order, but skill in treating "high-risk" fistulas requires patience, persistence, extensive experience, and access to facilities with more advanced capabilities. Ideally this should be at a specialist fistula center dedicated exclusively to the treatment of these injuries. A good case can be made for repairing obstetric fistulas in dedicated wards and specialist centers, rather than trying to integrate these patients into the general hospital population. First, because obstetric fistulas are not surgical emergencies, unless they are repaired in facilities where such surgery is the institution's exclusive concern, these women are always in danger of being bumped from the operating list for more urgent cases such as road traffic accidents, strangulated hernias, infected wounds, and so on. Second, because these women may be physically offensive to others from the loss of urine and/or feces that plagues their lives, they are often rejected by other patients and do not fit in well on general hospital wards (Wall 1998; Prevention of Maternal Mortality Network 1992). Because the real reasons (obstructed labor) they have sustained their injuries are often poorly understood by the communities from which they come (and often by themselves as well) women with fistulas may be further stigmatized by moral reproach from others who assume their affliction is the result of a hideous venereal disease or a punishment from God or the ancestral spirits. These women often do much better from a psychosocial perspective if they can live together, talk with each other, and recover from surgery as part of community bound together by their shared experience of suffering. Many women with fistulas do not realize that their situation is not unique until they find the company of other women with similar problems. Third, because women with fistulas are typically young, illiterate, impoverished, isolated from their families, and cast adrift in the wider society, they generally lack the social support and political influence that may be needed to navigate their way through the hospital system in order to receive proper care (Wall 1998; Prevention of Maternal Mortality Network 1992). These barriers can be eliminated by institutions whose sole mission is the care of such patients. Finally, special fistula programs are more likely to be able to muster the resources needed to deal with complicated cases and to maintain the level of expertise required to provide high-quality care.

Prevention of Obstetric Fistulas

Review of the obstetric fistula pathway (Fig. 17.3) reveals how deeply this problem is ingrained within the social, political, and economic structures of the societies where fistulas are prevalent. Because both the prevention (cesarean delivery) and the treatment (surgical repair) of fistulas are surgical interventions, the fistula problem can be solved only by the development of a robust medical infrastructure that can cope with acute problems as they arise and treat them appropriately after such damage has been done. This clearly will require long-term planning and the investment of substantial financial resources in all countries in which obstetric fistulas are found, but this is unlikely to happen until other cultural changes also take place.

First of all, eradication of the obstetric fistula will require that female children come to be valued just as much as male children in these societies. Girls must be given proper nutrition, health care (including vaccinations), and education during childhood so that they reach reproductive age fit enough to become healthy wives and mothers. Second, childbearing should be postponed until pelvic growth is complete. Early marriage should be discouraged. The number of early teenage pregnancies must be reduced, as these young women are at particularly high risk for developing obstructed labor. Abundant evidence suggests that the best way to do this is to provide equal educational opportunities for females, who will turn out to be better wives and mothers as a result. This will also require enhanced

family life education, frank discussions about reproductive physiology and sexual health, access to contraception and family planning information, and information concerning the prevention and treatment of sexually transmitted diseases. Gaining cultural acceptance for such programs may not be easy in all cultures. Third, harmful traditional medical practices (such as female genital cutting) should be eliminated. Although in some cases these practices are directly responsible for the creation of fistulas (such as *gishiri* cutting in northern Nigeria), in most cases these traditions are not direct causal factors; rather they are associated with fistulas because both the traditional cutting practices and the high prevalence of fistulas are markers of the low socioeconomic status of women and their relative lack of personal autonomy and political power in those societies where these practices and fistulas coexist. Fourth, a major effort must be made to make the male population of fistula-prevalent societies understand the direct stake that they themselves have in women's reproductive health. All males have important relationships with women as their sons, husbands, brothers, and fathers. The interests that men have in raising and being a part of strong, flourishing families are put in jeopardy in cultures in which women's health is neglected and their mothers, wives, sisters, and daughters are put at risk. Emphasizing this point is crucial for sustainable, long-term change.

Obstetric fistulas will be eliminated only when the principal root cause of the problem – obstructed labor – is eliminated. Since it is very difficult to predict with any precision which women are going to develop obstructed labor, the best preventive strategy is to insure that all women in labor are attended by a trained birth attendant who can detect abnormal labor and refer such cases to appropriate obstetrical facilities where they can be dealt with quickly and competently. Attaining this goal will require the gradual elevation of the general standards of obstetric care throughout the developing world, with a decreased emphasis on the use of traditional untrained birth attendants who do not possess adequate technical skills. Trained midwives who can evaluate the progress of labor, detect abnormalities, and provide appropriate triage during childbirth are required, with universal access to higher level referral when abnormalities in labor arise. There is good evidence from large multicenter trials that graphic recording of the progress of labor on a partograph decreases the number of prolonged labors, decreases unnecessary interference with normal labor, and enhances the appropriate triage and treatment of women with abnormalities of labor if use of such graphic records of labor is combined with an appropriate system of clinical analysis and prompt referral (World Health Organization 1994).

Conclusion

- Obstetric fistula is a devastating complication of childbirth in which obstructed labor produces an extensive crush injury to the soft tissues of the maternal pelvis, opening an abnormal passageway between the pregnant woman's vagina and her bladder and/or rectum. The fistula renders the afflicted woman totally incontinent of urine and/or feces. This problem is confined almost exclusively to women in impoverished, non-industrialized countries.
- The fistula problem is embedded in a complex social matrix in which low socioeconomic status

for women, early marriage and constricted life choices, female illiteracy, harmful traditional medical practices, and poor distribution of health-care services are intertwined. Together, all of these factors prevent timely access to emergency obstetric care when it is needed.

- The problem of obstetric fistulas has been largely neglected by the international public health community. Inadequate resources have been devoted to developing the infrastructure for obstetric care necessary to detect obstructed labor and to prevent it from becoming prolonged. Prompt access to emergency obstetric services must remain a high priority for maternal health worldwide.
- When obstetric fistulas arise, most can be repaired using "low-technology" surgical services at modest cost, but inadequate resources have been mobilized to treat women currently suffering from a fistula. Dealing with the backlog of unrepaired obstetric fistulas should be a high priority in the development of surgical services for women in non-industrialized countries. This can best be done by creating special surgical wards in general hospitals to treat "low-risk" fistulas and by creating specialist fistula referral centers in those parts of the world where fistulas are common.

Key Terms

Cephalopelvic disproportion (CPD)	Obstetric fistula	Traditional birth attendant
Cesarean section	Obstructed labor	Vesicovaginal fistula
Fetal malpresentation	Obstructed labor injury complex	Worldwide Fistula Fund
Fistula	Rectovaginal fistula	
Incontinence	Specialist fistula center	

Questions for Discussion

1. Define the following terms:

   a. Fistula.
   b. Obstetric fistula.
   c. Vesicovaginal fistula.
   d. Rectovaginal fistula.

2. Using the World Fistula Fund's pathways to the development of obstetric fistula, describe the biological, socioeconomic, and cultural factors that contribute to the development of the condition.
3. Outline and discuss measures (medical and nonmedical) for treatment, prevention, and eradication of obstetric fistula.

References

Arrowsmith S, Hamlin E, Wall L (1996) Obstructed labor injury complex: Obstetric fistula formation and the multifaceted morbidity of maternal birth trauma in the developing world. Obstetrical and Gynecological Survey, 51, 568–574

Dolea C, AbouZahr C (2003) Global Burden of Obstructed Labor in the Year 2000. Evidence and Information for Policy (EIP) Unit, World Health Organization. Geneva: World Health Organization. www.who.int/healthinfo/statistics/bod_obstructedlabour.pdf, cited 2 August 2008

Dumont A, de Bernis L, Bourvier-Colle MH et al. for the MOMA Study Group (2001) Cesarean section rate for maternal indication in sub-Saharan Africa: a systematic review. Lancet, 358, 1328–1334

Elkins TE, Wall LL (1996) Report of a pilot project on the rapid training of pelvic surgeons in techniques of obstetric vesico-vaginal fistula repair in Ghana and Nigeria. Journal of Pelvic Surgery, 2, 182–186

Holme A, Breen M, MacArthur C (2007) Obstetric fistulae: a study of women managed at the Monze Mission Hospital, Zambia. BJOG, 114(8), 1010–1017

Konje JC, Oladipo LA (2000) Nutrition and obstructed labor. American Journal of Clinical Nutrition, 72(Suppl), 291S–297S

Mathers CD, Loncar D (2006) Projections of global mortality and burden of disease from 2002 to 2030. PLoS Medicine, 3(11), e442

Moerman ML (1982) Growth of the birth canal in adolescent girls. American Journal of Obstetrics and Gynecology, 143(5), 528–532

Onolemhemhen OD, Ekwempu CC (1999) An investigation of sociomedical risk factors associated with vaginal fistula in northern Nigeria. Women's Health, 28(3), 103–116

Prevention of Maternal Mortality Network (1992) Barriers to treatment of obstetric emergencies in rural communities of West Africa. Studies in Family Planning, 23(5), 279–291

Smellie W (1752) A Set of Anatomical Tables, 2nd ed. London, England: Wilson & Durham

Thaddeus S, Maine D (1994) Too far to walk: maternal mortality in context. Social Science and Medicine, 38, 1091–1110

Wall L, Arrowsmith S (2007) The "continence gap": a critical concept in obstetric fistula repair. International Urogynecology Journal, 18(8), 843–844(2)

Wall LL (1998) Dead mothers and injured wives: the social context of maternal morbidity and mortality among the Hausa of northern Nigeria. Studies in Family Planning, 29(4), 341–359

Wall LL (2002) Fitsari 'dan Duniya: an African (Hausa) praise-song about vesicovaginal fistulas. Obstetrics and Gynecology, 100, 1328–1332

Wall LL, Karshima J, Kirschner C et al. (2004) The obstetric vesicovaginal fistula: characteristics of 899 patients from Jos, Nigeria. American Journal of Obstetrics and Gynecology, 190, 1011–1119

Wall LL, Arrowsmith SD, Briggs ND et al. (2005) The obstetric vesicovaginal fistula in the developing world. Obstetrical and Gynecology Survey, 60(Suppl 1), S1–S55

Wall L (2005) Hard questions concerning fistula surgery in third world countries. Journal of Women's Health, 14(9), 863–866

Wall L (2006a) Obstetric vesicovaginal fistula as an international public health problem. Lancet, 368, 1201–1209

Wall LL (2006b) The medical ethics of Dr. J. Marion Sims: a fresh look at the historical record. Journal of Medical Ethics, 32(6), 346–350

Weil O, Fernandez H (1999) Is safe motherhood an orphan initiative? Lancet, 354, 940–943

World Health Organization (WHO) (1994) Maternal health and safe motherhood programme. World Health Organization partograph in management of labour. Lancet, 344, 1399–1404

Chapter 18
Health Challenges for Women, Children, and Adolescents with Disabilities

Amy T. Wilson

Learning Objectives After reading this chapter and answering the discussion questions that follow, you should be able to

- Discuss the meaning and causes of disabilities.
- Present an overview of the global prevalence of disabilities among women, children, and adolescents.
- Discuss the relationship between poverty and disability.
- Appraise how local attitudes and beliefs frame society's perspective on disability and the effects these have on the health of women, children, and adolescents with disabilities.
- Evaluate international and national efforts and strategies to improve access to health and social care for women, children, and adolescents with disabilities.

Introduction

This chapter discusses the definition and causes of disability; global prevalence of disabilities; and the relationship between poverty and disability. Since one of the greatest barriers against access to appropriate health care for women and children with disabilities is negative societal attitude, this chapter examines how local concepts and beliefs frame a society's perspective of disability and how this perspective affects the status of women and children with disabilities. Another important barrier that women and children with disabilities face is the lack of national disability policies or laws or the

nonenforcement of such policies and laws where they exist. International and national efforts and strategies to improve inclusion and access to health and social care for women and children with disabilities are discussed.

The United Nations Convention on the Rights of Persons with Disabilities (2007) defines disability to include persons who have long-term physical, mental, intellectual, or sensory impairments which in interaction with various barriers may hinder their full and effective participation in society on an equal basis with others. The World Health Organization (2005) estimates that 600 million people, of which half are female and one-third are children, live with a mental, physical, or cognitive disability and that 70–80% of this population reside in developing countries. This amounts to nearly 200 million children who never reach their full cognitive potential (Msall and Hogan 2007). Of these, 80% live in impoverished rural areas. According to data from UNICEF (2007a), there is a wide variation among countries in the percentage of children with disability, ranging from 2% in Uzbekistan to 35% in Djibouti (Table 18.1).

Disparities in disability among countries can be explained by variations in largely preventable causes related to nutrition, exposure to environmental risks, accidents and conflicts, chronic infections, congenital impairments, and access to health-care services (Table 18.2). In the developed world, the prevalence of disability has been significantly reduced by health systems that address the causes of motor disabilities (WHO 2007).

Frequently, individuals with disabilities do not have the opportunity to attend school, work in the

A.T. Wilson (✉)
Gallaudet University, Washington, DC, USA

Table 18.1 Percentage of children aged 2–9 years with at least one disability, 2005

Country	Percentage
Djibouti	35
Central African Republic	31
Cameroon	23
Sierra Leon	23
Bangladesh	18
Mongolia	17
São Tomé and Príncipe	16
Ghana	16
Iraq	15
Jamaica	15
Montenegro	13
Thailand	12
Albania	11
Serbia	11
FYR Macedonia	10
Bosnia Herzegovina	7
Uzbekistan	2

Source: UNICEF (2007a)

Table 18.2 Preventable causes of disability

Disability	Associated health condition
Blindness	Vitamin A deficiency
Deafness	Measles, mumps, rubella, bacterial meningitis
Motor disability	Polio, cerebral palsy, iodine deficiency
Motor and cognitive disability	Accidents and injury

Source: Rasheed (1999)

formal marketplace, or live independent, fulfilling lives. Due to lack of appropriate services, they are forced to depend on their families and communities for physical and economic support. Women with disabilities can be treated differently according to why they are disabled, where they live, what their disability is, and what myths or beliefs may exist about their right to be wives and mothers. Both disabled women and children may confront social stigmatization and exclusion from family and community life as a result of just being different.

Although many poor people struggle to obtain appropriate health care, poor people with disabilities, and specifically women, are often the least able to access needed health care. Additional obstacles can include inaccessible public transport to health facilities, clinic buildings with steps but no ramps, lack of Braille or audio informational materials for blind people, and medical staff that are unable to communicate with their deaf clients. While poverty can lead to disability, disability is also a major cause of poverty. Having a disability can trigger social and economic difficulties for individuals, their families, their communities, and even countries. For children, lack of services appropriate to their needs can result in slower learning and difficulty progressing in school. These difficulties in childhood may lead to inability to live as independent adults later on. In addition, inaccessible environment often makes it difficult for adults with disabilities to secure employment, to perform a job as required, or to keep employment.

Without the right to appropriate education or access to employment, people with disabilities are effectively denied the right to become independent and contributing members of society. In order to improve the quality of life for people with disabilities, their families, and society as a whole, the global community needs to (a) standardize the terms concerning disability, (b) collect accurate and valid data about all aspects of people with disabilities in order to assist and monitor them (e.g., kind of disability, educational level, socioeconomic status), (c) create national programs, policies, and strategies for including people with disabilities, (d) increase and improve the health and rehabilitation services available to people with disabilities, and (e) promote the economic and social acceptance, inclusion, and empowerment of people with disabilities in their homes and national communities.

Disabled People's Organizations from around the world along with Member States of the United Nations met for over a period of 5 years to write the United Nations Convention for the Rights of People with Disabilities. Adopted on December 2006, it aims to protect and monitor the human rights of all persons with disabilities. It encourages, "... governments to work towards developing appropriate education policies and practices for children and adults with disabilities, to include persons with disabilities in strategies and plans aimed at eradicating poverty, promoting education and enhancing employment, and to take account of the right of persons with disabilities to housing, shelter,

Box 18.1 Articles 25 and 26 of the UN Convention for the Rights of People with Disabilities

Article 25 – Health: States Parties recognize that persons with disabilities have the right to the enjoyment of the highest attainable standard of health without discrimination on the basis of disability. States Parties shall take all appropriate measures to ensure access for persons with disabilities to health services that are gender-sensitive, including health-related rehabilitation. In particular, States Parties shall

(a) provide persons with disabilities with the same range, quality and standard of free or affordable healthcare and programmes as provided to other persons, including in the area of sexual and reproductive health and population-based public health programmes;

(b) provide those health services needed by persons with disabilities specifically because of their disabilities, including early identification and intervention as appropriate, and services designed to minimize and prevent further disabilities, including among children and older persons;

(c) provide these health services as close as possible to people's own communities, including in rural areas;

(d) require health professionals to provide care of the same quality to persons with disabilities as to others, including on the basis of free and informed consent by, inter alia, raising awareness of the human rights, dignity, autonomy and needs of persons with disabilities through training and the promulgation of ethical standards for public and private healthcare;

(e) prohibit discrimination against persons with disabilities in the provision of health insurance, and life insurance where such insurance is permitted by national law, which shall be provided in a fair and reasonable manner;

(f) prevent discriminatory denial of healthcare or health services or food and fluids on the basis of disability.

Article 26 – Habilitation and rehabilitation:

1. States Parties shall take effective and appropriate measures, including through peer support, to enable persons with disabilities to attain and maintain maximum independence, full physical, mental, social and vocational ability, and full inclusion and participation in all aspects of life. To that end, States Parties shall organize, strengthen and extend comprehensive habilitation and rehabilitation services and programmes, particularly in the areas of health, employment, education and social services, in such a way that these services and programmes

(a) begin at the earliest possible stage, and are based on the multidisciplinary assessment of individual needs and strengths;

(b) support participation and inclusion in the community and all aspects of society, are voluntary, and are available to persons with disabilities as close as possible to their own communities, including in rural areas.

2. States Parties shall promote the development of initial and continuing training for professionals and staff working in habilitation and rehabilitation services.

3. States Parties shall promote the availability, knowledge and use of assistive devices and technologies, designed for persons with disabilities, as they relate to habilitation and rehabilitation (p. 1).

Source: United Nations Enable (2007)

transport and supportive equipment" (United Nations Enable 2007). Two integral articles protecting the rights of people with disabilities in receiving appropriate health care are Article 25 and 26 (United Nations Enable 2007), which must be considered by Member States when writing health-care policies (Box 18.1). United Nations Conventions are international law and the countries that sign and ratify the convention have the legal responsibility to enforce them. National civil rights laws must reflect the articles agreed upon in the convention. Disabled People's Organizations and their advocates are working diligently to ensure that the articles in the convention are becoming national policy. In the past, strategies to assist those with disabilities focused on treating their medical problem. In current, transformative strategies, the disabled people advocate for themselves with health-care programs as allies alongside them, their families, and their communities.

Definition of Disability

Finding consensus on the definition of disability has been difficult, mainly because of the different medical and social perspectives from which people view disabilities. Historically, disability has been conceptualized as a medical problem caused by a disease, a trauma, or some other health condition. The disabled person was seen first and foremost as "disabled." Medical professionals attempted to cure the individual or change the person's behavior so that he or she would fit into the community as a "normal" person. Often children and adults with disabilities were institutionalized or put under custodial care where they were left to survive or receive rehabilitation. In this medical model, the person is seen as defective, and the role of how the social and physical environment may disable the individual is ignored. The political framework for this medical conceptualization of disability focused on reducing functional limitations and providing preventative health care.

The other conceptualization of disability is the social model, which classifies functioning and disability from the perspective of a person's life circumstances. This model considers how the environment influences whether a person with a disability is included in and able to gain access to, their family,

community, and society. As such, it underscores that society's failure to recognize the needs of people with disabilities marginalizes and excludes them from full integration into society. Rather than entirely focusing on cures or rehabilitation, the social model encourages the community to modify the environment so that all people can participate fully in all aspects of society. The political framework for a social conceptualization of disability calls for an attitudinal change by society to see people not as disabled, but different, to reduce the social, natural, and built environmental barriers, and to advocate for disabled persons' human rights rather than only lobbying for better health care.

To compare the two models, consider the case of deaf children. Historically, the medical model prescribed many arduous years learning to speech-read for these children. This "solution" placed the burden of disability on the child. Alternatively, the social model's approach would adapt the environment to respect and to include the child's difference by, for example, providing closed captioning or teachers fluent in sign language.

Disability-Adjusted Life Year (World Development Report)

Attempts to quantify the impact of disabilities vary widely depending on whether one believes that a disability is a health burden or a societal issue that must be addressed. In 1993, The World Bank addressed the definition of disability when it conducted a study concerning the global burden of disease in collaboration with the World Health Organization and the Harvard School of Public Health. One outcome of the collaboration was the disability-adjusted life year (DALY), a quantitative indicator of the state of the health of a country. The purposes of the DALY were to "(a) assist in setting health service priorities; (b) identify disadvantaged groups and target health interventions, and (c) provide a comparable measure of output for intervention, program, and sector evaluation and planning."

The DALY was created to calculate the total amount of healthy life lost by a person from either premature mortality, poor health, or some degree of disability, either physical or mental, during a specific period of time. A panel of experts weighed how diseases and disabilities affected mortality rates in order to create "disability weights." To calculate the burden of the disability/disease, one takes the predetermined disability weight and then multiplies it by the number of years lived in "that health state" and then adds the number of years lost due to that disease/disability. Theoretically, the DALY can help a country determine how to use funds more cost effectively and prioritize health interventions. For instance, if a country found that HIV/AIDS imposed the heaviest health burden on its populace, resources could be targeted to address HIV/AIDS.

Critics of the DALY argue that methods to collect data required to calculate disability are inefficient and require huge amounts of resources. Moreover, critics point out that the DALY itself and its disability weights include value judgments that have economic, political, and ethical implications. Its false assumptions include that disabilities affect quality of life across the globe – with no regard to individual health status or environmental factors – and that the medical diagnosis of the disability – not family circumstance, location, or access to health care – is the sole indicator of quality of life with a disability (Metts 2000).

In addition, the DALY equation and the disability weights imply that nondisabled persons are more valuable to society. However, health interventions and proper support can assist disabled people in participating in and contributing to society. For example, a wheelchair user may score very low on the DALY. However, this wheel chair user may be a brilliant woman, married with children, living in her own home, and earning an income and contributing to society as a computer software designer. Critics worry that because the DALY does not accurately portray the potential of disabled persons to contribute to society, policy decisions based on its framework may favor the application of scarce health resources to extend the lives of the able-bodied over those with a disability. The amount of funds officials will be willing to allocate to education, job training, social inclusion, health services, accessible architecture, transportation systems, and other support infrastructure for disability may be far less.

ICHS International Classification of Impairments, Disabilities, and Handicaps (WHO)

Another conceptual framework of disability is the International Classification of Impairments (ICIDH) and its newer version, the International Classification of Functioning, Disability and Health (ICF) (WHO 2003). The ICF differs from the DALY in that it is not quantitative and that it recognizes that a person's disability varies according to the degree to which the impairment affects his or her ability to function in the environment. The 1980 version of ICIDH (WHO 1980) was first in distinguishing "disability" from "impairment" and "handicap." While historically these three terms were used interchangeably, the move from a medical model to a social model requires that the definition of these terms be more clearly distinguished.

"Impairments" are the result of a disease or a disorder (such as cerebral palsy) which causes "a restriction or a lack of ability to perform an activity in a manner or within a range considered normal for a human being." A "disability" (such as lack of muscle coordination, which limits one's ability to do fine motor work) is a result of impairment and defined as a loss or an abnormality of anatomical, physiological, or psychological structure or function. "Handicaps" are the result of impairments and disabilities and are defined as disadvantages that a person experiences because society prevents or limits the role they would normally play in society depending upon their age, gender, and social/cultural factors. A woman with cerebral palsy may experience the handicap of not finding employment if a computer keyboard is not adapted to accommodate her ataxia. Impairment, such as a cleft lip, may not cause a disability but may be a handicap since it could limit a person's ability to relate socially.

The ICIDH also helped highlight for researchers and policy makers the role, power, and responsibility of society to become more accommodating for people with disabilities. For example, society can alter its attitudes toward disabilities and construct accessible classrooms, offices, hospitals, and other public spaces. Removing barriers to participation in family, community, educational, and vocational activities can then vastly improve economic, social, and health opportunities for people with disabilities. However, while the ICF serves to classify disabilities without regard to the ability of an individual to function in society, it does not allow for the quantification of the burden of disease and disabilities on a society. As a result, DALYs are still used in analyzing disease burdens on a society and in calculating the cost–benefit of proposed interventions.

Currently, the World Health Organization refers to the ICIDH as the International Classification of Functioning, Disability, and Health (ICF) and suggests using it in clinical settings, health services, or surveys and with individuals or at population levels. WHO (2007) writes that the ICF " …is a classification of health and health related domains that describe body functions and structures, activities and participation. The domains are classified from body, individual and societal perspectives" (WHO 2003). Table 18.3 provides an example of ICF model scenarios that describe both the disability

and its effect on a preschooler's life. The ICF recognizes that "since an individual's functioning and disability occurs in a context, the ICF also includes a list of environmental factors." As such, the World Health Organization has shifted in looking at disability from a medical model to a social model.

Disability in Developing Countries

Traditionally, in developed countries, people with disabilities were hidden from society and considered diseased or sick and in need of protection, treatment, and/or a cure. It was their families or welfare, health, religious, and charitable organizations that assumed responsibility for caring for these individuals by locking them away in institutions or sending them to special schools or sheltered workshops. Health care centered on developing prosthetics or providing rehabilitation in order to fix the disability without regard to the person's spiritual or psychological self. People with disabilities were not afforded the same

Table 18.3 ICF model scenarios in preschool children with physical disability in developing countries

Dimension	Definition	Girl, 3 years	Boy, 5 years	Girl, 4 years
Pathophysiology	Molecular/cellular mechanisms	Burns to face, chest, arms	Left cerebrovascular accident after severe dehydration	Hearing loss after cerebral malaria
Body structures and body functions	Organ structure/ function	Unable to lift arm above head or extend elbows	Hemiplegia; adaptive delays	Speech delays, 50db hearing loss
Activity (functional) strengths	Ability to perform essential activities: feed, dress, toilet, walk, talk	Runs well; memorizes songs and stories	Walks; very strong with left hand	Speech understood 50% of time
Activity (functional) limitations	Difficulty in performing essential activities	Unable to carry water from well	Cannot run; has lost animals during chores	Speech not understood by peers
Participation	Involvement in community roles typical of peers	Goes to church/ mosque	Helps in meal preparation	Loves to make baskets; herds animals
Participation restrictions	Difficulty in assuming roles typical of peers	Because of stigma, unable to leave hut for school	No soccer because he is considered "lame" by peers	No hearing aids available
Contextual factors	Attitudinal, legal, policy, and architectural facilitators	Has younger brother; minister at church encourages singing	Grandmother is positive influence; she encourages craft work	Audiologist is available in capital city (500 miles away); home village is not on bus route

Source: Msall and Hogan (2007)

civil and human rights that others enjoyed such as education, employment, freedom to marry, vote, drive, use their natural language (sign language), make decisions about their health care (could be sterilized against their will), or own property.

Although not yet fully equal, women with disabilities in developed countries, and in a few developing countries, enjoy richer, fuller lives than in the past. Unfortunately, the governments of many developing countries have not legally recognized the rights of their disabled citizens – or, if they do, these laws often are poorly enforced. In some instances, people with disabilities have been targets of genocide and infanticide (Supple 2007). In some cases, discrimination against children comes from within the family itself. Parents can decide not to feed or care for their disabled child as they would their able-bodied children. Parents can also make health decisions, such as sterilization and institutionalization, over the objections of their disabled child (Sullivan and Knutson 2000).

Today, in most developing countries, clinics, health centers, and hospitals are not accessible to people with disabilities. Common barriers include, but are not limited to, no ramps for people with motor difficulties, no materials in Braille, large print, or on tape for women with vision difficulties, no sign language interpreters for deaf people, no one who can explain information at an appropriate level to people with cognitive impairments, and no doctors or nurses trained or educated about the special health needs of people with disabilities. If a person with a disability is able to visit a clinic, there is still often the view that they are not normal and must be cured or rehabilitated. Women with disabilities report that medical personnel often ask questions about their disability even when they seek assistance for an entirely unrelated problem. For example, a woman's concern about sexually transmitted disease, the flu, or a lump in her breast may be ignored in favor of asking about her spinal cord injury.

Due in part to the lack of strong policies protecting the rights of people with disabilities, domestic and foreign charitable organizations have historically assumed the role of caretaker and continues to do so in recent years. Since the majority of these organizations are administered without the involvement or the participation of people with disabilities in the planning, running, or evaluation of their

programs, in developing countries, movement toward a socially empowering model of full integration of people with disabilities into society is still not prevalent. Nevertheless, a disproportionate share of disabilities is born by the poorest individuals in the developing world. The WHO estimates that 10% or 600 million people live with disabilities worldwide. Metts' World Bank study (2000) estimates that "half a billion disabled people are undisputedly amongst the poorest of the poor," while Elwan (1999) contends that 15–20% of the poorest in developing countries have disabilities. James Wolfensohn, former president of the World Bank, has said that "Unless disabled people are brought into the development mainstream, it will be impossible to cut poverty in half by 2015 or to give every girl and boy the chance to achieve a primary education by the same date – goals agreed to by more than 180 world leaders at the United Nations Millennium Summit in September 2000" (2002). Yet, disability is not mentioned specifically in any of the Millennium Development Goals and its role in contributing to other MDGs is largely ignored in the development framework (Secretariat of the African Decade for Persons with Disabilities 2007).

Since people with disabilities are marginalized by their community and discriminated against, it is difficult to gather data on the incidence, distribution, or trends of disability. Barriers to data collection include the different conceptualizations of disability throughout the world and the limited number of censuses, surveys, or health records which can reliably report the number of people with disabilities within a country. Eide and Loeb's (2006) literature review of existing studies concerning disability statistics showed the need to standardize measures since the data suffered from "poor quality, lack of comparability, and limited applicability." Historically, the United Nations Disability Statistics Database, or DISTAT, has amassed the largest amount of disability statistics assembled from individual countries' own national surveys, censuses, and administrative records from as early as 1970 and until 1995. Critics claim that the collected data are outdated, random, inadequate for a systemized analysis, and plagued by conceptual and definitional problems. For example, DISTAT reports data for Bangladesh from a 1987 demographic sample survey where interviewees were asked if anyone in the home was disabled and if so, were they blind, crippled, deaf and dumb, mentally handicapped, or other. Did the interviewees understand the terms given? Would the interviewer be able to explain the terms? How did their culture view disability? Would family members hide the person with a disability or even understand if a family member had a disability? Many concerns with the survey questions and design undermine the validity of the survey's findings. Because of the lack of reliable data, monitoring equality and opportunity for people with disabilities in receiving health care over time is relatively unfeasible.

However, interest in collecting valid data concerning disabilities is increasing. In 2001, the United Nations International Seminar on Measurement of Disability formed the Washington Group on Disability Statistics with the goal to standardize the collection of disability statistics in order to compare the data between countries. The United Nations Statistics Division annually collects country data such as: "... population size and composition, fertility, mortality, infant and fetal mortality, marriage and divorce" (United Nations 2006) in its Demographic Yearbook and in March 2006, added basic statistics on disability. The World Bank is currently working toward gathering disability statistics in partnership with other international organizations.

The Cycle of Poverty and Disability

Poverty Leads to Disability

Despite the inconsistency between how disability is defined and measured, and the questionable validity of the data that have been collected, one fact remains consistent – the strong link between poverty and disability. Poverty can lead to disability, and disability can lead to poverty. Poverty is a major factor in the increase in the number of people with disabilities throughout the world. Preventable communicable, perinatal, and maternal diseases, which cause disabilities, are regularly found in children of the poor. Malnutrition, lack of immunizations, contaminated injections, inadequate and poor health or medical care all contribute to disabilities. Refugees and people living in poorer rural areas are drawn to

overcrowded urban areas in search of employment and find themselves working in unregulated, unsafe work environments that put them at high risk of accident-related impairments (such as spinal cord injury, physical, and/or cognitive injuries due to neurotrauma, partial or complete amputation of limbs), diabetes, exposure to dangerous chemicals which can cause chronic respiratory or cardiovascular diseases, and cancer. Women may be injured as a result of violence from their employer or as a consequence of advocating for better working conditions. Poor people may have no recourse but to live in unsanitary conditions where they are exposed to pollutants in the air and water, debilitating diseases such as tuberculosis or leprosy and other infectious. The United Nations (2007) estimates that up to 25% of disabilities may be the result of injuries and violence such as child abuse, domestic abuse, youth violence, traffic accidents, falls, burns, war, and abandoned land mines, cluster bombs, chemicals, and bullets. Disabilities may also occur because uneducated poor people may be unaware of the high risks of passing on congenital disabilities when marrying within the family (for example, Down syndrome, deafness, muscular dystrophy), or that a woman has a higher risk of giving birth to a disabled child when over the age of 40, or if she has previously given birth to one or more children with a disability.

Disability Leads to Poverty

When disabled people are excluded from the opportunity to gain the skills they need to take care of themselves or denied the chance to generate their own income, they may slide into poverty. The UN states that only 2% of people with disabilities are able to access basic services within their communities. Marginalization from social institutions, which create and enforce policy concerning basic services, means that children and adults with disabilities do not attend school or receive vocational training, have lower expectations for themselves, are more vulnerable to exploitation and abuse, and are not included in economic development projects or programs offered by domestic or international organizations. Often times, a child or an elderly person with disabilities may be hidden away in their homes because of a family's shame, overprotectiveness, or a lack of knowledge on how to care for their disabled family member. The disabled person then becomes permanently dependent on the family that may then suffer economically if a wage earner needs to stay home to care for them. Some disabled children, adolescents, and adults, rejected by their families, become beggars or street workers who are even more excluded from society.

For women with disabilities, the results of marginalization can lower an already low ability to gain access to resources needed for a health life. In many countries, able-bodied women and girls have less access to resources or opportunities compared to able-bodied men and boys. Women and girls with disabilities often receive even less attention and care from their families and their communities. They are denied rehabilitation, good nutrition, access to maternal health care, or health care meant to prevent and treat illness. Only 1% of girls with disabilities in developing countries are enrolled in school and their literacy rate is under 5%. Girls who do attend school attend for a shorter amount of time than boys. In adulthood, women with disabilities do not have equal access to paid employment. Moreover, they are twice as unlikely to find work as their male counterparts and are often forced to work in the informal market. Globally, approximately 300 million women and girls with disabilities are doubly discriminated against because they live not only as females but also as females with disabilities.

Countering Negative Social Beliefs Toward People with Disabilities

Groce (2000) writes that various cultures assign a person's disability or "difference" to three major categories of social beliefs that are frequently negative: (a) *causality*: a cultural explanation which may stem from religious beliefs or folk medicine for why a difference occurs. For example, a mother who believes her child has a disability because of the evil eye cast her way during pregnancy may treat the disabled child differently than her other children. Another mother of a child with epilepsy may believe the disability to be caused by "spirits" and could think of her child in a negative manner. (b) *Valued*

and devalued attributes: Specific physical or intellectual attributes may be valued or devalued depending upon the society in which a child with a disability is born. For example, a "different" child may be accepted as a special gift from God, which leads to overprotection of the child. (c) *Anticipated role*: The role that people are expected to fulfill as adults in their community determines how they are accepted into their society. For example, the eldest adult son in a family may assume extra responsibilities or a young woman may be expected to bring wealth to her family through marrying someone of similar or higher status. The families may be concerned that because of the disability, the child would not be able to fulfill his or her anticipated role upon adulthood.

Finally, lack of understanding about the cause of a disability may lead to social exclusion. Some families with a disabled child are ostracized by their neighbors because of fear that the disability can spread to others or that associating with the child or her family will bring bad luck. All of these factors lead to discrimination toward people with disabilities and their families and prevent them from participating fully in the economic, social, educational, and political life of their communities.

For women and girls with disabilities, discrimination raises even more barriers to participation in society. If a baby girl is born with a disability and is allowed to live, she must contend with negative attitudes and beliefs about disability from her family and community. Often girls with disabilities are hidden within their homes where they care for children and relatives, cook, clean, and do daily chores. They have less access to health-care services, will not attend school or work, will be subject to physical abuse, sexual abuse and higher risk for HIV infection, will not receive rehabilitation services or HIV/AIDS education, testing, or access to clinical programs, and will receive less care and food in the home than her siblings (Werner 1999). Disabled women are discriminated against and remain marginalized and poor as a result of attitudinal, social, cultural, environmental, and economic barriers of society. They often have no rights to own or inherit land, to earn a fair wage, be promoted, or work without job discrimination.

The responsibilities and roles traditionally assigned to women for care of children and other family members mean that the experience of disability

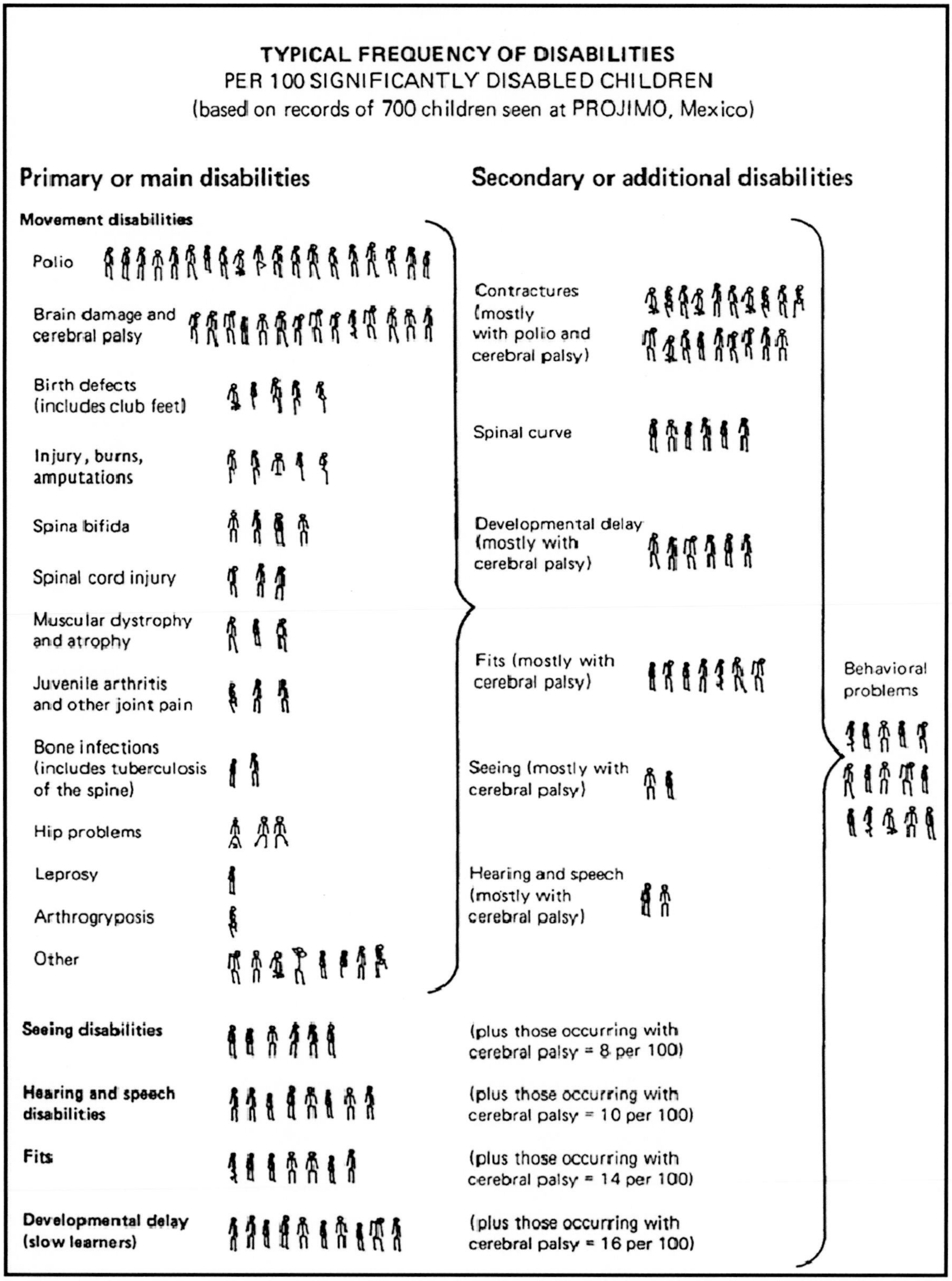

Fig. 18.1 Disabled village children disability frequency educational material. Source: Werner (1999)

is different for women than men. Some societies believe that women with disabilities are unable to fill the roles of a "good" wife and mother, thus assuming they are sexually inactive. As a result, societies may deny these women reproductive and maternal health care and HIV/AIDS/STD information. However, it has been shown that people with disabilities are as sexually active as their able-bodied peers, are able to and do become pregnant, are as frequently homosexual and bisexual as society as a whole, use drugs and alcohol, and are at higher risk of being victims of domestic and sexual abuse. Disregarding the sexual activity of disabled women, society keeps health care inaccessible to their special needs and denies the sexual and physical abuse they suffer. This cycle serves as an example of how societal beliefs and incorrect assumptions put women, their children, their partners, and families at greater health and economic risk.

Interventions aimed at educating local health-care workers on the nature of disabilities may help counteract the prevalence of negative societal beliefs toward disabled women and children, especially as they relate to health care. Below is a chart from *Disabled Village Children: A Guide for Community Health Workers, Rehabilitation Workers, and Families* (Fig. 18.1). This chart uses records of 700 children seen at PROJIMO, Mexico, between 1982 and 1985. It uses visuals, such as the little drawings of people, to show how many children might have each disability in a group of 100 significantly disabled village children. While the actual figures would be different depending on time and place, illustrative guides such as this one can be powerful tools in expanding local knowledge about disability.

A Changing Approach to Health Care for the Disabled Poor

Through time, a new perspective has emerged through the work of human rights advocates and Disabled People's Organizations where, as explained earlier in this chapter, people accept the social model of disability. This change may particularly improve the lives of women and children with disabilities.

Prevention, Increased Information, and Advocacy

Many childhood disabilities are preventable. Health care for low-income countries must incorporate strategies to address sources of disabilities, such as protein energy malnutrition, iodine deficiency, and infectious disease. Table 18.4 suggests some successful public health strategies for reducing the overall prevalence of disabilities and achieving a healthier society.

Table 18.4 Strategies for preventing disabilities and promoting disability awareness

Primary Level	Secondary Level	Tertiary Level
Increase immunization coverage	Screen for genetic disorders	Improve mother–child interaction to encourage better bonding and lower negative attitudes
Provide iodine, iron, zinc, and vitamin A supplementation through national programs	Screen for neonatal hypothyroidism	Provide better education and training for children in need
Develop school-meal programs	Identify intellectual and other disabilities in school and the community	Use different tools to improve hearing impairment
Improve parenting skills through schemes such as the Portage guide to home teaching	Increase level of awareness within the community; teachers to identify impairments	
Improve antenatal and postnatal care through programs such as Safe Motherhood		
Share information on birth spacing and harm of consanguineous marriage		

Source: Maulik and Darmstadt (2007)

Although little research has been done in the area of gender, development, and disability other than gathering statistics, international agencies are now beginning to recognize the need for more information (Singleton 2004). In 1997, disabled women from around the world began to organize and network at the International Leadership Forum, where women from 80 countries met in Washington, DC, as a follow up to the 1995 United Nations 4th World Conference on Women in Beijing. The purpose of the 1997 Forum was to monitor progress on the implementation of the Beijing Platform for Action. In addition, 10,000 women met at the United Nations "Beijing + 5: Women 2000 – Gender Equality, Development and Peace for the 21st Century." Among the participants were 65 women with disabilities from 31 countries who participated in the overall activities and in a training program. The nonprofit group Mobility International – USA holds Women's Institutes on Leadership and Disability and has published materials which document the many successes of women with disabilities from around the world (MIUSA 2007).

Community-Based Rehabilitation

Eighty percent of people with disabilities in developing countries live in rural areas where they have little or no access to schooling, health care, or vocational services. Most services are offered in large urban areas which may be difficult for people with disabilities to access because of transportation and communication barriers. About 30 years ago, the World Health Organization and UNESCO recognized this dilemma and noted that rehabilitation services were few and far between in rural areas. In response, the concept of Community-Based Rehabilitation (CBR) was created where services would be brought and taught to community and family members of those with disabilities. The goal was to integrate people with disabilities in their home communities, to begin educating the child as a toddler, to eliminate physical and social barriers in the community, to improve the health of the person with a disability, and to make them more independent socially and economically. CBR is the official approach used by many countries although not all CBR is the same. Some countries have set up centers where visits are made, while others have trained nonprofessionals to make home visits to train family and community members on how to do activities with their disabled child such as physical therapy, vocational training, games to stimulate their child's interest in the world around her, and using sign language with deaf children and adults. The ideal CBR program would be administered by people with disabilities and disabled trainers, but this is often not the case. The African Development Foundation lists both the pros and the cons of the CBR

Table 18.5 The achievements and limitations and risks of the CBR approach

Positive achievements	Limitations and risks
• Creates self-employment	• Becomes a top-down and technical project of community leaders, professionals, or the donors
• Builds up self-confidence and reduction of dependence and begging	• Does not rely on active participation and involvement of PWDs
• Positively changes community attitude	
• Integrates person with disabilities (PWDs) into social and economic development	• Competes for scarce community resources
• Encourages funders to support more community-based activities	• Emphasizes "fixing" children's disabilities, neglecting the vocational, educational, and employment components
• Empowers people with disabilities to display their talents within the society while participating in income-generating activities	• Creates suspicion among PWDs that they are being used by nondisabled persons
	• Undermines local initiatives
• Utilizes locally available resources	• Becomes politically motivated (e.g., a wheel chair donated to a deaf person by a politician who had no knowledge of the latter's needs)
• Creates sustainability by developing society's capability	
• Achieves the hitherto unreached	• Becomes difficult to coordinate because of lack of cooperation from the individual, family, or the community
	• Duplicates services from other programs

Source: African Development Foundation (2007)

approach to reaching people with disabilities in rural areas (Table 18.5).

A greatly modified and more holistic vision of CBR is being written through the collaboration of the International Labor Organization, the World Health Organization, UNESCO, Disabled People's Organizations, and 13 International Non-governmental Organizations. The new CBR guidelines, being field tested in 25 countries, contain five key domains which are necessary for all people to live with dignity and well-being and which reflect many of the core concepts found in the UN Convention on the Rights of People with Disabilities. The key components of the new CBR guidelines are health from existing health facilities, education from regular school or college, livelihood through traditional skills, income generation programs and micro-credit, social inclusion and participation through local cultural initiatives and community life, and empowerment (Khasnabis and Heinicke 2008). Rather than the older version of CBR which was medically focused, these CBR guidelines support including people with disabilities in all aspects of society, which can be seen in Fig. 18.2.

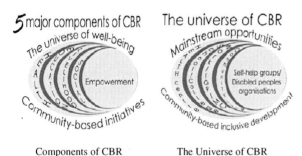

Components of CBR   The Universe of CBR

Fig: 18.2 The components and universe of CBR. Source: Khasnabis and Heinicke (2008)

Strategies and Health-Care Programs for Women with Disabilities

Development agencies are looking at poverty reduction programs, the human rights of women with disabilities, and long-term strategies to empower women with disabilities. These agencies must be aware that the resources and opportunities afforded to men are not granted to women. Not until these inequalities are balanced out, until women are represented in government institutions and can

participate in the creation of public policy, will their economic, educational, and legal rights be achieved. The health needs of women with disabilities will increasingly include problems beyond maternal health care, and health interventions must consider the unique characteristics of these women's lives that affect their ability to address these problems.

International health-care providers attempting to work with women and children with disabilities in developing countries must seriously consider effective strategies suggested by people with disabilities (Wilson 2006). A preliminary suggestion is that the organization's staff includes people with disabilities both domestically and in the host country. This change would necessitate a working environment that is accessible to all. MIUSA (2007) publishes a manual, funded by the United States Agency for International Development, which clearly describes how to make projects and programs inclusive both at home and abroad. The manual includes suggestions such as how to adapt technology for people with disabilities or how to make meetings, conferences, web sites, and information accessible to everyone.

Another suggestion for health care providers working with women and children overseas is that they work directly with organizations run by disabled women rather than organizations that may be taking care of women with disabilities rather than empowering them. While in some cases, women's disabilities may be so severe that this approach may not be possible, in many cases; international organizations can involve disabled women in the planning, implementation, and evaluation of the project or program. Often, Disabled People's Organizations (DPOs) are run by disabled men. Therefore, if no women's organization exists, the local DPOs should be encouraged to work with female members of the DPO either separately or in collaboration with the entire DPO. When possible, it is advisable to work directly with women who are disabled – they know themselves best.

In the case of working with children with disabilities, it is best to work directly with those who are affected by or live with the child. Parents are the best advocates for their children and have made the foremost impact on local and national policies throughout the world. Parents are often eager to fight for the rights of their children and to find them appropriate health care. In addition, adults who have grown up with the disability are also able to provide valuable insight and advocacy. Disabled adults may also be able to help parents and health-care workers better understand how a disabled child perceives their world and the services they receive. With age-appropriate support, disabled adolescents can advocate for themselves. As they are young enough to remember what it is like to be a child, they may, accordingly, have further firsthand insights to share on the needs of younger disabled children.

The health care provider must also understand (a) the many challenges and barriers that women with disabilities confront in their daily lives; (b) how different cultures respond to disability; and (c) how societies construct the meaning of disability. For example, a health-care worker would need to ask and answer questions such as, "In the majority culture, is being deaf perceived as either a negative or a positive attribute? Is there a religious belief that blindness is a gift, or punishment, from God?" Providers should also be trained and knowledgeable about the special health-care needs of women with disabilities and how best to care for them. (The best source for information on health care for women with disabilities in developing countries is "A Health Handbook for Women with Disabilities," which was developed with help of 40 different groups of women with disabilities in 27 countries around the world.) Health-care providers can be advocates and work alongside parents and women with disabilities to lobby local and national government agencies to write appropriate and fair health-care policies or to uphold existing ones.

Women and girls with disabilities in developing countries should be made aware that even small steps toward equal health care could make a big difference in their lives. Most often women and girls with disabilities are not taught about grooming and self health care since they are excluded from formal schooling and from the informal education of family conversations where information and experiences are shared by mothers, sisters, and aunts or by other women in the immediate community. Therefore, they may lack basic knowledge about proper care of their own body, about sexuality, pregnancy, childbirth and parenting, protection against sexual abuse, and against HIV/AIDS or STDs.

Women and girls with disabilities should be provided health education as well as the opportunity to learn more about their own disabilities and how to care for themselves. Only if women and girls with disabilities possess the knowledge about their own health care needs will they be able to take control over, and make informed decisions about, their own health and well-being. They can then educate their families, neighbors, and health-care providers about their needs.

Women and girls with disabilities or parents of children with disabilities could benefit from support groups. It is empowering for women to meet with one another to share their stories and experiences and to know there are others who understand what their lives are like. Women can share the knowledge they have learned with one another, plan social outings for their own pleasure, and to model to the community their "normalness," and open the group to others who may have no network outside of their home where they can make friends and learn social skills. They can also work with one another to bring attention to the unfair treatment of, or discrimination against, women and girls with disabilities in their community. Support groups sometimes become more formal women's organizations where members organize, learn leadership skills, start up small businesses, network with other disability organizations, request funding for small projects, and advocate for their civil and human rights both regionally and nationally.

Both support groups and more formalized women's organizations can work alongside health-care providers in being more "out" about their disability and increasing community awareness. Groups of women can make simple posters portraying aspects of their discrimination or things that should be changed in their environment. Empowered women can hold information sessions ("awareness events") for families, organize shows (handmade art, cooking, or a little play) for the immediate community, visit community services together, and work toward improving their assistance to people with disabilities. Instead of remaining isolated at home, women can support one another in joining community or church activities, in town or tribal meetings, and at family gatherings. They can play an active role in promoting change and changing attitudes about people with disabilities.

Health-care providers can learn from these disability groups as well as support them in creating appropriate materials (information, books, tools, trainings). Talk to them about their needs; let them educate you about their situation. Do not impose the changes without their involvement and direct participation. They may not be aware of the existing disability policies or health policies within their country or the UN Convention on Rights of people with disabilities. Health-care workers should teach them how to be advocates for themselves in getting appropriate health care and help them establish support groups and assist them in some of the activities mentioned above. Health service organizations should cooperate with other agencies that represent women and girls with disabilities and encourage them to lead the way in promoting the changes related to health care (topics such as establishing women health/body education, multileveled accessibility of the health-care system and information, education of professionals in health-care system, public awareness employment of women with disabilities in health-care system).

Incorporating Disability into MDG Strategies

Achieving MDGs will require an explicit disability dimension to be incorporated into these efforts. For example, the Secretariat of the African Decade for Persons with Disabilities (2002) asserts that the eradication of extreme poverty and hunger

(MDG #1) will be possible only through recognizing that disabled people and their families represent a very substantial proportion of the poor. A reduction in child mortality (MDG #4) must combat under-5 mortality of disabled children, which can be as high as 80% in some regions of Africa (UNICEF 2007b). Similarly, improvement in maternal health (MDG #5) will be achieved only by addressing the disabling impairments associated with pregnancy and childbirth, affecting up to 20 million women a year. To combat HIV/AIDS, malaria, and other diseases (MDG #6), we will need to account for the fact that disabled people are particularly vulnerable to these diseases (which are also a major cause of disabling impairments) (Secretariat of the African Decade for Persons with Disabilities 2007).

Conclusion

Meeting the unique health needs of women, children, and adolescents with disabilities in developing countries demands (a) a societal change in its attitudes concerning disability; (b) writing and enforcing health-care policies country by country; (c) empowering people with disabilities to advocate for their own health care personally and politically; and (d) comprehensive training for health-care practitioners in understanding how to communicate effectively with their disabled clients as well as to offer appropriate and accessible services to people with disabilities.

Key Terms

Able-bodied	Autonomy	Closed captioning
Abuse	Built environment	Cognitive disability
Access to health care	Cerebral palsy	Community-Based
Accidents	Chronic infections	Rehabilitation (CBR)
Amputation	Civil rights	Conflicts

Congenital impairments	Handicap	Poverty
Deaf children	Human rights	Quality of life
Dignity	Impairment	Rehabilitation
Disability	Inclusion	Sign language
Disability-adjusted life year (DALY)	Injuries	Social acceptance
	International Classification of Functioning, Disability and Health (ICF)	Social stigmatization
Disability weights		United Nations Convention on the Rights of Persons with Disabilities
Discrimination		
Disparities	International Classification of Impairments (ICIDH)	
Down syndrome		United Nations Disability Statistics Database (DISTAT)
Empowerment	Malnutrition	
Environmental risks	Marginalization	
Exclusion	Mobility	United Nations Enable
Exploitation	Motor disabilities	Violence
Gender	Muscular dystrophy	
Habilitation	Neurotrauma	

Questions for Discussion

1. Briefly discuss one major barrier to having a universally acceptable definition of disability.
2. Distinguish between the medical and social frameworks by which disability can be defined.
3. List any five causes of disability among women, children, and adolescents in less-developed countries.
4. In an essay of not more 1,000 words, describe the relationship between disability and poverty.
5. In what ways does disability affect access to health and social services for women, children, and adolescents in less-developed countries?
6. List any five strategies for improving the quality of life of women, children, and adolescents with disabilities. Discuss the potential barriers to implementing any of them.

References

African Development Foundation (2007) Community-based rehabilitation. In: African Development Foundation. http://www.adf.gov/SD&PWDch4.htm, cited 8 August 2008

Eide AH, Loeb ME (2006) Reflections on disability data and statistics in developing countries. In: B. Albert, In or out of The Mainstream? Lessons from Research on Disability and Development Cooperation. University of Leeds, Leeds England: The Disability Press

Elwan A (1999) Poverty and disability: a survey of the literature. Social Protection Discussion Series No. 9932. Social Protection Unit, Human Development Network, The World Bank. http://siteresources.worldbank.org/DISABILITY/Resources/280658-1172608138489/Poverty DisabElwan.pdf, cited 8 August 2008

Groce N (2000) Guest Editorial: Framing disability issues in local concepts and beliefs. Asia Pacific Disability Rehabilitation Journal, 10

Khasnabis C, Heinicke MK (2008) The participatory development of international guidelines for CBR. Leprosy Review 79: 17–29, http://www.lepra.org.uk/lr/Mar08/Lep17-29.pdf, cited 22 August 2008

Maulik P, Darmstadt G (2007) Childhood disability in low- and middle-income countries: Overview of screening, prevention, services, legislation, and epidemiology. Pediatrics, 120, S1–S55

Metts R (2000) Social Protection Discussion Paper No. 0007. World Bank. http://siteresources.worldbank.org/SOCIALPROTECTION/Resources/SP-Discussion-papers/Disability-DP/0007.pdf, cited 8 August 2008

MIUSA: Mobility International USA (2007) Institute on Leadership and Disability (WILD). http://miusa.org/wild, cited 8 August 2008

Msall M, Hogan D (2007) Counting children with disability in low-income countries: Enhancing prevention, promoting child development, and investing in economic well-being. Pediatrics, 120, 182–185

Rasheed S (1999) Major Causes and Consequences of Childhood Disability in Education Update, UNICEF. http://www.unicef.org/girlseducation/files/vol2disabileng.pdf, cited 8 August 2008

Secretariat of the African Decade for Persons with Disabilities (2002) Continental Plan of Action for the African

Decade of Persons with Disabilities. Pan-African Conference on the African Decade of Persons with Disabilities. Addis Ababa, Ethiopia. http://www.dpiafro.mr/ PDF%20FILES/Continental%20Plan%20of%20Action.pdf, cited 8 August 2008

Secretariat of the African Decade for Persons with Disabilities (2007) Moving from words to implementation in the struggle for human rights. Cape Town, South Africa. http://www.africandecade.org/reads/articles/disability-humanrights, cited 8 August 2008

Singleton T (2004) Gender and disability: a survey of Inter-Action member agencies: Findings and recommendations on inclusion of women and men with disabilities in international development programs. http://www.miusa.org/ publications/freeresources/media/genderdisabilityreport. PDF, cited 8 August 2008

Sullivan PM, Knutson JF (2000) Maltreatment and disabilities: a population-based epidemiological study. Child Abuse & Neglect, (10), 1257–1273

Supple C (2007) From prejudice to genocide: learning about the holocaust. Third Revised Edition. Staffordshire, England: Trentham Books

United Nations Children's Fund (UNICEF) (2007a) Children and the millennium development goals: progress towards a world fit for children. New York: UNICEF. http://www. unicef.org/worldfitforchildren/files/Children_and_the_ MDGs_Final_EN.pdf, cited 8 August 2008

United Nations Children's Fund (UNICEF) (2007b) Promoting the rights of children with disabilities. Innocenti Digest #13. New York: UNICEF Innocenti Research Center. http:// www.unicef-irc.org/publications/pdf/digest13-disability. pdf, cited 8 August 2008

United Nations Enable (2007) United Nations Convention on the Rights of People with Disabilities. New York: United Nations. http://www.un.org/disabilities/documents/convention/convoptprot-e.pdf, cited 8 August 2008

United Nations General Assembly A/61/611 (2007) United Nations Enable (December 6, 2006). http://www.un.org/ esa/socdev/enable/rights/convtexte.htm, cited 8 August 2008

United Nations Statistics Division (2006) Human functioning and disability. http://unstats.un.org/unsd/demographic/sconcerns/disability/disabmethodsDISTAT. aspx, cited 8 August 2008

Werner D (1999) Disabled village children: a guide for community health workers, rehabilitation workers and families. 5th Edition. Berkeley, CA: The Hesperian Foundation. http://www.dinf.ne.jp/doc/english/global/david/ dwe002/dwe00201.htm, cited 8 August 2008

Wilson A (2006) Studying the effectiveness of international development assistance from American organizations to deaf communities. American Annals of the Deaf, 150, 292–304. http://muse.jhu.edu/journals/american_annals_ of_the_deaf/v150/150.3wilson.html, cited 20 August 2008

Wolfensohn JD (2002) Poor, disabled and shut out. Washington Post, December 3. http://www.globalpolicy.org/soce con/develop/2002/1203disabled.htm, cited 8 August 2008

World Health Organization (WHO) (1980) International Classification of Impairments, Disabilities and Handicaps (ICF). A Manual of Classification Relating to the Consequences of Disease. Geneva: World Health Organization

World Health Organization (WHO) (2003) International Classification of Functioning, Disability and Health (ICF). Geneva: World Health Organization

World Health Organization (WHO) (2005) Disability, Including Prevention, Management and Rehabilitation. WHO Document #: WHA58.23. The Fifty-eighth World Health Assembly. Geneva: World Health Organization. http://www.who.int/gb/ebwha/pdf_files/ WHA58/WHA58_23-en.pdf, cited 8 August 2008

World Health Organization (WHO) (2007) International Classification of Functioning, Disability and Health (ICF). http:// www.who.int/classifications/icf/en/, cited 8 August 2008

Chapter 19
Unintentional Injuries in Children

William Pickett, Marianne Nichol, and John E. Ehiri

Learning Objectives After reading this chapter and answering the discussion questions that follow, you should be able to

- Identify key approaches for quantifying and measuring the burden of childhood injury.
- Discuss the contribution of injuries to global childhood mortality.
- Discuss the importance of analyzing childhood injury from a developmental perspective (i.e., according to developmental stages of children).
- Identify and appraise developmental, environmental, socioeconomic, and behavioral correlates of childhood injuries.
- Discuss factors related to inequity in childhood injury with regard to developed and less-developed countries.
- Assess the evidence base of interventions to prevent childhood injuries.

Introduction

Unintentional injuries are the leading cause of death for children in many developed countries, contributing more to potential life years lost than most other major causes of childhood illness combined. While infectious diseases and nutritional deficiencies still dominate the morbidity and mortality of children in developing countries, 98% of unintentional injuries occur in these parts of the world. Unfortunately, developing countries are also least equipped to prevent and manage injuries. Risk for unintentional injury varies by developmental stage, socioeconomic factors, environmental factors that protect or endanger the child, and characteristics of child behavior. Effective strategies for prevention must consider engineered changes to the physical environment and legislative regulation, in addition to educational interventions. Injury prevention is a growing field and, while disease surveillance is an established practice, effort is needed to create inexpensive and evidence-based prevention strategies for developing and developed nations.

With the advent of methods to control the development and spread of infectious disease, the prevention of childhood injuries has emerged as perhaps the leading public health challenge in some countries. There are few children in our world who do not feel the impact of injuries in their lives. Injuries happen frequently. They leave a substantial toll in terms of pain and suffering. The medical system and society in general incur great costs from injuries. In North America, as in many developed countries, once a child survives through infancy, injury becomes the leading potential cause of death until middle age. Injury also contributes more in terms of children's potential life years lost than cancer, cardiovascular disease, and other major causes of illness combined.

Within the past few decades, the epidemic of injuries has emerged as a major focus for prevention programs (WHO 2006). Once viewed and perhaps dismissed as unfortunate "accidents," health professionals have come to realize that injuries can be viewed conceptually as a disease with known causes, documented physical effects, and

W. Pickett (✉)
Department of Community Health and Epidemiology, Abramsky Hall, Queen's University, Kingston, Ontario, K7L 3N6, Canada

J.E. Ehiri (ed.), *Maternal and Child Health*, DOI 10.1007/b106524_19,
© Springer Science+Business Media, LLC 2009

predictable patterns of occurrence. Disease models and preventive thinking, originally developed for other causes of illness, have been adapted to childhood injury and have been helpful in establishing prevention initiatives and standardized treatment protocols. Through this process, a new collection of sciences emerged – those concerned with best practices for injury control.

Injuries in children may be more severe and have more lasting consequences than similar injuries in adults. Vulnerabilities include the potential for growth plate fractures that could result in disfigurement as the bone continues to grow, general organ immaturity that confers greater susceptibility to the harmful effects of environmental toxins, thin epidermis that increases the severity of burns, proportionately greater body surface area to volume that increases relative surface fluid loss after burns, smaller airways conferring greater risk for aspiration, and immunological immaturity that may complicate recovery from injury (Bartlett 2002).

Injury control scientists often categorize injuries into intentional and unintentional. *Intentional injuries* are those involving intentional harm to the victim and include not only injuries caused by others but also those due to self-harm. *Unintentional injuries* are those that have been traditionally called "accidents" (a term that is often discouraged these days because it implies that injuries are fatalistic in nature with no underlying causes). Because intentional and unintentional injuries have such different patterns and etiologies, they are rarely considered together.

This chapter will focus on unintentional injuries to children. The main purpose is to profile the occurrence of unintentional injuries in populations of children and to comment on their underlying determinants as well as possible approaches to prevention. In doing so, we present known disparities in childhood injury risk according to established social determinants, rates of fatal and traumatic injury across countries, leading external causes, and consequences of traumatic injury by age and sex. Current evidence surrounding the relative effects of different preventive approaches is summarized with suggested implications for prevention and future research.

Key Definitions

A number of technical terms are used in this chapter, and here, we provide operational definitions for the terms used repeatedly.

Injury Terms

Injury is defined as physical harm to the body caused by an acute physical, thermal, or chemical force. Studies of childhood injury typically use thresholds such as death, admission to hospital overnight, and presentation for medical treatment to make inferences about severity. *Trauma* is a term that is often used interchangeably with injury and refers to injuries that reach a certain threshold of severity based upon standard clinical criteria. *Unintentional injuries* are those injuries without known intentional causes. *Injury surveillance* is the routine monitoring, analysis, and interpretation of injury data for the purpose of informing prevention, treatment, and research efforts. This specialized form of disease surveillance provides evidence from which the problem of injury can be understood and addressed in an effective manner.

Child Development Terms

One focus of this chapter is to profile the occurrence of injury over *key developmental stages*. The latter simply refers to age groups that share common developmental characteristics and associated injury risks. Here, we have concentrated on infants (<1 year), preschoolers (1–4 years), young children (5–9 years), and adolescents (variably defined, depending upon the data source).

Descriptive Epidemiology Terms

There are also a number of standard epidemiological terms used in this chapter. The first of these is the term *risk for injury*, which is a per capita rate of injury occurrence (e.g., per 1,000 persons) within a population over a fixed period of time. A childhood injury rate can be interpreted as the probability that a child in a defined population will experience an injury during a relevant time period, typically 1 year. *Patterns of injury* refer to analyses that describe common characteristics associated with injury events (e.g., demographic, external causes, locations, timing, etc.) that are helpful for the planning of prevention efforts.

Measures of Disease Burden

Potential years of life lost (PYLL) refers to the cumulative number of potential years lost (average life expectancy minus age at death) attributable to a disease within a defined population. PYLL is a particularly important measure of disease burden for childhood injury because it captures the relatively long length of time between the disease event and the life expectancy in the absence of the event. A second measure of injury burden is the *economic cost of injury*. Economic costs are typically divided into two categories: *direct* and *indirect* costs. *Direct costs* refer to medical costs including treatment and rehabilitation. *Indirect costs* refer to productivity losses attributable to injuries and are calculated using measures such as goods and services that are not produced due to the injury, time lost from work, lost wages, lost benefits, and lost ability to perform household responsibilities.

Significance of Topic

In the past, injury surveillance projects have demonstrated the magnitude of the childhood injury problem relative to other health conditions. These studies have shown that it is important to use different data sources to examine the childhood injury problem, as the risks and patterns observed vary by severity of injury. For example, patterns of causes and consequences may differ substantially between fatal and nonfatal injuries. As well, traumatic injuries that require hospital-based medical care and rehabilitation are very different from other forms of fatal and nonfatal injury. Patterns of injury vary strikingly between different data sources and injury control scientists need to look at all available sources in order to obtain a complete composite picture.

Fatal Childhood Injuries

Rates of fatal childhood injury have been compared cross-nationally in order to demonstrate the magnitude and universal nature of the problem. One of the most notable recent reports of this kind is the *UNICEF Report from Rich Nations* (UNICEF 2001). This landmark report clearly shows that child deaths due to injury are universally important, despite striking variations in fatal injury risks across different societies. The authors were unable to obtain analogous data from countries without centrally, organized vital statistics registries; however, it is expected that rates from those nations would dwarf those depicted in Fig. 19.1. Among the countries examined, 4–6-fold differences in rates of fatal injury were observed. This suggests that environmental conditions leading to injury risks as well as approaches to childhood injury control vary widely between countries and cultures.

Boys consistently experience higher rates of fatal injury than girls. This is a finding that is almost always observed irrespective of data source or population under study. There are many arguments about why this pattern of injury exists. Some scientists would argue that the pattern is a natural phenomenon as boys are more likely to behave in manners that place them at increased risk. Others would attribute the pattern to the ways in which boys and girls are nurtured. For example, boys in developing countries are typically allowed more freedom than girls, which contributes to a higher incidence of falls, drowning, and motor vehicle crash injuries in boys (Bartlett 2002). However, girls in developing countries are more likely to experience burns attributable to time spent indoors and cooking (Krug et al. 2000). Irrespective of the explanation, variations in exposure exist between the sexes and these lead to differential injury risks. The result is an overall higher burden of injury experienced by boys.

Fig. 19.1 Injury deaths by gender and country. Source: UNICEF (2001)

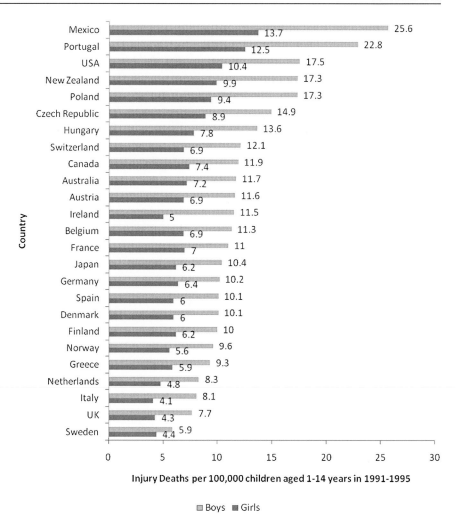

Nonfatal Childhood Injuries

Rates of nonfatal injury have also been examined in cross-national studies. The example provided in Fig. 19.2 highlights an international comparison of nonfatal injuries among adolescents in 35 (mainly European) countries (Pickett et al. 2005). These comparisons focus on childhood injuries requiring medical attention from a doctor or a nurse. In addition to being a major health problem, one should realize that experiences with injury are a normative part of growth and development. Figure 19.2 clearly depicts that most boys and a large percentage of girls from the general school systems experience one or more medically treated injuries each year. Differences between countries in the observed risks are mainly attributable to children reporting

multiple injury events, which in some cases is likely to reflect differences in access to medical care. Additional analyses of these cross-national data (not shown) indicate that nonfatal adolescent injuries result in major productivity losses assessed by time lost from school, work, or other usual experiences. They also lead to major direct costs attributable to emergency medical care, hospitalization, and post-injury rehabilitation.

Injury Pyramids

Injury control researchers often speak of fatalities as representing the "tip of the iceberg" or the "top of a pyramid" with respect to the magnitude of the

Fig. 19.2 Annual prevalence of medically treated injuries among adolescents in 35 countries. Source: Pickett et al. (2005)

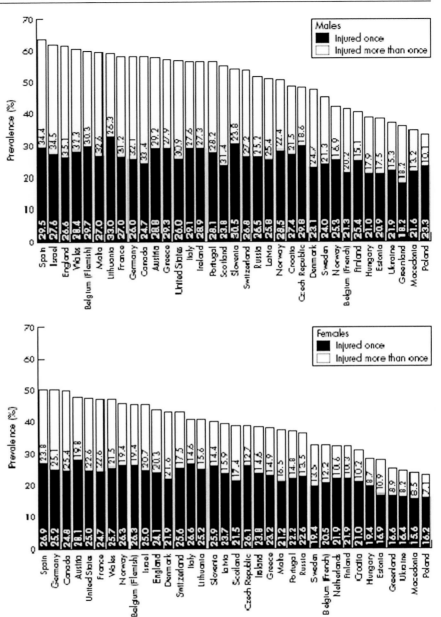

underlying problem. This concept has been illustrated using a diagram called an "injury pyramid." A good example of this concept is presented in Fig. 19.3 using national data compiled by the US Centers for Disease Control and Prevention (Fingerhut and Warner 1997). Among the general US population (all ages), for every death experienced due to injury, there are approximately 20 people hospitalized, 250 people who present to an emergency department, and 400 people who experienced an acute injury episode (1 to 20 to 250 to 400).

These ratios vary by demographic group and for different external causes of injury, and provide a rough illustration of the relative severities of different injury patterns. For children aged 5–14 years in the United States, the ratio is 1 death to 41 hospitalizations to 1,100 emergency department visits (no data on total injury events were provided). Similar injury pyramid ratios of 1 to 160 to 2,000 have been published for children aged 0–14 years in the Netherlands (UNICEF 2001) and 1 to 73 to 1,612 in Alberta, Canada (Spady et al. 2004). These ratios

Fig. 19.3 Injury pyramid
for the United States, 1995.
Source: Fingerhut and
Warner (1997)

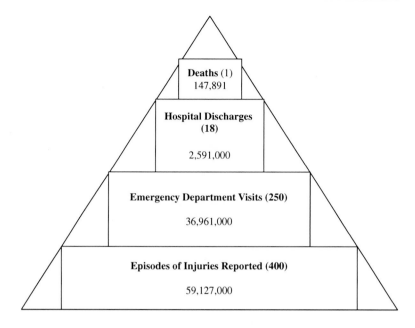

help to describe the extent and distribution of the problem. They are particularly informative for populations of children who experience enormous risks for both fatal and nonfatal injury.

Person Years of Life Lost

Person years of life lost (PYLL) provide another helpful measure describing the relative burden of injuries experienced in child populations. This statistic sums up the differences between the ages at which children die and their expected lifespan based upon life expectancy projections for their population. For example, if a child dies prematurely at the age of 10 due to an injury event, and their expected lifespan is 75 years, this injury has contributed 65 PYLL to an overall summary figure. In some countries, because injury is so heavily concentrated in children and young people, it is thought to contribute more PYLL than all other major causes of death including respiratory disease, cardiovascular diseases, and cancer. To illustrate, in 2004, unintentional injury was the leading cause of death in the United States in terms of years of potential life lost (PYLL), accounting for 19.1% of total PYLL due to premature death in the United States; all

combined cancers and heart disease on the other hand accounted for 16.2% and 12.2% of total PYLL, respectively (CDC 2005).

Economic Costs of Injury

Another important measure of disease burden that has been emphasized in recent years is the economic costs of injury and there is a growing literature in this field of study, particularly in North America. Much of this literature aims to demonstrate the enormous importance of injury as a health problem and is used as a tool for injury control practitioners to lobby for increased societal resources. For example, a recent US analysis estimated the lifetime costs attributable to childhood injury at 50.5 billion US dollars (Finkelstein et al. 2006). This estimate was broken down to 11.9 billion dollars in lifetime medical costs and 38.6 billion in total lifetime productivity losses. Among children 0–14 years of age, fatal, hospitalized, and nonhospitalized injuries accounted for 8.4, 8.4, and 33.8 billion dollars in total lifetime costs, respectively. These costs have obvious impact on societies and the individuals within those societies, and are a major burden that goes beyond the direct effects of pain and suffering.

Common Causes of Unintentional Childhood Injury

Childhood Injury from a Developmental Perspective

Analyses of the risks for injury experienced by children of different ages provide important information. Studying childhood injury from a developmental perspective is helpful for the design of focused prevention initiatives that are tailored to the needs of specific groups of children. This information is also helpful in setting priorities about the groups of children who are most at risk, assuming that larger childhood injury risks would be preferentially addressed over smaller ones. Many people have studied variations in injury experiences among children of different ages and hence developmental stages. One approach to such analyses is to examine the proportions of all deaths that are attributable to injury. According to the WHO (2006), the proportions of deaths attributable to injury increase as children age. Worldwide, injury accounted for approximately 1.5% of deaths observed among infants, 6% of deaths among preschoolers aged 1–4 years, 25% of deaths to children 5–9 years, and 31% of deaths to children 10–14 years of age.

A second approach to the profiling of injury risks across childhood developmental stages is to examine age-specific rates of injury. In the United States, the rate of unintentional injury remains relatively stable throughout childhood. According to the CDC (2005), the rate of unintentional injury in 2004 among those 0–4 years of age was 11,375 injuries per 100,000 persons. Similarly, the rate among those 5–9 years of age was 9,203 injuries per 100,000 persons and the rate among those 10–14 was 11,075 injuries per 100,000 persons. Among adolescents 15–19 years of age, the rate of unintentional injury in 2004 was 12,950 per 100,000 persons.

Annual rates of unintentional injury mortality are similar across age groups as well, except for a marked increase among those 15–19 years of age. The rate among those 0–4 years of age was 13.4 deaths per 100,000 persons in 2004 compared with 5.7 deaths per 100,000 persons and 7.3 deaths per 100,000 persons among those 5–9 and 10–14 years, respectively. The unintentional injury mortality rate among those 15–19 years of age in 2004 was 32.9 deaths per 100,000 persons (CDC 2005).

External Causes of Childhood Injury

Leading causes of injury-related death have been described for children of different ages. These are helpful in planning tailored injury control strategies. Table 19.1 provides such an analysis for children in the United States. The patterns observed here are typical of many developed nations (CDC 2003). Among the very young (infants <1 year), the leading causes of unintentional fatal injury include suffocation, followed by traffic crashes, drowning, fire, and flames. As children enter their preschool years, traffic crashes, drowning, fire and flames predominate. This pattern becomes more apparent as children enter into adolescence. This figure is also helpful in showing the relative importance of unintentional versus intentional (homicide, suicide) injury events as a cause of fatal injury, with noted variations between age groups.

Data from emergency department-based surveillance systems can also be used to examine developmental changes in patterns of nonfatal injury. Flavin and colleagues used a regional, population-based surveillance in Canada to identify leading external causes of acute injury in the very young (Flavin et al. 2006). Patterns observed among these nonfatal injuries were strikingly different than the above fatal injury patterns. Across all developmental groups examined (<1, 1–2, 3–4, 5–6 years), the leading external cause of nonfatal injury was falls. Falls have not been identified as a major contributor to fatal childhood injuries. Ingestion of foreign bodies, which occurs as a result of children's propensity to explore their environments using their mouths, was listed as the second leading cause of injury among the youngest age groups. Being struck by an object or a person was another leading cause

Table 19.1 Leading causes of injury death by age group highlighting unintentional injury deaths, United States – 2003

Rank	<1 year	1–4 years	5–9 years	10–14 years
1	Unintentional suffocation 619	Unintentional MV traffic 502	Unintentional MV traffic 597	Unintentional MV traffic 911
2	Unintentional MV traffic 144	Unintentional drowning 456	Unintentional fire/burn 137	Suicide suffocation 152
3	Homicide unspecified 135	Unintentional fire/burn 229	Unintentional drowning 126	Unintentional drowning 142
4	Homicide other spec. classifiable 100	Unintentional suffocation 159	Unintentional land transport 50	Homicide firearm 139
5	Unintentional drowning 58	Homicide unspecified 153	Homicide firearm 48	Unintentional land transport 81
6	Homicide suffocation 39	Unintentional pedestrian/ other 116	Unintentional suffocation 37	Unintentional fire/ burn 78
7	Undetermined suffocation 38	Homicide, other spec. classifiable 84	Unintentional other transport 21	Suicide firearm 73
8	Unintentional fire/burn 32	Unintentional fall 54	Homicide unspecified 18	Unintentional suffocation 44
9	Unintentional natural/ environment 20	Unintentional poisoning 49	Unintentional poisoning 18	Unintentional poisoning 43
10	Unintentional poisoning 20	Homicide firearm 40	Unintentional natural/ environment 17	Unintentional firearm 36

Source: CDC (2003)

in most age groups examined. Being struck by an object or a person and collisions with objects or people emerge as leading causes of injury in the older age groups and reflect the increasing mobility of children as they age. The rank order of patterns of childhood injury observed in US emergency departments is shown in Table 19.2 (CDC 2004).

The locations where injuries occur also vary as children age. Most injuries among the youngest age groups happen at home where parents or guardians are the responsible authority (Flavin et al. 2006). As children become older, they spend more time outside the home and consequently experience injuries in a more diverse array of locations such as daycare centers, schools, organized sports facilities, and occupational environments. These variations will have an obvious influence on the targeting of interventions to those responsible for the care of children.

Social Disparities and Vulnerable Populations

While very good literature exists to describe risks for childhood injury and immediate circumstances surrounding childhood injury occurrence, there is much to learn about underlying causes of injury to children. It has only been in the past two decades that research efforts have gone beyond basic descriptive efforts to the examination of determinants using modern study approaches. One etiological topic of emerging interest is the idea that there are underlying social determinants for health and illness and hence injury experiences are directly influenced by social disparities. This is supported by modern population health theory, which suggests that many diseases have underlying biological, physical, and social determinants. The result has been the identification of strong gradients

Table 19.2 National estimates of the 10 leading external causes of nonfatal injuries treated in hospital emergency departments, United States 2004, by age group

Rank	< 1 year	1–4 years	5–9 years	10–14 years
1	Unintentional fall 126,281	Unintentional fall 888,335	Unintentional fall 676,704	Unintentional fall 668,589
2	Unintentional struck by/ against 30,760	Unintentional struck by/ against 368,104	Unintentional struck by/against 404,124	Unintentional struck by/against 593,752
3	Unintentional other bite/ sting 12,753	Unintentional other bite/ sting 145,001	Unintentional cut/ pierce 115,886	Unintentional overexertion 272,797
4	Unintentional fire/burn 11,372	Unintentional foreign body 113,084	Unintentional pedal cyclist 101,891	Unintentional cut/ pierce 155,040
5	Unintentional foreign body 9,767	Unintentional cut/pierce 86,787	Unintentional other bite/sting 93,317	Unintentional pedal cyclist 140,063
6	Unintentional other specified 7,979	Unintentional overexertion 76,876	Unintentional MV – occupant 74,399	Other assault struck by/ against 116,670
7	Unintentional inhalation/ suffocation 7,801	Unintentional fire/burn 57,728	Unintentional overexertion 73,980	Unintentional MV – occupant 99,353
8	Unintentional MV – occupant 6,992	Unintentional other/ specified 49,446	Unintentional foreign body 58,303	Unintentional unknown/unspecified 95,311
9	Unintentional cut/pierce 6,152	Unintentional poisoning 47,402	Unintentional dog bite 52,568	Unintentional other transport 70,429
10	Unintentional poisoning 5,814	Unintentional unknown/ unspecified 47,076	Unintentional other transport 49,071	Unintentional other bite/sting 70,286

MV = Motor vehicle
Spec. = Specified
Source: CDC (2004)

in risk for poor health and some of these gradients have been demonstrated for different types of injury. To illustrate, higher risks for childhood injury are typically observed in association with poverty and mechanistically the hazardous social and physical environments and adult/child behaviors that are associated with poverty. One of the classic relationships demonstrated in multiple research contexts is risk for childhood injury and its association with socioeconomic status. Among young children, higher socioeconomic status is protective, whether measured in terms of household income, parental occupation, or parental education. Lower socioeconomic status is a risk factor and most studies of this issue show characteristic gradients in risk across socioeconomic strata.

In a recent analysis, Edwards and colleagues examined risks of fatal injury among British children aged 0–15 years of age according to eight household socioeconomic classes (Edwards et al. 2006). The results presented in Table 19.3 show a classic example of a "risk gradient" associated with social disparity, with children from lower social classes experiencing 2–12-fold risks for fatal injury compared with the highest socioeconomic class. These types of gradients are typically observed among young children and for serious traumatic events. Among adolescents, risk gradients may not be observed in all situations, depending on the type of injury outcome under study. Explanations for this typically focus upon population mixing and the lessening importance of the home environment as a key determinant. In addition, because sports

Table 19.3 Deaths from injury and poisoning and rates per year per 100,000 children aged 0–15 years by eight class NS-SEC, 2001. Example of a socioeconomic gradient in risks for fatal injury

NS-SEC	Deaths 2001– 2003*	Rate (95% CI) per year per 100,000 children
1. Higher managerial/ professional occupations	85	1.9 (1.6–2.4)
2. Lower managerial/ professional occupations	111	1.6 (1.3–1.9)
3. Intermediate occupations	59	2.9 (2.2–3.7)
4. Small employers/ own account workers	105	2.9 (2.4–3.5)
5. Lower supervisory/ technical occupations	91	2.7 (2.2–3.3)
6. Semiroutine occupations	148	4.0 (3.4–4.7)
7. Routine occupations	180	5.0 (4.3–5.8)
8. Never worked/long term unemployment	383	25.4 (22.9–28.1)
Total	1162	4.0 (3.8–4.2)

*Excludes one child for whom NS-SEC was missing
NS-SEC = National Statistics Socio-Economic Classification
Source: Edwards et al. (2006)

are a major cause of injury in adolescent populations and participation is in part driven by family wealth, relationships may be confounded by participation in sports.

There are other disparities in the occurrence of childhood injury in addition to those observed by socioeconomic status. Gradients in risk for child injury have been observed between rural and urban populations. Some of the most vulnerable populations of children are those that reside in remote geographic areas. Consequences of injuries in rural and remote areas are complicated by a lack of immediate access to trauma care. Even within these rural and remote areas, some populations are especially vulnerable.

Children on farms are one such group due to the unique nature of their residential environment. Farm-related injury accounts for up to 50% of occupational deaths among children. Starting at a young age, children on farms experience dramatic increases in risks for fatal injury and serious trauma compared with the general population (Brison et al. 2006). Among preschoolers, this occurs due to routine exposure to industrial hazards as children accompany adults during the course of farm work. Farm families may not have immediate access to childcare and there is a strong tradition of involving children in work at an early age. As children grow and develop, they experience additional risks due to their participation in agricultural work, including the risks associated with tractor and machinery operation, care of large animals, and working at heights. Farm children provide a classic example of a vulnerable group at high risk for injury due to the setting in which they grow up.

Childhood Injuries in Developing Countries

The vast majority of available data on the occurrence of childhood injuries are from developed countries. However, childhood injury poses an even greater burden to developing nations where nearly 98% of all worldwide childhood injuries are thought to occur (Taft et al. 2002). Children in such countries are five times more likely to die from injury prior to age 15 than children in developed countries. To illustrate, in 2000 the annual mortality rate due to injury among children in United States was 9.8 deaths per 100,000 persons. In Vietnam and South Africa, annual mortality rates due to injury were 38.1 and 44.3 per 100,000 persons, respectively. Causes of injury mortality in developing countries are consistent with those observed in industrialized nations, namely motor vehicle accidents, drowning, fire, poisonings, and falls (Taft et al. 2002). However, the problem exists at a much larger scale.

Despite the magnitude of the problem, injuries in developing countries are often ignored in prevention efforts because of the continuing higher prevalence of morbidity and mortality from nutritional deficiencies and infectious disease (Bartlett 2002). This means that while rates of injury are higher in developing compared with developed nations, they constitute a smaller percentage of overall illness and death. In addition, the view that injuries are "accidents" and occur randomly is pervasive and may impede the development of strategies to reduce them. In the last few decades, higher income countries have begun to devote more resources toward injury prevention and research, resulting in a 50% decrease in child injury deaths between 1970 and 1995 in the Organization for Economic Co-operation and Development (OECD) countries (UNICEF 2001). The opposite is more likely to be true in developing countries, where injury rates are actually increasing in response to growing motor vehicle traffic, migration of populations to unsafe urban areas, and the widening availability of products and drugs that are unregulated (Bartlett 2002).

Children in developing countries are a vulnerable population for unintentional injuries for a number of reasons. As with the example of children growing up on farms in developed nations, children who work are exposed to hazards in a workplace that is designed for adults. They may be expected to use tools or machineries that are inappropriate in size, complexity, or strength required (Bartlett 2002). Tasks that are complicated or require concentration may also put children at greater risk for injury, as mistakes and fatigue could increase the likelihood for injury (Bartlett 2002). Additionally, unsafe living conditions, a lack of safe play spaces, and inadequate childcare contribute to injuries in developing nations (Bartlett 2002).

Two important causes of injury-related mortality include deaths due to fire and flames and deaths to passengers of motor vehicles. In developed countries, prevention efforts such as improved construction codes, public education, emergency response and the wide use of smoke detectors are commonplace. In developing countries, substandard housing in combination with lack of electricity, and thus open flame cooking and use of heating fuels, is a main contributor to increased rates of injury due to fire (Taft et al. 2002). Older children are affected by increases in motor vehicle crashes that reflect rapid increases in vehicular traffic, particularly in urban areas of developing regions. Road travel hazards are compounded by poorly maintained roads and vehicles and additional pedestrian and cyclist traffic (Bartlett 2002). Child safety products remain prohibitively expensive in low-income countries and are not available for much of the population. In Vietnam, for example, the cost of a child safety car seat is equivalent to approximately 101 hours of work, whereas in the United States it is equivalent to 2.5 hours of work (Taft et al. 2002). A bicycle helmet, which in the United States requires 0.5 hours of work to purchase, requires 15.2 hours of work in Vietnam (Taft et al. 2002). Social inequity and poverty represent major barriers to the implementation of childhood injury prevention programs, both on the individual level (within countries) and cross-nationally.

Differences in risks for childhood injury observed between countries further highlight social inequity as a major determinant of health and the importance of initiatives such as the Millennium Development Goals which are trying to address such inequities between countries. In developed nations, injury rates have been declining due to prevention efforts; in low- and middle-income countries, lack of resources poses a significant barrier to such implementation (Taft et al. 2002).

Behavioral Risk Factors

One general risk factor for injury in childhood is risk-taking behavior. This has provided an additional focus for applied research. Among infants, the injury experiences are almost totally dependent upon the behavior of adults to minimize exposure to hazards in the home environment. As children grow and develop, experimentation with various risk-taking behaviors becomes normative and these in turn place children at risk. Most children are impulsive and curious. These are normative and often transient patterns of behavior, yet some patterns become engrained. When combined with unsafe physical environment, these behavioral patterns can have serious consequences.

As an extension of this concept, there has been considerable focus on the effects of adolescent risk taking in recent childhood injury control literature. Adolescents commonly experiment with a variety of adult behaviors as they enter high school. The influence of the peer group grows and many of these behaviors are performed in groups and are hence clustered in nature. Experimentation with smoking, alcohol, and other drugs are common examples of clustered risk behaviors, as are unprotected sexual intercourse and truancy from school. In isolation, such behaviors are modestly associated with a number of adverse health outcomes including childhood injury and psychosomatic health complaints. When these behaviors become part of a clustered phenomenon, this "multiple risk" pattern leads to substantial health problems.

Figure 19.4 provides an illustration of the concept of multiple risk behaviors and its association with injury. This comes from a cross-national study conducted among children aged 11–15 years in 12 countries (Pickett et al. 2002). Higher risks for injury were observed in association with the number of clustered risk behaviors that children reported. Injury risk gradients were observed in each of the 12 countries under study and within all demographic subgroups examined in each country. They were also observed for different injury outcomes. A lifestyle that includes engagement in multiple risk behaviors appears to be an important determinant of childhood injury. This pattern is generalizable to children from a wide variety of backgrounds and cultures. More recent analyses suggest that a strong and supportive environment does not necessarily mitigate the effects of these health risk behaviors on risk for injury.

Strategies for Prevention

The "gold standard" for evidence surrounding the effectiveness of injury prevention strategies is the randomized controlled trial. Yet, there are only a modest number of randomized controlled trials in existence for several key approaches to childhood injury prevention. Systematic reviews that synthesize all of the available evidence do exist (Ehiri et al. 2006a, b; Towner and Dowswell 2002; Towner et al. 2001), but they stress how inconclusive much of the existing evidence is with regard to many available prevention strategies.

Injury control scientists often refer to the "3 E's" for injury prevention, those being *educational* prevention strategies, *engineered changes* to physical environments, and the *enforcement* of regulations and legislation. The general sense is that all three strategies are helpful in preventing injuries, but there are serious limitations with those strategies that rely exclusively on education to promote behavioral change. Education is a necessary and important part of most injury prevention efforts. It may be quite effective in influencing behavior, but by itself, it is a generally unproven strategy in terms of affecting risk for childhood injury. In contrast, there is better evidence demonstrating the beneficial effect of comprehensive strategies that include engineered environmental changes and enforcement. The field has known this for years in the area of transportation injuries with major advances in prevention associated with better automobile design, drinking and driving legislation, and enforced traffic laws. However, many existing prevention efforts in the field of childhood injury control continue to be based upon education alone with the hopes of appropriate behavior change leading to injury risk reductions.

In a recent systematic review, Towner and colleagues (Towner and Dowswell 2002) updated the existing evidence surrounding the prevention of unintentional injuries to children. Following a search of the biomedical literature and contact with key informants, they compiled and reviewed evidence on evaluated intervention studies related to childhood injury prevention since 1992. Results were summarized according to various child environments, including interventions for road environments (pedestrian, bicycle, car passenger, and bus passenger injuries), home environments (burns and scalds, poisonings, fall prevention, and general home injuries), and leisure environments (aimed at drownings, play and leisure injuries). The amount of available evidence varied by topic and was often quite modest. In addition, less than a third of the studies used research designs where the evidence was rated as good/reasonable (Table 19.4). Many of the existing trials focused solely on behavior change as the primary outcome, while even fewer assessed the effects of interventions on injury outcomes.

Fig. 19.4 Associations
between numbers of health
risk behaviors and
adolescent injury. Source:
Pickett et al. (2002)

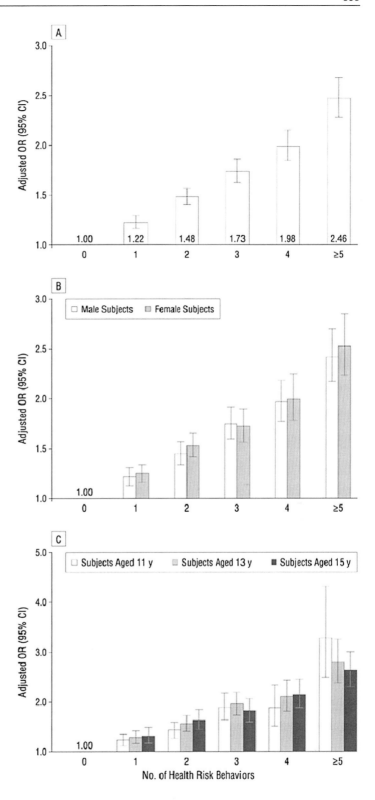

Table 19.4 Level of evidence in support of common interventions to prevent child injury

	(Good evidence***, reasonable evidence**, some evidence*)
Interventions in the road environment	
General	
– Area wide urban safety measure	Injury reduction**
– 20 mph zones	Injury reduction***
	Behavior change***
Pedestrian injuries	
– Education/enforcement aimed at driver	Behavior change*
– Education aimed at child/parent	Behavior change**
	Injury reduction*
Bicycle injuries	
– Bicycle training	Behavior change**
– Bicycle helmet educational campaigns	Behavior change***
– Bicycle helmet legislation	Behavior change***
	Injury reduction**
Car passengers	
– Child-restraint educational campaigns	Behavior change**
– Seat belt educational campaigns	Behavior change**
– Child-restraint loan schemes	Behavior change***
– Child-restraint legislation	Behavior change***
	Injury reduction**
Bus passengers	
– Education aimed at child	Behavior change*
Interventions in the home environment	
General	
– Product design	Injury reduction*
– Safety devices	Injury reduction*
Burns and scalds	
– Smoke detector promotion programs	Behavior change***
	Injury reduction***
– Tap water temperature reduction	Behavior change*
	Injury reduction*
– Parent and child education	Behavior change*
Poisoning	
– Child-resistant packaging	Injury reduction***
– Parent education	Behavior change*
Falls prevention	
– Window bars (education and environmental modification and legislation)	Behavior change**
	Injury reduction*
– Parent education	Injury reduction*
General campaigns	
– Parent education on hazard reduction	Behavior change**
Interventions in the leisure environment	
Drowning	
– Parent and child education	Behavior change*
– Adult supervision of public swimming pools, beaches, etc.	Injury reduction*
– Pool design and protection	Injury reduction*

Table 19.4 (continued)

Play and leisure injuries	
– Environment equipment – playground layout, equipment and surfacing	Hazard reduction*
– Training schemes for adult supervision	Little evidence
– Protective equipment	Injury reduction*
Community-based studies	
– Programs targeting a range of injury types in a range of different groups	Behavior change**
	Injury reduction**

Source: Towner et al. (2001)

The results presented in Table 19.4 demonstrate how much there is to learn about the effects of existing injury prevention methods and the uncertainty surrounding many popular approaches such as parental education. There is excellent evidence that enforced speed zones and traffic calming laws work. There is good evidence regarding the effectiveness of training and public campaigns aimed at promoting the use of bicycle helmet, child passenger seat, and installation of smoke detectors in promoting healthy behaviors. However, stronger evidence suggests that legislation is more effective in preventing associated injuries. The use of passive measures such as child-resistant packaging and window bars on apartment windows has proven effective as well. Yet these represent a relatively small number of proven successes and this area of evaluative study is ripe for further development.

Conclusion

Childhood injury research has evolved over the last few decades from a field that was dominated by descriptive study to a discipline that is beginning to embrace more sophisticated designs and the concepts of evidence-based practice. The science of injury surveillance is quite strong, particularly in the field of pediatrics. There is an excellent understanding of the magnitude of the childhood injury problem, what it looks like, and the burden that it imposes on modern society. Etiological research that examines possible determinants of childhood injury has been dominated by "risk factor" studies that quantify associations between physical and social exposures and the occurrence of injury. There is an ongoing need for more depth in this field, including studies that adapt

and test more sophisticated theoretical models of disease (injury) etiology and qualitative studies that provide additional insight into the occurrence of injury events. This appears to be naturally occurring as the science of injury control becomes multidisciplinary in nature, and each science influences the thinking of others. Major needs in the area of evaluative research remain. There is insufficient evidence surrounding the relative effects of different childhood injury control strategies on risks for injury and a dire need for randomized controlled trials and systematic reviews in this field. These types of efforts are emerging as the discipline of childhood injury control matures and these remain obvious priorities for research.

This chapter suggests some simple but important lessons for policy and practice. First, it is clear that the injury control field has put together some solid arguments about the magnitude of the childhood injury problem and the impact it has on society. These arguments need to be embraced by the public health system and government policy makers and childhood injury needs to be recognized for the major problem that it is.

Second, childhood injuries do not occur randomly within society. The vast majority of injuries worldwide occur in developing areas and injury rates within countries are higher among low-resource populations. Some groups tend to be especially vulnerable to specific forms of injury (i.e., young girls are more likely to be scalded while cooking than are boys). These groups need to be identified systematically and should potentially become targets for focused prevention strategies. There is a special need for inexpensive and practical interventions that could be implemented in developing as well as developed countries. Finally, it is clear that many traditional approaches to childhood injury prevention, while acceptable to society, have little or no evidence to support their ongoing use. This is particularly true for educational strategies aimed at behavioral change. As a society, we need to not only gather better evidence about the relative effects of the injury prevention strategies in common use, but also base our practices on what we know to be effective.

Key Terms

Accidents	Helmets	Premature death
Adolescence	Home environment	Preschoolers
Burden of injuries	Homicide	Scalds
Burns	Injury control	Smoke detectors
Child development	Injury pyramid	Social determinants
Child passenger seat	Injury risk gradients	Social disparities
Child-resistant packaging	Injury surveillance	Socioeconomic factors
Child safety	Intentional injuries	Speed zones
Childhood injuries	Legislation	Suffocation
Disfiguration	Life expectancy	Suicide
Drownings	Parental education	Traffic calming laws
Enforcement	Physical environment	Trauma
Engineered changes	Play spaces	Unintentional injures
Environmental factors	Poisonings	Vulnerable populations
Evidence-based prevention	Potential years of life lost (PYLL)	
Falls	Poverty	
Fire		

Questions for Discussion

1. What are injury pyramids? Of what value are they in childhood injury epidemiology?
2. Briefly explain the two approaches used in the analyses of childhood from a developmental perspective. What are the benefits of a developmental approach to childhood injury epidemiology?
3. What factors explain the disparities in childhood injuries by socioeconomic strata?
4. It is said that 98% of all worldwide childhood injuries occur in less-developed countries. What factors explain the increased vulnerability for children in less-developed countries?
5. With regard to injury prevention strategies, scientists often refer to the "3 E's." What do they mean by this? What are the limitations of childhood injury prevention strategies that rely solely on education?

References

Bartlett SN (2002) The problem of children's injuries in low-income countries: a review. Health Policy and Planning, 17(1), 1–13

Brison RJ, Pickett W, Berg R et al. (2006) Fatal agricultural injuries in preschool children: Risks, injury patterns and strategies for prevention. CMAJ, 174(12), 1723–1726

Centers for Disease Control and Prevention (CDC) (2003) Ten Leading Causes of Injury Death by Age Group Highlighting Unintentional Injury Deaths. Atlanta, Georgia: Centers for Disease Control and Prevention, National Center for Health Statistics. ftp.cdc.gov/pub/ncipc/10LC-2003/PDF/10lc-unintentional.pdf, cited 8 August 2008

Centers for Disease Control and Prevention (CDC) (2004) National Estimates of the Ten Leading Causes of Non-Fatal Injuries. Atlanta, Georgia: Centers for Disease Control and Prevention, National Center for Health Statistics. ftp.cdc.gov/pub/ncipc/10LC-2004/PDF/10lc-2004-nonfatal.pdf, cited 8 August 2008

Centers for Disease Control and Prevention (CDC) (2005) Web-Based Injury Statistics Query and Reporting System (WISQARS). Atlanta, Georgia: Centers for Disease

Control and Prevention, National Center for Health Statistics. www.cdc.gov/ncipc/wisqars, cited 8 August 2008

Edwards P, Roberts I, Green J et al. (2006) Deaths from injury in children and employment status in family: Analysis of trends in class specific death rates. British Medical Journal, 333(7559), 119

Ehiri JE, Ejere HOD, Magnussen L et al. (2006a) Interventions for promoting booster seat use in four to eight year olds traveling in motor vehicles. Cochrane Database of Systematic Reviews, Issue 1

Ehiri JE, Ejere HOD, Hazen AE et al. (2006b) Interventions to increase children's booster seat use: a review. American Journal of Preventive Medicine, 31(2), 185–192

Fingerhut LA, Warner M (1997) Injury Chartbook. Health, United States, 1996–1997. Hyattsville, Maryland: National Center for Health Statistics

Finkelstein EA, Corso PS, Miller TR (2006) Incidence and Economic Burden of Injuries in the United States. New York: Oxford University Press

Flavin MP, Dostaler SM, Simpson K et al. (2006) Stages of development and injury patterns in the early years: a population-based analysis. BMC Public Health, 18(6), 187

Krug EG, Sharma GK, Lozano R (2000) The global burden injuries. American Journal of Public Health, 90(4), 523–526

Pickett W, Schmid H, Boyce WF et al. (2002) Multiple risk behavior and injury: An international analysis of young people. Archives of Pediatric Adolescent Medicine, 156(8), 786–793

Pickett W, Molcho M, Simpson K et al. (2005) Cross national study of injury and social determinants in adolescents. Injury Prevention, 11(4), 213–218

Spady DW, Saunders DL, Schopflocher DP et al. (2004) Patterns of injury in children: a population-based approach. Pediatrics, 113(3 Pt 1), 522–529

Taft C, Paul H, Consunji R, Miller T (2002) Childhood Unintentional Injury Worldwide: Meeting the Challenge. Washington, DC: SAFE KIDS Worldwide

Towner E, Dowswell T, Jarvis S (2001) Updating the evidence, a systemic review of what works in preventing childhood unintentional injuries: Part 2. Injury Prevention, 7(3), 249–253

Towner E, Dowswell T (2002) Community-based childhood injury prevention: what works? Health Promotion International, 17(3), 273–284

United Nations Children's Fund (UNICEF) (2001) A League Table of Child Deaths by Injury in Rich Nations (Innocenti Report Card No. 2). Florence: UNICEF Innocenti Research Centre

World Health Organization (WHO) (2006) Child and Adolescent Injury Prevention: A WHO Plan of Action 2006–2015. Geneva: World Health Organization. http://www.capic.org.uk/documents/Childinjuryprevention_WHO2006_2015.pdf, cited 24 August 2008

Part IV
Programs, Policies, and Emerging Concerns

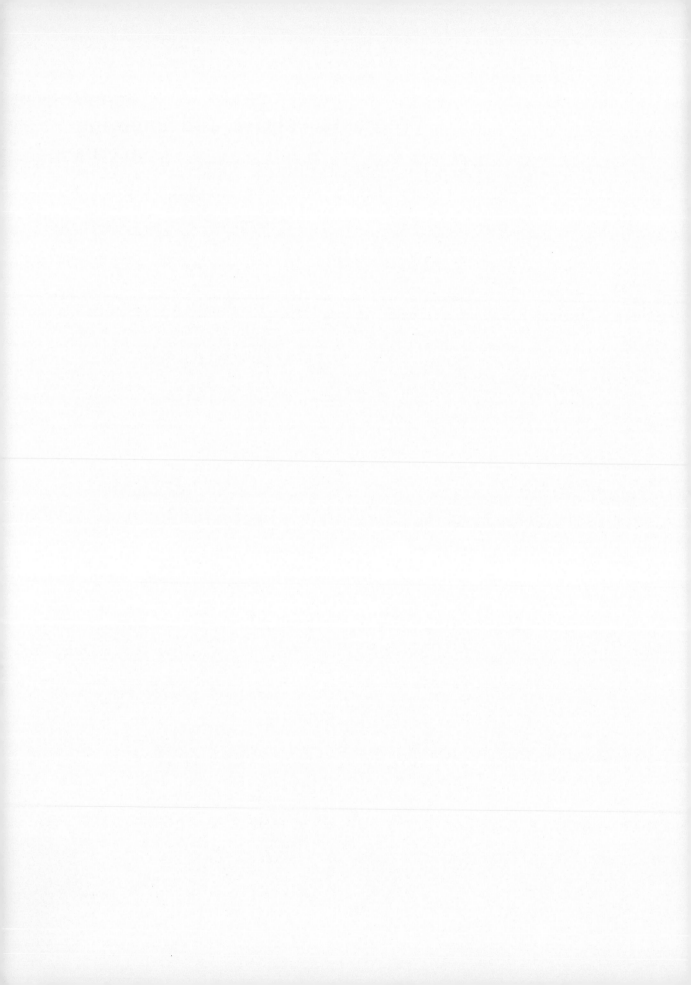

Chapter 20
Evidence-Based Maternal and Child Health

Alan Tita and John E. Ehiri

Learning Objectives After reading this chapter and answering the discussion questions that follow, you should be able to

- Present a synopsis of the status of evidence-based global maternal and child health practice and policy, with particular emphasis on developing countries.
- Discuss the methods, advantages and criticisms of evidence-based practice.
- Discuss relevant historical milestones in the emergence of the evidence-based maternal and child health movement.
- Identify and describe specific examples of maternal and child health interventions that are currently considered evidence based and evaluate research priorities relevant to achievement of maternal and child health-related Millennium Development Goals (MDGs).

Introduction

Evidence-based care has been defined as the conscientious, explicit and judicious use of current best evidence in making decisions about the care of individual patients or populations (Sackett et al. 1996). It shifts emphasis away from practice that is based solely on pathophysiological reasoning, experience, intuition, authoritarianism or conventional wisdom (Evidence-Based Medicine Working Group 1992) to one that emphasizes the use of systematic research

that involves explicit and rigorous application of essential processes outlined in Box 20.1 (Neilson 1998). Evidence-based care is dynamic; it evolves as new research is produced and older interventions debunked. This chapter presents a synthesis of the status of evidence-based global maternal and child health practice and policy, with particular emphasis on developing countries. It defines evidence-based care and examines its advantages, criticisms and methods. Relevant historical milestones in the emergence of the evidence-based maternal and child health movement are discussed. A selection of some specific maternal and child health interventions that are currently considered evidence based is presented, and research priorities relevant to achievement of the maternal and child health-related Millennium Development Goals (MDGs) are discussed. To set the chapter in proper context, maternal and child health is considered from the perspectives of two main practice domains (maternal and perinatal health, and infant and child health) that chronologically relate to the continuum of pregnancy, delivery and birth, and child development, taking into account, the overlap between maternal and child health issues during pregnancy and the neonatal period. Perinatal health as used in this chapter refers to both the intrauterine health of the viable foetus and the neonatal health.

Advantages of Evidence-Based Practice

Ever since the evidence-based care revolution was explicitly introduced in the early 1990s (Evidence-Based Medicine Working Group 1992), its principles have been adopted by a broad array of clinical

A. Tita (✉)
Obstetrics and Gynecology, University of Alabama, Birmingham, USA

Box 20.1 Key Processes in the Systematic Review of Research Evidence

- Clear objectives
- Explicit pre-stated criteria for including studies
- Identify all relevant published and unpublished studies
- Establish explicit study exclusion criteria
- Careful data abstraction
- Pooling of data from similar studies (meta-analysis) only where appropriate
- Description of results
- Drawing appropriate conclusions and
- Discussing implications for current practice and future research

Source: Adapted from Neilson (1998)

---

disciplines and by health-care planners, policy makers and evaluators. Because evidence-based practices and interventions are underpinned by research proving their efficacy or effectiveness, they are expected to lead to improvements in relevant health outcomes, the efficient delivery of health-care services and patient satisfaction. Widespread application of proven interventions or practices leads to cost savings by precluding the allocation of scarce resources, especially in developing countries, to unnecessary interventions (Neilson 1998).

Criticisms of Evidence-Based Practice

The growth in evidence-based care has not occurred without criticism. Five major attacks have been identified and addressed by leaders of the evidence-based care movement (Sackett et al. 1996). First, there is the assertion that everyone already practices evidence-based care. However, this is refuted by variations among practitioners in the provision of interventions for the same public health or clinical problems in the same setting. Second, some argue that evidence-based practice can be conducted only from academic ivory towers and armchairs, and busy practitioners cannot find the time to conduct systematic reviews of available literature to obtain

the best evidence. However, there is some evidence that practitioners can devote scarce time to selective, efficient problem-driven searching, appraisal and incorporation of best evidence into their practice (Sackett et al. 1996). In fact, not everyone is expected to have the training and expertise to conduct systematic reviews of research. There are resources such as the Cochrane Library, whose history is introduced later in this chapter, populated by experts who provide this service. Third, it is argued that evidence-based care is "cookbook" practice. This is refuted by the emphasis of evidence-based care on both practitioners' experience and consideration of the individual problem scenario in applying evidence. Fourth criticism is the contention that purchasers and managers can hijack evidence-based care to cut the cost of health care. While this is certainly possible, such a scenario would indicate a misuse of evidence-based care itself. In fact, correct use of evidence-based practices involving the most efficacious interventions may actually raise costs in some situations, while the avoidance of non-beneficial or harmful interventions will lead to cost savings in others. Finally, evidence-based care is criticized as being restricted to randomized controlled trials and meta-analyses. In response, it is important to emphasize that the purpose of evidence-based practice is to identify the best external evidence with which to answer practical questions – regardless of research methodology. For example, the best evidence about a diagnostic test may be available from properly conducted cross-sectional studies, while the best information regarding prognosis may be gleaned from cohort studies.

In developing countries, several barriers may account for the low practice of evidence-based care. These include limited resources, lack of political foresight to invest in evidence-based practices, unethical promotion of drugs by pharmaceutical companies, corruption, traditional training of health professionals which does not offer requisite skills and over-dependence on scientific information from developed countries which may not be relevant or applicable to developing countries. One study of barriers to the practice of evidence-based reproductive health care in sub-Saharan revealed that plain lack of awareness of evidence-based interventions and lack of materials and supplies necessary to implement these evidence-based interventions were by far the two most prevalent barriers (Tita et al. 2005). On the whole, few studies have actually assessed determinants and barriers associated with evidence-based practice of clinical medicine in general or maternal and child health care in particular in developing countries.

Research Methods and Hierarchy for Evidence-Based Care

Organizations such as the Cochrane Collaboration, the United States Preventive Services Task Force (USPSTF) and the Canadian Task Force on Periodic Examination use comparable systems to grade the quality of evidence, the internal validity of studies and the strength of recommendations arising from the research. The USPSTF, for example, has traditionally graded the quality of evidence according to a hierarchy based on research designs as outlined in Box 20.2 (US Preventive Services Task Force 2008).

It is evident from the USPSTF grading that experimental designs (randomized controlled trials), particularly with respect to the evaluation of therapeutic (or public health) interventions, are accorded the strongest weight. Although not explicitly included in this framework, systematic reviews and meta-analyses of randomized controlled trials, therefore, provide better evidence than do individual trials and have been given a Grade 0 category by some. Basic science studies, involving animals, for example, are not included in grading systems but have been accorded a Grade IV category by others. Thus, despite their importance in illuminating pathophysiological mechanisms, the value of basic science studies as an evidence basis for human or population-based intervention is low. Recognizing that evidence from a well-conducted observational study could be of better quality than evidence from a poorly conducted clinical trial, additional grading for the internal validity of each study is incorporated. The strength of recommendations is also graded, for example, from A to D, indicating a range from strong evidence for benefit (Level A) to strong evidence for ineffectiveness or harm (Level D) (U.S. Preventive Services Task Force 2008).

> ### Box 20.2 USPSTF Grading of Evidence by Research Design
>
> Grade I
>
> Evidence obtained from at least one properly designed, randomized controlled trial
>
> Grade II-1
>
> Evidence from well-designed controlled trials without randomization
>
> Grade II-2
>
> Evidence from well-designed cohort or case–control analytic studies, preferably from more than one centre or research group
>
> Grade II-3
>
> Evidence from multiple time series with or without the intervention. Dramatic results in uncontrolled experiments (such as the results of the introduction of penicillin in the 1940s) could also be regarded as this type of evidence
>
> Grade III
>
> Opinions of respected authorities, based on clinical experience, descriptive studies and case reports, or reports of expert committees
>
> Source: US Preventive Services Task Force (USPSTF) (2008)

Evidence-Based Maternal and Perinatal Health

Evidence-based medicine and obstetrics. The historical development of evidence-based maternal and perinatal health care can be traced back to the history of evidence-based obstetric care (King 2005). Although the term evidence-based medicine appears to have been first coined by Gordon Guyatt of McMaster University in Canada in 1990 (King 2005), the movement towards evidence-based care pre-dated this use. As early as 1972, Archie Cochrane in the United Kingdom emphasized the need for careful evaluation of health care interventions, especially through randomized controlled trials in his monograph, *Effectiveness and Efficiency, Random Reflections on Health Services* (Cochrane 1972). The principles he set out in this text were straightforward. He suggested that because resources would always be limited, they should be used to provide equitably, those forms of health care that had been shown in properly designed evaluations to be effective. In particular, he stressed the importance of using evidence from randomized controlled trials (RCTs) because these were likely to provide much more reliable information than other sources of evidence. Cochrane's simple propositions were soon widely recognized as seminally important by lay people as well as by health professionals. In 1979, he wrote, "It is surely a great criticism of our profession that we have not organized a critical summary, by specialty or sub-specialty, adapted periodically, of all relevant randomized controlled trial" (Cochrane 1979).

Taking up the challenge already in 1974 and recognizing the lack, and non-use of good evidence in obstetric care, Ian Chalmers, based at the time in Cardiff, UK, initiated a project to accomplish the systematic identification and collection of controlled trials in obstetric and perinatal medicine. These efforts by Chalmers and colleagues were given added impetus when in 1979, Archie Cochrane awarded a wooden spoon to Obstetrics as the specialty with the worst use of randomized trials (best available evidence) to inform its practices (the wooden spoon is a figurative trophy due to who ever comes last in any contest). Chalmers subsequently established the National Perinatal Epidemiology Unit in Oxford and continued the development of the perinatal trials registry. By 1985, over 3,500 reports of trials were included. Chalmers, Enkin and Keirse collaborated in the production of the groundbreaking publication *Effective Care in Pregnancy and Childbirth* [http://www.childbirthconnection.org/article.asp?ClickedLink=194&ck=10218&area=2], which appeared in 1989, with an introduction from none else than Archie Cochrane (Chalmers et al. 1989). The text was a compilation of reviews of existing clinical trials addressing various perinatal topics. This enterprise effectively put obstetrics at the forefront of the evidence-based medicine movement. In his introduction, Cochrane referred to this publication as a real milestone in the history of randomized trials and in the evaluation of care and suggested that other specialties should copy the methods used. His encouragement and the endorsement of his views by others led to the opening of the first Cochrane Centre (in Oxford, England) in 1992 and the founding of The Cochrane Collaboration in 1993. These

steps have led to major advances in the development of evidence-based obstetric care in the developed world. A chronological account of the history of the Cochrane Library can be found here: http://www.cochrane.org/consumers/docs/01Cochrane5min.ppt#263,2,Slide 2.

The proliferation of clinical trials in Obstetrics as a result of the work of Cochrane, Chalmers and their colleagues included hallmark and influential perinatal trials such as the Collaborative Eclampsia and Magpie trials coordinated from Oxford (Box 20.3), the Term PROM, Post Term and Term Breech trials from Canada, and multiple trials from the Maternal Fetal Medicine Units Network in the United States. At the same time, there was the introduction and proliferation of the methodology of rigorous assessment of evidence through systematic reviews. This ultimately led to the Cochrane Pregnancy and Childbirth Database of Systematic Reviews, a vital component of the pregnancy and childbirth section of the Cochrane Library, with systematic reviews continuously updated as new trials are published.

Unfortunately, the growth of evidence-based care in developed countries was not accompanied by a similar growth in the developing countries. Maternal and perinatal mortality remain disproportionately high in developing countries, particularly those in sub-Saharan Africa (WHO 2004). Attempts to resolve these serious public health problems have been punctuated by at least two important initiatives: the Safe Motherhood Initiative and the Averting Maternal Death and Disability initiative.

The Safe Motherhood Initiative (see Chapter 22) arose from a Safe Motherhood conference convened in Nairobi, Kenya, in 1987 by the World Bank, the World Health Organization and the United Nations Fund for Population Activities (Mahler 1987). The purpose of the conference was to address the neglected problem of over 500,000 maternal deaths that occurred annually (99% in developing countries). The ensuing Safe Motherhood Initiative aimed to reduce maternal mortality in developing countries by 50% in one decade. The four-part strategy identified to achieve this lofty goal involved:

1. adequate primary care, including food for females and universal family planning;
2. good prenatal care, including nutrition and early identification and referral of high-risk patients;

Box 20.3 Collaborative Eclampsia and Magpie Trials

The Collaborative Eclampsia Trial and the Magpie Trial are two of the most important (and largest) obstetric trials ever conducted. Both were led by Lelia Duley at the Resource Centre for Randomized Trials at the Oxford Institute of Health Sciences.

– *The Magpie Trial* was a randomized placebo-controlled trial in 33 countries that evaluated whether or not pregnant women with pre-eclampsia, and their babies, benefit from magnesium sulphate. The study involving over 10,000 women found that women who were allocated magnesium sulphate had a 58% lower risk of eclampsia than those allocated placebo. Also, it is likely that magnesium sulphate reduces the risk of maternal death. There were no short-term substantive harmful effects to mother or baby (The Magpie Trial Collaborative Group 2002).
– *The Collaborative Eclampsia Trial* was set up to determine which, if any, of the following anticonvulsants should be used to treat women with eclampsia: diazepam, phenytoin or magnesium sulphate. This clinical trial, conducted in 12 different countries across three continents, concluded that magnesium sulphate was superior to the other two treatments (Duley 1995).

As a result of this pioneering research, countless numbers of young mothers were and will be saved from death or disability, especially in developing countries where the risk of eclampsia can be 20 times that of industrialized countries (Duley 1995).

3. assistance of a trained person at all births;
4. access to essential elements of obstetric care for women at higher risk.

An appraisal after one decade indicated no major progress in reducing maternal mortality and suggested that the magnitude of the problem was worse than originally thought. However, awareness of the problem was enhanced and an understanding of major causes of mortality increased. The Averting Maternal Death and Disability (AMDD) program originated out of the Mailman School of Public Health at Columbia University in 1999 under the leadership of the late Alan Rosenfeld, and Deborah Maine (Maine and Rosenfield 2001). Through their seminal article in the Lancet titled *Maternal Mortality – A neglected tragedy. Where is the M in MCH?* they were influential in generating the awareness that led to the Safe Motherhood Initiative. The AMDD advocates that focus on emergency obstetric care is the strategy most likely to lead to the greatest reduction in maternal mortality.

The Institute of Medicine, through the Board on Global Health of its Committee on Improving Birth Outcomes, has also weighed in with suggested strategies on solving the problem of safe motherhood in 2003. In the publication, *Improving Birth Outcomes: Meeting the challenge in the developing world*, [http://www.nap.edu/catalog.php?record_id=10841] they proposed the following prioritized recommendations for immediate improvement of birth outcomes:

- Every delivery, including those at home should be attended by a skilled birth attendant such as a midwife, a nurse or a physician.
- Essential obstetric and neonatal care should be accessible to address all complications of childbirth that cannot be managed by a skilled attendant.
- Postpartum care should be available during the critical first hours following childbirth and over the first month.
- Reinforcement of pre-conceptional and antenatal care through family planning services to women and men of reproductive age and several other interventions (Bale et al. 2003).

More recently in late 2006, through a series of papers published in the Lancet as part of the build-up to the 20th anniversary of the Safe Motherhood Initiative, the Lancet Maternal Health Steering Group also advocated the strategy involving professionalization of maternity care as the absolute priority (Campbell and Graham 2006).

All of these initiatives and strategic positions by influential groups have certainly been useful in increasing awareness and renewing commitment to the problem of maternal health. In addition, some of the individual interventions proposed have a proven evidence base. However, the strategies have generally been premised on problem analyses that indicate a high plausibility for their effectiveness. Unfortunately, from an evidence-based practice standpoint, these proposals are often implemented without a careful evaluation of their actual effectiveness, especially through cluster-randomized trials, which usually represent the best source of evidence in such circumstances (Tita et al. 2007). Arguments have been proffered that some of the individual interventions are already proven in clinical trials and that it may therefore be unethical to conduct further trials to test strategies offering them. However, it is uncertain that a package of several competing interventions, especially when implemented within a resource-constrained system, necessarily leads to improved outcomes. In fact, the persistent high rates of maternal mortality and morbidity give credence to the uncertainty surrounding the effectiveness of proposed strategies so far. It is therefore, crucial and ethical that proposed strategies to improve maternal health and mortality be underpinned by strong evidence, ideally from cluster-randomized trials evaluating such strategies.

Current Evidence-Based Maternal and Perinatal Interventions

Evidence-based practice is dynamic; new interventions are adopted and others discarded as new evidence accumulates from research. It is therefore impossible to cite an exhaustive list of evidence-based interventions. Nevertheless, the most pertinent resource for evidence-based maternal health care relevant to developing as well as developed countries is the World Health Organization Reproductive Health Library [http://apps.who.int/rhl/en/]. It is an electronic database of systematic reviews from the Cochrane Database accompanied by commentaries and information on implications for practice (Box 20.4).

Based on the results of the systematic reviews, interventions are categorized in the WHO RHL according to their effectiveness or lack thereof, into six categories: beneficial, likely beneficial, with a trade-off, of unknown effectiveness, likely to be ineffective and likely to be harmful. Selected maternal and perinatal interventions listed in the 2006 version of the WHO Reproductive Health Library as beneficial or likely beneficial, and their effects, are listed in Box 20.5.

Knowledge Gaps, Research Priorities and Implications for the MDGs

The Millennium Development Goal #5 to improve maternal health has the reduction of maternal mortality ratio in developing countries by 75% by 2015 as its main objective. Clearly, there are evidence-based interventions aimed at alleviating individual factors that contribute to the high rates of maternal mortality. As already outlined, these high rates have remained unchanged in spite of multiple remedial initiatives and strategies premised on analyses of the underlying barriers and causes (Tita et al. 2007). This analysis approach is analogous to pathophysiological reasoning in clinical medicine, which does not always lead to effective therapy. Therefore, before strategies proposed as part of initiatives to reduce maternal mortality are widely adopted, their effectiveness should be established through cluster-randomized trials or other methods deemed suitable for the situation. Consequently, research to evaluate and validate interventions that are individually effective against major causes of maternal mortality should be prioritized. Given the variations in settings in the developing world, the local reality should be considered in designing and evaluating such strategies. Finally, research should continue to develop additional interventions against causes of maternal mortality. Examples of such interventions include those to primarily prevent pre-eclampsia/eclampsia, haemorrhage and obstructed labour.

Box 20.4 Evidence-Based MCH Resources

1. *The World Health Organization Reproductive Health Library*: The WHO Reproductive Health Library (RHL) is a resource that puts the best research evidence available from systematic reviews into practical context for use to improve health outcomes. Started in 1997, the RHL is available both on CD-ROM and Online, and is published in several languages including French, Spanish and English. It is Cochrane-based and regularly updated with new evidence and additional resources on an ongoing basis online, and with CDs published annually. It is available free to developing country workers on CD-ROM or on the Internet and to workers in developed countries for an annual fee. Internet link: http://www.who.int/rhl/en/

2. *The Cochrane Library* and the *Cochrane Pregnancy and Child Birth Database*: The Cochrane Library contains high-quality, independent evidence to inform health care decision making from systematic reviews, particularly of clinical trials. These are considered the gold standard in evidence-based health care. Found within this Library is the Pregnancy and Childbirth Database which focuses on maternal and child health clinical and public health issues. The Cochrane Library (http://www3.interscience.wiley.com/cgi-bin/mrwhome/106568753/HOME) is available to readers in low-income countries at no cost and can be accessed either directly or through the Health InterNetwork Access to Research Initiative (HINARI). The HINARI program, http://www.who.int/hinari/en/, set up by the WHO and several major publishers, provide health workers and researchers with access to published research information. Individuals in about 113 countries have access to nearly 4,000 journals through this initiative.

3. *Better Births Initiative*: The Better Births Initiative aims to ensure that clinical policies and procedures used in essential obstetric services are grounded in reliable research evidence. It is targeted at health-care providers and assists them in understanding research evidence, making decisions about best practice, and establishing implementation procedures to assure change. It is aimed at middle- and low-income countries, where resources for health care are limited and better services will reduce maternal mortality. Internet link: http://www.liv.ac.uk/evidence/BBI/home.htm

4. *The Lancet Neonatal Survival, Child Survival, and Maternal Survival Series*: Although falling within the sphere of Level III (expert review) evidence, the series of papers on each of these three areas provide an instructive overview of each target area. Currently available evidence-based interventions are also discussed in some of the papers. The series are important because they likely represent the mainstream orientation of actions to address each of these problem areas. The papers in these series can be traced through a PubMed or MedLine search.

Evidence-Based Infant and Child Health

Information on the precise historical development of evidence-based childcare is sparse. However, there is evidence that efforts at improving child health, and the progress made, have historically exceeded those of maternal health. Jim Grant, the late director of the United Nations International Children's Fund (UNICEF), launched the revolution in child survival with widespread international support in 1982 (UNICEF 1996). In 1990, this international commitment was again reaffirmed at the World Summit for Children in New York, USA. As already discussed, progress made in infant and child health led to a seminal paper that called for attention to the "M" in MCH (Rosenfield and Maine 1985). In contradistinction to maternal and perinatal health, over the last two decades following Jim Grant's initiative, there has been a reduction in average global child mortality, albeit with a recent stagnation in a few countries severely affected by the HIV/AIDS pandemic. Better understanding of

Box 20.5 Beneficial and Likely Beneficial Maternal and Perinatal Health Promotion Intervention

Beneficial Interventions
- Active management of the third stage of labor (involving administration of medications to promote uterine contraction after delivery of the baby) to decrease blood loss.
- Use of antibiotics for preterm, pre-labour rupture of membranes to prolong pregnancy and reduce maternal and infant infections.**
- Administration of prophylactic antibiotics to women undergoing caesarean section to reduce post-operative infections.
- Use of antibiotic treatment of asymptomatic bacteriuria to prevent pyelonephritis in pregnancy and to reduce preterm delivery.**
- Administration of corticosteroids to women with impending preterm delivery to reduce neonatal mortality and morbidity related to prematurity.*
- Use of external cephalic version at term to reduce rates of breech delivery and cesarean section.**
- Injection of saline solution with oxytocin into the umbilical vein to reduce the need for manual removal of placenta.
- Administration of magnesium sulphate over other anticonvulsants to women with eclampsia to prevent recurrent seizures.
- Administration of magnesium sulphate to women with pre-eclampsia to reduce eclampsia and maternal death.
- Induction of labor after 41 completed weeks of gestation to reduce perinatal death and cesarean section.*
- Routine supplementation with iron and folate during pregnancy to prevent maternal anemia.
- Routine periconceptional supplementation with folate to reduce neural tube defects.*
- Provision of social support to women in labor, to reduce the need for pain relief and operative vaginal delivery and enhance their labor experience.
- Use of combination injectable contraceptives to prevent unwanted pregnancies.
- Use of emergency contraception after unprotected intercourse to prevent unwanted pregnancy.
- Use of medical methods involving RU-486, misoprostol and methotrexate for safe first trimester abortion.
- Use of tubal sterilization by minilaparotomy, where laparoscopy is not available to definitively prevent unwanted pregnancy.
- Administration of intrapartum Nevirapine followed by a single dose within 72 hours to the newborn to reduce mother-to-child transmission of HIV infection.*
- Regular use of condom to reduce HIV transmission particularly in sero-discordant couples.
- Routine screening during pregnancy and treatment of syphilis to decrease congenital syphilis.*
- Administration of long- or short-course Zidovudine to reduce the risk of mother-to-child transmission of HIV infection.*

Likely beneficial interventions

- Use of prophylactic antimalarials or presumptive treatment during pregnancy in women of low parity in endemic areas to decrease low-birth-weight babies and maternal anaemia.**
- Use of prophylactic antimalarials or presumptive treatment during pregnancy in endemic areas to decrease recurrent malaria.
- Use of breast and nipple stimulation at term to reduce post-term pregnancy.*
- Early use of antibiotics in women with intra-amniotic infection to prevent postpartum complications.

- Use of exclusive breastfeeding up to 6 months to reduce morbidity and possibly mortality due to diarrheal infections.*
- Use of orally and rectally administered misoprostol after other uterotonics to reduce further blood loss.
- Use of manual or electric vacuum aspiration over rigid curettage to treat incomplete abortion.
- Education about contraceptive use to increase contraceptive use up to 6 months postpartum.
- Use of levonorgestrel or mifepristone over Yuzpe regimen (birth control pills) for more effective emergency contraception.
- Use of erythromycin or amoxicillin to treat genital chlamydia during pregnancy.**
- Use of broad-spectrum antibiotics to treat gonorrhoea treatment during pregnancy.**

*Perinatal interventions
**Maternal and perinatal interventions
Source: World Health Organization (2006)

these gains has been attributed to the pioneering work of Moseley and Chen, who proposed a framework for studying child survival in developing countries (Mosley and Chen 1984). They postulated that underlying socioeconomic factors affect child survival through five key proximate determinants: maternal factors, nutritional deficiency, environmental exposures, injury and self-efficacy (personal illness control). This framework served as a backbone for the development of child survival programs. While the reduction in child mortality coincided with the implementation of child survival programs involving use of evidence-based interventions such as immunization, oral rehydration therapy for diarrhoea, and the improvement in health and nutrition of women and their children, few efforts were made to document the actual effectiveness of the program strategies and to identify components that actually work. One strategy that has received considerable programmatic evaluation from its onset is the Integrated Management of Childhood Illnesses (IMCI) (Chapter 27). Overall, the strategy has not yielded consistent improvements in childcare as expected. This is due to multiple barriers, which have led to sub-optimal implementation. Nevertheless, over 100 countries have already adopted IMCI as the primary approach to improving child health, and its implementation is ongoing (Ingle and Chetna 2007).

Furthermore, the trend indicating decreased child mortality conceals serious disparities within and between countries. In Brazil, for example, data indicate a sixfold disparity in child mortality rates between the richest 10% and the poorest third (Victora et al. 2000). Other reports from several developing countries also demonstrate significant deficits in the proportion of children reached by individual evidence-based interventions.

Overall, a review of the historical background of child survival programs reveals that proven individual interventions are used without specific evaluation of the effectiveness of different strategies utilized to deliver these interventions to large populations. This situation is similar to that of maternal and perinatal health, with the major difference that the child health efforts nevertheless coincide with improvements in child mortality. In the next section, we present some of the individual interventions with an evidence basis.

Current Evidence-Based Infant and Child Interventions

Notwithstanding improvements in child mortality, over 10 million children under 5 years of age continue to die annually. The vast majority occur in developing countries including over 40% in sub-Saharan Africa and about 35% in south Asia. It has been estimated that 90% of

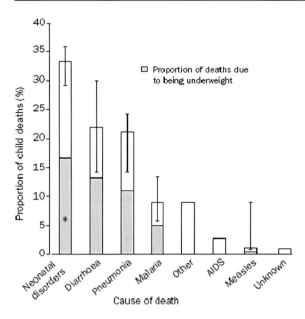

Fig. 20.1 Leading clinical causes of under-5 child mortality

Knowledge Gaps, Research Priorities and Implications for the MDGs

The Millennium Development Goal #4 to improve child health has the reduction of child mortality by two-thirds of 1990 levels by the year 2015 as prime objective. However, as is still the case with maternal health targets, there is still much to be accomplished. Improvements noted over the years in child mortality have occurred without close evaluation and monitoring for effective strategies. Therefore, the main priority in this area is the need for research to evaluate and identify strategies that are effective in producing measurable benefits. In addition, strategic programming should take into consideration, the local reality. Such programming requires a solid base of epidemiological information on local causes of child mortality and their distribution within the population. Therefore, observational research in this area is needed. Further research, including basic and clinical trial research, is needed to develop other relevant evidence-based interventions such as vaccines for malaria and for microbes causing pneumonia and diarrhoea, and to plan interventions to prevent and treat malnutrition.

child mortality is attributable to just a few clinical conditions (Fig. 20.1) (Black et al. 2003). Besides neonatal complications, diarrhoea, pneumonia, malaria and AIDS account for over 50% of deaths, while malnutrition interacts with these clinical conditions to produce the majority of deaths (Black et al. 2003).

It is therefore evident that key interventions for each of these conditions are needed. The Cochrane database of systematic reviews remains the leading single source of reliable reviews of evidence on a wide range of interventions that address child health problems. *Evidence Based Child Health*, a quarterly publication of the Cochrane Child Health Field based in Australia, publishes prioritized summaries of some of these systematic reviews with commentaries. Also, a number of common child health problems are addressed in *Clinical Evidence*, an electronic compendium of evidence-based clinical interventions issued and regularly updated by the British Medical Journal (BMJ) Publishing Group. Some of the currently available effective interventions are shown in Table 20.1. Interventions affecting neonatal health have been previously listed under maternal and perinatal interventions (Box 20.5).

Conclusion

As in clinical medicine, the need for maternal and child health interventions to be evidence based is intuitive. Unfortunately, this has not been the historical reality. Policies should be based on the best available evidence and warrant systematic reviews of applicable clinical trials and/or observational studies, as appropriate. When strategies are designed based on situational analyses, it is vital that their implementation include demonstration projects or action research using preferably cluster-randomized trials to verify their effectiveness. Many available evidence-based interventions are not reaching those in need. While development of additional evidence-based interventions is important, findings ways to reach individuals and families with already validated, evidence-based interventions remains an abiding global health challenge.

Table 20.1 Selected evidence-based interventions to promote child health

Intervention	Source	Summary of evidence
Oral zinc for treating acute persistent diarrhoea in children	Lazzerini and Ronfani (2008)	In areas where diarrhoea is an important cause of child mortality, research evidence shows zinc is clearly of benefit in children aged 6 months or older
Antiretrovirals for reducing the risk of mother-to-child transmission (MTCT) of HIV infection	Volmink et al. (2007)	Short courses of antiretroviral drugs are effective for reducing mother-to-child transmission of HIV and are not associated with any safety concerns in the short-term
Efficacy and safety of cesarean delivery for prevention of mother-to-child transmission (MTCT) of HIV-1	Read and Newell (2005)	Elective Cesarean Section is an efficacious intervention for the prevention of MTCT among HIV-1-infected women not taking antiretroviral drugs or taking only Zidovudine
Vaccines for preventing influenza in healthy children	Jefferson et al. (2008)	Influenza vaccines are efficacious in children older than 2, but little evidence is available for children under 2 years of age
Vitamin A for preventing acute lower respiratory tract infections in children up to 7 years of age	Chen et al. (2008)	Vitamin A supplements prevent acute lower respiratory tract infections in children with low serum retinol or those with poor nutritional status
Antibiotics for preventing complications in children with measles	Kabra et al. (2008)	Antibiotics may be beneficial in preventing complications such as pneumonia, purulent otitis media and tonsillitis in children with measles
Neuraminidase inhibitors for preventing and treating influenza in children	Matheson et al. (2007)	Neuraminidase inhibitors are effective in shortening illness duration in healthy children with influenza, but efficacy in "at-risk" children remains to be proven. Oseltamivir is also effective in reducing the incidence of secondary complications and may be effective for influenza prophylaxis
Vitamin A for treating measles in children	Huiming et al. (2005)	Two doses of vitamin A were associated with a reduced risk of mortality and pneumonia-specific mortality in children under the age of 2 years
Chemoprophylaxis and intermittent treatment for preventing malaria in children	Meremikwu et al. (2008)	Prophylaxis and intermittent treatment with antimalarial drugs reduce clinical malaria and severe anemia in preschool children
Interventions to improve water quality for preventing diarrhoea	Clasen et al. (2006)	Interventions to improve water quality are generally effective in preventing diarrhoea, and interventions to improve water quality at the household level are more effective than those at the source
Hand washing for preventing diarrhoea	Ejemot et al. (2008)	Hand washing can reduce diarrhoea episodes by about 30%. This significant reduction is comparable to the effect of providing clean water in low-income areas
Rotavirus vaccine for preventing diarrhoea	Soares-Weiser et al. (2004)	Rhesus rotavirus vaccines (particularly RRV-TV) and the human rotavirus vaccine 89-12 are efficacious in preventing diarrhoea caused by rotavirus and all-cause diarrhoea
Insecticide-treated bed nets (ITNs) and curtains for preventing malaria	Lengeler (2004)	ITNs are highly effective in reducing childhood mortality and morbidity from malaria

Key Terms

Abortion	Effectiveness	Nevirapine
Allocation of resources	Efficacy	Oxytocin
Amoxicillin	Emergency contraception	Patient satisfaction
Analytic studies	Emergency obstetric care	Perinatal mortality
Antenatal care	Erythromycin	Placebo
Archie Cochrane	Evidence-based care	Postpartum care
Averting maternal death and disability initiative	Family planning	Postpartum complications
	Folate	Pre-conception
Better Births Initiative	Gonorrhoea	Pre-eclampsia
Birth outcomes	Harmful interventions	Prophylactic antibiotic
Breech delivery	Intra-amniotic infection	Randomized controlled trials
Caesarean section	Iron	RU-486
Case-control studies	Laparoscopy	Safe motherhood initiative
Chlamydia	Levonorgestrel	Skilled attendant
Clinical trials	Low birth weight	Syphilis
Cluster-randomized trial	Magnesium sulphate	Systematic reviews
Cochrane Pregnancy and Child Birth Database	Magpie trials	The Cochrane Library
	meta-analysis	Trimester
Cohort studies	Methotrexate	Tubal sterilization
Collaborative eclampsia trial	Mifepristone	Uncontrolled experiments
Condom	Minilaparotomy	Unnecessary interventions
Cookbook practice	Misoprostol	Vaginal delivery
Corticosteroids	Mother-to-child transmission	Zidovudine
Cost savings	Neural tube defects	

Questions for Discussion

1. What is evidence-based practice and what are its limitations?
2. In an essay of about 1,000 words, present an argument to counter the five criticisms of evidence-based practice.
3. What are the major barriers against the implementation of evidence-based maternal and child health services in developing countries?

References

Bale JR, Stoll BJ, Lucas AO (2003) Improving Birth Outcomes: Meeting the challenge in the developing world. Board on Global Health (BGH), Institute of Medicine (IOM). Washington, DC: National Academy Press.

Black RE, Morris SS, Bryce J. (2003) Where and why are 10 million children dying every year? Lancet, 361: 2226–2234

Campbell OM, Graham WJ (2006) Strategies for reducing maternal mortality: getting on with what works. Lancet, 368: 1284–1299

Chalmers I, Enkin MW, Keirse MJNC (eds.) (1989) Effective care in pregnancy and childbirth. Oxford University Press.

Chen H, Zhuo Q, Yuan W et al. (2008) Vitamin A for preventing acute lower respiratory tract infections in children up to seven years of age. Cochrane Database of Systematic Reviews, Issue 1

Clasen T, Roberts I, Rabie T et al. (2006) Interventions to improve water quality for preventing diarrhea. Cochrane Database of Systematic Reviews, Issue 3

Cochrane AL (1972) Effectiveness and Efficiency: Random Reflections on Health Services. London: Nuffield Provincial Hospitals Trust

Cochrane AL (1979) 1931–1971: a critical review, with particular reference to the medical profession. In: Medicines for the Year 2000. London: Office of Health Economics

Duley L (1995) Which anticonvulsant for women with eclampsia? Evidence from the Collaborative Eclampsia Trial. Lancet, 345: 1455–1463

Ejemot RI, Ehiri JE, Meremikwu MM et al. (2008) Hand washing for preventing diarrhea. Cochrane Database of Systematic Reviews, Issue 1

Evidence-Based Medicine Working Group (1992) Evidence-based medicine. A new approach to teaching the practice of Medicine. Journal of the American Medical Association, 268: 2420–2425

Huiming Y, Chaomin W, Meng M (2005) Vitamin A for treating measles in children. Cochrane Database of Systematic Reviews Issue 4

Ingle GK, Chetna M (2007) Integrated management of neonatal and childhood illness: an overview. Indian Journal of Community Medicine, 32(2): 108–110

Jefferson T, Rivetti A, Harnden A et al. (2008) Vaccines for preventing influenza in healthy children. Cochrane Database of Systematic Reviews, Issue 2

Kabra SK, Lodha R, Hilton DJ (2008) Antibiotics for preventing complications in children with measles. Cochrane Database of Systematic Reviews, Issue 3

King JF (2005) A short history of evidence-based obstetric care. Best Practice & Research Clinical Obstetrics & Gynaecology, 19: 3–14

Lazzerini M, Ronfani L (2008) Oral zinc for treating diarrhoea in children. Cochrane Database of Systematic Reviews, Issue 3

Lengeler C (2004) Insecticide-treated bed nets and curtains for preventing malaria. Cochrane Database Systematic Reviews, Issue 3

Mahler H (1987) The safe motherhood initiative: a call to action. Lancet, 1: 668–670

Maine D, Rosenfield A (2001) The AMDD program: history, focus and structure. International Journal of Gynaecology and Obstetrics, 74: 99–103, discussion 104

Matheson NJ, Harnden AR, Perera R et al. (2007) Neuraminidase inhibitors for preventing and treating influenza in children. Cochrane Database of Systematic Reviews, Issue 1

Mosley WH, Chen LC (1984) An analytic framework for the study of child survival in developing countries. Population and Development Review, 10: 25–45

Meremikwu MM, Donegan S, Esu E (2008) Chemoprophylaxis and intermittent treatment for preventing malaria in children. Cochrane Database of Systematic Reviews, Issue 2

Neilson JP (1998) Evidence-based intrapartum care: evidence from the Cochrane library. International Journal of Gynecology and Obstetrics, 62 (Suppl. 1): S97–S102

Read JS, Newell ML (2005) Efficacy and safety of cesarean delivery for prevention of mother-to-child transmission of HIV-1. Cochrane Database Systematic Reviews, Issue 4

Rosenfield A, Maine D (1985) Maternal mortality – a neglected tragedy. Where is the M in MCH? Lancet, 2: 83–85

Sackett DL, Rosenberg WM, Gray JA et al. (1996) Evidence-based medicine: what it is and what it isn't. BMJ, 312: 71–72

Soares-Weiser K, Goldberg E et al. (2004) Rotavirus vaccine for preventing diarrhoea. Cochrane Database of Systematic Reviews, Issue 1

Tita AT, Selwyn BJ, Waller DK et al. (2005) Evidence-based reproductive healthcare in Cameroon: population-based study of awareness, use and barriers. Bulletin of the World Health Organization, 83: 895–903

Tita AT, Stringer JS, Goldenberg RL et al. (2007) Two decades of the safe motherhood initiative: time for another wooden spoon award? Obstetrics and Gynecology, 110(5): 972–976

The Magpie Trial Collaborative Group (2002) Do women with pre-eclampsia, and their babies, benefit from magnesium sulphate? The Magpie Trial: a randomised placebo-controlled trial. Lancet, 359(9321): 1877–1890

U.S. Preventive Services Task Force (2008) Ratings: Strength of Recommendations and Quality of Evidence: Guide to Clinical Preventive Services. Third Edition: Periodic Updates, 2000–2003. Agency for Healthcare Research and Quality, Rockville, MD http://www.ahrq.gov/clinic/3rduspstf/ratings.htm, cited 29 July 2008

United Nations Children's Fund (UNICEF) (1996) The state of the world's children: fifty years for children. http://www.unicef.org/sowc96/1980s.htm, cited 29 July 2008

Victora CG, Vaughan JP, Barros FC et al. (2000) Explaining trends in inequalities: evidence from Brazilian child health studies. Lancet, 356(9235): 1093–1098

Volmink J, Siegfried NL, van der Merwe L et al. (2007) Antiretrovirals for reducing the risk of mother-to-child transmission of HIV infection. Cochrane Database Systematic Reviews, Issue 1

World Health Organization (WHO) (2004) Neonatal and Perinatal Mortality. Department of Making Pregnancy Safer. Geneva: World Health Organization. http://whqlibdoc.who.int/publications/2007/9789241596145_eng.pdf, cited 28 July 2008

World Health Organization (WHO) (2006) Beneficial and harmful care: beneficial forms of care. The WHO Reproductive Health Library, No. 9, Update Software Ltd, Oxford

Chapter 21
A Global Perspective on Teen Pregnancy

Andrew L. Cherry, Lisa Byers, and Mary Dillon

Learning Objectives After reading this chapter and answering the discussion questions that follow, you should be able to

- Discuss the problem of teen pregnancy from a global perspective, and identify regional and cross-national themes, trends, progress, and challenges.
- Describe social, economic, and cultural determinants of teenage pregnancy and review the gaps in knowledge and research priorities.
- Evaluate programs and policies designed to reduce the health, economic, and social risks associated with teen pregnancy.

Introduction

Adolescence (ages 10–19 years) is a period of transition, growth, exploration, and opportunities. It is a period when young people have increased interest in sex, with attendant risks of unintended pregnancies, health risks associated with early childbearing, abortion outcomes, and sexually transmitted infections, including HIV/AIDS. Adolescents who have unintended pregnancy face a number of challenges, including abandonment by their partners, inability to complete school education (which ultimately limits their future social and economic opportunities), and increased adverse pregnancy outcomes.

A.L. Cherry (✉)
School of Social Work, University of Oklahoma, Tulsa, OK, USA

Children born to adolescent mothers are more likely to have low birth weight and to be victims of physical neglect and abuse. Because teenagers have higher risks of adverse pregnancy outcomes compared to their adult counterparts (Chen et al. 2007), health care for them and their babies is more costly (Miller 2000). Death rates for teenage mothers and their babies are higher in less developed countries, the rates are at epidemic proportions. Thus, the birth of a child to a mother who has only just left childhood herself is a cause for concern across countries and cultures. This chapter discusses the problem of teen pregnancy from a global perspective and explores regional and cross-national themes, trends, progress, and challenges. Social, economic, and cultural determinants are discussed. Programs and policies designed to reduce health, economic, and social risks among pregnant teens are reviewed and gaps in knowledge and research priorities are identified. To set the discussion in specific regional contexts, the chapter examines the situation in North America (represented by the United States), Europe and Central Asia (represented by United Kingdom and Russia), East Asia and the Pacific (represented by Vietnam and Japan), South Asia (represented by India), Central and South America (represented by Mexico), Africa (represented by Nigeria), and Middle East and North Africa (represented by Egypt). These countries were purposively highlighted because they are known to drive trends in teen pregnancy rates in their respective regions and globally.

Cross-national studies provide different views on teenage pregnancy and the social, intellectual, and moral forces that sustain and restrain teen

J.E. Ehiri (ed.), *Maternal and Child Health*, DOI 10.1007/b106524_21,
© Springer Science+Business Media, LLC 2009

pregnancies. Teenagers who engage in premarital sex do so in the broader context of their societies' cultural and socioeconomic environment. Essentially, all negative consequences that result from a teen birth have as their sequel public attitude, political policy, and poverty. To provide a common understanding, definitions of some terminologies used in teenage pregnancy research, and which are frequently referenced in this chapter, are presented in Box 21.1.

Although many countries have experienced significant declines in the rates of teenage pregnancy since the mid-1990s, current rates remain unacceptably high in many countries and regions of the world. According to available data (UNFPA 2005)

- Adolescent girls account for 11% of all births (15 million a year).
- Teen birth rates vary between a low of 29 per 1,000 in Europe and 58 per 1,000 in Asia to a high of 130 per 1,000 in Africa.

- Girls aged 15–19 from the lowest socioeconomic groups are three times more likely than their economically better-off peers to give birth in adolescence and have twice as many children.
- Of the 260 million girls and young women aged 15–19, about 11% (29 million) lack access to effective contraceptive protection.
- Of the 29 million girls who lack contraceptive protection, 16.2 million are married and say they want to delay childbirth; 9.8 million are unmarried and sexually active; 3.2 million are adolescents, both married and unmarried, who use traditional methods. As shown in Table 21.1, Canada's teenage birth rate is six times that of Japan or Switzerland and more than twice that of Sweden and Finland. However, Canada's rate is significantly lower than that of the United States and slightly lower than the rate in the United Kingdom.

Box 21.1 Key Definitions

Teenage pregnancy: Generally speaking, teenage pregnancy is a term used to refer to a situation where girls become pregnant when they have not reached legal adulthood. Thus, the definition of teen pregnancy varies from country to country and from culture to culture. Whereas industrialized countries use age to define teen pregnancy, many less developed countries tend to define teen pregnancy as a problem mostly when the teenage girl is unmarried. In the United States, teen pregnancy is defined as a minor becoming pregnant. The term "minor" is used to refer to a person who is under the age in which one legally assumes adulthood and is legally granted rights afforded to adults in society. Depending on the jurisdiction and application, this age may vary, but is usually marked at either 18 or 21. In the United Kingdom, a woman is said to be a pregnant teenager if she falls pregnant before the age of 18.

Reproductive health: Refers to the biological, psychological, and social aspects of female and male sexual and reproductive behavior. Reproductive health services include the provision of information, contraceptives, and abortion and postabortion services.

Socioeconomic risk: An economic and/or social factor that increases the vulnerability of the teen mother and her child to poor outcomes in the biological, psychological, and/or social areas of life. These factors operate on the level of the individual, family, community, and nation. Examples of individual and familial socioeconomic risks include ignorance, low educational attainment, and low expectations for the future, unemployment, and poverty. Community and national factors include inadequate housing, neighborhood deprivation, permissive social norms, limited job opportunities, and lack of access to health care.

Table 21.1 Adolescent fertility rates for selected countries, 2005 (per 1,000 females aged 15–19 years)

Country	Pregnancy rate	Abortionrate	Birth rate	Death rate per live birth	Maternal mortality rate
United States	68	22	46	6.5	7 in 100,000
Canada	37	17	20	4.8	1 in 100,000
United Kingdom	42	20	22	5.2	13 in 100,000
France	12	7	5	4.3	10 in 100,000
Germany	14	3	11	4.2	8 in 100,000
Sweden	24	17	7	2.8	1 in 100,000
Israel	24	9	15	6	5 in 100,000
Russian Federation	100	55	45	18	55 in 100,000
India	70	25	45	65	450 in 100,000
Japan	9.6	6	3.6	3.3	45 in 100,000
Vietnam	103	83	20	20	170 in 100,000
Brazil	110	40	70	33	74 in 100,000
Mexico	86	24	62	24	100 in 100,000
Egypt	65	20	45	33	170 in 100,000
Nigeria	125	25	100	88	530 in 100,000

Sources: AGI (1998); UNFPA (2005)

Regional and Country-Specific Perspectives

North America

United States of America

Early pregnancy and childbearing are pressing concerns for adolescent health in the United States. About 31% of American women become pregnant before the age of 20. Nearly 13% of the sexually active American men between the ages of 15 and 19 report that they have fathered a pregnancy (Suellentrop and Flanigan 2006). Teen pregnancy rates vary widely by race and ethnicity. In 2002, the pregnancy rate for non-Hispanic white teens was 49 per 1,000 of girls 15–19 years of age. The pregnancy rate for Hispanic teens was 135.2. For African-American teens it was 138.9 (Ventura et al. 2006). Approximately 80% of teenage pregnancies are unintended. In 2002, they accounted for one-fifth of all accidental pregnancies in the United States (Finer and Henshaw 2006; National Campaign to Prevent Teen Pregnancy 2006). There were over 760,000 pregnancies to women under the age of 20 in 2002 and about 420,000 births to teens in 2004. The rate of teen childbearing in the United States has fallen steeply from 96 births per 1,000 girls aged 15–19 in 1950 to 49 in 2000 (Fig. 21.1).

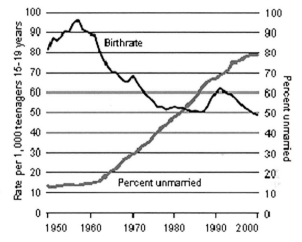

Fig. 21.1 Trend in teenage pregnancies in the United States, 1950–2000. Source: CDC, National Center for Health Statistics (2001)

Birth rates also fell steadily throughout the 1960s and 1970s and were fairly steady in the early 1980s. They rose sharply between 1988 and 1991, before declining throughout the 1990s. In recent years, this downward trend has occurred among teens of all ages and races. In spite of these declines, the United States still has one of the highest teen pregnancy and birth rates in the industrialized world (Fig. 21.2).

Rates of teen pregnancy in the United States are two to six times higher than those in most of Western Europe including France, Holland, Denmark, and Sweden (Hoffman 2006). Negative

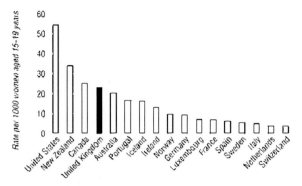

Fig. 21.2 Teenage pregnancy rates in selected high-income countries, 1998. Source: Tripp and Viner (2005)

consequences for both the mother and the child go beyond pregnancy and child birth. It is estimated that teenage pregnancy costs the United States between $7 and $9 billion annually (Hoffman 2006; National Campaign to Prevent Teen Pregnancy 1997). In the United States as in many other industrialized countries, teens can be classified into two broad categories in terms of their attitudes toward pregnancy, namely those with no intention of getting pregnant and who never planned on teen parenting and those that actually want to become pregnant. Evidence shows that teens who desire to become pregnant are often those with low expectations for their future, low self-esteem, alienation from their own family, and a history of sexual abuse or poor parenting (Stevens-Simon et al. 2005). For these teens, pregnancy is often seen as a way to bring meaning to their lives.

Research evidence has shown that age of first sexual intercourse is an important determinant of pregnancy risk; 46% of teenage girls and 22% of teenage boys who engage in their first sexual experience before the age of 15 have been involved in a pregnancy. For teens who engage in their first sex experience at age 15 or older, the risk declines to 25% and 9% for girls and boys, respectively (Suellentrop and Flanigan 2006). Teens that use contraception during their first sexual experience are less likely to experience a pregnancy; 27% of teen girls and 12% of teen boys who used contraception at first sex have been involved in a pregnancy. For teens that did not use contraception at first sex, 43% of girls and 18% of boys have been involved in a pregnancy (Suellentrop and

Flanigan 2006). Teenage girls with older partners are more likely to become pregnant than those with partners closer in age. A study by Darroch et al. (1999) showed that 6.7% of girls aged 15–17 have partners 6 or more years older. The pregnancy rate for this group was shown to be 3.7 times as high as the rate for those whose partners are no more than 2 years older (Darroch et al. 1999). Similarly, the greater the number of sex partners, the more likely teens are to be involved in a pregnancy; as a study by Suellentrop and Flanigan (2006) showed, 37% of teen girls and 18% of teen boys with three or more partners have either experienced or have been involved in a pregnancy. With less than two partners, only 25% of teen girls and 9% of teen boys have either experienced or have been involved in a pregnancy.

Teen mothers and their children are more likely to live in poverty (Crosby and Holtgrave 2006). Compared to teenagers from higher income families, teenagers from low-income families are more sexually active and less likely to use contraception correctly (AGI 1998). Teens from low-income families make up 38% of all females who are between the ages of 15 and 19; yet, these teens account for 73% of all pregnancies in that age group (AGI 1998). About 60% of these teens live in poverty at the time of the birth (AGI 1994). They are less likely to complete their school education; more likely to face limited career and economic opportunities, and less likely than older women to obtain timely prenatal and postnatal care (Ganesh 2005). These and other factors contribute to the result that babies born to teenagers are more likely to be preterm and have low birth weight. Babies of teenage mothers are also at greater risk of serious and long-term illness, developmental delays, and death in the first year of life compared to infants of older mothers (WHO 2004).

Public perception about teen pregnancy and childbearing in the United States is that problems associated with a teenage pregnancy should fall on the shoulders of the teen moms and their parents (Mauldon and Delbanco 1997). It is perceived that the teenage mother made the choice of becoming pregnant, and therefore, it is her responsibility to provide for herself and her child. A large number of people believe that only minimum resources should be provided to teenage mothers and their children.

Increasing resources to teenage mothers, they argue, would only encourage young women to become pregnant and give birth. A substantial proportion of the public does not want to pay for services needed to level the playing field for teenage mothers and their children compared to all other older mothers and their children. Public attitude in the United States toward childhood and teenage pregnancy is based in part on the religious and moral principles brought over by settlers from Western Europe in the 1600s. At the time, the most important sanction was not children or teenagers giving birth, but whether the young girl was married or not. Early colonial church records indicate that if a young woman became pregnant out of wedlock, she would confess her transgression and marry the father if possible (Ravoira and Cherry 1992).

In the 20th century, however, this view and response to pregnancy and childbirth out of wedlock changed rather rapidly beginning with the sexual revolution of the late 1960s and early 1970s (Lynch 2005). Many longheld ideas and attitudes were altered. There was also a shift in the view of pregnant teens. Instead of teen pregnancy being viewed as a moral issue, policy makers, service providers, and the public began to view it as a systems issue (Arney and Bergen 1984). Historically, one major influence on teen pregnancy rates in the United States was the legalization of abortion in 1973 (*Roe vs. Wade* 1973) (Supreme Court of the United States 1973). Twenty-nine% of the 757,000 pregnancies to teens (15–19 years) in 2002 resulted in abortion (Ventura et al. 2006). The 1973 legalization of abortion gave pregnant teenagers access to legal abortions for unwanted pregnancies without parental consent. By the end of the 20th century this right of teenage girls to an abortion without parental consent was scaled back by both federal and state legislation (AGI 2008). In 2008, the majority of states require parental notification or consent of one or sometimes both parents. Currently, only 15 states and the District of Columbia allow a minor to seek an abortion without parental consent (AGI 2008). In addition to parental consent, many other factors affect a woman's access to abortion services in the United States. Limited services are one of the major barriers. Providers are only available in 16% of all the counties in the country (Henshaw and Finer 2003). This means an adolescent must travel

and deal with a limited number of providers that perform only a certain number of abortions annually. Travel, especially across states, entails cost and safety issues for teenage girls. The cost of the abortion itself is out of pocket since federal funds do not pay for abortion unless incest, rape, or an endangerment to the mother's life is involved. The final barrier is the anti-abortion sentiment in the United States. A young woman needing an abortion must consider the possibility of confronting pro-life protesters outside doctors' offices and clinics when seeking an abortion. A great deal of stigma is still associated with being a teen mother in the United States.

Programs to prevent unintended pregnancy among teenagers have taken many forms in the United States, ranging from sex education in schools, provision of free condoms, family planning services, and faith-based initiatives to increase abstinence. Currently, prevention policy and funding is focused on promotion of abstinence. Although abstinence-only programs have been show to be ineffective in reducing teen pregnancies and preventing sexually transmitted infections (STIs) among teenagers (Santelli et al. 2006), they emerged as the cornerstone of current policy in the United States under the Bush administration. According to recent data from Alan Guttmacher Institute (2006):

- Eighty-six percent of public school districts that have a policy to teach sex education require that abstinence be promoted.
- About 35% require abstinence to be taught as the only option for unmarried people and either prohibit the discussion of contraception altogether or limit discussion to its ineffectiveness; the other 51% have a policy to teach abstinence as the preferred option for teens and permit discussion of contraception as an effective means of preventing pregnancy and sexually transmitted illnesses (STIs).
- More than half of the districts in the southern United States with a policy to teach sex education have an abstinence-only policy, compared with one in five of such districts in the Northeast.
- There are three federal programs dedicated to funding restrictive abstinence-only education: Section 510 of the Social Security Act, the Adolescent Family Life Act's teen pregnancy

prevention component, and Community-Based Abstinence Education (CBAE). The total funding for these programs in 2006 was $176 million.

- Federal law establishes a stringent eight-point definition of "abstinence-only education" which requires programs to teach that sexual activity outside of marriage is wrong and harmful – for people of any age. The law also prohibits programs from advocating contraceptive use or discussing contraceptive methods except to emphasize their failure rates (Dailard 2002). Federal guidelines now define sexual activity to include any behavior between two people that may be sexually stimulating, which could be interpreted as including kissing or hand-holding (Dailard 2006).

- There is currently no federal program dedicated to supporting comprehensive sex education that teaches young people about both abstinence and contraception (Dailard 2006).

Europe and Central Asia

England, United Kingdom

The teenage pregnancy rates vary greatly across Europe. England has the highest rate of teenage pregnancy and STI among adolescents in Western Europe. The rate of teenage pregnancy in England is triple the rate for Germany and France (Fig. 21.3) and six times higher than the rate in the Netherlands (Tripp and Viner 2005). In 2005 it was estimated that 42 of every 1,000 pregnant women were teenagers. This figure was more than three times the rate for France and Germany in the same year. Rates of teenage pregnancy fell during the 1970s and 1980s in many European countries including the UK. The rate of decline was much slower in relative to her neighbors (Fig. 21.4).

In England, less than 33% of teens are sexually active before they are 16. However, half of those who are sexually active use no contraception the first time they engage in intercourse (AGI 2002). As a result, 39,286 teen pregnancies were recorded in 2002 (AGI 2002). In 1999, over 15,000 pregnant girls under 18 years of age opted for an abortion (AGI 2002). In England, at the beginning of the 21st century, 90% of all teenage mothers have their babies outside marriage. There is pronounced concern among the public about the high rate of teen pregnancy, unwed births, and the number of teens who contract sexually transmitted diseases. Before World War II, little thought was given to teen pregnancy, and for the most part, unintended pregnancy was handled using "homes for unwed mothers" and adoption (Justin 2005).

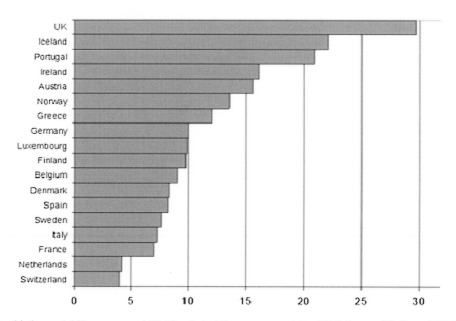

Fig. 21.3 Live births per 1,000 women aged 15–19, selected European countries, 1996. Source: Wellings (2007)

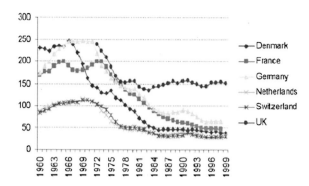

Fig. 21.4 Age-specific fertility rates in women aged 20 years and younger from selected European countries. Source: Wellings (2007)

Today, however, almost everyone in England may know of a teenage girl who has given birth to a child out of wedlock. Out of wedlock births to teenagers are socially unacceptable in England but because 90% of teenage girls are not married when giving birth, public health and social services have accepted the reality of the phenomenon.

The trend in England is to view teen pregnancy as a "personal responsibility" issue (AGI 2002). Based on this paradigm and the logical programming that follows, it will be difficult for English health and social service providers to use the more pragmatic models that have worked in other Western European nations. It is likely that officials will continue to use poorly developed sexual education curricula and blame the teenage girls and boys for the high rate of teen pregnancy. Efforts to address the serious problems faced by teenagers at risk of unintended pregnancy are hampered by lack of recognition of the diversity of modern England by politicians and public officials. For example, in England, there are no comprehensive statistics on either live births or abortions by ethnic group (AGI 2002). The mother's ethnic group is not recorded if the pregnancy is aborted or during the birth registration. Information is collected on the mother's country of birth, but this does not identify the specific ethnicity. Although official surveys recognize three ethnic minorities whose teenage girls are at increased risk of becoming a teen parent, Bangladeshis, Afro-Caribbean, and Pakistanis (AGI 2002), there is no way of identifying the extent of teen pregnancy by ethnic group. This can hinder the understanding of teen pregnancy because for

these groups, the tradition of early childbirth within marriage has a common history. A 1994 survey of Pakistani and Bangladeshi women in their twenties who had given birth in their teens found that over 90% were or had been married, compared with 55% for native English women (Health Education Authority 1994). Surveys have also reported that Pakistani and Bangladeshi women are least likely of all ethnic groups to have had sex before the age of 16 (Wellings et al. 1994). In addition, the relationship between low socioeconomic status and early pregnancy appears to be strong for these ethnic minority groups. For example, 41% of Afro-Caribbeans, 82% of Pakistanis, and 84% of Bangladeshis have incomes less than half the national average compared with 28% of English nationals (Policy Studies Institute 1997). Some individuals in ethnic minority groups are at risk, especially if they are excluded from school or are in a foster care situation. Other advocates point out that sexual health services were typically not designed in a way that would reach specific ethnic minority groups (Department of Health 1999).

A sexually active teenager who does not use contraception has a 90% chance of conceiving over the first year of sexual activity and of contracting a sexually transmitted infection. In a single act of unprotected sex with an infected partner, teenage girls in England have a 1% chance of acquiring HIV, 30% risk of getting genital herpes, and 50% chance of contracting gonorrhea (Nicoll et al. 1999). Chlamydia affects English teenage girls more than any other age group (Nicoll et al. 1999). It is the leading cause of ectopic pregnancy and can lead to infertility. It can cause discharge and pain, but is usually asymptomatic, so the sufferer may never know they are infected. Diagnoses of Chlamydia in Genito-Urinary Medicine clinics for 16–19-year-olds rose by around 53% between 1995 and 1997. This age group also had the highest diagnostic rates (1,035 per 100,000) in 2001 (Nicoll et al. 1999).

England is unique in that it continues to value the involvement of the parent, but tolerates the adolescent's decision to terminate her pregnancy. The ultimate authority does not lie with the teenager, however, but with the practitioner. Before performing an abortion, practitioners are required to attempt to persuade the teenager to contact her parents about her desire to abort her pregnancy. If she refuses, the practitioner can perform the abortion if the teenager is deemed capable of understanding the implications and potential complications of the procedure. It can be assumed that there is much variability in terms of individual practitioners' attempts to dissuade teenagers from seeking an abortion (Wellings 2001). According to a report by Wellings (2001), slightly over half of teenagers who are 16 years old and younger terminate their pregnancy. According to the report, this statistic has changed little since the 1970s. For young people in their twenties, over a third of conceptions end in abortions, and this figure is rising. Furthermore, it was noted that one in ten 16–19-year-old girls who have had an abortion have had one earlier, and 2% have had both an abortion and a birth. Pregnant teenagers are also 1.5 times more likely than women who are in their twenties to have an abortion at 13 weeks or later. Nevertheless, abortion ratio (the proportion of pregnancies that are terminated) is low in the UK compared with other European countries (Wellings 2007). However, it has been on the rise and is beginning to approximate more to the European picture (Wellings 2007). This is in contrast to the situation in the United States, where the abortion ratio is very low and falling.

There has been research into factors that influence a teenager's decision to have an abortion. Moore et al. (1996) report that "... a greater influence seems to be young women's perceptions of their future prospects. Those who have higher education aspirations are more likely to have abortions, and students tend to have more abortions than non-students."

While affluent areas in England have high rates of teenage pregnancy, it is the poorer areas that have the highest rates. The Department of Health's (2001) report on strategies to reduce teen pregnancy makes several good points about teen pregnancy. It identifies economic barriers, lack of social support systems, lack of education about sex and preventive measures, and lack of skills needed for decision making regarding relationships and unwanted pregnancy (Department of Health 2001).

Russian Federation

Teenagers that live in the Russian Federation countries of the former Soviet Union have been living through some of the most extreme and rapid changes any group of teens has ever experienced. The downfall of the Soviet Union was followed by a decade of deteriorating infrastructure, a major increase in poverty, and an overall decrease in quality of life (Singh and Darroch 2000). Over the last 25 years, in most industrial countries around the world, there has been a decline in teen birth rates, with the exception of Russia. Adolescent birth rates, which fell between 1970 and 1995 in most Western countries (Singh and Darroch 2000), rose by 54% in Russia. A comparative study of teen pregnancy rates in developed countries (Singh and Darroch 2000) showed that Russia has one of the highest teen pregnancy rates (more than 100 per 1,000) of all industrialized countries.

Unintended adolescent pregnancies are common in the Russian Federation in part because of the limited availability of accurate and confidential information on contraception and a reluctance to discuss sexual issues openly at home or to provide sex education at school. In Russia, teens receive the same reproductive services as adults. As data on teen fertility are not collected separately, few official statistics are available on teen pregnancy and birth rates. Even so, the statistics kept by the Ministry of Public Health and other agencies about services provided to people by age and sex can reveal a great deal. In 1997, according to official marriage records in Moscow, 305 girls, who were 16 years of age, were married. Among 16-year-old boys, only 26 were married. There were 867 Moscow girls who were married at 17 years of age and only 120 married boys of the same age. These numbers suggest that teenage girls tend to marry males who are older than they are.

In Moscow, according to official reports (UNICEF 1999), 75 girls under the age of 15 became mothers in 1996. Girls who were 16 years of age gave birth to 315 babies. For three of the 16-year-old mothers, it was their second child. Seventeen-year-old Moscow girls gave birth to 864 babies. For 16 of them, it was their second child. Among Moscow girls under the age of 15, there were 71 legal abortions in 1996. Girls between the ages of 15 and 19 had 10,536 abortions the same year. This was a drop from a 1994 high of more than 12,000 abortions performed on Moscow adolescents (UNICEF 1999). Available data show that at least 56.1% of adolescent pregnancies end in abortion (Singh and Darroch 2000). In 1996, there were 2,700,000 legal abortions recorded in Russia as a whole. Teenage girls accounted for about 270,000 or a tenth of these abortions. The number of abortions officially reported does not account for illegal abortions. Some experts suggest that abortions in the country are probably more than 25% under-reported and does not account for illegal abortions.

It is believed that poverty plays a significant role in teen pregnancies in Russia. A lack of educational and job opportunities result in girls and boys seeking other paths to self-fulfillment. Inadequate health services for the poor also contribute to the problem. Russian teens face inadequate family planning services and little school-based sexuality education (UNICEF 1999). There is a lack of choice between effective birth control methods. Abortion has traditionally been the way Russian teenage girls and women controlled their reproductive lives (RAND 2001). This method was supported by the central government in part because of cost and the reliability of abortion. To increase the use of other methods, a mass education campaign is needed to correct years of misinformation by the central government health service (Cohen 1997).

East Asia and the Pacific

In East Asia as in other regions of the world, teen child birth is highly correlated with the level of each country's socioeconomic development and varies from a low fertility rate of 1.39 per 100 among 15- to 19-year-old girls in Japan to a high of 60 per 100 in Thailand (Table 21.2).

In much of East Asia and the Pacific region, premarital sexual activity is considered uncommon. A survey conducted by East-West Center (1997) in the Philippines showed that most sexual activity takes place within the context of a committed rather than a casual relationship. Reported levels of premarital sex are higher than many have assumed, but most premarital sexual activity, particularly for women, appears to be initiated at some point during a process that leads to formal marriage. Indeed, the very definition of what is premarital is not always entirely clear.

However, early initiation of marriage is high and adolescent pregnancy rates are high. In countries where early marriage is common, fertility rates tend to be high (Singh and Samara 1996). In many Asian cultures, childbearing is highly valued, and

Table 21.2 Age-specific fertility (15–19 years) in selected countries of the EASP region

Country	Births/100 women aged 15–19 years
Cambodia	23
China	5
Democratic People's Republic of Korea	5
Indonesia	45
Japan	1.39
Lao People's Democratic Republic	51
Malaysia	29
Mongolia	38
Myanmar	36
Philippines	41
Republic of Korea	4
Singapore	8
Thailand	60
Vietnam	35

Source: Mehta et al. (1998)

newly married couples are often under pressure from their family and community to have children shortly after marriage. As contraceptives are becoming more widely used among older women of reproductive age, fertility has become concentrated among young married women (Singh and Samara 1996). Rapid economic, social, and demographic changes have led to changes in adolescent sexuality in the region. A trend toward increasing age of marriage has led to a perceived increase in the acceptance of premarital sex among young people. Limited information is available on the sexual patterns of unmarried adolescents. However, recent studies (Cherry et al. 2001) have found that attitudes and behaviors toward sex are becoming more open to sexual activity before marriage and at an earlier age. While pregnancy outside of marriage is still rare in much of the region, it is more common in the Pacific area and is considered an emerging problem needing special attention. In some South Pacific countries, adolescent mothers constitute over 10% of the total births (House and Nasiru 1999).

Social and cultural restrictions on adolescent premarital sexuality lead many teenagers to terminate their pregnancies to avoid detection by their elders. Abortions are common, and due to socio-cultural factors and financial restraints, these abortions are often performed secretly in unsafe conditions by unqualified providers (Mehta et al. 1998).

Japan

Japanese adolescent girls have the lowest pregnancy and birth rates in the world; only 4 girls per 1,000 (15–19 years) give birth in Japan. It is even lower for girls between the ages of 15 and 17. They give birth to 1.1 children per 1,000 girls. The low birth rate can be attributed to a number of factors. However, it is no coincidence that Japan's young people lead the world in the use of condoms for protection against unwanted pregnancy and STIs (Bankole et al. 1998). The teen abortion rate in Japan is among the 10th lowest in the world (Cherry et al. 2001). The adolescent abortion rate in 2005 was approximately 6 per 1,000 (see Table 21.1). Even so, there is concern about Japanese teenagers using abortion as a way to control births. In 1995, around 1.2 million Japanese women had an abortion (Shirk 1997).

A woman may seek an abortion to save her own life, eliminate risks to her physical health, if rape or incest was involved, and for economic or social reasons. Japan has a unique situation due to its 1948 Eugenic Protection Law (Ota 1967) which allowed abortion in the case of hereditary or mental disease not only in the mother or father but also in fourth-degree relatives. The national goal was the prevention of a genetically inferior population. Abortions rose to a high of 1,170,000 compared to 1,731,000 births. These stipulations were taken out in 1996 mainly due to the influence of disability rights organizations (United Nations 2002).

An important long-term social problem that will continue to affect Japanese girls and young women is the general status of women in Japan. In Tokyo, prostitution is legal as long as a pimp is not involved (Yayori 1999). A man can legally have sex with a child as long as he or she is over the age of 12 and consents (Reitman 1996). Furthermore, incest is not a crime unless it is a rape (Reitman 1996). Internationally, Japan is known as the largest market for enslaved women in the world (Yayori 1999).

Nonetheless, Japan is essentially a secular society where religion is not a central factor in daily life; even so, certain religious traditions and practices are very important. Buddhism has contributed a great deal to the religious and social life of Japan. It has had a tremendous influence on the arts, social institutions, and philosophy (Buckley 1998). These traditions define Japanese society, and most Japanese people affirm some religious affiliation (Picken 1994). Today, young women in Japan often talk of being disillusioned with married life. They spend long hours at home alone while their husbands are away at work. They are also burdened with the care and demands of older relatives. They are finding it increasingly difficult to accept the long-established role of mother and wife based on the competing demands of tradition and a modern world. In response, Japanese women are determined to develop a role for themselves that combines motherhood, self-fulfillment, and social usefulness. In spite of their efforts, Japanese culture continues to celebrate male dominance and female submissiveness (Miyazaki 1999).

One interesting variation on the small family theme that is seen in most developed and developing countries is the choice of gender of the only child. In countries such as China and India, where there is pressure to reduce family size, the desire is to have a male child. In Japan, however, this phenomenon is not true; a large proportion of couples in Japan want a female child. Parents in Japan believe girls will have more options than boys in the future (Women Envision 1999).

Vietnam

Much like other developing countries in this region of the world, early in its history, the Vietnamese society adopted the patriarchal family as the basic social institution. With the introduction of Confucian culture, societal norms were defined in terms of the duties and obligations of a family to a father, a child to a parent, a wife to a husband, and a younger brother to an older brother. They believed the welfare and continuity of the family group were more important than the personal interests of any one individual. In the first decade after World War II, the vast majority of North and South Vietnamese clung tenaciously to traditional Confucian customs and practices. This attitude changed, however, with the introduction of Communism. The Communists criticized the traditional concept of family as remnants left over from the failed feudal system that resulted in their third world status.

The concept of teen pregnancy in Vietnam is rarely mentioned as a separate issue from the overall high birthrate. In the larger society, it is considered normal for girls in Vietnam to marry at 13 or 14 years of age and begin to have children before they are 16. Moreover, teen pregnancy is not considered a major concern in Vietnam; rather it is the high poverty rate and the extensive use of child labor that are considered problematic. Poverty, along with the possibility of added family income from working children, tends to pressure mothers to bear more children.

Modern contraception was introduced in Vietnam on a limited scale in the 1960s, but it took 20 years before family planning was actively promoted to reduce the rapid population growth. The highest intrauterine device (IUD) prevalence rate in the world is found in Vietnam, where it became the method of choice when the country launched its two-child policy in the early 1980s (Johansson et al. 1998). Contraceptive services and legal abortion are provided free of charge through an extensive public health network. In some provinces in Vietnam, particularly in the north of the country, various incentives and fines are applied to ensure compliance with the two-child norm. As in other countries, laws to reduce the fertility rates in Vietnam resulted in an increase in abortion rates. The annual rate of adolescent abortions is over 100 per 1,000 (Table 21.1). This puts the total number of abortions at 2.5 per woman, one of the highest reported rates of induced abortion worldwide (Johansson et al. 1998).

Abortion has been available on request in Vietnam since 1975. There are no criminal codes associated with performing an abortion on a minor female. In 1989, a national law established free abortion services through the public health services and created support for sick leave related to abortion. The Survey Assessment of Vietnam Youth (Ministry of Health, Vietnam, 2003), a nationally representative study of youth in Vietnam conducted in 2003, indicates that the abortion rate is very low for married adolescents aged 15–19. It has been estimated that the inclusion of unmarried adolescents would greatly increase the abortion%age.

SAVY (Ministry of Health, Vietnam 2003) found that 7.2% of the females reported having an abortion.

South Asia

India

In the late 1990s it was estimated that 42,000 babies were born every day in India and that 4 women died out of every 1,000 live births. This is an average of about 40 women per day (Cherry et al. 2001). Currently, 70 (per 1,000) adolescent females aged 15–19 are estimated to become pregnant with 45 (per 1,000) giving birth (Cherry et al. 2001). Problems for Indian women begin at birth. Boys are considered more desirable. Traditionally, sons remain in their parents' home even after marriage. Girls are often seen as a burden, as they not only leave the family when married but also need an adequate dowry. Consequently, girls may be fed less if there is insufficient food, and their education is neglected. Clinics in India advertise pregnancy testing to determine the sex of the fetus. In many instances, abortions are performed if it is a female (Cherry et al. 2001). Although such practices are now illegal, they still occur (Cherry et al. 2001). In 2006, for the first time in India since the law against sex selection abortions (the Female Foeticide Law) was passed in 1994 a doctor was sentenced to jail and fined for using ultrasound technology to determine the sex of an unborn child for purposes of abortion (White 2006).

For the urban, middle-class adolescent girl in cities such as Delhi and Bombay, life is materially more comfortable. She is more likely to be given an education. Once married, however, she is still expected to be a mother and homemaker. Like her village counterpart, if she fails to provide a son the consequences can be severe. Reports continue to describe girls burning to death in kitchen fires, most of which have been identified as either suicide or murder (Shaha and Mohanthy 2006; Jutla and Heimbach 2004). The best data available are from the 1992 to 1993 National Family Health Survey of India (International Institute for Population Sciences 1995) which indicates that girls are breastfed for shorter periods than boys and are less likely to be vaccinated or to receive treatment for diseases such as diarrhea, fever, and acute respiratory infections. Hence, child mortality in the 0–4 years age group is 43% higher for females (at 42 per 1,000) than for males (29 per 1,000) (Sen 1994). India's National Family Planning initiative has contributed to increased awareness about family planning, contraceptives, and available medical services. According to the Department of Family Planning statistics, the percentage of females either sterilized or fitted with an IUD increased from 10.4% in 1971 to 44.1% in 1991 (Department of Family Welfare 1990–1991). Most of this increase has been achieved through sterilization of women with a mean age of 31. These women have on average 3.3 living children (Department of Family Welfare 1990–1991). This profile has changed little over the years. This means that India's Family Planning has not been very successful in recruiting teenage girls or younger couples, and it has not been able to popularize the use of safer forms of birth control, like the condom (Zodgekar 1996).

An abortion in India can be performed if any one of six criteria are met: (1) to save the life of the woman, (2) to preserve the physical health of the woman, (3) to preserve the mental health of the woman, (4) in cases of rape or incest, (5) fetal impairment, or (6) for social or economic reasons. Abortions performed to ensure a male child is a serious problem in India. The decade 1991–2001 saw a decline in the birth of girls per 1,000 as compared to boys from 945 to 927. Some states have more pronounced declines such as Punjab (875 to 793) and Haryana (879 to 820). The statistics were accompanied by some poignant statements which reflected that it may become impossible to make up for the missing female babies (UNFPA 2003).

It is difficult to report findings related to abortion that go beyond the mere reporting of its legality. Estimates of the adolescent abortion rate are 45 per 1,000 (Table 21.1). The stigma of having an abortion creates barriers to studying why Indian women seek abortion and the actual services they receive. Nevertheless, a recent study of decision making, reasons for seeking an abortion, variation in provider services, and the young women's awareness of the legality of abortion provides some data

on these behaviors (Kapilashrami n.d.). The findings suggest that there is a lower level of decision making related to abortion for adolescents (below the age of 20) in comparison to women that were between the ages of 21 and 24, and older. Spacing of children was the main reason for seeking an abortion. Sex selection is the reason given for one out of every eight abortions. Age and being married played a major role in differentiating trends in girls and young women. The younger the woman, the more likely the doctor was to insist on spousal consent even though the law does not require spousal involvement. Unmarried adolescents faced a higher cost for a private sector abortion than for married teenagers (Ganatra and Hirve 2002). A finding that puts into question the effectiveness or lack of public education about abortion is that 60% of the adolescents that received an abortion did not know that abortion was legal even for unmarried women (Ganatra and Hirve 2002).

Legalizing abortion does not by itself guarantee safe abortion. Abortion has been legal on broad grounds in India for almost 30 years; yet, many women, especially in rural areas, cannot access a legal abortion. Authorized facilities that provide safe abortions services are inadequate in number, and some women have found their treatment by government health professionals to be degrading (Kapilashrami n.d.). As a result, women frequently go outside the authorized system and obtain an illegal abortion, many of which are unsafe.

Central and South America

The Pan American Health Organization (PAHO) states clearly and in numerous ways that poverty greatly increases the risks of pregnancy among Latin American adolescents between the ages of 15 and 19 years (PAHO 2000). PAHO bases it conclusion on studies that show that about 70% of pregnant teens come from the most disadvantaged groups in Latin American, such as those girls living in rural areas of their country. Poverty and teen motherhood in Central and South America has serious consequences for the children of these teen moms. The children are likely to be undernourished; they are less likely to attend school, and show poorer motor skills than children of adult women (UNICEF 2008). In Chile and Mexico, approximately 75% of women who gave birth before the age of 20 are the children of teen mothers themselves (Cherry et al. 2001). The number of teen pregnancies is similar in the countries that are found in the Central and South American regions of the world. The teen pregnancy rates in South America vary from a low of 56 per 1,000 teens (15–19 year) in Chile to a high of 101 per 1,000 teen girls in Venezuela. In Central America, the rates vary from a low of 91 per 1,000 in Panama to a high of 149 per 1,000 in Nicaragua (Gatti 1999).

Mexico

Like most developing countries, Mexico is committed to reducing its population growth and improving its public health (Po 1997). Mexico is a developing nation sharply divided by income and education. While a middle class is developing in the cities, there remains widespread poverty and sharp divisions between the wealthy educated elite and the poor. Among urban residents, 40% have incomes below the poverty level. More revealing, a large%-age of government employees can be classified as having incomes below the poverty level. Many areas of Mexico are experiencing a significant industrial boom. Industrialization with the promise of high pay and steady work is drawing the young from the depressed and rural countryside to the urban areas. The wages and benefits from industry (most often multinational corporations) have fueled a consumer movement in Mexico like none it has ever witnessed. This prosperity has also created a major cultural conflict. Although a traditional agrarian culture has characterized family life in Mexico for almost 500 years, these agrarian traditional roles for men and women do not fit with the pragmatism of commerce. Women are working outside the home more often; they are becoming better educated, and especially in affluent urban areas the young women are cosmopolitan. Most importantly, women bring home a paycheck.

In modern Mexico traditional family values have given way to family economics. This is especially true when the traditional way of life results in the subjugation of girls and women. Today in Mexico,

women have economic value that far exceeds the value of their fertility. The meaning of these events is even more understandable when it is remembered that women in Mexico did not have basic civil rights or the right to vote until the mid-1950s. This left Mexican women powerless in family relationships, their community, and in legal matters. They had difficulty in making their husbands share the responsibility for contraception and childcare and were often left destitute if their husband for whatever reason was no longer in the home.

From a national perspective, these traditional ideals of the past, early marriage, childbirth, and large families do not fit with the demands of a growing industrial complex. They do not fit with the increasing awareness of ecological and population stressors. High birth rates, while prized in traditional agrarian cultures in Central and South America, are seen as deleterious to the environment and the economy of these developing industrial states. The industrial sites that are rapidly being developed in Central and South America are largely owned by multinational corporations. These industrial sites are similar to the *maquiladora* plants and factories that have been built along the border between Mexico and the United States. These factories typically owned by firms in the United States profit greatly from the labor of Mexican girls and young women they hire. Today there are more than 4,000 such plants employing almost 1 million workers in Mexico. Almost 80% of these plants are located along the border. Since the 1970s, the majority of workers at these assembly plants have been girls and young women.

While it is legal to hire adolescents when they turn 16, and some children work legally with their parent's permission, or with permission obtained from local authorities at the age of 14, it is common for girls as young as 12 (with false documents) to be working for some of the largest multinational companies in Mexico. To obtain and keep their jobs at many plants, the adolescent girls and young women are required to submit to medical examinations and pregnancy tests to prove that they are not pregnant. Among Mexican adolescents under the age of 20, over 500,000 become pregnant each year. Of these, 380,000 adolescents gave birth; the other 120,000 lose their babies through abortion or medical complications (Cherry et al. 2001). Between 300,000 and

600,000 women of all ages have clandestine abortions each year. The government-run National Health System reported that four women die every day in Mexico from maternity-related causes, and 40% of these women die from the consequences of induced abortion. Contraceptive use has been low among sexually exposed adolescents in Mexico. One study of adolescents living in Leon, Mexico, found that male students scored higher on knowledge of sexuality but that female students had a greater knowledge of contraception. Both males and females among the lower socioeconomic class scored lower on knowledge of sexuality, contraception, and sexually transmitted diseases than those of the middle and upper classes (Huerta-Franco et al. 1996).

"Contraceptive use among women without education who live in rural areas is under 30% among women from urban areas with six or more years of schooling, the contraceptive use exceeds 75%" (Cherry et al. 2001). Among adolescents, the IPPF report noted that although 68% of adolescents ask for contraceptives, only 29% use them. At the turn of the 21st century, adolescents were giving birth to more than 500,000 children a year in Mexico. Adolescent childbirths tend to be unplanned, and the younger the mother is, the less likely she is to be married. Unmarried adolescent mothers face social ostracism at all social levels. They have insufficient family support and no financial support from the government. If a girl becomes pregnant, there is intense pressure for her to marry, even if she thinks that a forced marriage would end up in severe marital conflict and divorce (AGI 1994). The consequences of not marrying would limit her prospects of marrying again in the future.

Teenagers in Mexico who become pregnant often find themselves alone and facing a major crisis. The pregnancy rate for adolescents in 2005 was 86 per 1,000 (see Table 21.1). In Mexico, contraceptives are often difficult to acquire, especially for the rural or urban poor. In addition, abortion is illegal throughout Mexico. Still, 24 per 1,000 adolescents sought an abortion in 2005 (Ross-Fowler 1998). These circumstances often lead to sad choices for all involved (Ross-Fowler 1998).

Because abortion is illegal in Mexico, the woman and the person performing the abortion are both faced with imprisonment (AGI 2000). The Federal District and most of the 31 states in Mexico permit legal abortions if it endangers a woman's life or if the pregnancy was the result of rape. The abortion must be performed within 12 weeks of gestation. The Federal District specifies additional conditions related to termination of a pregnancy. A person can receive 6–8 years in prison if they inflict physical or moral violence that results in the end of a pregnancy. The most restrictive states only allow abortion in the case of rape. Other states consider fetal defects and the woman's health as a legitimate reason to seek an abortion. Chiapas in 1991 passed a law that would have expanded legal abortion to include a woman who was single or in certain cases where seeking an abortion was a couple's decision. Later in that same year, the state legislature suspended the law (AGI 2000).

Sub-Saharan Africa

The African continent is generally divided into two parts: the north, which is located above the Sahara Desert, and the sub-Saharan countries that are located below the Sahara Desert (the world's largest desert). The majority of Africans live in sub-Saharan Africa. Sub-Saharan Africa includes the countries of Ethiopia, Somalia, Uganda, Angola, Cameroon, Ghana, Nigeria, the Democratic Republic of the Congo, South Africa (including the homelands: Botswana, Lesotho, Namibia, Transkei, and others), and a number of islands, the largest of which is Madagascar. In the mid-1980s, there was widespread concern that the population explosion taking place in sub-Saharan Africa would destabilize the entire continent of Africa. The number of adolescents giving birth was far too high for both wed and unwed adolescent girls in much of sub-Saharan Africa. At that time, great emphasis was placed on programs that provided effective contraception methods to slow down the population growth (Metz 1991). In 2000, there was continued concern over the high number of adolescents becoming pregnant; however, of greater concern was the spread of HIV infection, especially among adolescents and teenagers. Botswana, the country in the sub-Sahara with the world's highest HIV infection rate reports that 36% of adults were infected in the year 2000. Deaths from

AIDS dropped the life expectancy of people born in Botswana from 71 to 39 years of age. It was also the first time that the United States Census Bureau predicted that a country's population would drop because of AIDS (Haney 2000).

Even in the face of this most devastating pandemic, in Africa as elsewhere, more teenage girls are enrolled in school and delaying the birth of their first child. In some rural areas, however, large families with 4–10 children is still the norm, large families for the most part are viewed as more of a burden than a help. Traditional values based on an agrarian culture have been replaced with urban attitudes and ideas. In the past, adolescent childbearing was confined to marriage; today, early childbearing increasingly occurs outside of marriage. Rapid social changes as a result of Western influence, commerce, and knowledge of the world outside of sub-Saharan Africa have convinced large numbers of teenage girls that adolescent pregnancy could be hurtful to their health and future and to the future of the child they may deliver. Consequently, although sexual activity has increased slightly, births among adolescent girls are not increasing in most sub-Saharan African countries. The rate of unintended births has either leveled off or is declining. Nevertheless, as a region, most sub-Saharan Africa still has the highest rates of adolescent pregnancies in the world (Amazigo et al. 1997).

Nigeria

Nigeria has the largest population of any country in Africa, an estimated 131 million people (UNICEF 2008). Despite having the largest population in Africa, Nigeria has one of the lowest HIV/AIDS infection rates in sub-Saharan Africa. Nevertheless, rapid increase in HIV infection is imminent, if sexual behaviors do not change. Young married men in Nigeria like in other sub-Saharan African nations are drawn to industrial areas where work is available and where they can provide for their wife and children back home. At first they tend to return home every 2 or 3 weeks with their earnings and renew their relationship with their wives and children. Overtime, however, the men tend to return home less often. While away from their families, many men become involved in sexual relationships

with women in the urban areas. These relationships often involve unprotected sex (UNICEF 2008). This leads to the men contracting STIs and HIV/AIDS which are then taken back home to their wives. In Nigeria, 15- to 29-year-olds accounted for 63% of all AIDS cases among females between 1986 and 1995.

In the year 2000, slightly over 40% of Nigerians live in an urban area, twice the number that lived in cities in 1970. Nigeria has a long history of urban development, particularly in northern and southwestern regions. A vast number of these urban areas were important cities many centuries before the Europeans arrived. Lagos was colonial Nigeria's capital and is today the leading port city. It is one of the largest cities in the world (Metz 1991). In 2003, about 66% of Nigerian girls aged 15–19 had weekly access to at least one of the three main types of media – newspapers, radio, or television, and about 10% had access to all three types. However, 34% did not have any media exposure in the average week (AGI 2004).

Between 1980 and 2003, the birthrate among Nigerian girls aged 15–19 decreased by 27% (from 173 to 126 births per 1,000 girls this age) and remained relatively stable in 2005 at 125 per 1,000. Nonetheless, 46% of women nationally and about 70% of those in some regions still give birth before their 20th birthday (National Population Commission (NPC), Federal Republic of Nigeria and ORC Macro 2003). Prenatal care by a doctor or nurse-midwife during pregnancy, at delivery, and during postpartum (within 2 months of delivery) vastly improves birth outcomes. In Nigeria, only half of young women aged 15–24 who have given birth receive prenatal care. Young women in rural areas are much less likely than those in urban areas to have professional care during their pregnancy (40% vs. 78%). Less educated women (under 7 years of education) are also much less likely to have had professional care than more educated young women (39% vs. 81%). The likelihood of a young woman receiving obstetric care during delivery is even poorer. Only 30% of young women aged 15–24 giving birth are attended by a trained health professional (Singh et al. 2004).

The inadequacy of Nigeria's maternal and child health services has tragic consequences. The rate of infant mortality is high (88 deaths per 1,000 births), as is the rate of maternal mortality (533 maternal deaths per 100,000 live births) (WHO 2004). One study found that 72% of all deaths among young women under the age of 19 were due to the consequences of unsafe abortions (Shane 1997). Many other young women who survive unsafe abortion suffer complications leading to infertility (Shane 1997). Nigerian abortion laws in the northern states are different from abortion laws in the southern states. In the northern states, where the population is predominantly Muslim, abortion is only allowed when it is needed to save the life of the woman. In the southern states where the population is predominantly Christian, three exceptions permit legal abortion: to save the life of the woman, to preserve her mental health, or to preserve her physical health. Two physicians must certify that the pregnancy constitutes a danger to the woman's life in both the northern and southern states. Fines for individuals performing an illegal abortion are 14 years of imprisonment. The woman receiving the abortion also faces this length of time in prison. There is a harsher sentence for those performing an illegal abortion if the woman dies. Induced abortion is a major cause of maternal morbidity. Girls between 15 and 19 years of age make up the highest risk group (Shane 1997).

The widespread use of injectable contraceptives and the pill, which is common among sub-Saharan African women, is in great part due to the limited range of methods provided by government programs. Government services promoted methods that required minimal education, little client involvement, and few follow-up services. These forms of contraception, however, do not protect the woman or man from STIs, including HIV/AIDS. In rural areas, social conditions are poor and there are limited educational and job opportunities for adolescents, especially girls. Marrying at a young age and having children while still in her teens is a social expectation and may seem to be a more certain route to social standing than education. However, having children early can have negative consequences because young mothers are often physiologically immature and lack access to adequate health care. Due to the lack of government-sponsored programs that disseminate educational materials on various types of birth control, 58% of Nigerian females use the form of birth control that is most familiar to them, injectable implants (Amazigo et al. 1997).

Middle East and North Africa

Middle East and North Africa is considered a region with strong family values and conservative, patriarchal culture. A woman's virginity at marriage is highly valued, and women are often sheltered from sexual situations. This conservatism can benefit a young woman's well-being, but can also serve as a barrier for young women accessing reproductive health information and services. This region is not what it was a generation ago; young people are spending more years in school and are marrying later. Many girls are reaching puberty sooner due to improved nutrition, and the period of unmarried adolescence is growing longer, leading to longer period of risk for unintended adolescent pregnancy. As Fig. 21.5 shows, births to teenagers aged 15–19 years range from a low of 7 per 1,000 in Tunisia to a high of 93 per 1,000 in Yemen (DeJong et al. 2007).

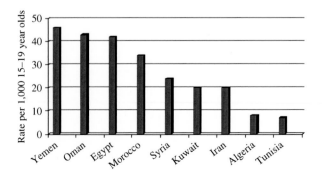

Fig. 21.5 Births per 1,000 women aged 15–19, selected countries, 2004. Source: World Bank (2006)

Early marriage is still common in some of the areas of the region. Average age at first marriage usually occurs between 17.9 and 24.3 years of age (Ozcebe and Akin 1995). However, in Syria, 25% of girls are married by age 19, in Algeria 10% are married between 15 and 19 years of age, and in Egypt 14% of young women are married before age 20. Early marriage often leads to early pregnancy and associated biological risks. As young men are usually valued greater than young women, young women often do not receive the health care and attention they need during pregnancy (Ozcebe and Akin 1995). Additionally, young women are often married to older men who have had prior sexual relations and may be carriers of sexually transmitted infections (Ozcebe and Akin 1995).

Throughout the region, there is a lack of access to information and services that deal with sexual and reproductive health (DeJong et al. 2007). Discussion of sex is taboo and there is a belief that talking openly about sexual health may encourage young women to have premarital sex. This creates an obstacle to informed discussion. However, as the risk of STIs, adolescent pregnancy, and unsafe abortion increases, steps have been made in some nations toward sexual health education. Algeria, Iran, Morocco, Tunisia, and Bahrain have recently included human reproduction and health education in their national school curriculum (Dejong et al. 2007). Iran has developed a reproductive health curriculum for high schools and requires all university students to take a course that includes reproductive health. High schools and universities are also beginning to develop extra-curricular reproductive health awareness activities across the region (Dejong et al. 2007).

Egypt

The nations in the region above the sub-Sahara are represented in this section by Egypt. National Policy for Youth in Egypt encourages "healthy development," which means that overall health is integrated with education, psychological development, skills training, work, and legal protection for youth. The five health areas emphasized in the youth policy are basic nutrition, preparation for puberty and marriage, negative and risky behaviors, prevention and treatment of health problems, and social and psychological development. Education is free and compulsory in Egypt, but only 58% of adults can read (U.S. Department of State 2007). Gender roles continue to change in Egypt for both boys and girls. At times, these role changes occur faster than attitudes. The gap between what is perceived as socially "right" and what is "reality" fuels the conflict over the change in the role of Egyptian women and girls. Although girls are valued for their fertility, during childhood, male siblings receive preferential treatment. In one study (Ragheb and Guirgis 1998), the average number of doctor visits was 1.6 for boys vs. 0.9 for girls. Additionally, the better educated the mother is, the more likely that her daughter will be attending school (Ragheb and Guirgis 1998). Both boys and girls clearly prefer segregated gender roles, but they have come to believe that decision making should be shared. Many more adolescent girls than boys, however, think decisions concerning contraceptives, health care, and the wife working outside the home should be as much their decision as their husbands (Ragheb and Guirgis 1998).

In a national survey of Egyptian adolescents in 1998 (Digges 1999) both boys and girls agreed that a wife should get her husband's permission for everything she does (girls 89% and boys 91%). They agreed that the husband should know about pregnancies, childbirth, and any birth complications (girls 89% and boys 93%). And, most adolescents agree that the wife should keep trying to have a male baby, even if she was satisfied with the number of children she had (girls 81% and boys 80%) (Digges 1999).

The number of adolescent girls who marry began to fall in the 1990s. Yet, despite the decline, it is still high in rural Upper Egypt. The median age of first pregnancy is 17.6 years of age, which indicates that 50% of adolescent girls become pregnant before they turn 18. One of the reasons for the young age at first pregnancy is that less than 16% of married adolescent girls use a contraceptive and which typically only after the first birth, which most often happens in the first year of marriage (Digges 1999). There are about 45 stillbirths per 1,000 live births and 74 infant deaths per 1,000 live births in Egypt (Sahar 1999). Eighty percent of adolescents believe that the best place to have a child was in a government hospital, although actual delivery of Egyptian children is split about 50% in a government hospital and 50% at home (Qayed and Waszak 1999). Almost all older adolescent girls in Egypt are familiar with "family planning" and most have a positive attitude about contraception. However, knowledge of specific methods varies. For instance, 53% of adolescent girls and younger women are familiar with injectables as compared to 21% of older women. Also, 92% of all adolescent females and women know about "intrauterine devices" (IUD), compared to 79% of males (Qayed and Waszak 1999).

Among adolescent wives in Egypt, the use of contraception increases as the number of children increases. A study by Qayed and Waszak (1999) showed that 15% of those with one child were using contraception, compared with 79% of those with four or more children (Qayed and Waszak 1999). The majority of Egyptian women, over 90%, have used contraception at some point in their lives. At any given time, 80% will be using a contraception method. The intrauterine device (IUD) continues to be the most popular method.

Abortion is legal if it is determined that a continued pregnancy will pose a risk to the mother's life. This allowance is not officially in the penal code, but it is an accepted practice. A woman, however, must obtain certification from three doctors that her life is in danger. A woman's right to seek an abortion alone is denied with the legal codes that demand a husband's consent. The only allowable exception to a husband's consent is if a doctor deems that the abortion is necessary. More than one-third of women who experience an unintended pregnancy said they tried to terminate their pregnancy through abortion. Due to its illegality, many women sought clandestine or unsafe abortions. Women need information on the risks of unsafe abortion, and physicians need training in treating abortion complications (Kader and Maklouf 1998).

Although there are no government statistics on the number of abortions performed annually in Egypt, in studies of females being admitted to Egyptian hospitals, 19% or one in five females were admitted for treatment of an induced or spontaneous abortion (Huntington et al. 1998).

In this study, it was shown that 86% of the pregnancies were terminated at 12 weeks. At least 14% of the women admitted were suffering from excessive blood loss, and 5% had one or more infections. Based on these numbers, the abortion rate in Egypt is estimated to be somewhere around 15 per 100 pregnancies. Treatment for complications from unsafe abortion requires a substantial amount of Egyptian health-care resources (Huntington et al. 1998). Others have argued that stillbirths and miscarriages are more common among adolescent and teenage mothers and can be mistaken for and tend to increase the abortion estimates. In 2005, 20 per 1,000 adolescent females sought abortion (Table 21.1).

In Egypt, other North African countries, and in Arab countries, teenage pregnancy is common (65 per 1,000) (Table 21.1). The difference between teenagers who are pregnant or parenting is that in almost all cases the teen mom is married. In Egypt as in many other countries in the region, most girls marry in their teens. Then, because of societal pressures to prove their womanhood and to increase their status, many girls become pregnant soon after marriage. Yet, few of these married adolescents know about or understand the concept of reproductive health (Sallam et al. 1998). Even so, contraceptive use has increased among adolescent wives and young married women from 24% in 1980, to 30% in 1984, and 48% in 1991 (USAID 2000).

Traditionally, Egyptian men have preferred that their wife (almost always an adolescent) have a child as soon after marriage as possible. Hence, at least 50% of adolescent girls who marry are pregnant the first time within 4 months of being married. Consequently, very high rates of stillbirth and infant death are found among married adolescent girls. In the early 1970s, there was little hope that family planning would work in Egypt. The average family had eight children. Any suggestion that population growth was a problem attracted protests from religious and political leaders. In 1970, only about 8% of women used any kind of contraceptive.

In Egypt and other societies in which female chastity at marriage is of paramount importance, unmarried pregnant adolescent girls will often commit suicide or may be murdered by family members. In some cases, she might be relegated to a life of prostitution (Gordon 1991). Most near Eastern societies place great value on female chastity at marriage (Gordon 1991). Adolescent and teen pregnancy in Egypt is a concern because of the young age at which wedded adolescent girls give birth to their first child and the number of times they will become pregnant during their lifetime. Few girls in Egypt become pregnant before marriage. If an unmarried girl does become pregnant and does not marry quickly, the consequences can be, and often are, disastrous for the girl (Shawky and Milaat 2000).

Conclusion – Research Priorities

This section has two inter-related purposes: (1) to describe the aspects of research that will lead to the most relevant global knowledge of teen pregnancy and (2) to identify topics for research focus. Addressing these two areas will guide the development and sustainability of evidence-based policies and practices for teen mothers and their children. The first aspect of relevant research is context. Collaborative research internationally and within the countries is the only viable route for future research. For example, we know that Western European countries experience a low rate of teen pregnancy. One proposed reason for these low rates is the holistic orientation of these nations to adolescent sexuality. This means that adolescent sexuality is viewed as an integral part of a young person's well-being. A topic for international consideration is to test this approach to adolescent sexuality in other countries. The most obvious argument against the development of this type of research relates to cultural congruence with the obvious question of how Western European approaches can be replicated and tested within countries that do not promote adolescent sexuality. In order to address this barrier, the focus must be not on the approach but on the underlying value. While specifics of the Western European approach such as national advertising campaigns related to sexual health and the provision of contraceptive products to minors do not currently correspond to every nation's level of

openness, the underlying value of holism can apply. Sexuality as just one aspect of wellness presents a holistic orientation to the self that can potentially translate into nations based on a collectivist orientation to the self, family, and community. This presentation may create an openness and freedom in tailoring approaches within countries. Key to the success of this development is the inclusion of researchers and service providers within the country and policy officials. Another subject of study would be the change processes for countries that have the most restrictive policies related to female reproductive decision making. For example, Colombia has recently liberalized its abortion law (AGI 2006). The process of change within this highly restrictive country would inform other changes related to policies regarding teen sexual health.

As mentioned in the previous section, effort to include previously under-researched groups is critical to address the health of each nation's adolescent populations. A priority area should be in-depth research of indigenous peoples, rural residents, and populations that are disenfranchised and who often carry a greater burden of risk factors and negative outcomes. A contemporary area of research within at-risk populations is the identification and study of individuals that have avoided negative outcomes. Research of the decisions and social networks of these "resilient" individuals would create knowledge of a neglected group that could lead to interventions for the larger at-risk populations. The inclusion of males as a population of study is another critical piece to the future research agenda. While childbearing is a female reality and parenting is considered a female responsibility, the influence of males needs further study in order to inform prevention of teen pregnancy and/or interventions of existing families involving teen parents.

The course of research across all areas of interest tends to be cross-sectional. This research should continue in an international multi-site context to enhance comparisons within and across nations. An important topic for research would relate to the economic outcomes associated with basic reproductive health provision in the immediate and long term. The reliability and validity of measures across nations and even within nations is also an issue for research.

Finally, some saw the worldwide decline in teen pregnancy as a result of effective pregnancy prevention programming. Others attributed the decline to religious campaigns promoting abstinence. Still others interpreted it as confirmation that globalization has taken roots. Researchers saw the phenomenon as an opportunity that could provide information on events and characteristics that coalesced to cause this cross-national change in a teenage girl's sexual behavior. The cross-national themes identified in this chapter provide a platform on which

research can test the themes, where knowledge can be developed around the themes, and where understanding of this phenomenon can go beyond the individual teenage girl's reasons for becoming pregnant. Today's adolescents are the next generation of parents, workers, and leaders. To fill these roles to the best of their ability, they need the guidance and support of their family and their community. They also need governments that are committed to their health, development, education, and well-being.

Key Terms

Abstinence	Gonorrhea	Prostitution
Abstinence-only policy	Incest	Rape
Abuse	Infertility	Reproductive health
Adolescence	Intrauterine device	Roe vs. Wade 1973
Adverse pregnancy outcomes	Low birth weight	Sex education
Age of sexual intercourse	Low-income families	Sexual revolution
Anti-abortion	Miscarriage	Socioeconomic risk
Birth rates	Neglect	Sterilization
Chastity	Obstetric care	Stillbirths
Chlamydia	Population growth	Teen birth rates
Condoms	Postnatal care	Teen pregnancy
Contraception	Poverty	Unprotected sex
Faith-base	Premarital sex	Unsafe abortion
Family planning	Prenatal care	Virginity
Gender	Pro-life	

Questions for Discussion

1. What are the risk factors for unintended pregnancy among adolescents?
2. Outline and discuss the health, economic, and social consequences of unintended teenage pregnancy.
3. Which programs are known to be most effective in reducing unintended teenage pregnancies and why?
4. What factors account for the disparity in teen pregnancy rates between the United States and Western European countries?
5. It is known that England has higher rate of teen pregnancy compared to other countries in Western Europe, e.g., triple the rate in Germany and France. Outline and discuss the factors that account for these disparities.

References

Alan Guttmacher Institute (AGI) (1994) Women and reproductive health in Latin America and the Caribbean. http://www.popline.org/docs/122206, cited 2 August 2008

Alan Guttmacher Institute (AGI) (1998) Into a New World: Young Women's Sexual and Reproductive Lives. New York: Alan Guttmacher Institute

Alan Guttmacher Institute (AGI) (2000) Abortion Surfaces as Key Issue in Mexican Politics. Washington, DC: Author. The Guttmacher Report on Public Policy, 3(5). http://www.guttmacher.org/media/index.html#news5, cited 2 August 2008

Alan Guttmacher Institute (AGI) (2002) Teen pregnancy: trends and lessons learned. http://www.guttmacher.org/pubs/tgr/05/1/gr050107.pdf, cited 2 August 2008

Alan Guttmacher Institute (AGI) (2004) Early Childbearing in Nigeria: A Continuing Challenge. Research in Brief (2). Washington DC: Alan Guttmacher Institute. http://www.guttmacher.org/pubs/rib/2004/12/10/rib2-04.pdf, cited 2 August 2008

Alan Guttmacher Institute (AGI) (2006) Colombia liberalizes abortion law. In The News. http://www.guttmacher.org/media/index.html#news5, cited 2 August 2008

Alan Guttmacher Institute (AGI) (2008) State policies in brief: parental involvement in minors' abortions. http://www.guttmacher.org/statecenter/spibs/spib_PIMA.pdf, cited 2 August 2008

Amazigo U, Silva N, Kaufman J et al. (1997) Sexual activity and contraceptive knowledge and use among in-school adolescents in Nigeria. International Family Planning Perspectives, 23, 28–33

Arney W, Bergen B (1984) Power and visibility: the invention of teenage pregnancy. Social Science Medicine, 18(1), 11–19

Bankole A, Singh S, Haas T (1998) Reasons why women have induced abortions: evidence from 27 countries. International Family Planning Perspectives, 24(3), 117–127, 152

Buckley R (1998) Japan Today. 3rd Ed. Cambridge, England: Cambridge University Press

Chen XK, Wen SW, Fleming N et al. (2007) Teenage pregnancy and adverse birth outcomes: a large population based retrospective cohort study. International Journal of Epidemiology, 36(2), 368–373

Cherry AL, Dillon ME, Rugh D (2001) Teenage Pregnancy: A Global View. Westport, CT: Greenwood Press

Cohen SA (1997) The Role of Contraception in Reducing Abortion. Washington, DC: Alan Guttmacher Institute

Crosby RA, Holtgrave DR (2006) The protective value of social capital against teen pregnancy: a state-level analysis. Journal of Adolescent Health, 38(5), 556–559

Dailard C (2002) Abstinence promotion and teen family planning: the misguided drive for equal funding. The Guttmacher Report on Public Policy, 5(1), 1–3

Dailard C (2206) Legislating against arousal: the growing divide between federal policy and teenage sexual behavior, Guttmacher Policy Review, 9(3), 12–16

Darroch JE, Landry DJ, Oslak S (1999) Age differences between sexual partners in the United States. Family Planning Perspectives, 31(4), 160–167

Dejong J, Shepard B, Roudi-Fahimi F et al. (2007) Young People's Sexual and Reproductive Health in the Middle East and North Africa. Washington, DC: Population Reference Bureau. http://www.prb.org/pdf07/MENAYouthReproductiveHealth.pdf, cited 2 August 2008

Department of Family Welfare (1990–1991) Family welfare programme. In: India Year Book, pp. 257–263. Delhi, India: Department of Family Welfare

Department of Health (1999) Me, Survive, Out There ? New Arrangements for Young People Living and Leaving Care, Department of Health Consultation Paper, June 1999. London, England: Department of Health

Department of Health (2001) The National Teenage Pregnancy Strategy (2001–2010). Teenage Pregnancy Unit. London, England: Department of Health. http://www.everychild-matters.gov.uk/health/teenagepregnancy/about/, cited 24 August 2008

Digges D (1999) Adolescence in profile: the country's first national survey of a critical demographic group indicates some gains in education but ongoing, endemic poverty. Egypt: The Cairo Times, (3) 5

East-West Center (1997) Survey sheds new light on marriage and sexuality in the Philippines. Program on Population Asia-Pacific Population Policy #42.http://www2.east-westcenter.org/pop/misc/p&p-42.pdf, cited 2 August 2008

Finer LB, Henshaw SK (2006) Disparities in rates of unintended pregnancy in the United States, 1994 and 2001. Perspectives on Sexual and Reproductive Health, 38(2), 90–96

Ganatra B, Hirve S (2002) Induced abortions among adolescent women in rural Maharashtra, India. Reproductive Health Matters, 10(19), 76–85. http://www.jstor.org/sici?sici=0968-8080(200205)10%3A19%3C76%3AIAAAWI%3E2.0.CO%3B2-0&cookieSet=1, cited 24 August 2008

Ganesh D (2005). An update on teen pregnancy. The Internet Journal of Gynecology and Obstetrics, 5(1)

Gatti D (1999) Population-Latin America: child exploitation cuts across class divisions. Inter Press Service English News Wire

Gordon D (1991) Female circumcision and genital operations in Egypt and the Sudan: a dilemma for medical anthropology. Medical Anthropology Quarterly, 5, 3–14

Haney DQ (2000) AIDS toll in Africa to soar, experts say. Miami Herald, p.A.1

Health Education Authority (1994) Analysis of health education and lifestyle survey. London: UK Department of Health

Henshaw SK, Finer LB (2003) The accessibility of abortion services in the United States, 2001. Perspectives on Sexual and Reproductive Health, 35(1), 16–24. http://www.guttmacher.org/pubs/psrh/full/3501603.pdf, cited 24 August 2008

Hoffman SD (2006) By the numbers: the public costs of teen child bearing. http://www.teenpregnancy.org/costs/pdf/report/BTN_Executive_Summary.pdf, cited 2 August 2008

House W, Nasiru I (1999) Fertility patterns of adolescent and older women in pacific island countries: programming implications. UNFPA Country Support Team: Office for the South Pacific, Discussion Paper No. 20

Huerta-Franco R, Diaz de Leon G, Mmalacara J (1996) Knowledge and attitudes toward sexuality in adolescents and their association with the family and other factors. Adolescence, 31, 179–192

Huntington D, Nawar L, Hassan EO et al. (1998) The post abortion caseload in Egyptian hospitals: a descriptive study. International Family Planning Perspectives, 24(1), 25–31

International Institute for Population Sciences (1995) National family health survey 1992–1993. http://www.nfhsindia.org/data/india1/iaintro.pdf, cited 2 August 2008

Johansson A, Nguyen TL, Hoang TH et al. (1998) Population policy, son preference and the use of IUDs in North Vietnam. Reproductive Health Matters, 6(11), 66–76

Justin RG (2005) Women helping women – four generations of women's health. John Hopkins Advanced Studies in Medicine, 5(6), 319–320

Jutla RK, Heimbach D (2004) Love burns: an essay about bride burning in India. Journal of Burn Care and Rehabilitation, 25(2), 165–170

Kader A, Maklouf H (1998) Social and behavioral outcomes of unintended pregnancy. Draft report prepared for the Women's Studies Project. Research Triangle Park, NC: Family Health International. http://www.fhi.org/NR/rdonlyres/efbroyf6jl67qqxqkqx4g4qo44frebjlb3nmzhalafy7faok7zx7oligjkrcyv2z35kdgwhfvfjqap/egypt4s.pdf, cited 24 August 2008

Kapilashrami MC (n.d.) Socio-demographic problems of unsafe abortion: consortium on national consensus for medical abortion in India http://www.aiims.edu/aiims/events/Gynaewebsite/ma_finalsite/report/1_1_2.htm, cited 2 August 2008

Lynch E (2005) Sexual revolution. Nursing Standard, 20(8), 20–21

Mauldon J, Delbanco S (1997) Public perceptions about unplanned pregnancy. Family Planning Perspectives, 29(1), 25-9-40

Mehta S, Groenen R, Roque F (1998) Adolescents in changing times: issues and perspectives for adolescent reproductive health in the ESCAP region. Population and Social Integration Section, Emerging Social Issues Division of the United Nations Economic and Social Commission for Asia and the Pacific. http://www.unescap.org/esid/psis/population/icpd/sec7.asp, cited 2 August 2008

Metz HC (1991) Nigeria, a country study. Library of Congress, Federal Research Division. http://lcweb2.loc.gov/frd/cs/, cited 2 August 2008

Miller FC (2000) Impact of adolescent pregnancy as we approach the new millennium. Journal of Pediatric and Adolescent Gynecology, 13(1), 5–8

Ministry of Health, Vietnam (2003) The survey assessment of Vietnam youth. http://www.unicef.org/vietnam/Questionnaire.pdf, cited 2 August 2008

Miyazaki T (1999) Representation of women in Japan's media. In changing lenses-women's perspectives on media (electronic version)

Moore KA, Miller BC, Sungland BW et al. (1996) Adolescent sexual behavior, pregnancy and parenthood: a review of research and interventions. Washington DC: Child Trends

National Campaign to Prevent Teen Pregnancy (2006) General facts and statistics. http://www.teenpregnancy.org/resources/data/genlfact.asp, cited 2 August 2008

National Center for Health Statistics (2001) Births to teenagers in the United States, 1940–2000. National Vital Statistics Report, 49:10

National Population Commission (NPC), Federal Republic of Nigeria, and ORC Macro (2003) Nigeria Demographic and Health Survey 2003. Calverton, MD, USA: ORC Macro

Nicoll A, Catcpole M, Cliffs S et al. (1999) Sexual health of teenagers in England and Wales: analysis of national data. BMJ, 318, 1321–1322

Ota T (1967) The Prohibition of induced abortion and the eugenic protection law. The Milbank Memorial Fund Quarterly, 45(4), 467–471

Ozcebe H, Akin A (1995) Adolescent health: a Middle East and North African perspective. International Journal of Gynecology and Obstetrics, 51(2), 151–157

Pan American Health Organization (PAHO) (2000) Sexual and reproductive health. http://www.paho.org/English/AD/FCH/CA/sa-sexualidad.htm, cited 2 August 2008

Picken SD (1994) Essentials of Shinto. CT: Westport. Greenwood

Po Z (1997) Population: reproductive health rights lacking in Latin America. Inter Press Service English News Wire

Policy Studies Institute (PSI) (1997) Fourth national survey of ethnic minorities. London, England: PSI

Qayed M, Waszak C (1999) Reproductive health among adolescents and youth in Assuit Governate, Egypt. Family Health International. http://www.fhi.org, cited 2 August 2008

Ragheb S, Guirgis W (1998) Family size and gender equity in childrearing. Summary of Final Report Prepared for The Women's Studies Project Family Health International and the Research Management Unit of The National Population Council, Cairo, Egypt. http://www.fhi.org/NR/rdonlyres/eox7rckoqigrwxbo3cixadgny7osuchc2i5aorvpvyzloanu3ubqa6bg4ibke2wsmlyvjf7mtssxmn/egypt3s.pdf, cited 24 August 2008

RAND (2001) Improvements in contraception are reducing historically high abortion rates in Russia. http://www.rand.org/pubs/research_briefs/RB5055/index1.html, cited 2 August 2008

Ravoira L, Cherry AL (1992) Social Bond and Teen Pregnancy. Westport, Connecticut: Praeger, Press

Reitman V (1996) Japan's new growth industry: Schoolgirl prostitution [Electronic version]. Wall Street Journal

Ross-Fowler G (1998). Population: Reports on Reproductive Rights. Off Our Backs. New York: Center for Reproductive Law and Policy

Sahar E (1999) Transitions to Adulthood: A National Survey of Adolescents in Egypt. Cairo, Egypt: The Population Council, Regional Office for West Asia and North Africa

Sallam SA, Mahfouz AAR, Dabbous IN (1998) Reproductive health of adolescents married women in squatter areas in Alexandria. Research Management Unit, Institutional Development Project, National Population Council. http://www.fhi.org/NR/rdonlyres/emefaub66keeu3m6cyqzy4q2zvplhmwyib4zvnj4dah4myhoe3bf2bgxes7q5h5hqrygkr4v6ys4gn/egypt5s.pdf, cited 24 August 2008

Santelli J, Ott MA, Lyon M, et al. (2006) Abstinence and abstinence-only education: a review of U.S. policies and programs. Journal of Adolescent Health, 38(1), 72–81

Sen A (1994) Population policy: authoritarianism versus co-operation. Social Change, 24(3–4), 20–35

Shaha KK, Mohanthy S (2006) Alleged dowry death: a study of homicidal burns. Medical Science Law, 46(2), 105–110

Shane B (1997) Family Planning Saves Lives. 3rd ed. Washington, DC: Population Reference Bureau

Shawky S, Milaat W (2000) Early teenage marriage and subsequent pregnancy outcome. Eastern Mediterranean Health Journal, 6(1), 46–54

Shirk M (1997) Temples show Japan's ambivalence toward abortion. St. Louis Post-Dispatch. March, p. 3A

Singh S, Audam S, Wulf D (2004) Early Childbearing in Nigeria: A Continuing Challenge. Research in Brief #2. New York: The Alan Guttmacher Institute. http://www.guttmacher.org/pubs/rib/2004/12/10/rib2-04.pdf, cited 24 August 2008

Singh S, Darroch JE (2000) Adolescent pregnancy and childbearing: levels and trends in developed countries. Family Planning Perspectives, 32(1), 14–23

Singh S, Samara R (1996) Early marriage among women in developing countries. International Family Planning Perspectives, 22(4), 148–158

Stevens-Simon C, Sheeder J, Beach R Harter S (2005) Adolescent pregnancy: do expectations affect intentions? Journal of Adolescent Health, 37(3), 243

Suellentrop K, Flanigan C (2006) Science says: pregnancy among sexually experienced teens. http://www.teenpregnancy.org/works/pdf/Science_Says_23.pdf, cited 2 August 2008

Supreme Court of the United States (1973) 410 U.S. 113 Roe v. Wade. Appeal from the United States District Court for The Northern District Of Texas. No. 70-18 Argued: December 13, 1971 – Decided: January 22, 1973

The National Campaign to Prevent Teen and Unplanned Pregnancy (1997) Whatever happened to childhood? The problem of teen pregnancy in the United States. Washington, DC. www.teenpregnancy.org/resources/reading/ppt/shortweb.ppt, cited 2 August 2008

Tripp J, Viner R (2005) Sexual health, contraception, and teenage pregnancy. British Medical Journal, 330(7491), 590–593

United Nations Children's Fund (UNICEF) (1999). After the fall: The human impact of ten years of transition. The United Nations Children's Fund (UNICEF). http://www.unicef-icdc.org, cited 2 August 2008

United Nations Children's Fund (UNICEF) (2008) State of the world's children: child survival. http://www.unicef.org/sowc08/index.php, cited 2 August 2008

United Nations Development Programme (UNDP) (2002) Abortion Policies: A Global Review. Volumes I, II, III. New York: United Nations

United Nations Fund for Population Activities (UNFPA) (2003) Missing: Mapping the Adverse Child Sex Ratio in India. New York: United Nations

United Nations Fund for Population Activities (UNFPA) (2005) State of world populations 2005. Chapter 5: The Unmapped Journey: Adolescents, Poverty and Gender. New York: UNFPA. http://www.unfpa.org/swp/2005/english/ch5/chap5_page1.htm, cited August 8, 2009

U.S. Department of State (2007). Egypt. http://www.state.gov/r/pa/ei/bgn/5309.htm, cited 2 August 2008

United States Agency for International Development (USAID) (2000) Breaking Egypt's Contraceptive "plateau." U.S. Agency for International Development. Washington DC: United States Agency for International Development (USAID). http://www.usaid.gov/regions/ane/newpages/perspectives/egypt/fmplng.htm, cited 2 August 2008

Ventura SJ, Abma JC, Mosher WD (2006) Recent trends in teenage pregnancy in the United States, 1990–2002. Health E-stats. Hyattsville, MD: National Center for Health Statistics. http://www.cdc.gov/nchs/products/pubs/pubd/hestats/teenpreg1990-2002/teenpreg1990-2002.htm, cited 2 August 2008

Wellings K (2001) Country Report for Great Britain: Teenage Sexual and Reproductive Behavior in Developed Countries. Occasional Report # 6. New York: Alan Guttmacher Institute

Wellings K (2007) Reducing the rate of teenage conceptions. BMJ Health Intelligence. http://healthintelligence.bmj.com/hi/do/public-health/topics/content/teenage-pregnancy/index.html, cited 24 August 2008

Wellings K, Field J, Johnson AM, Wadsworth J (1994) Sexual Behavior in Britain: The National Study of Attitudes and Lifestyles. London: Penguin Press

White HW (2006) Abortion doctor on India jailed under female foeticide law. http://www.lifesitenews.com/ldn/2006/mar/06032906.html, cited 2 August 2008

Women Envision (1999) Preference for baby girls: A two-way deal in Japan and America. Women Envision, 76:6

World Bank (2006) World Development Report 2006 – Equity and Development. Washington, DC: World Bank http://siteresources.worldbank.org/INTWDR2006/Resources/477383-1127230817535/082136412X.pdf, cited 2 August 2008

World Health Organization (WHO) (2004) Maternal Mortality in 2000: Estimates Developed by WHO, UNICEF and UNFPA. Geneva: United Nations Children's Fund (UNICEF) and United Nations Fund for Population Activities (UNFPA)

Yayori M (1999) Women in the New Asia. London: Zed Books

Zodgekar AV (1996) Family welfare programme and population stabilization strategies in India. Asia-Pacific Population Journal, 11(1), 3–24

Chapter 22
Progress and Challenges in Making Pregnancy Safer: A Global Perspective

Monir Islam

Learning Objectives After reading this chapter and answering the discussion questions that follow, you should be able to

- Discuss global trends and distribution of maternal and infant mortality.
- Identify the impact of HIV/AIDS, malaria, and tuberculosis on maternal and neonatal morbidity and mortality.
- Appraise the challenges of ensuring equitable and sustainable reduction in adverse pregnancy and birth outcomes.
- Analyze strategies and techniques for improving of current maternal and child survival programs.

Introduction

Each year, there are at least 3.2 million stillborn babies, more than 4 million neonatal deaths, and more than half a million maternal deaths worldwide. The vast majority of these deaths are preventable, and countries with the highest burdens of maternal and neonatal morbidity and mortality are those which currently appear to be making the least progress in reducing these rates. Inequities in morbidity and mortality rates are increasing both between and within countries. Thus, for all the very real progress that has been made, the world is far from eliminating avoidable suffering and premature mortality among women of reproductive age. As

shown in Chapters 12, 14, and 15, malaria, tuberculosis, and HIV/AIDS have significant negative impact on maternal mortality, which can reverse the progress made over the decades. The challenge ahead is to refocus program content and to shift from development of new technologies to the establishment of viable organizational strategies that build health system infrastructure and ensure effective and efficient continuum of care. Strategies for improvement include revising the structure and content of current maternal and newborn health programs, developing funded national implementation plans to achieve universal coverage for maternal and newborn health-care services, and initiating action to muster the political commitment needed to achieve and sustain these systems and programs. Much of the challenge, in fact, is to accommodate both programmatic and systemic concerns which are organizational rather than technical problems.

During the early years of the 20th century, standard maternity care among well-to-do women in Europe, North America, and Japan consisted of home deliveries with regular, frequent visits by an obstetric specialist (Loudon 1992). The arrival of modern obstetric care during the late 1930 s did not alter this practice, but gradually moved the whole process to institutional settings. Women were kept in the hospital for 10 or more days following delivery, depending on whether the birth was normal or complicated. Today, many women with uncomplicated childbirth are discharged within a day or two, and sometimes, even as little as a few hours after childbirth. This is possible, given the availability of postpartum follow-up and care by skilled health-care providers. Antenatal care is a relatively new concept, as services became generally

M. Islam (✉)
Department of Making Pregnancy Safer, World Health Organization, Geneva, Switzerland

J.E. Ehiri (ed.), *Maternal and Child Health*, DOI 10.1007/b106524_22,
© Springer Science+Business Media, LLC 2009

available only following World War II. Today, pregnant women in most developed countries receive an integrated package of antenatal, childbirth, and postpartum care.

Maternal health-care services in developing countries, by contrast, have followed a very different path. Overall, antenatal care tends to be the primary service to receive resources and is widely implemented within maternal health programs. Today in developing countries, most pregnant women visit antenatal care services at least once during pregnancy (WHO 2003). By contrast, childbirth care (in health facilities or at home) and access to emergency obstetrics and newborn care services are far less available or accessible (WHO 2003). In many settings, systematic and regular postpartum follow-up and care are not available at all (WHO 2003). Even when women have access to skilled care at the time of childbirth or are able to deliver in a health facility, they are often discharged within a matter of hours and not seen again by a health professional until a considerable time afterward. Therefore, an integrated package of care is not available to most pregnant women in developing countries.

The Magnitude of the Problem

Box 22.1 provides a glossary of definitions of terminologies that are frequently used in this chapter. The prevalence of maternal mortality is currently estimated at 529,000 deaths per year (WHO 2004), which equals a global ratio of 400 maternal deaths per 100,000 live births. In the last decade alone, about 7 million women died during pregnancy, childbirth, or the postpartum period. However, progress in averting maternal deaths and improving women's health has been significant.

In areas where there is no access to health care to avert maternal deaths, "natural" mortality is approximately 1,000–1,500 maternal deaths per 100,000 live births. This estimate is based on historical studies and data from contemporary religious groups who do not intervene in childbirth (Van Lerberghe and De Brouwere 2001). If women were still experiencing "natural" maternal mortality rates today – if health services were

discontinued, for example – then the maternal death toll would be four times its current rate. This means that three-quarters of all possible maternal deaths worldwide are currently avoided. However, great inequalities persist between regions and populations, as maternal deaths are even more inequitably spread than newborn or early childhood deaths. In developed countries, nearly all the "natural" maternal mortality is averted, while only two-thirds is averted in Southeast Asia and the Eastern Mediterranean region. This proportion drops to only one-third in African countries (WHO 2005). Only 1% of maternal deaths occur in the developed world. Maternal mortality ratios range from 830 per 100,000 live births in many African countries to 24 per 100,000 live births in many European countries. Of the 20 countries with the highest maternal mortality ratios, 19 are in sub-Saharan Africa. Regional rates may also mask large disparities between countries in the same region (Fig. 22.1).

Maternal mortality varies between and within regions, countries, and populations. Regions with low overall mortality rates, such as the European region, also contain countries with high mortality rates. Within a single country there can be striking inequities and differences between population groups, with national figures masking substantial internal variations based on geography, economics, and social status. Rural populations suffer higher mortality rates than urban populations, and within urban populations mortality is higher in urban slums. Mortality rates vary widely by ethnicity and/or socioeconomic status, and remote areas can have disproportionate death tolls. The main differences in maternal mortality between the world's regions are not simply explained by variations in economic growth. For example, Vietnam, Sri Lanka, and Cape Verde have achieved much lower levels of maternal mortality than Yemen and Côte d'Ivoire, despite being matched on gross national income per head.

Risk factors for maternal mortality have been studied extensively. For example, McCarthy and Maine (1992) proposed a framework of determinants: distant factors such as individual, family, and community status interacting with intermediate factors such as the mother's health status, reproductive status, access to health services, and health behaviors. The distant determinants act on the intermediate factors, which

Box 22.1 Definition of Terms

Maternal death: The death of a woman while pregnant or within 42 days of termination of pregnancy, irrespective of the duration and site of the pregnancy, from any cause related to or aggravated by the pregnancy or its management, but not from accidental or incidental causes.*

Maternal conditions: A maternal death is one for which the certifying physician has designated a maternal condition as the underlying cause of death. Maternal conditions are those assigned to pregnancy, childbirth, and the puerperium, ICD-10 codes A34, O00–O95, O98–O99.*

Maternal mortality ratio: The number of maternal deaths per 100,000 live births. The maternal mortality rate is a measure of the likelihood that a pregnant woman will die from maternal causes. The number of live births used in the denominator is a proxy for the population of pregnant women who are at risk of a maternal death.*

Natural maternal mortality: Death of women caused by a naturally occurring disease process that is not mediated by obstetric factors.*

Obstetric complications: Disruptions and disorders of pregnancy, labor and delivery, and the early neonatal period. Examples of such complications include prenatal drug exposure, poor maternal nutrition, minor physical anomalies (or MPAs: indicators of fetal neural maldevelopment, occurring near the end of the first trimester), and birth complications.

Birth rate: Calculated by dividing the number of live births in a population in a year by the midyear resident population.*

Infant mortality rate: Calculated by dividing the number of infant deaths during a calendar year by the number of live births reported in the same year. It is expressed as the number of infant deaths per 1,000 live births.*

Neonatal mortality rate: The number of deaths of children under 28 days of age, per 1,000 live births.*

Post-neonatal mortality rate: The number of deaths of children that occur between 28 days and 365 days after birth, per 1,000 live births.*

Perinatal mortality rate: The sum of late fetal deaths plus infant deaths within 7 days of birth divided by the sum of live births plus late fetal deaths, per 1,000 live births plus late fetal deaths.*

Stillbirth: When fetal death occurs after 22 weeks of pregnancy (March of Dimes 2008).

Skilled health professional: An accredited health professional – such as a midwife, doctor, or nurse – who has been educated and trained to proficiency in the skills needed to manage normal (uncomplicated) pregnancies, childbirth, and the immediate postnatal period and in the identification, management, and referral of complications in women and newborns (WHO 2005).

Antenatal care: Appointments at clinics or hospitals for pregnant women, relating to their pregnancy.

Postpartum care: Encompasses management of the mother, newborn, and infant during the postpartum period which includes the 6-week period after childbirth.

Emergency obstetrics: Emergency care given directly before, during, or after childbirth including blood transfusions, improved surgical procedures and anesthesia, rapid transport to medical facilities, and rapid response within those facilities (Fortney 2001).

Fertility rate: The total number of live births, regardless of age of mother, per 1,000 women of reproductive age, 15–44 years.*

Total fertility rate (TFR): Shows the potential impact of current fertility patterns on reproduction, that is, completed family size. The TFR indicates the average number of births to a hypothetical cohort of 1,000 women, if they experienced throughout their childbearing years the age-specific birth rates observed in a given year.*

*Source: CDC, National Center for Health Statistics (2007)

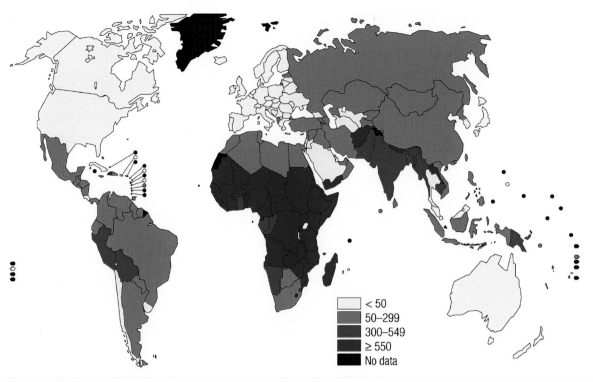

Fig. 22.1 Global situation of maternal mortality. Source: WHO (2005)

interact with unknown or unpredicted factors to lead to outcomes that include pregnancy, obstetric complications, and death or disability. This framework brings up a number of important implications. One is that distant determinants like socioeconomic status (SES) and education must act through other determinants in order to affect pregnancy outcomes. In other words, although many studies suggest correlations between high SES and/or education with lower maternal mortality (van Egmond et al. 2004), these factors do not directly effect maternal survival. McCarthy and Maine (1992) illustrate this point by looking at high mortality among people with religious opposition to medical care and the period of "interventionist obstetrics." Both cases involve people with high education and SES having higher mortality rates than people with lower education and lower SES. Another important point made by McCarthy and Maine (1992) is that even in developed countries, obstetric complications are very difficult to predict, with the majority occurring in women without any known risk factors.

Castro et al. (2000) studied risk factors for maternal mortality in Mexico using a qualitative approach. They identified maternal deaths from hospital records

and interviewed relatives to determine the factors leading to the death. They decided to classify the risk factors under the three-delay framework, in which delay in deciding to seek help (under-estimation of warning signs and their severity, opposition to care by partner, poor impression of health services, lack of money), delay in getting to a health facility (physical isolation of community, insufficient transportation, having to travel to multiple facilities), and delay in receiving care from that health facility (poor quality of care from providers, insufficient resources) are the main contributors to maternal death.

A number of other indirect causes for maternal mortality are often mentioned. These include the "four too's" – too young, too old, too few births (referring to primipara), and too many births (parity greater than four) (Aliyu et al. 2005a,b; Ronsmans and Campbell 1998; McCarthy and Maine, 1992) – and comorbid conditions such as malaria (Granja et al. 1998), micronutrient deficiencies including Vitamin A (Christian et al. 2000), iron and calcium (Villar et al. 2003), severe anemia (Brabin et al. 2001), lack of antenatal care (Sibley at al. 2004), and unsafe abortion (Goyaux et al. 2001; Jewkes et al. 1997; Johnson et al.

2002; Rahman et al. 2001). A knowledge, attitude, and practices (KAP) survey in Afghanistan (van Egmond et al. 2004) found a positive correlation between education and antenatal care, institutional delivery, skilled attendance at birth, and use of family planning. Ronsmans and Campbell (1998) provide evidence against the assumption that closely spaced births are a risk factor for maternal mortality. However, they only compared the current birth outcome with the previous birth outcome, so the interaction of close birth spacing for more than two pregnancies is a possibility.

Risk factors for maternal mortality also include factors that interfere with the provision of care for life-threatening complications experienced during pregnancy. Early complications are typically associated with abortions (much more so than miscarriage, possibly due to the illegality, stigma, and method of inducing abortion), with the remainder of complications clustering around birth and the period immediately following.

Between 11 and 17% of maternal deaths happen during the act of childbirth itself and between 50 and 71% occur during the postpartum period. Risk tends to be concentrated on the childbirth, and many postpartum deaths are a direct result of what happens during birth. Therefore, particular attention is warranted during the hours and sometimes days that are spent in labor and giving birth. These are the critical hours when a joyful event can suddenly turn into an unforeseen crisis. The postpartum period, despite its heavy death toll, is often neglected (Dhakal et al. 2007). Mothers and their newborns are most prone to complications during the first week of the postpartum period. About 45% of postpartum maternal deaths occur during the first 24 hours after birth,

and more than two-thirds occur during the first week after birth. The global toll of postpartum maternal deaths is accompanied by the large and often overlooked number of stillbirths and early newborn deaths.

Maternal deaths result from a wide range of indirect and direct causes. The largest share of deaths is attributable to direct causes (Table 22.1). These occur following complications of pregnancy and childbirth, or are caused by interventions, omissions, incorrect treatment, or events that result from these birth complications. The five major direct causes of maternal deaths are hemorrhage, infection, eclampsia (unsafe), abortion, and obstructed labor. The rates of maternal mortality depend on whether these complications are treated adequately and in a timely manner. Serious complications early in pregnancy are generally the result of abortions, often illegal and performed under unsafe conditions. These account for approximately 12% of all maternal deaths (Khan et al. 2006). Prevention of unsafe abortions is possible through the use of contraceptives to prevent unwanted pregnancies that would lead to abortion and the legalization of abortion, which would permit women to have an abortion from a skilled provider.

Maternal deaths due to indirect causes represent 16.7% of the global total (Khan et al. 2006). They may be caused by diseases (pre-existing or concurrent) that are not complications of pregnancy, but rather complicate pregnancy or are aggravated by it. These include malaria, anemia, HIV/AIDS, and cardiovascular disease. The disease role in maternal mortality varies from country to country, according to the epidemiological context and the effectiveness of the health systems' response. Of the 136 million women who give

Table 22.1 Incidence of major complications of childbirth worldwide

Complication	Incidence (% of live births)	Number of cases per year	Case-fatality rate (%)	Maternal deaths in 2000	Main sequelae for survivors	DALYs lost (000)
Postpartum hemorrhage	10.5	13,795,000	1	132,000	Severe anemia	4,418
Sepsis	4.4	5,768,000	1.3	79,000	Infertility	6,901
Pre-eclampsia and eclampsia	3.2	4,152,000	1.7	63,000	Not well evaluated	2,231
Obstructed Labor	4.6	6,038,000	0.7	42,000	Fistula, incontinence	2,951

Source: AbouZahr (2003)

birth each year, some 20 million (approximately 15%) experience pregnancy-related illness after birth. The list of morbidities is diverse, ranging from fever to psychosis, and the range of care responses needed is equally varied. For women who almost die in childbirth, recovery from organ failure, uterine rupture, fistulas, and/or other severe complications can be long, painful, and leave lasting complications. Other, non-life-threatening illnesses can be frequent as well. Some of these postpartum problems are temporary, but others can become chronic illnesses. These include urinary incontinence, uterine prolapse, pain following poor repair of episiotomy and perineal tears, nutritional deficiencies, depression and puerperal psychosis, and mastitis. Even less is known about these morbidities than about maternal deaths. They are difficult to quantify, owing to problems with definitions and inadequate records (WHO 2005). More reliable information on the range of maternal morbidities is an important step toward better planning of services and improved care around childbirth.

Mother and Newborn Outcomes Are Closely Linked

Neonatal mortality is the death of an infant within 28 days of birth. Reliable conclusions on global trends are not available given the short period of time that neonatal mortality has been measured. However, WHO estimates from 1995 to 2000 suggest that most countries in the Americas, Southeast Asia, Europe, and the Western Pacific have made some progress in reducing the infant mortality rate. Improvements have been less marked in the Eastern Mediterranean region (although regional averages mask variations between countries), and the African region has experienced an increase in its neonatal mortality rate (WHO 2008).

Of the 136 million babies born every year, 3.3 million are stillborn and 4 million die during the first month of life (WHO 2005). Ninety-eight% of these deaths occur in low-income and middle-income countries. Neonatal deaths contribute to about 40% of all deaths in children under-5 globally and more than half of all infant mortality. Globally, the largest numbers of newborns die in the Southeast Asian region (WHO

2005). This region has 1.4 million newborn deaths and a further 1.3 million stillbirths each year (WHO 2005). While the actual number of deaths is highest in Asia, the rates for both neonatal deaths and stillbirths are greatest in sub-Saharan Africa (Pathmanathan et al. 2003). Of the 20 countries with the highest neonatal mortality rates, 16 are in sub-Saharan Africa (Pathmanathan et al. 2003) (Fig. 22.2).

The gap between rich and poor countries is widening: neonatal mortality is now 6.5 times lower in high-income countries than in low-income countries (Tinker and Ransom 2002). The lifetime risk for a newborn baby to die is now approximately 1 in 5 for countries in Africa, compared with 1 in 125 in developed countries (Tinker and Ransom 2002). Obstetric complications, particularly in labor, account for as many as 58% of stillbirths and early neonatal deaths (Kusiako et al. 2000). Intrapartum risk factors increase the likelihood of perinatal or neonatal death more than pre-pregnancy or antenatal factors. Likewise, the repercussions for children who survive the death of their mothers can be staggering. In Nepal, for example, infants of mothers who died during childbirth were 6 times more likely to die in the first week of life, 12 times more likely to die between 8 and 28 days, and 52 times more likely to die between 4 and 24 weeks (Katz et al. 2003). While early infant deaths were attributable to obstetric complications, later deaths were explained by an absence of appropriate childcare and nutrition (WHO 2005).

The health and survival of newborns is closely linked to that of their mothers. First, because healthier mothers have healthier babies; second, because where a mother gets no or inadequate care during pregnancy, childbirth, and the postpartum period, her baby also receives little or no care. Both mothers and newborns have a better chance of survival if they have skilled care during childbirth and access to emergency care services (Tinker and Ransom 2002).

The Progress and Reversal in Reduction of Maternal and Newborn Mortality

Maternal: Industrialized countries halved their maternal mortality in the early 20th century by providing professional midwifery care during childbirth and further reduced it to current historical lows by improving

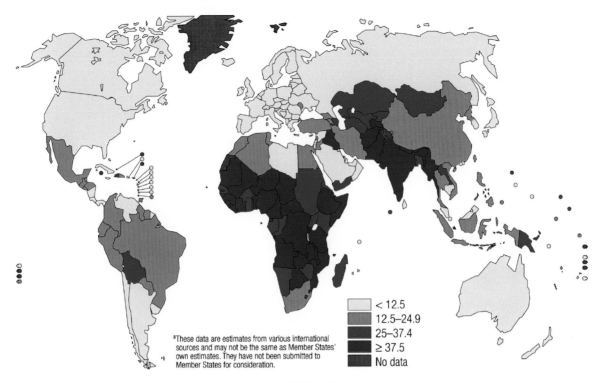

Fig. 22.2 Global patterns for newborn mortality. Source: WHO (2005)

The legend in the figure:
- < 12.5
- 12.5–24.9
- 25–37.4
- ≥ 37.5
- No data

aThese data are estimates from various international sources and may not be the same as Member States' own estimates. They have not been submitted to Member States for consideration.

access to emergency obstetric care after World War II (Loudon 1992). Quite a few developing countries have done the same over the last few decades. One of the earliest and best-documented examples is Sri Lanka, where maternal mortality levels were compounded by malaria. Maternal deaths had remained well above 1,500 per 100,000 live births in the first half of the 20th century despite 20 years of antenatal care (WHO 2005). In this period, midwifery was professionalized, but access remained limited. Beginning in 1947, mortality rates dropped in correlation to improved access and the development of health-care facilities in the country. This brought mortality ratios down to between 80 and 100 deaths per 100,000 live births by 1975 (WHO 2005). Improved management and quality of care further lowered mortality rates to less than 30 in the 1990 s, according to a Ministry of Health time series (Kusiako et al. 2000).

Malaysia also has a long-standing tradition of professional midwifery (since 1923). Maternal mortality was reduced from more than 500 per 100,000 live births in the early 1950 s to around 250 per 100,000 live births in 1960 (Katz et al. 2003). The country then gradually improved survival of mothers and newborns by introducing a maternal and child

health program. A district health-care system was introduced and midwifery care was increased through a network of "low-risk delivery centers" that were supplemented by high-quality referral care, all with close and intensive quality assurance. This brought maternal mortality rates below 100 per 100,000 live births by around 1975 and then to below 50 per 100,000 by the 1980 s (Katz et al. 2003).

Until the 1960 s, Thailand had maternal mortality rates well above 400 per 100,000 live births, which is the equivalent of those in the United Kingdom in 1900 or the United States in 1939 (WHO 2005). During the 1960 s, traditional birth attendants were gradually substituted by certified village midwives, 7,191 of whom were newly registered within a 10-year period. This aided in a reduction in the mortality rate to 200 per 100,000 live births (WHO 2005). During the 1970 s, the registration of midwives was stepped up with 18,314 new registrations. Midwives became key figures in many villages, proud of their professional and social status. Mortality dropped steadily and caught up with the mortality in Sri Lanka by 1980. The main effort then went into strengthening and equipping district hospitals. Within 10 years, from 1977 to 1987, the number of beds in small community

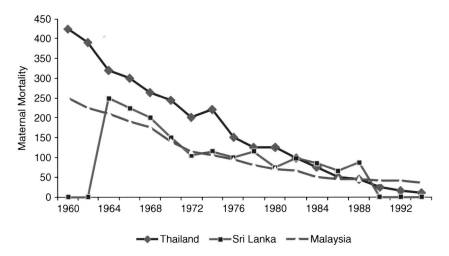

Fig. 22.3 Maternal mortality since the 1960 s in Malaysia, Sri Lanka, and Thailand. Source: WHO (2005)

hospitals quadrupled, from 2,540 to 10,800, and the number of doctors in these districts rose from a few hundred to 1,339. By 1990 the maternal mortality rate dropped below 50 per 100,000 live births (WHO 2005) (Fig. 22.3).

More recent improvements have occurred in Egypt, Honduras, and China. Egypt reduced its maternal mortality rate by more than 50% in 8 years, from 174 in 1993 to 84 per 100,000 live births in 2000. This was accomplished through major efforts to promote safer motherhood which doubled the proportion of births attended by a doctor or nurse and improved access to emergency obstetric care (Van Lerberghe and De Brouwere 2001). Honduras brought maternal deaths down from 182 to 108 per 100,000 between 1990 and 1997 by opening and staffing 7 referral hospitals and 226 rural health centers (Danel 1998). They also increased the number of health personnel and skilled birth attendants. China reported a large decline in the maternal mortality rate over three decades from approximately 1,500 per 100,000 live births in 1950 to 100–200 in rural areas in 1980, with the majority of childbirths occurring in facilities with easy access to emergency care (Pathmanathan et al. 2003). Botswana, Cape Verde, Cuba, Costa Rica, Jamaica, Mauritius, and South Africa followed a similar path to increase skilled care during childbirth and timely access to lifesaving emergency care.

The above examples illustrate that long-term initiatives to provide skilled care during childbirth and timely access to emergency care produce substantial decreases in maternal mortality. Unfortunately, the opposite is true as well. Systematic breakdown in access to skilled care can rapidly result in an increase in unfavorable outcomes. In Malawi, a catastrophic shortage of staff in maternity units resulted in deterioration of the quality of care within health facilities. Between 1989 and 2001 the proportion of deaths associated with deficient health care increased from 31% to 43%. The chances of Malawi women giving birth in a safe environment diminished accordingly, and the maternal mortality rate increased from 752 maternal deaths per 100,000 live births to 1,120 per 100,000 in 2000, according to the Demographic and Health Survey (WHO 2005). In Tajikistan, economic upheaval following the break up of the Soviet Union and independence in 1991, compounded by civil war, led to a startling erosion of the capacity of the healthcare system to provide accessible care. This resulted in a tenfold increase in the proportion of women giving birth at home with no skilled assistance and a subsequent increase in maternal mortality (Falkingham 2003). Similarly in Iraq, sanctions during the 1990 s severely disrupted previously well-functioning healthcare services, and maternal mortality ratios increased from 50 per 100,000 in 1989 to 117 per 100,000 in 1997 (UNICEF 1998). The maternal mortality rate was as high as 294 per 100,000 in central and southern parts of the country. Iraq also experienced a massive increase in neonatal mortality during this period, from 25 to 59 per 1,000 between 1995 and 2000 (WHO 2005).

In addition to breakdown in access to skilled care, HIV/AIDS, malaria, and TB during pregnancy have an impact on maternal mortality. These indirect causes can reverse progress made over decades. Zimbabwe's story of maternal mortality has taken a detour on its road to success. In 1989–1990, a community-based study in urban Harare and rural Masvingo reported a maternal mortality ratio of 85 per 100,000 and 168 per 100,000, respectively. The Zimbabwe Demographic and Health Surveys showed a rise in this rate from 283 in 1994 to 695 per 100,000 in 1999 (Pathmanathan et al. 2003). According to the same surveys, skilled care during childbirth increased from 69% in 1994 to 73% in 1999. The cesarean section rate increased from 6% to 6.7% during that same period (Pathmanathan et al. 2003). The most likely explanation for this increase in the maternal mortality rate is a change in the causes of maternal mortality. In the University Teaching Hospital in Lusaka, Zambia, a year prospective study in 1996–1997 found that indirect causes contributed to 58% of the maternal deaths. Malaria, tuberculosis, AIDS, and unspecified chronic respiratory infections were the leading causes of maternal mortality (Ahmed et al. 1999).

Newborns: Early newborn survival is directly linked to maternal health and survival. Consecutive household surveys from 34 developing countries show that most countries have experienced a decrease in neonatal mortality rates over recent decades (Lawn et al. 2005). Much of the progress in child survival has been made in the late neonatal period, with little improvement in the first week of life. This mirrors the historical experience of many developed countries, where neonatal mortality (and particularly early neonatal mortality) did not decrease until years after a decline in post-neonatal and childhood mortality had been achieved (Koblinsky 2003). In many countries, neonatal mortality has decreased at a slower rate than either post-neonatal or early childhood mortality. Inadequate investment in maternal health services is the likely reason for this deficit. Household surveys also suggest that there has been reversal and stagnation in newborn mortality across sub-Saharan Africa since the beginning of the 1990 s. Indeed, the actual number of deaths has increased substantially in the African region (WHO 2005). In only 5 years, the dramatic drop in deaths in Southeast Asia means that Africa has the highest neonatal mortality rate in the world, with almost 30% of newborn deaths worldwide (WHO 2005).

The reversal of progress in neonatal health in sub-Saharan Africa is both concerning and unusual. Historically, declines in child mortality have often reversed when the social context deteriorated. Within Europe, these reversals often affected older children and remained modest for neonatal mortality (Lawn et al. 2005). The causes of the poor progress in reducing both neonatal and later childhood deaths in sub-Saharan Africa are likely to be many and complex. As demonstrated in Chapter 7 (conflicts and maternal and child health), economic decline and conflicts are likely to have played significant roles through their disruptive effect on access to health services. The impact of the HIV/AIDS epidemic on mortality is less established for newborns than for children in the post-neonatal period. Infants born to HIV-positive mothers are more likely to be stillborn, premature, and/or have very low birth weights (Ticconi et al. 2003). Countries that make a deliberate and sustained effort to provide professional childbirth care, supported by timely emergency care facilities with quality services, can improve maternal and newborn survival dramatically.

Significant Progress Has Been Made in Coverage of Antenatal Care Services

In spite of the controversies regarding the impact of prenatal visits on birth outcomes, there is sufficient evidence which supports the fact that prenatal visits have a positive effect on birth outcomes in less developed countries (Brown et al. 2008; Raatikainen et al. 2007). Early entry to antenatal care is important for early detection and treatment of adverse pregnancy-related outcomes. Periodic health check-ups during the antenatal period are necessary to establish confidence between the woman and her health-care provider in order to individualize health promotional messages and to identify and manage any maternal complications or risk factors. Antenatal visits are used to provide essential services that are recommended for all pregnant women, such as tetanus toxoid immunization and the prevention of anemia through nutrition education and provision of iron/folic acid tablets (WHO 1994). A WHO Technical Working Group recommended a minimum of four antenatal visits for a woman with a normal pregnancy (WHO 1994). This was not intended to imply that countries where pregnant women receive more than the minimum number of visits should reduce that number. Rather, the objective was to focus on the content of care and to set a basic, essential standard for quality for all countries. Problems may arise at different times during pregnancy, so the assessment of risk factors and complications must be an ongoing process throughout pregnancy, labor, delivery, and the postpartum period. Some women will require more visits than others. The WHO recommended that pregnant women in developing countries should seek antenatal care within the first 4 months of pregnancy (WHO 1994). In developed countries such as the United Kingdom and the United States, antenatal care is recommended within the first 12 weeks of pregnancy (American Academy of Pediatrics 2007; National Institute for Health and Clinical Excellence 2003). The WHO recently recommended a reduction in the number of antenatal visits in developed countries because of evidence suggesting that having fewer antenatal visits does not affect the outcomes of care, other than women's satisfaction levels (Villar et al. 2001). However, women are still advised to attend antenatal care early and even earlier than previously recommended. In high-income and middle-income countries today, use of antenatal care by pregnant women is almost universal, except among marginalized groups such as migrants, ethnic minorities, unmarried adolescents, the very poor, and those living in isolated rural communities (Sloan et al. 2002). Even in low-income countries, coverage rates for antenatal care (at least for one visit) are often quite high and often much higher than use of a skilled health-care professional during childbirth. There were noticeable increases in the use of antenatal care in developing countries during the 1990 s (WHO 2005). The greatest progress was seen in Asia, mainly as a result of rapid changes in a few large countries such as Indonesia. Significant increases also took place in the Caribbean and Latin America, although countries in these regions already had relatively high rates of antenatal care. In sub-Saharan Africa, by contrast, antenatal care use increased only marginally over the decade (although levels in Africa are relatively high compared with those in Asia) (Fig. 22.4).

While antenatal care coverage has improved significantly in recent years in terms of increased access and use of antenatal visits, it is generally recognized that the antenatal care services currently provided in many parts of the world fail to meet the recommended standards. The proportion of women who are obtaining the WHO-recommended minimum of four visits is too low. A huge potential thus remains insufficiently exploited, for example, by using antenatal care as a platform for programs that tackle nutrition, HIV/AIDS, sexually transmitted infections,

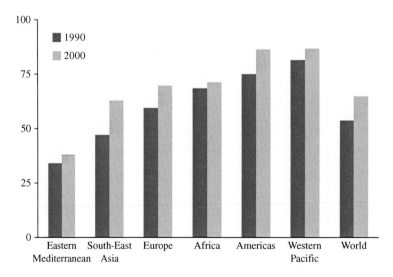

Fig. 22.4 Antenatal care is a success story: uptake and demand are on the increase. Source: WHO (2005)

malaria and tuberculosis, among others. Diseases and other health problems can often complicate or become more severe during pregnancy. Many women have their first consultation late in pregnancy, whereas maximum health benefits require early initiation of antenatal care. Antenatal care is given by doctors, midwives and nurses, and many other cadres of health workers (Koblinsky 2003). Little is known about the capacities of non-professional workers such as traditional birth attendants to deliver the known effective interventions during pregnancy.

Skilled Care During Childbirth and Lifesaving Emergency Care Is Increasing

Globally the availability of nationally representative data on skilled attendants at birth is high with data for 93.5% of all live births. From this we know that 61.1% of births worldwide are attended by a professional who, at least in principle, has the skills to assist. Data from 58 countries that account for 76% of births in the developing world show that the use of a skilled attendant at delivery (the key feature of first-level care) increased significantly, from 41% in 1990 to 57% in 2003. This is a 38% increase in the number of women with a skilled birth attendant between 1990 and 2003 (WHO 2007). The greatest improvements occurred in Southeast Asia (from 34% in 1990 to 64% in 2003) and North Africa (from 41% in 1990 to 76% in 2003). These trends represent an increase in the number of women with a skilled birth attendant of more than 85% in both regions. Hardly any change was observed, however, in sub-Saharan Africa, where rates remained among the lowest in the world at around 40% (WHO 2007). Within these regional averages, there are significant differences between countries and between urban and rural areas, which often represent rich and poor sections of the population (WHO 2005). Almost all of the increases in births with a skilled attendant are driven by increases in the presence of medical doctors at birth. In fact most regions, with the exception of sub-Saharan Africa, show decreasing use of other types of professional assistance. There is a marked increase in the proportion of deliveries that take place in health-care facilities, both in rural and urban areas.

This tendency toward increased use of professional maternal and newborn care services should not give rise to excessive optimism. There are many countries where hospitals with trained professional staff exist, and yet mortality remains staggeringly high. In 1996, for example, Brazzaville, Congo, had a maternal mortality ratio of 645 per 100,000 live births (Belgrade, Serbia and Montenegro Statistical Office 2004), despite having a university hospital and additional health-care facilities. Adequate care is not merely having a hospital with trained clinicians, but requires a conducive environment with appropriate and timely supplies, along with quality management, supervision, and referral facilities (Ehiri et al. 2005).

Rates of caesarean section are one method for gauging access to care when complications arise during childbirth. The overall caesarean birth rate for developing countries stands at 12% (8.5% if China is excluded), with large variability between and within countries (WHO 2005). Rural caesarean rates are often less than a third of urban rates, and many countries, particularly in sub-Saharan Africa, still have rural rates much lower than the recommended 5% minimum (WHO 2005). These data imply a continuing shortfall of lifesaving emergency obstetric care services in many countries. However, since 1990, overall caesarean rates have been increasing (WHO 2005). Outside Africa increases of 2–5% per year are common and have taken place in both urban and rural areas where rates are now well above 10%. Private-sector caesarean section rates are higher and in some cases are increasing at an alarming rate (WHO 2005). With cesarean section rates climbing, it is possible that excessive surgical intervention during childbirth will actually lead to an increase in maternal mortality in these regions, given complications from surgery.

Postpartum and Postnatal/Newborn Care Need More Attention

While the need for immediate postpartum care is widely acknowledged, later postpartum care is often completely forgotten and/or neglected. The poor coverage of care in the postpartum period is reflected in the limited data available on a global level. Less than one in three developing countries report national data on postpartum care and even in countries with existing data the levels of coverage are often as low as 5% (Islam 2007). Despite the burden of morbidity during this period, uptake of postpartum care in developing countries is usually extremely low. Typically, it is less than half the uptake of antenatal or delivery care. Estimates based on the limited available data indicate an overall use of postpartum care below 30% for developing countries (Lawn et al. 2005). In many low-income countries, even where the proportion of institutional deliveries is already high or is increasing, women are often discharged less than 24 hours after giving birth (Lawn et al. 2005). However, more than half of maternal deaths and many newborn deaths occur after this period. In areas where the majority of births take place at home, postpartum care may be unavailable or women may not know that services exist.

Many service providers and families focus on the well-being of the new baby and may not be aware or able to assess the importance of women's complications, such as postpartum bleeding. Where childbirth is under professional supervision, be it at home or in a health facility, women are usually expected to attend a postpartum/postnatal checkup at a health facility 6 weeks after delivery. This may not be enough care to be effective. Women may not attend because they do not know that the service is available to them. They may not perceive any benefit in attending or the opportunity costs of attending may be too high (Masuy-Stroobant 1997). Health staff themselves may not feel empowered or skilled in providing postpartum/postnatal interventions. Apart from some countries, such as Sri Lanka, rates of postnatal visits among women are low and inequitably spread. The structures that exist are often not fully suited to the needs of poor women who require increased first-level care as well as easy-to-reach backup facilities for complications. In most areas, there are severe shortages of trained health workers with the capability to diagnose, refer, and treat these problems. Recent evidence has also shown that early postnatal care (within the first day and first week after birth) is highly effective in reducing newborn mortality. Countries are now beginning to make concerted efforts to work toward a continuum of care from early pregnancy through the postpartum/natal period. This is done by creating synergies between maternal and child health services and increasing the emphasis on provision of postpartum/neonatal care.

Inequities in Progress: The Rich–Poor Divide

There is ample evidence of inequities in the risk of maternal death between and within developed and developing countries, irrespective of the stage of development or the condition of the health system. Differences in maternal mortality between urban and rural areas within poor countries are substantial. In Egypt, the maternal mortality rate was over twice as high in the nomadic frontier region than in the metropolitan region, 120 vs. 48 deaths per 100,000 (Ronsmans and Graham 2006). In Afghanistan the differences were even more striking, with a mortality of 418 per 100,000 in the capital city of Kabul, compared with 6,507 per 100,000 in the remote district of Ragh (Bartlett et al. 2005). Data from selected population-based studies in sub-Saharan Africa are in accord with these urban–rural patterns. A link between poverty and maternal health has been clear for more than a century. Figure 22.5

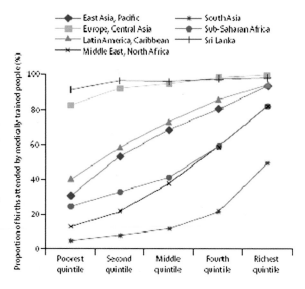

Fig. 22.5 Rich poor divide: birth attended by medically trained people by wealth quintile and regions. Source: Lancet Maternal Survival Series (2006)

shows data for the poverty gradient in comparison to access to maternal health-care services. Sri Lanka is a country that shows equitable use of health professionals for births across all population groups. However, in Peru, for example, the estimate for the poorest group is in excess of 800 maternal deaths per 100,000 live births compared with less than 130 per 100,000 for the richest quintile – a greater than six-fold difference (Ronsmans and Graham 2006). Some societal factors contributing to inequities are group characteristics such as ethnicity, caste, race, or emigrant populations, whereas others are individual and include marital status or social standing (Ronsmans and Graham 2006).

Achieving Millennium Development Goals

The Millennium Declaration set out eight specific Millennium Development Goals (MDGs), each with its own numerical targets and indicators for monitoring progress. These goals give special priority to the health and well-being of women, mothers, and children. The target set for MDG-5 is a 75% reduction in the global maternal mortality ratio between 1990 and 2015. The evidence suggests that a reduction of 75% is achievable with a 25-year time frame, similarly to the way some industrialized countries halved their maternal mortality rate in the late 19th century (mostly through the provision of skilled health-care professionals at birth). Evidence from several transitional countries also suggests that a 75% decline can be achieved. As discussed earlier, during the last 40 years Thailand, Malaysia, and Sri Lanka have substantially reduced their maternal mortality, which is now comparable to many industrialized countries. However, reliable trends are not available for many countries with high levels of maternal mortality, and some investigators believe there is little to suggest any progress, especially in sub-Saharan Africa.

Seventy-five countries contribute to 96% of all maternal and 92% of all neonatal deaths globally. Therefore, it is possible to envision various scenarios for scaling-up services, taking into account the specific circumstances in each country. At present, some 43% of mothers and newborns receive some

care, but not the full range of what they need to avoid the majority of risk of maternal death (WHO 2005). Adding up the optimistic (but also realistic) scenarios for each of the 75 countries would give access to the full package of first-level and backup care to 101 million mothers (some 73% of the expected births) in 2015 and to their babies. If these scenarios were implemented, the MDG for maternal health would be reached in every country and the reduction of maternal and perinatal mortality globally would be well on the way. Unfortunately achievement of MDGs does not reflect equity or universal coverage of care. Therefore, in almost all countries, the rich population would achieve MDGs but not the poor population. It is also clear that achievement of MDG-4 (Reduction of Child Mortality) will not be possible without substantial advances for the newborn. This is related to improvement of maternal health. Without much improvement in the control and treatment of malaria and HIV/AIDS in pregnancy, MDG-6 (related to HIV/AIDS, malaria, and TB) will not be achievable. Therefore, maternal health programs provide a unique strategic opportunity to achieve all three health-related MDGs (WHO 2005).

Challenges

Reduction in maternal and neonatal mortality does not require new technologies or new knowledge of effective interventions. We know what needs to be done to save the lives of mothers and newborns. The challenges are how to deliver services and scale up interventions particularly to those who are vulnerable, hard to reach, marginalized, and/or excluded. Effective health interventions exist for mothers and babies, and several proven means of distribution are available. However, none of them will work if political will is absent where it matters most: at national and district levels (Van Lerberghe and De Brouwere 2001). In many of the countries experiencing stagnation and reversal (particularly in sub-Saharan Africa), barriers to the uptake of health benefits are a critical source of exclusion for many pregnant women. Often services simply do not exist or cannot be reached. For example, lack of access to facilities where major obstetric interventions can be performed is the prime reason why large numbers of mothers in rural areas are excluded from lifesaving care during childbirth. But there are many other barriers to the uptake of health benefits. These include service use that is often constrained because of women's lack of decision-making power, the low value placed on women's health, and the negative or judgmental attitudes of family members.

Policy challenges differ between countries that are close to universal health-care access (where exclusion is limited) and those where exclusion is pervasive. The countries where exclusion is limited to a small and marginalized proportion of the population are usually on track or at least are slowly progressing toward the reduction of maternal and newborn mortality. These are countries with well-developed health systems, although they may not always be health systems with an optimal range of technical interventions. Examples of countries in this group include Brazil, Colombia, and the Dominican Republic. For these countries, the challenge is targeting mothers and newborns that are currently excluded from the possibility of claiming entitlements. This tackles the roots of social exclusion, removes the barriers to uptake of health services, responds appropriately to their needs, and offers them financial protection from the consequences of illness and obtaining care. Most of the countries that showed limited progress in mortality reduction, stagnated, or went into reversal in regard to maternal mortality show patterns of massive exclusion or queuing. Such countries include Bangladesh, Chad, and Ethiopia. These countries typically have weak, low-density, and fragile health systems. Complex emergencies, in addition to high poverty rates and HIV/AIDS, lead to additional constraints on health systems development. The main challenge is to build and implement primary health care as the vehicle for maternal, newborn, and child health care, with timely access to emergency lifesaving services.

By the mid-1990 s, many countries were creating district health systems within the context of a primary health-care approach. They defined a minimum package of services and established a system for timely supply of drugs and equipment. However, as in the years after the Alma-Ata declaration, funding often did not follow. This was particularly true in sub-Saharan Africa. In the bleak economic environment, financing remained a real barrier to progress. With a decrease in gross domestic product per capita in real terms between 1990 and 2002, total health expenditure in many African countries stagnated or decreased. Public health expenditure remained below US $10 per person. Up to 1999, per capita was stagnant and external assistance did not make up for this.

Civil service regulations and structural adjustment policies often leave little flexibility to improve working conditions in the public sector, especially in terms of salaries and incentives. As a result, many health workers have moved to the private sector or to other countries. Data from Ghana, Zambia, and Zimbabwe show that losses of health workers from the public health sector continued or accelerated during the 1990 s. The stringent budgetary measures under structural adjustment programs also imposed ceilings on personnel recruitment. Even in countries with unemployed health professionals, such as Zambia, governments often were not able to hire additional staff (U.S. Agency for International Development 2003).

Absenteeism was another major issue that affected the already scarce human resources within health-care services. In Burkina Faso, for example, absenteeism of health district doctors in seven rural districts in 1997 varied between 30% to more than 80%. Vacancy rates for doctors in Ghana increased from 43% in 1998 to 47% in 2002. Over the same time period vacancy rates for registered nurses rose from 26 to 57% (Dovlo 2003). Much of the absenteeism was related to inadequate working conditions, insufficient salaries, and declining staff morale. In a number of countries, however, the HIV/AIDS epidemic aggravated this acute human resource crisis. Data are scarce but suggest that besides contributing to absenteeism, HIV/AIDS may cost Africa's health systems one-fifth of their employees over the next few years (Tawfik and Kinoti 2001). The absence of adequate measures to protect health workers against HIV/AIDS and the stress of caring for HIV/AIDS patients are additional factors motivating migration of health-care employees.

The shortage of health personnel is the most visible aspect of the human resources crisis in sub-Saharan Africa. The figures are stark: in Zimbabwe, of the 1200 physicians trained during the 1990 s, only 360 remained practicing in the country in 2001. Ghana's loss of 328 nurses in 1999 was the equivalent of its annual output (U.S. Agency for International Development 2003). More than half of the health professionals in Zimbabwe, Ghana, and South Africa are thinking of migrating to other countries. At the same time, 35,000 South African nurses are not employed in the health sector and two-thirds of the health workforce in Swaziland is working in the private sector.

Other challenges are how to address the issues of deteriorating infrastructure, stock-out of drugs, dwindling supplies and equipments, lack of transport, ineffective referral to and availability of 24 hour quality services, particularly emergency obstetric care services and weak management systems. Part of the task ahead is political. Maternal, newborn, and child health cannot be reduced to a set of programs delivered to a target population. Rather, mothers and children must be in a position to claim entitlements as their right. This implies an adjustment of macro-level health policies and resource mobilization, at the country level and internationally. Three issues need urgent attention: the funding of the health sector, the human resource crisis, and the accountability of health systems and providers to their clients. Politically, the problem of scaling up looks very different. Political solutions emphasize the speed and visibility of results, affordability, buy-in of professional groups, and the importance of existing hierarchies and structures, however fragile. Political solutions also take into account the views and demands of the electorate.

A new era of strategic thinking for maternal and neonatal health should start with a realistic needs assessment of present care coverage and move forward by understanding supply constraints that have blocked progress in developing countries for over 20 years. Currently, only half the world's women receive care from a skilled professional while giving birth, and they often do not receive the quality of care they need. Even fewer women receive the full package of care from pregnancy to the end of the postpartum period. For those who are able to access care, the message is clear: women need protection, standards need to be improved, care must be respectful, and the health personnel who attend them need to be remunerated and managed properly if they are to remain in service.

Most countries facing major maternal and newborn health and survival challenges have yet to develop national strategies for increasing access to adequate health care or to translate these strategies into investment plans that are endorsed by political authorities. There are three distinct, but related, work strategies that must be taken up to develop such comprehensive strategies: first, national health authorities need to revisit the structure and content of maternal and newborn health programs; second, they need to plan the scaling up of services within a health system that is able to respond to current needs; and third, they need to enter the political arena to muster the political commitment to universal coverage of maternal and newborn health services. The task ahead is also one of refocusing program content. For too long attention has been directed toward the development of technologies, rather than toward embedding these in viable organizational strategies. Strategies need to ensure a continuum of care through pregnancy, childbirth, and the postpartum/postnatal period and include the home, community, and health facilities. Much of the challenge, in fact, is to accommodate both programmatic and systemic concerns: an organizational rather than a technical problem.

Key Terms

Antenatal care	Distant factors	Fertility rate
Birth outcomes	Eclampsia	Hemorrhage
Birth rate	Emergency obstetric services	Home delivery
Caesarean section	Episiotomy	Indirect causes
Direct causes	Family planning	Infant mortality rate

Intermediate factors	Obstetric care	Stillbirth
Interventionist obstetrics	Obstetric complications	Total fertility rate (TFR)
Maternal death	Obstructed labor	Traditional birth attendants (TBAs)
Maternal health programs	Perinatal mortality rate	Uncomplicated care
Maternal mortality ratio	Post-neonatal mortality rate	Unsafe abortion
Maternity care	Postpartum care	Urinary incontinence
Midwifery care	Postpartum death	Uterine prolapsed
Miscarriage	Pregnancy outcomes	Uterine rupture
Neonatal mortality rate	Prenatal mortality rate	
Newborn care services	Severe anemia	
Newborn outcomes	Skilled health professionals	

Questions for Discussion

1. It is said that sustainable reduction in maternal and infant mortality will require emphasis on establishment of viable organizational strategies that build health systems infrastructure and ensure effective and efficient continuum of care. Do you agree with this statement? Justify your position in about 1,000 words, citing specific country examples as appropriate.
2. Draw a flow chart to illustrate McCarthy and Maine's (1992) framework for determinants of maternal mortality, noting distant factors, intermediate factors, and unknown/unpredicted factors.
3. Briefly explain what you understand by Castro et al.'s (2000) "three delays" framework for classifying risk factors for maternal mortality.
4. It is said that both mothers and newborns have a better chance of survival if they have a skilled attendant at birth, and access to emergency services. Briefly explain what this means. What are the implications for reduction of maternal mortality in less developed countries?
5. In an essay of about 1,000 words, describe the major barriers against efforts to significantly reduce global maternal and neonatal mortality.

References

AbouZahr C (2003) Global burden of maternal death and disability. In: Rodeck C, ed. Reducing Maternal Death and Disability in Pregnancy. Oxford: Oxford University Press, pp. 1–11

Ahmed Y, Mwaba P, Chintu C et al. (1999) A study of maternal mortality at the University Teaching Hospital, Lusaka, Zambia: the emergence of tuberculosis as a major non-obstetric cause of maternal death. The International Journal of Tuberculosis and Lung Disease, 3(8), 675–680

Aliyu MH, Salihu HM, Keith LG et al. (2005a) Extreme parity and the risk of stillbirth. Obstetrics and Gynecology, 106(1), 446–453

Aliyu MH, Salihu HM, Keith LG et al. (2005b) Hyper-fertility and fetal morbidity outcomes trends in birth to fertile mothers by race/ethnicity and maternal age in the United States. Journal of the National Medical Association, 97(6), 799–804

American Academy of Pediatrics (2007) Guidelines for Perinatal Care (6th Edition). Washington, DC: American Academy of Pediatrics/American College of Obstetricians and Gynecologists (ACOG). http://www.acog.org/bookstore/Guidelines_for_Perinatal_Care_Sixth_Edition_P262.cfm, cited 27 August 2008

Bartlett LA, Mawji S, Whitehead S et al. (2005) Where giving birth is a forecast of death: maternal mortality in four districts of Afghanistan, 1999–2002. Lancet, 365(9462), 864–870

Belgrade, Serbia and Montenegro Statistical Office (2004) Statistical pocket book 2004

Brabin BJ, Hakimi M, Pelletier D (2001) An Analysis of Anemia and Pregnancy-Related Maternal Mortality. American Society for Nutritional Sciences, 131, 604–615

Brown CA, Sohani SB, Khan K et al. (2008) Antenatal care and perinatal outcomes in Kwale district, Kenya. BMC Pregnancy Childbirth, 10(8), 2

Castro R, Campero L, Hernandez B et al. (2000) A study on maternal mortality in Mexico through a qualitative approach. Journal of Women's Health and Gender-based Medicine, 9(6), 679–690

Centers for Disease Control and Prevention (CDC) (2007) NCHS Definitions. Atlanta, Georgia: Center for Disease Control and Prevention (CDC), National Center for Health Statistics. http://www.cdc.gov/nchs/datawh/nchsdefs/rates.htm#maternal, cited 8 August 2008

Christian P, West KP, Khatry SK et al. (2000) Night Blindness During Pregnancy and Subsequent Mortality among Women in Nepal: Effects of Vitamin A and ß-Carotene Supplementation. American Journal of Epidemiology, 152(6), 542–547

Danel I (1998) Maternal Mortality Reduction, Honduras, 1990–1997: A Case-Study. Atlanta, GA: Centers for Disease Control and Prevention. http://wbln0018.worldbank.org/LAC/lacinfoclient.nsf/6f1c77f445edaa6585256746007718fe/2f153269dab5f9838525685c006b532b/$FILE/WBCASE5.pdf, cited 8 August 2008

Dhakal S, Chapman GN, Simkhada PP et al. (2007) Utilisation of postnatal care among rural women in Nepal. BMC Pregnancy Childbirth, Sep. 3, 7, 19

Dovlo D (2003) The brain drain and retention of health professionals in Africa. A case study. Paper presented at: Regional Training Conference on Improving Tertiary Education in Sub-Saharan Africa: the things that work! Accra, 23–25. http://www.medact.org/content/health/documents/brain_drain/Dovlo%20-%20brain%20drain%20and%20retention.pdf, cited 8 August 2008

Ehiri JE, Oyo-Ita AE, Anyanwu EC et al. (2005) Quality of child health services in primary healthcare facilities in Calabar, Southeastern Nigeria. Child Care: Health and Development, 31(2), 181–191

Falkingham J (2003) Inequality and changes in women's use of maternal healthcare services in Tajikistan. Studies in Family Planning, 34, 32–43

Fortney JA (2001) Emergency obstetric care: the keystone in the arch of safe motherhood. International Journal of Gynecology and Obstetrics, 74, 95–97

Goyaux N, Alihonou E, Diadhiou F et al. (2001) Complications of induced abortion and miscarriage in three African countries: a hospital-based study among WHO collaborating centers. Acta Obstetricia et Gynecologica Scandinavica, 80, 568–573

Granja AC, Machungo F, Gomes A et al. (1998) Malaria-related maternal mortality in urban Mozambique. Annals of Tropical Medicine and Parasitology, 92(3), 257–263

Islam M (2007) The safe motherhood initiative and beyond. Bulletin of the World Health Organization, 85(10), 733–820

Jewkes RK, Fawcus S, Rees H et al. (1997) Methodological Issues in the South African Incomplete Abortion Study. Studies in Family Planning, 28(3), 228–234

Johnson BR, Ndhlovu S, Farr SL et al. (2002) Reducing Unplanned Pregnancy and Abortion in Zimbabwe through Postabortion Contraception. Studies in Family Planning, 33(2), 195–202

Katz J, West KP Jr, Khatry SK et al. (2003) Risk factors for early infant mortality in Sarlahi district, Nepal. Bulletin of the World Health Organization, 81, 717–725

Khan KS, Wojdyla D, Say L (2006) WHO analysis of causes of maternal death: a systematic review. Lancet, 367, 1066–1074

Koblinsky MA (2003) Reducing Maternal Mortality: Learning from Bolivia, China, Egypt, Honduras, Indonesia, Jamaica, and Zimbabwe. Washington, DC: World Bank. http://books.google.com/books?hl=en&id=7I9-NjYv-YkC&dq=Koblinsky++Reducing+Maternal+Mortality&printsec=frontcover&source=web&ots=M5Sc8mXnf9&sig=RQemDreh1tp9RmpQoDqBW7bYkWQ#PPP1,M1, cited 8 August 2008

Kusiako T, Ronsmans C, van der Paal L (2000) Perinatal mortality attributable to complications of childbirth in Matlab, Bangladesh. Bulletin of the World Health Organization, 78, 621–627

Lawn J, Zupan J, Knippenberg R (2005) Newborn survival. In Jamison, D. et al. (2nd eds.), Disease Control Priorities in Developing Countries. New York: Oxford University Press

Loudon I (1992) Death in childbirth: an international study of maternal care and maternal mortality, 1800–1950. Oxford: Clarendon Press

Masuy-Stroobant G (1997) Infant health and child mortality in Europe: lessons from the past and challenges for the future. In: Corsini C, Viazzo PP, eds. The Decline of Infant and Child Mortality: The European Experience 1750–1990. The Hague: Kluwer Law International/Martinus Nijhoff

McCarthy J, Maine D (1992) A framework for analyzing the determinants of maternal mortality. Studies in Family Planning, 23(1), 23–33

National Institute for Health and Clinical Excellence (NICE) (2003) Clinical guideline # CG62. Antenatal care: routine care for the healthy pregnancy woman. National Collaborating Center for Women's and Children's Health. National Institute for Health and Clinical Excellence (NICE) and UK National Health Services (NHS). http://www.nice.org.uk/nicemedia/pdf/CG62FullGuidelineCorrectedJune2008.pdf, cited 26 August 8, 2009

Pathmanathan I, Liljestrand J, Martins JM et al. (2003) Investing in maternal health: learning from Malaysia and Sri Lanka. Washington, DC: World Bank

Raatikainen, K, Heiskanen N, Heinonen S (2007) Under-attending free antenatal care is associated with adverse pregnancy outcomes. BMC Public Health, 7(147), 268

Rahman M, DaVanzo J, Razzaque A (2001) Do better family planning services reduce abortion in Bangladesh? Lancet, 358, 1051–1056

Ronsmans C, Campbell O (1998) Short Birth Intervals Don't Kill Women: Evidence from Matlab, Bangladesh. Studies in Family Planning, 29(3), 282–290

Ronsmans C, Graham WJ (2006) Maternal mortality: who, where, when and why? Lancet, 368, 1189–1200

Sibley LM, Sipe TA, Koblinsky M (2004) Does traditional birth attendant training increase use of antenatal care? A review of the evidence. Journal of Midwifery and Women's Health, 49(4), 298–305

Sloan FA, Conover CJ, Mah ML et al. (2002) Impact of medicaid managed care on utilization of obstetric care: evidence from TennCare's early years. Southern Medical Journal, 95(8), 811–821

Tawfik L, Kinoti SN (2001) The Impact of HIV/AIDS on the Health Sector in Sub-Saharan Africa: The Issue of Human Resources. Washington, DC: United States Agency for International Development, Bureau for Africa, Office of Sustainable Development, SARA Project. http://www.vitalneeds.com/documents/AIDS-Africa-Health-Care-Personnel/2001%20HIVAIDS%20Impact%20on%20-Health%20Sector%20in%20Sub%20Saharan%20Africa%20II.pdf, cited 8 August 2008

Ticconi C, Mapfumo M, Dorrucci M et al. (2003) Effect of maternal HIV and malaria infection on pregnancy and perinatal outcome in Zimbabwe. Journal of Acquired Immune Deficiency Syndromes, 34, 289–294

Tinker A, Ransom E (2002) Healthy mothers and healthy newborns: the vital link. Washington, DC: Save the Children/Population Reference Bureau

United Nations Children's Fund (UNICEF) (1998) Situation analysis of children and women in Iraq. New York: UNICEF

United States Agency for International Development (USAID) (2003) The health sector human resources crisis in Africa: an issue paper. Washington, DC: United States Agency for International Development, Bureau for Africa, Office of Sustainable Development, SARA Project. http://www.hrhresourcecenter.org/node/33, cited 8 August 2008

Van Egmond K, Bosmans M, Naeem AJ et al. (2004) Reproductive Health in Afghanistan: Results of a Knowledge, Attitudes and Practices Survey among Afghan Women in Kabul. Disasters, 28(3), 269–282

Van Lerberghe W, De Brouwere V (2001) Of blind alleys and things that have worked: history's lessons on reducing maternal mortality. In: De Brouwere V and Van Lerberghe W, eds. Safe Motherhood Strategies: A Review of the Evidence. Antwerp, ITG Press

Villar J, Ba'aqeel H, Piaggio G et al. (2001) WHO antenatal care randomised trial for the evaluation of a new model of routine antenatal care. Lancet, 357, 1551–1564

Villar J, Merialdi M, Gulmezoglu AM et al. (2003) Nutritional interventions during pregnancy for the prevention or treatment of maternal morbidity and preterm delivery: An overview of randomized controlled trials. Journal of Nutrition, 133, 1606–1625

World Health Organization (WHO) (1994) Antenatal Care. Report of a Technical Working Group, 1994 – WHO/FRH/MSM/968 1994. Geneva: World Health Organization. http://www.who.int/reproductive-health/publications/MSM_96_8/index.html, cited 8 August 2008

World Health Organization (WHO) (2003) Antenatal Care in Developing Countries: Promises, Achievement, and Missed Opportunities. http://www.childinfo.org/files/antenatal_care.pdf, cited 8 August 2008

World Health Organization (WHO) (2004) Maternal Mortality in 2000: Estimates Developed by WHO, UNICEF and UNFPA. Geneva, World Health Organization. http://www.reliefweb.int/library/documents/2003/who-saf-22oct.pdf, cited 8 August 2008

World Health Organization (WHO) (2005) World Health Report 2005: Make Every Mother and Child Count. http://www.who.int/whr/2005/whr2005_en.pdf, cited 8 August 2008

World Health Organization (WHO) (2007) Skilled Attendants at Birth: 2007 updates. http://www.who.int/reproductive-health/global_monitoring/skilled_attendant.html#results, cited 8 August 2008

World Health Organization (WHO) (2008) The World Health Report: Progress and Some Reversals. http://www.who.int/whr/2005/chapter5/en/index2.html, cited 8 August 2008

Chapter 23
Global Immunization Challenge: Progress and Opportunities

Rebecca Affolder, Michel Zaffran, and Julian Lob-Levyt

Learning Objectives After reading this chapter and answering the discussion questions that follow, you should be able to

- Outline important milestones in the emergence of vaccines as a means of disease control and prevention.
- Discuss factors that underpin the disparity in access to vaccines between rich and poor countries.
- Identify and appraise innovative options for financing vaccine development, and for ensuring wider access to new and underused vaccines in developing countries.
- Evaluate strategies for ensuring sustainability in vaccine development, management, and access.
- Outline priorities for future research, policy, and practice with regard to vaccine development, procurement, and access.

Introduction

Vaccines, having been developed over the last 200 years to become one of the most cost-effective and successful public health interventions, are one of the most exciting technologies in the world today. Yet every year, around 2.5 million children die from diseases that can be prevented by currently available or new vaccines. Vaccines have the potential to erase some of the most glaring global health inequities which currently shape the lives of millions. Often the most vulnerable – women, children, and

adolescents in even the poorest countries, could be protected against life-threatening and debilitating disease within a generation. This chapter presents a historical perspective on the emergence of vaccines as a means of disease control and prevention over the past two centuries. Beginning with discovery of smallpox vaccine by Edward Jenner in 1796, the chapter identifies important milestones in widespread use of vaccines in global health, including

- The smallpox eradication initiative of the World Health Organization in 1970s, the Child Survival Revolution, and the Expanded Program on Immunization (EPI) of the 1980s
- The United Nations Millennium Summit of 2000 and the resulting global commitment to the Millennium Development Goals (MDGs)
- The International Conference on Financing for Development held in Mexico in 2002 and the corresponding financial commitments from high-income nations to support achievement of MDGs
- Establishment of the Global Alliance for Vaccines and Immunization in 2000 to accelerate access to new and underused vaccines in poor countries

Inequity in access to vaccines between rich and poor countries and the underpinning factors are discussed, including lack of safety and quality assurance systems in poor countries, focus of research and development on rich nations' priorities, and the diversion of scarce resources to other emerging global health priorities. Various innovative options for financing wider access to new and underused vaccines in poor countries are explored, including the role of the International Finance Facility for Immunization (IFFIm), the Advanced Market

R. Affolder (✉)
GAVI Alliance Secretariat, 2 Chemin des Mines, 1202 Geneva, Switzerland

J.E. Ehiri (ed.), *Maternal and Child Health*, DOI 10.1007/b106524_23,
© Springer Science+Business Media, LLC 2009

Commitment (AMCs), the Heavily Indebted Poor Countries (HIPCI) and Multilateral Debt Relief (MDRI) initiatives, and the Debt Buy-Down program of the World Bank. Issues of sustainability in vaccine development, procurement, and management are discussed as are priorities for future research, policy, and practice.

The first immunization – and the origin of a smallpox vaccine – is believed to have been in 1796 (Table 23.1) when British physician Edward Jenner administered fluid from a cowpox lesion obtained from a milkmaid named Sarah Nelmes

Table 23.1 Timeline of vaccine discoveries and global events

Date	Vaccine target	Research strategy
1796	Smallpox (Jenner)	Use of related animal virus
1881	Anthrax	Chemical attenuation
1885	Rabies (Pasteur)	Chemical attenuation
1896	Cholera	Inactivated whole organisms
1896	Typhoid	Inactivated whole organisms
1896	Plague	Inactivated whole organisms
1923	Diphtheria (D)	
1926	Pertussis (wP)	Inactivated whole organisms
1927	Tetanus (T)	Use of toxoids
1927	Tuberculosis (BCG)	Passage in vitro
1935	Yellow fever	
1936	Influenza	Inactivated whole organisms
1955	Polio (IPV)	Inactivated whole organisms
1957	DTPw	
1958	Polio (OPV)	
1961	DTIPV	
1963	Measles (M)	Passage in vitro
1965	*SMALLPOX ERADICATION UNIT AT WHO CREATED*	
1966	DTPIPV	
1967	Mumps (M)	
1969	Rubella (R)	Cell culture passage w/cold adaptation
1971	MMR	
1972	Meningococcus	Use of toxoids
1974	*Expanded Programme on Immunization*	

Table 23.1 (continued)

Date	Vaccine target	Research strategy
	(EPI) DEFINED AND LAUNCHED	
1976	Pneumococcus	
1979	*SMALL POX ERADICATION CERTIFIED*	
1981	Acellular Pertussis (aP)	
1981	Hepatitis B (HB)	
1984	Universal childhood Immunization Goal (UCI) LAUNCHED	
1984	Varicella (V)	
1986	rDNA HB	
1988	H. influenzae b (Hib)	Protein-conjugated capsular
1988	*GLOBAL POLIO ERADICATION INITIATIVE LAUNCHED*	
1991	Hepatitis A (HA)	
1993	DTPwIPVHib	
1994	DTPa	
1996	DTPwHB	
1996	HBHA	
1997	DTaP-Hib	
1997	DTaP-IPV-Hib	
1998	Lyme	
1998	Rotavirus	
1999	DTaP	
1999	HATy	
2000	DTaP-HB-IPV	
2000	DTaP-HB-IPV-Hib	
2000	Meningococcus C conjugate vaccine.	
2000	Pneumococcus conjugate vaccine	
2000	*GLOBAL ALLIANCE FOR VACCINES AND IMMUNIZATION (GAVI) LAUNCHED*	
2003	Influenza (LAIV) Cell culture passage w/ cold adaptation	
2006*	HPV vaccine that protects against infection with four HPV genotypes was licensed; a second vaccine that protects against two HPV genotypes is likely to be licensed soon.	

*WHO (2007a)
Sources: Andre (2003); Plotkin (2005)

to a 13-year-old boy named James Phipps. Jenner later found that the boy was "secure" to smallpox virus (Andre 2003). Louis Pasteur later coined the term vaccine in reference to the Latin word for cow: vacca.

Records of a similar medical approach can be found in Chinese literature dating back to the eleventh century and linked with the fight against the smallpox virus (Plotkin 2005). According to the National Library of Medicine (U.S. National Library of Medicine 2002), the practice of variolation, where small scabs of tissue containing smallpox were inhaled causing the individual to contract the disease in a mild form, reduced the mortality rate among those exposed to the disease to 1–2% as opposed to 30% when individuals contracted the disease naturally. By 1700, the practice of variolation as a response to smallpox had expanded to India, Africa, and throughout the Ottoman Empire. Variolation was first practiced in Europe by 1717 and, by 1721, in the American colonies (U.S. National Library of Medicine 2002).

The immunization field grew in the 19th and 20th centuries, with major breakthroughs in the mid- to late 20th century through discovery of vaccines that protect against such diseases as influenza, polio, and yellow fever (Table 23.1). Prior to the development of such vaccines, the loss of life from disease is illustrated in some staggering figures. For example, the influenza (or "Spanish flu") outbreak of 1918–1919 resulted in more deaths than enemy fire in World War I (Plotkin 2005). The period of 1974–2000 can be considered a second phase in the history of immunization. The World Health Organization (WHO) launched the Expanded Program on Immunization (EPI) in 1974, expanding the smallpox eradication effort which was focused on one single vaccine into an infant program of six vaccines (against diphtheria, pertussis, tetanus, poliomyelitis, measles, and tuberculosis). At the time, less than 5% of the world's children were immunized against these six diseases. Meanwhile, an increased degree of population mobility, for example, through commercial air travel, helped bring about the recognition that infectious disease prevention required a coordinated, global effort.

The EPI launch marked an important turning point: immunization became an international public good. In response to a 1977 World Health Assembly challenge (World Health Assembly 2003), immunization coverage rose over the next decade, with the United Nations Children's Fund (UNICEF) declaring 80% of the world's children under the age of 13 immunized against tuberculosis, polio, and measles by 1990 (Hardon and Blume 2005).

A number of global initiatives contributed to the progression of immunization coverage rates in the 1980s. UNICEF, with the support of other international organizations, launched the "Child Survival Revolution" in 1982 (UNICEF 1996). This initiative comprised four interventions for reducing mortality: growth monitoring, oral rehydration, breastfeeding, and immunization (GOBI). At the same time, WHO led major vertical programs to combat vaccine-preventable disease, diarrhea, and acute respiratory infections (Hardon and Blume 2005). The Universal Childhood Immunization (UCI) Goal was launched in 1984 to catalyze efforts toward universal immunization coverage. UCI aimed at accelerating EPI, capitalizing on the success in mobilizing support. As a result of these dedicated efforts, child mortality declined in many countries (Hardon and Blume 2005).

Yet, despite the overall success of accelerating immunization coverage in the period described above, significant disparities are apparent (Fig. 23.1). The expansion in coverage was largely in developed countries with large populations. One hundred and seven countries did not reach the immunization coverage of 80%, and the declaration of success did not reflect the uneven coverage within many countries – where some of the most vulnerable children in hard-to-reach areas were missed. A great success for some masked the growing divide in access between North and South.

The characteristics of the North/South divide, which remains the current global situation, developed during the 1990s. A gap in the routine immunization schedules for children in developed and developing countries emerged as new vaccines, including those for hepatitis B, Haemophilus influenzae b (Hib), varicella, pneumococcal, meningococcal, and combination formulations became a routine part of the immunization schedule for children and adolescents in high-income countries

Fig. 23.1 Global number of unimmunized children under 5 years of age. Source: WHO/UNICEF coverage estimates 1980–2007, August 2008

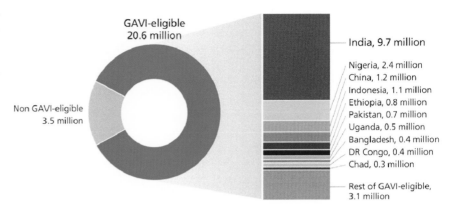

(Hardon and Blume 2005). Research and development priorities favored those products targeting developed countries. Vaccine quality and safety, taken for granted in many countries with robust regulatory agencies, fell behind in many countries lacking an effective quality assurance program for medical products. Quality and safety issues also point to the weakness of health delivery systems in many poor countries which limited the effective rollout of routine immunization. The gap in financial commitment to maternal and child health – which underpins and drives the North/South divide in access to immunization – widened over the 1990s as scarce resources were diverted to other emerging global health priorities. Many developing countries struggled to improve or even maintain their immunization rates. The end of the decade saw an overall decline in global immunization and vaccine production, and particularly among the poorest populations in the poorest parts of the world.

The new millennium set the stage for a major shift in the global response to the growing inequities between North and South. Under the leadership of the then UN Secretary General Kofi Annan, the UN Millennium Summit, the largest-ever gathering of world leaders, was convened at the United Nations Headquarters in New York, USA, in September 2000 (United Nations Development Program 2003). At the close of the summit, world leaders unanimously adopted the "United Nations Millennium Declaration" taking on a clear obligation to act through commitment to the Millennium Development Goals (MDGs) (United Nations 2006). These goal comprised a set of time-bound

and measurable goals and targets for combating poverty, hunger, disease, illiteracy, environmental degradation, and discrimination against women. Corresponding financial commitments from the developed world in the form of aid, trade, debt relief, and investment were made at the International Conference on Financing for Development in Monterrey, Mexico (IFAD 2007).

As part of a renewed commitment to poverty reduction and human development, the international community moved to address the growing inequalities in immunization and the unacceptable toll of infectious disease in developing countries. Marking the start of a "third phase" in the history of immunization, the Global Alliance for Vaccines and Immunization (now the GAVI Alliance) was launched in January 2000 to accelerate access to new and underused vaccines in the poorest countries. GAVI, an innovative public/private partnership, brought together the major stakeholders in immunization in order to achieve global immunization targets. These stakeholders included national governments, UNICEF, WHO, The World Bank, the Bill and Melinda Gates Foundation, the vaccine industry, public health institutions, and nongovernmental organizations (GAVI Alliance 2008a). Soon after GAVI's launch its mandate came to include action on the child mortality target of the Millennium Development Goals – namely, a 2/3 reduction of the under-5 mortality rate by 2015 (GAVI Alliance 2008b).

In the years since GAVI's launch, overall DTP3 coverage increased from 64% in 1999 to 73% in 2005 in GAVI-eligible countries, i.e., those with a gross national income (GNI) of less than $1,000 per capita. The figures are more pronounced in the WHO African region where DTP3 coverage increased from 48% (1999) to 73% (2007) and has overtaken Southeast Asia (66% in 2007), which is now the region with most unimmunized children (WHO 2007b). Much of this increase in DTP3 coverage has been attributed, through independent evaluation, to the Immunization Services Support provided by GAVI to strengthen immunization delivery systems and infrastructure (Lu et al. 2006).

In terms of new and underused vaccine introduction, the cumulative achievement of the poorest countries to improve coverage is impressive (GAVI Alliance 2008b). Over 5 years, 88.5 million additional children were immunized against HepB3 (2000–2005). Four and a half million additional children were immunized against yellow fever in 2005, equaling a cumulative 13.1 million additional children immunized over 5 years against yellow fever. An additional 4.5 million additional children were immunized with Hib vaccine in 2005, equaling a cumulative 13.2 million additional children immunized with Hib vaccine over 5 years.

Critical to these improvements has been the ability of the GAVI Alliance to raise new and additional resources – providing funds to introduce new and underused vaccines, improve injection safety, improve immunization delivery services, and strengthen health systems. GAVI-supported countries are continuing to produce impressive results (GAVI Alliance 2008a). Despite the exciting results, we must not lose sight that the key challenges remain gaining better data on disease burden to stimulate demand and ensuring the affordability and long-term sustainability of new vaccine introduction. Until prices become more affordable, slow uptake of new vaccines in the poorest countries remains inevitable. How this challenge can be better addressed through innovative approaches is covered in the discussion on funding challenges below.

The GAVI Alliance is but one element of a growing complexity of agencies working on maternal and child health issues; while it maintains a niche focus, this requires close collaboration with partners in the broader global health community. The launch of the Global Immunization Vision and Strategy (GIVS) in 2005 (WHO/UNICEF 2005) provided a critical overarching framework that exhibits the need for coordinated mix of instruments and approaches.

These approaches may be in the form of highly successful vertical campaign strategies for the global eradication of polio and control of measles, delivery of basic vaccines in conflict environments, or in the longer-term efforts to create sustainable markets for new and underused vaccines in the poorest countries. GIVS was approved by the member states of WHO and the Executive Board of UNICEF in 2005. It sets out a plan to address the global immunization challenges over the decade 2006–2015 and strives to act with equity and gender equality, in addition to personal ownership, partnership, and responsibility. Placing immunization firmly within the health system strengthening agenda, GIVS "aims to sustain existing levels of vaccine coverage, extend immunization services to those who are currently unreached and to age groups beyond infancy, introduce new vaccines and technologies, and link immunization with the delivery of other health interventions and the overall development of the health sector" (WHO/UNICEF 2005). The vision and goals of GIVS are a world in 2015 that highly values immunization and that has equal access to immunizations for all. This world would also support sustainable interventions in diverse social situations, changing demographics and economies, as well as being a world that will put vaccines to the best global health and security use.

Addressing the Key Challenges: Funding, Sustainability, Equity

Funding

Following the launch of GIVS in 2005, a WHO/UNICEF study examined the cost, financing, and impact of immunization programs in the 72 poorest countries (WHO/UNICEF 2005). Implementation of GIVS would protect more than 70 million children in the world's poorest countries against the 14 major childhood diseases by 2015. The estimated total price tag for immunization activities for 2006–2015 in these countries is US $35 billion, one-third of which would be spent on vaccines and two-thirds of which would be spent on immunization delivery systems. The study concluded that spending on immunization will need to rise from

US $2.5 billion per year (2006) to US $3.5 billion by 2010 and US $4 billion by 2015 (WHO/UNICEF 2005).

National budgets will ultimately fund vaccines and health services. The challenge will be to grow and sustain financing from domestic resources. How will the poorest countries reach this point? Donor funding in the interim and the growth of poor economies will determine the ability of countries to finance their health sectors. To illustrate the additional sums required, it is worth noting that the Report of the Commission for Africa (2005) recommended that donors spend around 40% of the Commission's proposed US $75 billion package for Africa to strengthen health systems and ensure a satisfactory response to HIV and AIDS by 2010. This call for additional spending is supported by analysis which shows that many countries will be able to work within a substantially increased spending envelope for health (Foster 2005). Yet donor aid remains volatile. In health, the shortcomings of traditional aid – from poor allocation to an absence of a results-focused, coordinated effort among donors – have clearly, if not tragically, been illustrated over the last decades (Radelet and Levine 2007).

Innovative financing mechanisms provide a way to overcome some of the current limitations of aid while mitigating the political risks that many donors associate with significantly scaling up finance to developing countries, for example, through transfers such as budget support. Global Funds and Partnerships such as GAVI have shown that innovative solutions to development challenges, including raising additional finance for development, can be generated by bringing together public and private stakeholders, including the civil society. GAVI provides the leverage so that both donor and developing country governments can employ new and innovative funding strategies – such as performance-based grants and co-financing (long-term subsidy agreements) for new vaccines – which characterize GAVI as an instrument for innovative financing. While it is too early to make any conclusive statement on the long-term market-shaping impact of GAVI, an independent study states that "emerging suppliers view the GAVI market as attractive and credibility-building, with the added economic advantage of alignment with domestic or middle-income markets. This is thanks to the significant size and growth of GAVI, as well as the price levels it has provided" (Boston Consulting Group 2005).

As a catalyst for further innovation in finance, GAVI has had a critical role in developing two further mechanisms for financing vaccine introduction and development: the International Finance Facility for Immunization (IFFIm) and Advance Market Commitments (AMCs). The IFFIm, launched in 2006, is a pilot of the larger International Finance Facility (IFF) that was originally proposed by the Government of the United Kingdom in 2005 to double global aid for development and to accelerate the availability of funds through the GAVI Alliance in 70 of the poorest countries around the world. The mechanism takes long term (20 years), legally binding commitments from donors (IFFIm 2008) and borrows against them for 10 years in the capital markets, producing upfront finance and thus stabilizing a portion of aid flow to developing countries. Because of the innovative "frontloading" funding program, an anticipated IFFIm investment of US $4 billion is expected to prevent 5 million child deaths between 2006 and 2015 and more than 5 million future adult deaths from hepatitis B-related liver disease. Advance Market Commitments (AMCs) provide legally binding promises, usually offered by governments or other financial entities, to guarantee a viable market if a vaccine is successfully developed. This ensures revenues will be generated from the newly developed vaccine that will match those of other comparable medicines. AMCs speed the development of new vaccines by enabling biotech and pharmaceutical companies to successfully invest in vaccine development (IAVI 2005).

Beyond the clear benefit of providing long-term, predictable finance to countries, allowing them to make longer-term budgeting and planning decisions, the predictable funding for immunization through IFFIm has the potential to leverage significant market benefits by allowing bulk purchasing of vaccines. The predictability and legally binding nature of the financial commitment provides strengthened negotiating power and the ability to negotiate longer-term arrangements with suppliers, generating lower prices and therefore more vaccines for the same envelope of funds.

A second market-shaping innovative mechanism – an "advance market commitment" (AMC) pilot for a pneumococcal vaccine – was launched in February 2006. An AMC is a financial commitment to subsidize the future purchase, up to a pre-agreed price, of a currently unavailable vaccine – if an appropriate vaccine is developed and providing the demand exists when the vaccine is finally produced. By guaranteeing that the funds will be available to purchase vaccines once they are developed and produced, the AMC mimics a secure vaccine market and takes away the risk that countries will not be able to afford a high-priority vaccine, addressing current market failure: vaccines that would prevent millions of deaths facing long delays before they are developed, tested, and produced for use in the poorest developing countries.

By establishing a valuable market, AMCs provide incentives for private investment in the development of vaccines against neglected diseases. Such a *"pull mechanism"* is not an alternative, but is highly complementary to other public and philanthropic interventions in the health sector and, more generally, in development aid. AMCs will be most effective when combined with *push* interventions because of the network effects of the increased number of scientific researchers working on the target diseases as well as the enhanced probability that scientific research swiftly translates into the production of effective and safe vaccines. Push interventions include public and philanthropic funding of research through academia, public–private partnerships, and other bodies. The private resources mobilized by successful AMCs would act in synergy with initiatives to expand immunization (e.g., GAVI and IFFIm) and strengthen health systems.

The success to date of raising funds through innovative financing instruments will continue to catalyze more thinking on both innovative means for raising and delivering development aid and how to better align these new instruments with more traditional aid streams. Debt relief is an emerging area in innovative financing for health which could usefully be applied to accelerate sustainable vaccine introduction. The two major broad initiatives for debt relief are the Heavily Indebted Poor Countries Initiative (HIPC) and Multilateral Debt Relief Initiative (MDRI) programs.

The *HIPC Initiative* was launched by the International Monetary Fund (IMF) and the World Bank in 1996 and aims to reduce debt for heavily indebted poor countries that face unsustainable debt burdens, that are pursuing reform programs, and that have developed a poverty reduction strategy paper. The HIPC estimates providing debt assistance in the amount of US $68 billion dollars in debt relief, funded by bilateral creditors and multilateral lenders, to a total of 32 countries (Table 23.2). An additional nine countries are eligible for the HIPC initiative and may wish to use the debt relief services in the future (International Monetary Fund 2007a). HIPC debt relief represents only a relatively small share of government spending (about 5% for Burkina Faso between 2001 and 2004). However, where social expenditures also represent but a small part of the government budget, HIPC debt relief can have a considerable impact on social sectors. Several HIPCs are using HIPC funds to scale up immunization financing. For example, in Benin, in 2004, 22% of the EPI program was funded by HIPC resources (International Monetary Fund 2008).

Table 23.2 Four generic categories of vaccines in relation to disease burden and reliability of markets

| Category of vaccine | Developing countries | | Industrialized countries | | |
	Disease burden	Current markets	Disease burden	Current markets	Examples
Global market vaccines	Large	Small	Large	Large	Hib conjugate; HepB; Rotavirus
Industrialized market vaccines	Small	Small	Large or moderate	Moderate	Lyme disease
Impeded vaccines	Large	Small	Large	Large	RSV
Developing market vaccines	Large	Small	Small	Small	Malaria; tuberculosis; typhoid; Shigella

Source: WHO (2000)

Taking the HIPC a step further, the Multilateral Debt Relief Initiative (MDRI) was launched by the group of eight industrialized countries (G8) in 2005 and will provide 100% cancellation of debt owed by HIPCs to the International Development Association (IDA), to the African Development Fund (AfDF), and to the IMF (International Monetary Fund, 2007b). This program enacts up-front, irrevocable debt cancellation for eligible countries (Table 23.2). The main objective of the MDRI is to enable HIPCs to mobilize funding for poverty reduction programs in order to reach the Millennium Development Goals. The intent is that additional resources made available through debt relief should be allocated to poverty alleviation programs. But as there is no formal obligation to allocate resources relieved by the MDRI to any specific sector, competition between departments for the use of these extra resources is likely. Potential impact of the MDRI on health system strengthening and on financing immunization programs could be significant. As annual amounts of debt service relief will be significant in many HIPCs, especially around 2020–2030, a small percentage of these resources could have a reasonable impact on the health sector and in particular on immunization financing.

The GAVI Alliance partners are currently exploring options for using debt relief – in the form of an International Development Association (IDA) buy-down – to specifically support countries' vaccine programs. In addition, a number of bilateral debt relief programs may also offer an opportunity for targeted debt relief. IDA buy-downs are currently being explored as new innovative financing mechanisms for vaccines. IDA is member of the World Bank Group. It provides long-term loans (also called concessional loans or credits) and grants to the poorest of the developing countries, particularly those that are severely constrained by conflict, epidemics, and debt. A buy-down refers to a third party paying off all or part of a specific IDA credit on behalf of the government upon successful achievement of pre-determined performance indicators. The World Bank began an IDA buy-down pilot in 2003, when it provided the governments of Nigeria and Pakistan with roughly $48 million in IDA credits for the purchase of vaccine to help achieve the global polio eradication objective. The Bill and Melinda Gates Foundation, Rotary

International, and the United Nations Foundation agreed to pay off the IDA credits upon successful achievement of the performance indicators, in this case receipt and distribution of vaccine and specified polio immunization coverage levels.

Innovative financing, while not a magic bullet, will nonetheless offer a range of new possibilities for countries to help reach the significant increases in finance required to meet the MDGs. Ultimately, the real test will be whether the donor community is successful in working together to ensure traditional aid is aligned to a mixed instrument approach. This has been done before. Bangladesh, one of the poorest countries in the world, has achieved the most radical improvements in reproductive health the world has ever seen. This has impacted significantly on women's and child mortality and morbidity, their social status and economic growth – despite poverty, poor governance, political upheaval, and an apparent lack of any potential for economic growth in the early years. The key was that for 20 years from the mid-1970s, through a mixture of aid instruments, donors and multilateral agencies provided substantial, predictable but coordinated financial and technical support for salaries, a radical expansion in the workforce (notably paramedics), associated infrastructure, and "expensive" reproductive commodities which the government delivered through state and civil society structures.

Sustainability

It has become clear that new technologies such as vaccines or antiretrovirals (ARVs) for HIV have the potential to deliver a generational leap in achieving the MDGs. The health gains made in Europe over 150 years could be achieved in Africa over a 10–20-year period (WHO/UNICEF 2005). Of the more than 10 million annual child deaths, an estimated 25% could be avoided through immunization with existing and newly developed vaccines such as pneumococcal and rotavirus vaccines. Procurement of essential health commodities is an area where this can be carried forward without risk to macroeconomic stability. Yet without basic health systems – essential for the sustainable availability of medical products – the poor will never access these benefits.

Despite evidence of the cost-effectiveness of vaccines in particular and the economic and social benefits of health in general, the track record of national and donor budget allocations to date is not good. GAVI-eligible countries have very modest health budgets, with government health spending across Africa, for instance, averaging $13–$21 per capita and with many countries below $10. Responding to the needs of poor countries by investing in the critical foundation for the delivery of basic health services requires a long-term view. While vertical approaches have been effective at raising the profile and funding levels for vaccines, countries must now be supported to move systematically to introducing the full range of vaccines in immunization programs as part of integrated maternal and child health services. With expensive new vaccines coming to market (for example, three doses each of pentavalent (DTP-HepB-Hib), rotavirus, and pneumococcal conjugate vaccines could amount to more than US $35 per child) it is clearly no longer appropriate to focus on financial sustainability of a single product in isolation from broader system sustainability.

Moving toward a truly sustainable planning framework will not be a simple endeavor, yet it represents an exciting opportunity for the GAVI Alliance partners. One challenge will be to gather the information on demand and future prices required by countries to inform longer-term planning and decision making. UNICEF's commitment and global procurement ability over the years has brought great benefits in terms of quality, security, and better prices for such long established vaccines as BCG, DPT, measles, and polio. But it has become clear that this procurement model is most effective in mature markets with overcapacity and competition, and notably capacity in countries located in emerging markets (e.g., India, Brazil, Indonesia, and Cuba).

New or combination vaccines such as DTP-HepB-Hib challenge the established means of procurement, where cost limits the ability of donors to deliver affordable products to the poorest parts of the world. It is only through competition that the prices of new vaccines will become affordable to the poorest countries. Clearly the key to success will be the ability to mobilize additional donor funds, but to use those funds in such a way that the vaccine market is shaped to promote competition and to bring prices within reach of the poorest countries.

Beginning in 2007, GAVI support shifted toward national co-financing (as opposed to GAVI providing vaccines free). This is based on the intent by the GAVI alliance partners to ensure that GAVI financial support is seen by all stakeholders as time limited and to ensure that countries move to a fuller ownership of their immunization program, including the introduction of new vaccines. Co-financing therefore aims at supporting and stimulating evidence-based priority-setting within the immunization program and within the health sector more generally. Financial commitments, however small, also generally require a higher level of government engagement. Through this approach, which will be evaluated in 2010, GAVI Alliance partners are working to help countries to be on a trajectory of eventual independence from GAVI support, acknowledging, however, that, for most of the GAVI-eligible countries this is likely to require a very long time

Over the next decade, the ability of developing countries to achieve sustainable introduction of new technologies will be largely dependent on how donor funds are provided, particularly whether there is a shift toward long-term, predictable aid and if innovative financing instruments are appropriately aligned and taken to scale. The other key determinant will be sustained political support for health and for vaccines by developing country governments. Guyana is an example of a country that has been highly successful in achieving high immunization coverage and is the first GAVI-supported country to fully finance the purchase of pentavalent vaccine from its national budget (United Nations 2007). Guyana's continuing success is in part due to a very strong political commitment at the highest levels to finance the national immunization program, including efforts to protect it from economic shocks and shifts in donor priorities. More broadly, there has been a remarkable growth in the health budget from US $6.5 per capita in 1991 to US $61 in 2006 (excluding overseas development assistance). This accounts for 10% of national expenditure, while the government's goal is to reach 15% (Ministry of Health, Guyana 2002; Editorial, PharmacoEconomics and Outcomes News, 2007).

The Ministry of Health China/GAVI Hepatitis B Vaccination Project is another example of where political commitment and clear financial partnership have brought remarkable results through a 5-year US $76 million project, co-funded equally by the Government of China and the GAVI Alliance. Hepatitis B virus (HBV) is endemic in China where over one-third of the world's HBV carriers reside. In 1999–2000, it was estimated that HBV was responsible for 280,000 deaths annually, over one-third of the global death toll estimated to be between 600,000 and 700,000. Since 2002, China has immunized 19.1 million children in the country's poorest and most remote western and central provinces against hepatitis B, reducing their risk of developing a deadly and common liver cancer. In the western provinces, the campaign, with technical guidance from WHO and UNICEF, has reached almost 80% of newborns with a birth dose of vaccine in 2005, up from 47% in 2002 (World Health Organization 2006, China – GAVI Project Annual Reports).

From an equity point of view, GAVI's condition of support to the Ministry of Health, China, was that vaccines be made available at no cost (removing the previous charge). This policy was subsequently adopted across China for all vaccines.

Equity

While the spread of HIV and AIDS has led to recent discourse on health as a global security issue, most arguments – and certainly those related to maternal and child health – have at their root the principle of equity and the belief that health is a basic human right. Equity in health has been defined (for measurement and operationalization) as "the absence of systematic disparities in health (or in the major social determinants of health) between groups with different levels of underlying social advantage/disadvantage – that is wealth, power or prestige" (Braveman and Gruskin 2003). The 2004 World Development Report, *Making Services Work for Poor People*, noted that "the concern for equity is either a social choice or based on the notion that health is a human right" (World Bank

2004). As an ethical or social justice issue, equity in health is therefore a critical element for consideration and measurement, particularly when looking at the trade-offs and choices made around financial sustainability issues discussed in the previous section.

Many of the disparities in health result from social determinants such as poverty, access to services, education, gender, and ethnicity. Harnessing the potential of new medical technologies, such as vaccines, to reach underserved groups will take concerted effort and in some cases, explicitly defined political choices. New vaccines against human papilloma virus (HPV) provide the opportunity for such a political choice: to ensure that all women, rather than just those in wealthy countries, are provided with a vaccine that will prevent most cervical cancer cases. HPV vaccines, as the first vaccines to focus primarily on women's health, provide the global health community an unprecedented opportunity to tackle a key neglected women's health issue – one which especially impacts on the poorest women.

Cervical cancer is not difficult to prevent; yet, it affects an estimated 490,000 women each year and leads to more than 270,000 deaths (Ferlay et al. 2006). It is largely a disease of poor women who have limited access to health services; about 85% of women dying from cervical cancer live in developing countries (Fig. 23.2) (Ferlay et al. 2006). The lack of effective cervical cancer prevention interventions – part of a regular medical checkup for women in wealthy countries – is a major factor in the high rates of cervical cancer among poor women. If current trends in women's health continue, there are projected to be over 1,000,000 new cases of HPV annually by the year 2050 (Boyle 2004).

Many challenges must be addressed before HPV vaccine can reach the millions of girls and young women who would benefit from it, especially those living in the developing world where the need is greatest. With the right combination of scientific, educational, and financing efforts, HPV vaccine could become available globally within a few years. Accelerating access to HPV vaccine could make cervical cancer – the second most common cancer among women worldwide – a rarity in just a few decades.

Fig. 23.2 Global burden of morality from cervical cancer, 2002. Source: Ferlay et al. (2006)

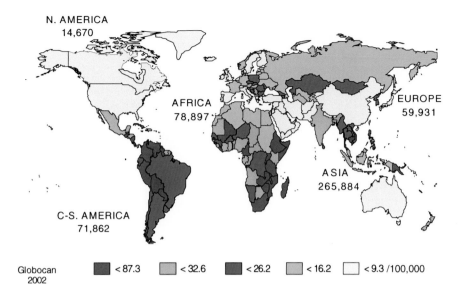

N. AMERICA
14,670

AFRICA
78,897

EUROPE
59,931

ASIA
265,884

C-S. AMERICA
71,862

Globocan 2002   ■ < 87.3   □ < 32.6   ■ < 26.2   ▨ < 16.2   □ < 9.3 /100,000

Another social determinant of health is where one lives. Within large developing countries, such as India, Nigeria, or China, there are significant inequities in the population's health. Disparities in access to, and utilization of, services within these countries are often a result of factors such as geography, social barriers, conflict, and weak governance. Of the 28 million children that missed out of immunization in 2005 more than 75% live in 10 countries (Fig. 23.1). India and Nigeria stand out as countries with the largest number of unimmunized children in the world.

Reaching MDG 4 will thus require a significant increase in investment in immunization – both domestic and external – in countries with large numbers of unimmunized children who account for more than half of all vaccine-preventable deaths among children less than 5 years of age. With some states or regions in some of these countries being equal or larger in population to many countries, a fresh state- or region-based approach will likely be required, with a focus on the poorest. For example, child and maternal mortality rates in the poorest eastern provinces of China equal or exceed those found in much of Africa (World Bank 2005). Despite economic growth, equity is worsening. National political commitment in such countries will be key. A program approach, tailored to country-specific challenges, will be required. Additional

long-term finance (domestic and global) will be critical to support that political commitment. New technology, including new and better vaccines, will be vital.

Vaccine Research Priorities

Which Vaccines for the Future?

Research and development for vaccines and other essential health commodities point to another disparity between North and South and constitute a market failure. Priorities in the global allocation of resources for vaccine research and development do not match the global burden of death and disease. Few resources are allocated to tackling diseases that disproportionately affect people in developing countries; new vaccines are therefore expensive and out of the reach of the poor. This discrepancy between need and reality is illustrated in Table 23.2, illustrating that normal market mechanisms do not work for the poor.

Among the vaccines currently under development, the three most needed today in terms of their potential public health impact are for AIDS, TB, and malaria. Jointly, these diseases account for over 5 million deaths per year or around 50%

of all infectious disease deaths. The total investment in vaccines against these diseases is far lower than their importance as dictated by disease burden and it will probably take at least 5–10 years before a vaccine against any of these diseases is available. In the past two decades, advances in biotechnology have resulted in the licensure of new vaccines such as Hib, acellular pertussis, HepB, and attenuated varicella. Most of the basic scientific breakthroughs have been generated in research institutions in the public sector whereas the cost for clinical development is borne by the pharmaceutical industry. This requires heavy investments that need to be recouped from profits. The markets needed to recoup these investments are in industrialized countries that can afford to buy.

The evolving disease burden in developing countries will bring new diseases into prominence while sometimes allowing old ones to resurface. This will influence priorities for vaccine research (Table 23.3). The Severe Acute Respiratory Syndrome (SARS) epidemic, the outbreak of avian influenza, and the emergence of bioterrorism threats such as Anthrax have led to new research avenues for vaccines against these infections. The threat of a reassorted influenza pandemic virus strain has highlighted the need for more resources and attention to the development and distribution of effective flu vaccines.

vaccine delivery strategies where non-professionals can administer vaccines. New administration routes such as oral, nasal, and transcutaneous are currently being explored. One option currently being explored through collaboration by WHO, PATH, and the Serum Institute of India is focusing on the development of a measles aerosol vaccine that could make a big difference in eliminating this disease by facilitating administration, during mass campaigns (Burger et al. 2008). The measles aerosol vaccine is useful in situations where the availability of trained medical personnel, who can safely administer injections, is limited. Immunogenically in studies, the aerosol vaccine was proven effective >80% of the time among infants <9 months of age and 86–100% among infants >9 months and school-aged children (Henao 2000). This vaccine continues to be tested in clinical trials in order to find the most appropriate and effective aerosol delivery method.

Another interesting option is the concept of using plant-derived or edible vaccines that involve encoding protective antigens from pathogens into transgenic plants (Mor et al. 1998). The plants are processed so that they can deliver a uniform dose of vaccines. Human clinical trials have been conducted with bananas and raw potatoes, which showed encouraging antibody responses (Sala et al. 2003). Plant-derived vaccines are formed when a gene

Table 23. 3 New vaccines required

Non-questionable vaccines	Close to or already licensed vaccines (but not totally suited to the developing country burden of disease)	Neglected vaccines	Others	New threats
HIV, TB, Malaria	Meningococcus, Streptococcus pneumonia, Rotavirus Human papilloma virus	Shigella, Dengue, Japanese encephalitis, Leishmaniasis, Schistosomiasis, Cholera	Respiratory Syncytial virus, Herpes simplex, Enterotoxigenic Escherichia coli	SARS, Anthrax, Smallpox, pandemic influenza

Source: WHO/UNICEF (2005)

New Vaccine Administration Routes

Alternative administration routes for vaccines would greatly contribute to improving immunization program safety and potentially reduce the quantity of contaminated waste which needs to be safely disposed. This could help avoid needle transmission of blood-borne pathogens and ease

is integrated with a plant nucleus or chloroplast genome. This transforms higher plants (e.g., tobacco, potato, tomato, and banana) into bioreactors for the production of subunit vaccines for oral or parental administration (Sala et al. 2003). The potential advantage of this technology could include thermostability, low investment needs, multivalency, and oral administration.

New Immunization Technologies

New technologies that strengthen vaccine delivery are under development. Priority is given to such technologies that will (a) expand access, (b) improve safety, and (c) cut the cost of immunization programs. They include the following five technologies:

(i) *"Sharps" processing*: The increased use of auto-disable (AD) syringes (syringes which lock themselves after a single injection) has greatly improved the safety of immunization programs by avoiding the reuse of contaminated syringes and reducing risks of transmission of blood-borne pathogens such as hepatitis B, hepatitis C, and HIV (Lloyd 2000). This success is, however, highlighting another problem which the health sector is facing, that of the handling of contaminated medical waste. In the case of immunization, this is mainly related to the disposal of used syringes and needles (these syringes represent between 5 and 10% of all injections given in the health sector but nevertheless the push to introduce AD syringes is increasing the pressure on immunization programs to tackle this challenge). Sharps are rarely disposed of at the point of use. Since sharps are transported to the point of destruction, the risk of infection from accidental exposure to sharps must be minimized. Four different technologies are being explored for this purpose: corrosive disinfectants, thermoprocessing, needle destruction, and plastic melting (Lloyd 2000). However, none of these options is currently sufficiently developed to be put into use in the field.

(ii) *Monodose pre-filled devices*: Vaccine wastage constitutes a considerable cost to immunization programs. Monodose presentations eliminate wastage and the risk of contamination. When the monodose is pre-filled into an injection device, it increases quality and safety at the point of use. UniJect® is one such device that has been tested with HepB and tetanus toxoid (TT) (Lloyd 2000). Village health workers can administer it. Currently, major obstacles reside in the cost of the device and the need for additional cold storage space when multidose presentation is exchanged for monodose, but ultimately, the objective would be to provide an increasing number of immunizations with monodose preparations that would not require increased cold chain capacity.

(iii) *Needle-free injections*: Needle-free injectors deliver vaccine at high velocity into the skin without penetration of a needle, thereby reducing the risk of transmission of blood-borne pathogens (WHO 2007c). Technologies are being developed for both mono- and multidose presentations. Multidose injectors available have not been found safe and new models are under development. There are several monodose models available; however, they are not feasible for large-scale programs because of regulatory obstacles and high cost (WHO 2000).

(iv) *Thermostable vaccine*: Vaccine distribution and storage without a cold chain would considerably simplify the delivery system, reduce cost, and allow for integrated supply mechanisms. Removal of vaccines from the cold chain should be the highest priority for technology research. Sugar glass drying is one such technology that has shown great promise (Lloyd 2000). It can be used to produce multivalent vaccines that are completely heat stable, except under extreme climatic conditions. The high cost of regulation/licensing and the uncertainty about market prospects in industrialized countries have so far impeded the development and use of this technology.

Vaccine Management

Vaccines are delicate products that are easily destroyed if handled incorrectly. Vaccine management spans a spectrum of aspects involving the use and disposal of vaccines, from the manufacturers to the end-users, for which plans must be in place and regularly updated to ensure an effective and efficient service delivery including (i) inventory and forecasting; (ii) stock control; (iii) in-country distribution; (iv) storing and handling; (v) equipment replacement; (vi) procedures for the use of vaccine; (vii) monitoring of vaccine storage; (viii) transport management; and (ix) operational management. All of these areas would benefit significantly from research efforts to find alternative and innovative approaches. For instance, the heavy reliance on the cold chain remains a major economic and logistical burden on programs. The possibility of taking greater advantage of the real thermostability of vaccines and the increasing use of the Vaccine Vial Monitor by taking vaccines "out of the cold chain" is a field which has only begun but could potentially revolutionize immunization delivery (Table 23.4). Vaccine Vial Monitors are heat-sensitive circular labels, no wider than a centimeter, that change color as vaccines are exposed to heat. They are time–temperature indicators used to (i) ensure that the vaccines have not been damaged by excessive exposure to heat, (ii) identify weaknesses in the cold chain, and (iii) take vaccines beyond the cold chain to reach out to children who have no access to fixed health facilities. Health workers can use the Vaccine Vial Monitor color to tell if the vaccine has been overexposed to heat and whether or not it is safe for immunization. This indicator cuts down on the uncertainty of vaccine safety due to potential temperature changes during transport along the cold chain. Therefore, the vaccine vial monitor reduces waste.

Conclusion

Immunization remains one of the most cost-effective of all public health interventions. Maternal and child health-related MDGs will be difficult to meet without significantly scaling up the coverage of existing vaccines and successfully introducing new pipeline products – ensuring that research and development priorities are aligned with the diseases for which preventative technologies are needed most. Financing this effort, however, poses a considerable challenge. A serious commitment to closing the North/South divide and meeting MDGs will require a joint approach that involves increased investment by developing country governments and better, more stable aid flows from donors. Increased investment, particularly in the social sector, will be critical to finance costs such as system building that require large amounts of sustained finance. In-kind investments in commodities can be scaled up rapidly without major concerns around absorptive capacity or macroeconomic stability. Long-term, predictable aid flows are also needed to reduce volatility and provide increased certainty over future budget flows to enable better planning in countries.

As a global community, we must start approaching our work from a perspective that evaluates who is taking on the burden of risk – it clearly should not be the poorest countries. Risk analysis is a common tool in the private sector – companies only take decisions based on the probable level of risk it implies for them. Yet the donor community consistently places the poorest countries in a position where it is very difficult for them to make choices of how or whether to radically scale up access to basic services. The donor community, including the GAVI Alliance and the international financial institutions, needs to develop strategies to reduce financial and political risks. This means adjusting processes and requirements to support the long-term integrated plans of developing countries. The financial risks of development strategies must be more equitably shared between donors and national governments. Development will be led by developing countries when they are enabled to plan ahead;

Table 23. 4 New vaccines required

Commodity	Trends/developments	Implication for logistics systems
Vaccines	■ GAVI is expanding access to new vaccines and financing vaccine development ■ New vaccine delivery technology may reduce reliance on cold chain ■ Increased focus on safe injection, new injection equipment, and better disposal of sharps ■ Shift from donations to purchases	■ Newer vaccines often require more storage space and additional training for staff ■ Reduced dependence on cold chain may make it more feasible to integrate vaccine logistics with other commodities ■ New technology may also reduce vaccine waste ■ More staff, training, and systems are needed to manage procurement

when donors act on their recognition of the importance of predictable and long-term aid flows to meet the MDGs. Development will only happen when poor and vulnerable people are ensured equitable access to basic services. Accelerating the sustainable introduction of new and underused vaccines is part of realizing this ambition.

Key Terms

Acellular pertussis	Haemophilus influenza vaccine (Hib)	Rotavirus vaccine
Advance market commitment (AMC)	Hepatitis B vaccine (HBV)	Severe Acute Respiratory Syndrome (SARS)
Attenuated varicella	Human papilloma virus (HPV) vaccine	Smallpox
Auto-disable (AD) syringes	Immunization coverage	Tetanus toxoid (TT)
Bacille Calmette-Guerin (BCG)	Immunization delivery systems	Vaccine distribution
Breastfeeding	Immunization programs	Vaccine management
Cervical cancer	Immunization rates	Vaccine market
Child Survival Revolution	Influenza	Vaccine production
Cold chain	International Finance Facility for Immunization (IFFIm)	Vaccine quality
Cold chain capacity	Measles aerosol vaccine	Vaccine safety
Diphtheria, pertussis, tetanus vaccine (DPT)	Oral rehydration therapy (ORT)	Vaccine vial monitor
Expanded Program on Immunization (EPI)	Pneumococcal conjugate vaccines	Vaccines
Global Alliance for Vaccines and Immunization (GAVI)	Polio	Variolation
Global immunization targets	Population mobility	Vertical programs
Growth monitoring		Yellow fever

Questions for Discussion

1. What factors account for the disparity in immunization coverage between developed and less developed countries?
2. What is the GAVI Alliance? How does its mission compare with those of Global Immunization Vision Strategy (GIVS)?
3. What major barriers confront the GAVI Alliance and GIVS in their efforts to ensure equity in access to new and underused vaccines in developed and less developed countries?
4. In a narrative of about 1,000 words, describe the meaning and mission of the following initiatives:

   a. International Finance Facility for Immunization (IFFIm).

   b. Advance Market Commitments (AMCs).
5. How successful are IFFMs and AMCs in accomplishing their mission?
6. Outline and discuss potentially viable strategies for ensuring sustainability in procurement, access, and uptake of vaccines in less developed countries. What are the major barriers?
7. What should be the priorities for future vaccine research and development globally? Provide justification for your position.

References

Andre F (2003) Vaccinology: past achievements, present roadblocks, and future promises. Vaccine, 21, 7–8; 593–595

Boston Consulting Group (2005) Global vaccine supply: the changing role of suppliers. Report to the External Stakeholder Advisory Board Meeting. http://www.gavialliance. org/resources/Global_Vaccine_Supply_Sept05.pdf, cited 2 August 2008

Boyle P (2004) Cervical cancer prevention: current situation. EUROGIN International Expert Meeting on HPV Infection and Cervical Cancer Prevention. Nice, France

Braveman P and Gruskin S (2003) Defining equity in health. Journal of Epidemiology and Community Health, 57(4), 254–258

Burger JL, Cape SP, Braun CS et al. (2008) Stabilizing formulations for inhalable powders of live-attenuated measles virus vaccine.Journal of Aerosol Medicine, 21, 1–10

Editorial (2007) Developing countries are providing cofinance for life-saving vaccines. PharmacoEconomics and Outcomes News, 531, 11

Ferlay J, Bray F, Pisani P et al. (2006) GLOBOCAN: Cancer incidence, mortality and prevalence worldwide. IARC CancerBase, 5:2. Lyon, France: IARC Press

Foster M (2005). Fiscal space and sustainability: towards a solution for the health sector. High Level Forum on Health MDGs. Paris, France. http://www.hlfhealthmdgs. org/Documents/WHOConferenceReportENG.pdf Cited 2 August 2008

GAVI Alliance (2008a) Innovative partnership. http://www. gavialliance.org/about/in_partnership/index.php, cited 2 August 2008

GAVI Alliance (2008b) Strategy. http://www.gavialliance. org/vision/strategy/index.php, cited 2 August 2008

Hardon A, Blume S (2005) Shifts in global immunization goals (1984–2004): Unfinished agendas and mixed results. Social Science and Medicine, 60, 345

Henao AM (2000) An overview of aerosol immunization, meeting of the WHO steering committee on new delivery systems. http://www.who.int/vaccine_research/diseases/measles/en/aerosol.pdf, cited 2 August 2008

International Fund for Agricultural Development (IFAD) (2007) International conference on financing for development – statement by Lennart Båge, President of IFAD. http://www.ifad.org/events/op/2002/ffd.htm, cited 2 August 2008

International Finance Facility for Immunization Company (IFFIm) (2008) Financial background. http://www.iff-immunisation.org/02_financial_background.html, cited 2 August 2008

International AIDS Vaccine Initiative (2005) Advance market commitments: helping to accelerate AIDS vaccine development. http://www.iavi.org/viewfile.cfm?fid = 35155, cited 2 August 2008

International Monetary Fund (2007a) Debt relief under heavily indebted poor countries (HIPC) initiative. http://www.internationalmonetaryfund.org/external/np/exr/facts/hipc.htm, cited 2 August 2008

International Monetary Fund (2007b) The multilateral debt relief initiative (MDRI). http://www.imf.org/external/np/exr/facts/mdri.htm, cited 2 August 2008

International Monetary Fund (2008) Benin: third review under the three-year arrangement under the poverty reduction growth facility, request for waiver of nonobservance of a performance criterion, and request for extension of the arrangement; IMF Country Report 08/19. http://www.imf.org/external/pubs/ft/scr/2008/cr0819.pdf, cited 2 August 2008

Lloyd J (2000) Technologies for vaccine delivery in the 21st century. Geneva: World Health Organization. http://whqlibdoc.who.int/hq/2000/WHO_V&B_00.35.pdf, cited 2 August 2008

Lu C, Michaud CM, Gakidou E et al. (2006) Effect of the global alliance for vaccines and immunization on diphtheria, tetanus, and pertussis vaccine coverage: an independent assessment. Lancet, 68(9541), 1088–1095

Ministry of Health, Guyana (2002) Guyana financial immunization sustainability plan 2002. Brickdam, Georgetown: Ministry of health/Ministry of Finance. http://www.who.int/immunization_financing/countries/guy/en/guyana_fsp.pdf, cited 2 August 2008

Mor TS, Gomez-Lim MA, Palmer KE (1998) Perspective: edible vaccines – a concept coming of age. Trends in Microbiology, 6(11), 449–453

Plotkin S (2005) Why certain vaccines have been delayed or not developed at all. Health Affairs, 24(3), 631.

Radelet S, Levine R (2007) Can we build a better mousetrap? Three new institutions designed to improve aid effectiveness. In Bill Easterly (ed.) Reinventing Foreign Aid. Cambridge, MA: MIT Press

Sala F, Rigano MM, Barbante A et al. (2003). Vaccine antigen production in transgenic plants: strategies, gene constructs, and perspectives. Vaccines, 21(7–8), 803–808

United States National Library of Medicine (2002) Smallpox a great and terrible scourge. http://www.nlm.nih.gov/exhibition/smallpox/sp_variolation.html, cited 2 August 2008

United Nations Children's Fund (UNICEF) (1996) The state of the world's children 1996: The 1980s: Campaign for child survival. http://www.unicef.org/sowc96/1980s.htm, cited 2 August 2008

United Nations Development Programme (2003) Human Development Report: Millennium Development Goals: A Compact among Nations to End Human Poverty. New York: Oxford University Press

United Nations (2006) The millennium development goals report. http://mdgs.un.org/unsd/mdg/Resources/Static/Products/Progress2006/MDGReport2006.pdf, cited 2 August 2008

United Nations (2007) Developing countries join GAVI Alliance and WHO to "co-finance" vaccines for poor children. http://www.maximsnews.com/107mnunmay16gavialliancevaccinespoorestnationscommitfunds.htm, cited 2 August 2008

World Bank (2004) The 2004 World Development Report – Making Services Work for Poor People. New York: World Bank. http://www-wds.worldbank.org/external/default/WDSContentServer/IW3P/IB/2003/10/07/000090341_20031007150121/Rendered/PDF/268950PAPER0WDR02004.pdf, cited 27 August 2008

World Bank (2005) China's progress toward the health MDGs. http://siteresources.worldbank.org/INTEAPREGTOPHEANUT/Resources/502734-1129734318233/BN2-MDG-final.pdf, cited 2 August 2008

World Health Organization (WHO) (2000) Proceedings of the first global vaccine research forum. Montreux, Canada, June 7–9. http://www.who.int/vaccine_research/documents/en/GVRF2000.pdf, cited 2 August 2008

World Health Organization (WHO) (2003) Traditional medicine. The Fifty-sixth World Health Assembly (WHA56.31) Geneva: World Health Organization. http://www.who.int/gb/ebwha/pdf_files/WHA56/ea56r31.pdf, cited 2 August 2008

World Health Organization (WHO) (2006) China immunises millions of children against Hepatitis B in historic collaboration between government and GAVI Alliance. http://www.prnewswire.com/cgi-bin/stories.pl?ACCT = 104&STORY = /www/story/07-25-2006/0004402683& EDATE = , cited 2 August 2008

World Health Organization (WHO)/United Nations Children's Fund (UNICEF) (2005) Global immunization strategy (2006–2015). Geneva, Switzerland: WHO. http://www.who.int/immunization/givs/Q_and_A_EN.pdf, cited 2 August 2008

World Health Organization (WHO) (2007a) WHO IVB Human Papillomavirus & HPV Vaccines: Technical information for policy-makers and health professionals

World Health Organization (WHO) (2007b) WHO Report on GAVI Progress 2000–2006 & Projected Achievements 2007–2010.

World Health Organization (WHO) (2007c) Immunization safety. http://www.who.int/immunization_safety/en/, cited 2 August 2008

Chapter 24
Adolescent Health

Elizabeth Lule and James Rosen

Learning Objectives After reading this chapter and answering the discussion questions that follow, you should be able to

- Define adolescence and discuss the rationale for interest in health issues of concern to adolescents by governments and international health agencies.
- Analyze major health problems of adolescents and identify global and regional disparities in specific conditions that contribute to the burden of disease among adolescents.
- Appraise the effectiveness of programs to address adolescent health problems.
- Discuss gaps in adolescent health policy and programs and identify future priorities.

Introduction

Adolescence is as much a stage of development as it is a specific age range. The transitions that mark this period of life do not conform to a standard timetable. Nonetheless, this chapter will use the standard World Health Organization (1998) definition of adolescents as those people between the ages of 10 and 19. Individual countries and different organizations may use somewhat different age categories to define adolescence. This chapter will, as often as possible, use data for the 10–19 age group, although not all data conform to this specific age range.

The current world population of adolescents aged 10–19 is 1.2 billion, the largest ever (UNFPA 2003; United Nations 2006a). This total is projected to peak in the year 2030 at about 1.3 billion (UNFPA 2003; United Nations 2006a), with about 90% living in developing countries. However, as Fig. 24.1 shows, trends in the growth of this age group vary markedly by region. The population of adolescents has already peaked in the developed world and in East and Southeast Asia, while the adolescent population will not peak until 2015 in Latin American and the Caribbean and until 2030 and 2035 in South Central Asia and South Central Asia, respectively. In sub-Saharan Africa, the population of adolescents will still be growing in 2050 (UNFPA 2003; United Nations 2006a).

Improving adolescent health is a challenge everywhere. However, this chapter will focus on the developing world since that is where the vast majority of adolescents live and where access to health care is limited. Because of the relative paucity of rigorous intervention research from the developing world, this chapter will also draw on evidence from more rigorously evaluated and researched programs on adolescent health in the developed world.

The Importance of Adolescent Health

Recent reviews (World Bank 2006a; National Research Council and Institute of Medicine 2005; Lule et al. 2006; Birdsall et al. 2001) have highlighted several reasons why countries have an interest in healthy adolescents, including the following:

E. Lule (✉)
AIDS Campaign Team for Africa (ACTafrica) The World Bank, 1818 H Street NW, Washington DC 20433, USA

J.E. Ehiri (ed.), *Maternal and Child Health*, DOI 10.1007/b106524_24,
© Springer Science+Business Media, LLC 2009

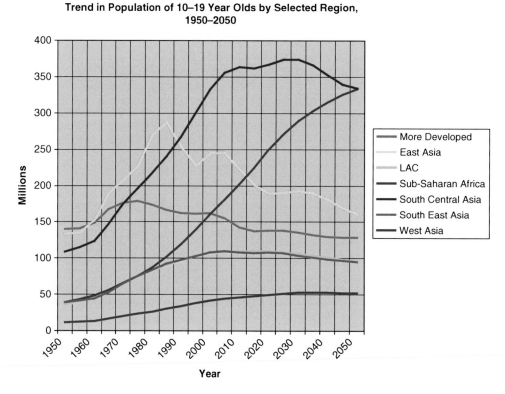

Fig. 24.1 Trend in Population of 10–19-year-olds by selected region, 1950–2050. Source: United Nations (2006b)

The size of the adolescent cohort: As noted, the current generation of adolescents is the largest ever. They constitute one of every five persons. Adolescents are entitled to the universal human rights that other age groups enjoy and under which those groups are protected through various international agreements.

Making the most of the demographic dividend: The demographic transition completed or underway in most countries increases the proportion of productive individuals relative to dependents, which creates a window of opportunity conducive to economic growth. Countries that astutely exploit this demographic dividend through investments in education, skills, and health of the working-age population while simultaneously creating a favorable macroeconomic policy climate can experience economic growth.

Prevention is cheaper than cure: The disease burden in adolescence is largely preventable and acting now to encourage healthy adolescent behaviors will avoid future loss from death and illness. Countries can save money by investing in preventive behaviors.

Adolescent health affects economic prosperity: By reducing HIV infection in young people, countries can lessen the devastating social and economic impact of HIV/AIDS. Encouraging young people to postpone marriage and childbearing can foster a reduction in family size and a slowing of population growth, which, when combined with investments in health and education, can contribute to higher economic growth and incomes.

Adolescent health investments can reduce poverty: Death and illness exacerbates poverty by disrupting and cutting short school opportunities, by weakening or killing young people in the prime of their working lives, or by placing heavy financial and social burdens on families and society. Keeping adolescents healthy can help individuals and families out of poverty.

Improving adolescent health will help accelerate achievement of the MDGs: Better adolescent health will directly or indirectly contribute to achieving most of the eight Millennium Development Goals (MDGs) (Table 24.1).

Table 24.1 The path to achieving the MDGs runs through adolescence

Millennium Development Goals	Indicator	Adolescent-focused activities to achieve the goal
Goal 1: *Eradicate extreme poverty and hunger*	Proportion living on less than $1 a day	Preventing teen pregnancy
	Proportion of people who suffer from hunger	Reducing HIV infection in youth
Goal 2: *Achieve universal primary education*	Net enrolment ratio in primary education	Gender equity in school enrollment.
	Proportion of pupils starting grade 1 who reach last grade of primary	Prevention of teen pregnancy
	Literacy rate of 15–24 year-olds, women and men	Infrastructure development and maintenance to ensure quality education.
Goal 3: *Promote gender equality and empower women*	Ratio of girls to boys in primary, secondary, and tertiary education	Educating girls
	Among 15–24-year-olds, ratio of literate females to literate males	Changing social norms to promote gender equity
Goal 4: *Reduce child mortality*	Infant death rate	Preventing high-risk pregnancies to young mothers and reducing adolescent malnutrition
Goal 5: *Improve maternal health*	Maternal mortality ratio (to the extent that young mothers are at higher risk of pregnancy-related death and disability)	Improving maternal care for pregnant adolescents
	Proportion of births attended by skilled health personnel	Expanding post-abortion care for youth
	Contraceptive prevalence rate	Expanding youth access to information and services for pregnancy prevention
Goal 6: *Combat HIV/AIDS, malaria, and other diseases*	HIV prevalence among 15–24-year-old pregnant women	Expanding youth-specific HIV prevention and care efforts
	Prevalence and death rates associated with tuberculosis and malaria	Educating youth how to identify the symptoms of TB and get care for themselves, friends, and family members
		Preventive malaria treatment for pregnant adolescents
Goal 7: *Ensure environmental sustainability*	Proportion of population with sustainable access to an improved water source	Investing in the human capital of young people, leading to lower fertility and less pressure on natural resources
Goal 8, target 16: *Develop and implement strategies for decent and productive work for youth*	Unemployment rate of 15–24-year-olds	Carrying out policies and programs to expand youth employment

Source: Rosen (2004)

Common Influences on Adolescent Health

Researchers have identified many factors that either increase (risk factor) or decrease (protective factor) the chances that an adolescent will have unhealthy behaviors. These factors operate at the individual, family, institutional, and community level and include feelings of self-efficacy, attitudes and behaviors of friends, connectedness with parents and other influential adults, and involvement in the community. A recent exhaustive review of quantitative studies conducted in developing countries (Blum and Mmari 2005) found

several common factors that can protect youth from risky sex. These include connectedness to parents and parental expectations about school, marriage, and sexuality; factors in the school environment such as connectedness, family life education, and academic performance; expectations and attitudes of sexual partners and peers; and feelings of self-efficacy and self-control.

One study in Zambia (Magnani et al. 2002) which sought to identify risk and protective factors influencing exposure of Zambian youth to HIV revealed that level of education and current school attendance were protective with regard to initiation of sexual intercourse. Living with both birth parents and having knowledge about AIDS was protective against ever having had sex. However, knowledge about using condoms was a risk. Knowing peers that had had sex was associated with a higher probability of ever having had sex among youth (males and females). Youth who engaged in higher risk activities (drinking alcohol and using drugs) were also more likely to have had sex. Communication with the first close friend about reproductive health issues was associated with higher levels of sexual activity, likely reflecting the influences of peers.

Studies in developed countries also reveal the importance of multiple influences on sexual behavior. For example, Kirby et al. (2005) analyzed research on adolescent sexual and reproductive health in the United States and identified over 400 factors that affect one or more sexual behaviors (the initiation of sex, frequency of sex, number of sexual partners, use of condoms, and use of other contraceptives) or

consequences of those behaviors (pregnancy, childbearing, or a sexually transmitted infection). Those factors most amenable to change by programs that directly address sexual and reproductive health issues involve sexual beliefs, values and attitudes, skills and behaviors of teens regarding having sex, using condoms and other methods of contraception, and avoiding pregnancy and HIV and other STIs (Table 24.2). Evidence from qualitative studies on the factors influencing young people's sexual behavior further underlines the importance of social expectations and the influence of sexual partners (Marston and King 2006).

Studies focusing on such other domains of adolescent health as mental health have equally demonstrated the role of multiple factors (Patel et al. 2007), including psychological factors (e.g., sexual physical, emotional abuse, and neglect), family factors (e.g., family conflict and poor family discipline), school factors (failure of schools to prove appropriate

Table 24.2 Risk and protective factors most amenable to change directly by pregnancy and STD prevention agencies, United States

	Risk factor	Protective factor
Family		Greater parent/child communication about sex and condoms or contraception especially before youth initiate sex
Peer	Peers' pro-childbearing attitudes or behavior	Positive peer norms or support for condom or contraceptive use
	Permissive values about sex	Peer use of condoms
	Sexually active peers	
Individual	More permissive attitudes toward premarital sex	Greater feelings of guilt about possibly having sex
	Perceiving more personal and social benefits (than costs) of having sex	Taking a virginity pledge
	Greater frequency of sex	Greater perceived male responsibility for pregnancy prevention
	Having a new sexual relationship	Stronger beliefs that condoms do not reduce sexual pleasure
	Greater number of sexual partners	Greater value of partner appreciation of condom use
	Previous pregnancy or impregnation	More positive attitudes toward condoms and other forms of contraception
	History of recent STD	More perceived benefits and/or fewer costs and barriers to using condoms
		Greater self-efficacy to demand condom use
		Greater self-efficacy to use condoms or other forms of contraception
		Greater motivation to use condoms or other forms of contraception
		Greater intention to use condoms
		Greater perceived negative consequences of pregnancy
		Greater motivation to avoid pregnancy, HIV, and other STDs
		Older age of first voluntary sex
		Discussing sexual risks with partner
		Discussing pregnancy and STD prevention with partner
		Previous effective use of condoms or contraception

Source: Kirby et al. (2005)

environment to support attendance), and community factors (community disorganization) (Table 24.3). These findings demonstrate the role of multiple individual, community, and sociocultural factors in adolescent health.

In addition to sharing many root causes, studies have shown that many of the health problems of adolescents are inter-related. Mental illness is associated with substance abuse, violence, and sexual and reproductive health problems (Patel et al. 2007). Problem drinking is a factor in many fatal traffic crashes and in suicide (WHO 2007d). Gender-based violence is associated with poor reproductive health outcomes and suicide (WHO, 2005a). Poor nutrition leads to problems in pregnancy and childbirth (Behrman et al. 2004).

Major Adolescent Health Problems

Overall Burden of Death and Disability

Tables 24.4 and 24.5 summarize the main causes of death and disease burden in adolescents aged 10–19. From the immediate death and disability standpoint, adolescence is easily the healthiest time of life (Fig. 24.2).

Death and disability rates for the 10–19 age group are lower than for any other cohort. Moreover, many signs point to the fact that young people as a group (at least in developing countries) have gotten healthier over time (National Research Council and Institute of Medicine 2005). Yet, many behaviors or conditions that begin or occur

Table 24.3 Selected risk and protective factors for mental health of children and adolescents

	Risk factors	Protective factors
Biological		
	Exposure to toxins (e.g., tobacco, alcohol) in pregnancy	Age-appropriate physical development
	Genetic tendency to psychiatric disorder	
	Head trauma	Good physical health
	Hypoxia at birth and other birth complications	Good intellectual functioning
	HIV infection	
	Malnutrition	
	Substance abuse	
	Other illnesses	
Psychological		
	Learning disorders	Ability to learn from experiences
	Maladaptive personality traits	Good self-esteem
	Sexual, physical, emotional abuse and neglect	High level of problem-solving ability
	Difficult temperament	Social skills
Social		
Family	Inconsistent care-giving	Family attachment
	Family conflict	Opportunities for positive involvement in family
	Poor family discipline	Rewards for involvement in family
	Poor family management	
	Death of a family member	
School	Academic failure	Opportunities for involvement in school life
	Failure of schools to provide appropriate environment to support attendance and learning inadequate or inappropriate provision of education	Positive reinforcement from academic achievement
	Bullying	Identity with school or need for educational attainment
Community	Transitions (e.g., urbanization)	Connectedness to community
	Community disorganization	Opportunities for leisure
	Discrimination and marginalization Exposure to violence	Positive cultural experiences
		Positive role models
		Rewards for community involvement
		Connection with community organizations

Source: Patel et al. (2007)

Table 24.4 Conditions causing greater than 1% of adolescent deaths

Condition	Percent of total
Lower respiratory infections	11.2
Road traffic accidents	10.0
Self-inflicted injuries	6.0
Maternal conditions	4.8
Violence	4.8
Tuberculosis	4.0
HIV/AIDS	3.9
Falls	1.4
Protein–energy malnutrition	1.3
Nephritis and nephrosis	1.1
Ischemic heart disease	1.0
Cerebrovascular disease	1.0
Cirrhosis of the liver	1.0

Source: Mathers (2009)

Table 24.5 Conditions causing greater than 1% of adolescent DALYS

Condition	Percent of total
Mental Illness*	18.59
Maternal conditions	6.69
Road traffic accidents	6.07
Lower respiratory infections	5.43
Asthma	3.53
Violence	3.42
Self-inflicted injuries	3.18
Alcohol use disorders	2.94
Falls	2.90
Tuberculosis	2.10
HIV/AIDS	1.87

* Includes unipolar depressive disorders, schizophrenia, and bipolar disorder.
Source: Mathers (2009)

during adolescence – for example, tobacco and alcohol use, poor eating habits, sexual abuse, and risky sexual behaviors – have long-term health consequences whose toll in death and illness is not counted during the adolescent years.

In fact, as Figs. 24.3 and 24.4 show, 28% of the disease burden and over 50% of premature deaths among persons 15 and over are linked to behaviors or conditions that begin or occurred during adolescence.

Adolescence-rooted risk factors are currently a greater problem in wealthier countries, largely because of the relatively greater impact of smoking and diet-related risks in those countries. Nonetheless, the impact of these risks is projected to expand rapidly in many poorer countries as their epidemiologic profiles converge with those of the developed countries (Mathers and Loncar 2006). Through this lens, adolescent health problems comprise problems and risk behaviors that affect their immediate health and well-being and those that have longer-term health impacts. The following sections analyze some of the main contributors to adolescent health problems.

Mental Disorders

Mental disorders, including unipolar depressive disorders, schizophrenia, bipolar disorder, self-

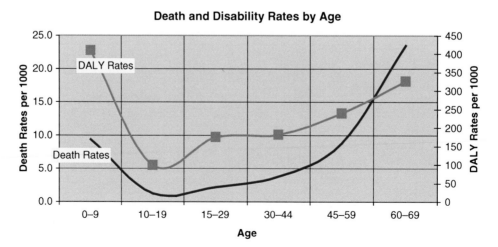

Fig. 24.2 Rates of death and disease burden by age. Source: WHO (2007a)

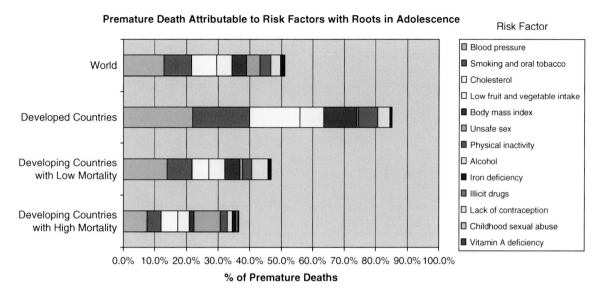

Fig. 24.3 Premature deaths attributable to risk factors with roots in adolescents. Source: WHO (2007a)

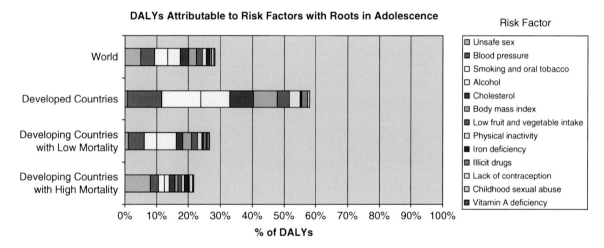

Fig. 24.4 DALYS attributable to risk factors with roots in adolescence. Source: WHO (2007a)

inflicted injuries, and alcohol use disorder, account for about one-fourth of the disease burden among 10–19-year-olds (Table 24.5) and affect between 20 and 25% of young people in any given year (Patel et al. 2007). Suicide is the third leading cause of death among young people worldwide, accounting for 6% of deaths (Table 24.4). No clear trend has emerged in the prevalence of mental disorders in adolescence (Patel et al. 2007). Many of the mental health problems of the young are both preventable and treatable. Like other health problems that begin during

adolescence, lack of attention to mental health during the adolescent years can result in lifelong disability and consequences that continue far into adulthood. For this reason, prevention and treatment are especially critical during the adolescent years.

Intentional and Unintentional Injuries

Both intentional and unintentional injuries are major causes of death and disease burden in adolescents. Detailed discussion about injuries among MCH populations is presented in Chapter 18. Intentional violence accounts for 4.8% of all deaths and 3.4% of DALYs in adolescents worldwide. A major contributor to violence is homicide. Homicide as a proportion of all deaths varies widely by region, among males, ranging between 2.4% in Southeast Asia and 33.2% in the Americas. The same proportion among females aged 15–29 is significantly lower (Fig. 24.5). Homicide rates in both males and females have trended upward in recent years (WHO 2002). Non-fatal youth violence results in between 20 and 40 victims in need of hospital care for every youth who dies from homicide (WHO 2002).

Unintentional injuries caused by road crashes are the second leading cause of death among adolescents, accounting for 10% of all deaths, and the third leading cause of disability-adjusted life year (DALYs), accounting for 6% of DALYs (Tables 24.4 and 24.5). Adolescent males are more than twice as likely as females aged 10–19 to die from road traffic injuries (WHO 2007d). Relative to adults, adolescents are particularly vulnerable to road traffic injuries because of their emotional and social immaturity, their small size (for younger adolescents), their lack of driving experience, their greater propensity to mix driving with alcohol and drug use, their tendency toward greater risk-taking, their relatively infrequent use of safety devices such as crash helmets and seat belts, and their tendency to

work in often-hazardous public transport jobs (WHO 2007d).

Diet, Nutrition, and Exercise

Nutritional deficiencies in adolescent girls contribute to problems in pregnancy and childbirth and increase the disease burden related to the maternal conditions. They account for 5% of all deaths in adolescents (Delisle et al. 2001). Malnutrition may also increase risk of HIV transmission, including from mothers to their infants, compromise antiretroviral therapy, and hasten the onset of full-blown AIDS (World Bank 2006a). Many adolescents in developing countries suffer from chronic undernutrition which delays growth and physical maturation and increases pregnancy-related health problems (Behrman et al. 2004). Iron deficiency leading to anemia is the most common micronutrient deficiency in adolescence (World Bank 2003). Surveys show that almost 40% of adolescent girls are anemic (Table 24.6). Poor dietary and exercise habits that begun in childhood and adolescence are at the root of many chronic diseases such as cardiovascular disease and diabetes that are major killers among adults in the developed world, and now, of increasing importance in developing countries (Adeyi et al. 2007). High cholesterol, low fruit and vegetable intake, overweight, and physical inactivity account for one in five deaths worldwide (Fig. 24.3). Young people are increasingly overweight and obese (National Research Council

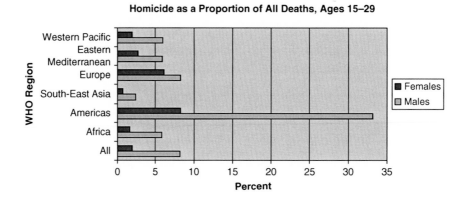

Fig. 24.5 Homicide as a proportion of all deaths in the 15–29 age group. Source: WHO (2002)

Table 24.6 Anemia status of adolescent girls 15–19, mid-1990s–2005

Country (year of survey)	Mild anemia(%)	Moderate anemia(%)	Severe anemia(%)	Any anemia(%)
Sub-Saharan Africa				
Benin (2001)	42.1	21.6	1.5	65.2
Burkina Faso (2003)	37.6	13	1.3	51.9
Cameroon (2004)	34.7	10.2	0.7	45.6
Congo (Brazzaville) (2005)	42.3	13.6	0.5	56.5
Ethiopia (2005)	16.6	7.4	0.9	24.8
Ghana (2003)	37.3	7.9	0.7	45.9
Guinea (2005)	29.4	17.8	3.7	50.9
Lesotho (2004)	20.7	8.4	0.4	29.5
Madagascar (2003/2004)	35.6	8.3	4	47.9
Malawi (2004)	28.9	10.5	2.7	42.2
Mali (2001)	39.5	20.4	2.3	62.2
Rwanda (2005)	18	6.8	4.1	29
Senegal (2005)	41.5	15.9	3.1	60.5
Tanzania (2004)	33.6	14.6	0.8	49
Uganda (2000/01)	17.6	6.3	0.6	24.5
North Africa/West Asia/Europe				
Armenia (2000)	8	0.9	0	8.9
Armenia (2005)	17.3	3.3	0.7	21.4
Egypt (2000)	24.5	5.2	0	29.7
Egypt (2005)	36.3	8.6	0	44.9
Jordan (2002)	15.8	4	0.3	20
Moldova, Republic of (2005)	21.7	2.1	0.1	23.9
Central Asia				
Kazakhstan (1995)	38.8	6.4	0.4	45.6
Kazakhstan (1999)	25.8	6	0	31.9
Kyrgyz Republic (1997)	25.2	5.9	0.7	31.9
Turkmenistan (2000)	33	4.1	0.5	37.6
Uzbekistan (1996)	45.3	10.4	0.6	56.3
South and Southeast Asia				
Cambodia (2000)	49.7	8.4	0.4	58.5
India (1998/1999)	36.3	17.8	1.9	55.9
Latin America and Caribbean				
Bolivia (1998)	17.7	4.5	0.7	22.9
Bolivia (2003)	27	3.8	0.1	30.9
Haiti (2000)	36.7	16.5	4.7	57.9
Honduras (2005)	14.8	1.7	0.3	16.8
Peru (1996)	27.2	3.8	0.1	31
Peru (2000)	24.5	4.5	0.2	29.2
Unweighted Average	29	9	1	39

Source: Demographic and Health Surveys (2008)

and Institute of Medicine (2005), and physical activity is on the decline (MacKay and Mensah 2004).

Tobacco, Alcohol, and Drug Use

Although tobacco use accounts for little disease burden in the adolescent years, its impact in adulthood is huge. Half of the roughly 300 million young people smoking today will eventually die from tobacco use (WHO 2001b). By 2030, tobacco is projected to be responsible for about 8.3 million deaths per year worldwide, or about 10% of total deaths, more than any other cause (Mathers and Loncar 2006). Most adult smokers worldwide begin smoking in adolescence or earlier (Jha et al. 2006). An estimated 10.5% of young men and 6.7% of young women aged 13–15 are currently smoking cigarettes, according to 132 surveys conducted between 1999 and 2005 (American Legacy Foundation 2002). About double these%ages are using some type of tobacco product (Fig. 24.6). Rates of tobacco use are lowest in Southeast Asia and the Western Pacific and highest in the Americas and Europe.

Alcohol use disorders in adolescents aged 10–19 currently account for about 3% of all DALYS (Table 24.4). The earlier young people start drinking, the more likely they are to suffer alcohol-related problems later in life (WHO 2001a). Most of this disease burden stems from periodic heavy drinking rather than chronic drinking (Ahlström et al. 2004). Surveys of in-school adolescents aged 13–15 years in 18 countries showed that 25% of boys and 15% of girls have had at least one heavy drinking episode (WHO 2004). Rates of heavy drinking range from 1% of girls in Tajikistan to 47% of girls in Zambia (Table 24.7). Alcohol-attributable DALYs for all ages worldwide account for 3.6% of the total DALYs (Rehm et al. 2006). Internationally, the trend is that youth start drinking alcohol earlier (WHO 2001a). Drinking, particularly heavy drinking, among youth is also on the increase (WHO 2004).

Sexual and Reproductive Health

Health problems associated with sexual and reproductive health such as maternal conditions and HIV/AIDS account for almost 10% of both deaths and disease burden in adolescents (Tables 24.4 and 24.5). Moreover, unsafe sex, an adolescent-rooted reproductive health risk factor, accounts for 4.3% of premature deaths worldwide and is the single leading risk factor worldwide for DALYs later in life (Figs. 24.3 and 24.4). In high-mortality developing countries, unsafe sex is the leading risk factor for premature death (Kirby et al. 2006). Several important trends are influencing sexual and reproductive health in adolescents. Worldwide, both boys and girls are experiencing puberty at an earlier age (National Research Council and Institute of Medicine 2005). Meanwhile, age at first marriage has gradually increased in most regions, with the exception of Latin America (Mensch et al. 2003). The majority of young people initiate sexual activity during adolescence (Table 24.8). Contrary to popular belief, today's adolescents are not having sex at earlier ages than before in most countries (National Research Council and Institute of Medicine 2005). There is even recent evidence that very early sexual initiation is on the decline in sub-Saharan Africa (UNAIDS 2006). However, premarital sex is increasing in most countries where data are available, largely because of increases in the age at first marriage (National Research Council and Institute of Medicine 2005).

Teen pregnancy, associated risk factors, and intervention programs are discussed in detail in Chapter 21. Rates of contraceptive use among

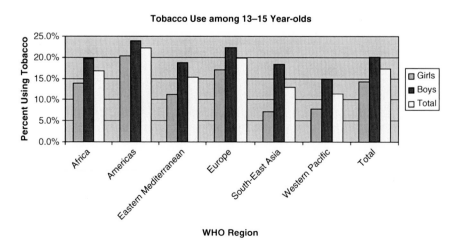

Fig. 24.6 Tobacco use worldwide. Source: Mochizuki-Kobayashi et al. (2006)

Table 24.7 Percent of students aged 13–15 reporting episodes of heavy drinking*

Country (year of survey)	Total	Boys	Girls
Sub-Saharan Africa			
Botswana (2005)	21	25	17
Kenya (2003)	20	24	15
Namibia (2004)	32	35	29
Senegal (2005)	5	7	2
Swaziland (2003)	19	24	16
Tanzania (2006)	6	8	3
Zambia (2004)	43	39	47
Zimbabwe (2003)	19	24	15
Latin America and the Caribbean			
Cayman Islands (2007)	28	28	28
Chile-Metropolitan (2004)	26	26	26
Guyana (2004)	28	40	18
Uruguay (2006)	31	33	29
Venezuela-Barinas (2003)	20	26	15
Middle East and North Africa			
Lebanon (2005)	14	21	7
Morocco (2006)	4	5	2
Tajikistan (2006)	2	2	1
Asia			
China–Beijing (2003)	8	12	5
Philippines (2003)	19	26	14
Median	19	25	15

*Heavy drinking = drank so much alcohol that they were really drunk one or more times during their life.
Source: Global School-Based Student Health Surveys (2007)

both married and unmarried adolescents are still quite low (Table 24.8). Moreover, substantial proportions of young women are not using contraception even though they are sexually active and do not want to have a child. A study of women in 53 developing countries found that this unmet need for contraception was highest in younger women aged 15–24 years (Fig. 24.7) (Sedgh et al. 2007).

Adolescent pregnancy and childbearing remains a problem in many countries (see Chapter 21). Rates of adolescent childbearing have dropped in most regions in the past three decades (Bearinger et al. 2007), but remain high, especially in Africa. Moreover, childbearing before age 16, which greatly increases the risk of negative health consequences, remains a problem in some regions (Table 24.8). Pregnant women under 20 bear a disproportionate burden of pregnancy-related death and illness. The roughly 15 million adolescent girls aged 15–19 that give birth each year account for about 11%

of births worldwide. Yet adolescent girls face health risks during pregnancy and childbirth, accounting for 15% of the Global Burden of Disease for maternal conditions and 13% of all maternal deaths (WHO and UNFPA 2006). Compared to women in their twenties and thirties, women under 20 years have a higher risk of dying from maternal causes (National Research Council and Institute of Medicine 2005). In countries where abortion is legally restricted, unsafe abortion is an important source of mortality and morbidity for young women. An estimated 14% of all unsafe abortions (about 2.5 million abortions per year) are to adolescents aged 15–19 years (Shah and Ahman 2004). As Fig. 24.8 shows, unsafe abortion is far more concentrated among adolescents in Africa than in other regions; adolescents aged 15–19 in Africa account for about 25% of unsafe abortion in the region versus less than 10% in Asia and about 15% in Latin America and the Caribbean.

Table 24.8 Indicators of sexual and reproductive behaviors among adolescents and youth by gender and age group, late 1990s to early 2000s

A. Sexual activity	Females, 20–24 Percent who initiated before age			Males, 20–24 Percent who initiated before age		
Region	15	18	20	15	18	20
East/Southern Africa	17	57	77	14	45	65
West and Middle Africa	21	59	77	12	40	61
Caribbean/Central America	13	44	62	31	70	84
South America	9	41	61	31	73	87
Former Soviet Asia	1	20	53	na	na	na
Middle East	na	na	Na	na	na	na
South and Southeast Asia	na	na	Na	na	na	na

B. Marriage	**Females, 20–24** **Percent who married before age**		**Males, 20–24** **Percent who married before age**	
Region	18	20	18	20
East/Southern Africa	37	55		14
West and Middle Africa	45	60		12
Caribbean/Central America	35	53		22
South America	23	38		14
Former Soviet Asia	16	50		na
Middle East	23	40		na
South and Southeast Asia	42	60		na

C. Childbearing	**Percent of females aged 20–24 who had a child before age**		**Percent of males who ever fathered a child at age**	
Region	16	18	15–19	20–24
East/Southern Africa	9	27	2	24
West and Middle Africa	13	31	2	13
Caribbean/Central America	7	22	2	27
South America	4	16	3	23
Former Soviet Asia	0	4	na	na
Middle East	3	11	na	na
South and Southeast Asia	9	24	na	na

D. Contraceptive Use	**Percentage of sexually active females aged 15–19 using contraception**	
Region	**All**	**Unmarried**
East/Southern Africa	21	28
West and Middle Africa	20	26

Table 24.8 (continued)

A. Sexual activity	Females, 20–24 Percent who initiated before age		Males, 20–24 Percent who initiated before age
Caribbean/Central America	24	na	
South America	28	38	
Former Soviet Asia	25	na	
Middle East	na	na	
South and Southeast Asia	na	na	

Source: National Research Council & Institute of Medicine (2005)
na = not available

Fig. 24.7 Unmet need for contraception by age group and region. Source: Sedgh et al. (2007)

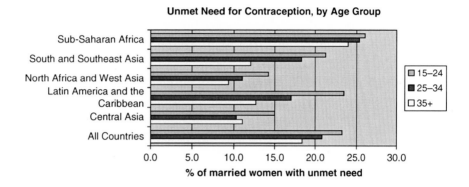

Fig. 24.8 Distribution of unsafe abortion by age. Source: Shah and Ahman (2004)

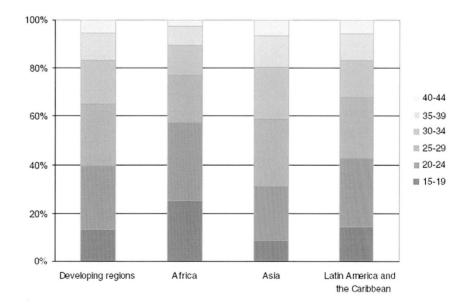

The complications associated with abortion are the reason why maternal conditions are among the highest contributors to DALYs in adolescents.

HIV/AIDS and Other Sexually Transmitted Infections

HIV/AIDS remains a serious threat to the immediate health of adolescents. Worldwide, HIV/AIDS accounts for 4% of deaths and about 2% of DALYs in adolescents (Figs. 24.3 and 24.4). Young people continue to be at the center of the HIV/AIDS epidemic. People under 25 (including children through mother-to-child transmission) account for roughly half of all new HIV infections (UNAIDS 2006). In Africa and the Caribbean, the epidemic disproportionately affects young women, with infection rates for young women two to three times higher than for young men (Table 24.9). Prevalence trends in HIV infection among young people are mixed. According to UNAIDS (2006), 6 of 11 countries reporting HIV/AIDS data showed a drop of 25% or more in prevalence in the 15–24 age group between 2000/2001 and 2004/2005 (UNAIDS 2006).

Table 24.9 HIV prevalence among 15–24-year-olds by region and sex, 2005

Region	Young women (15–24) rate (%) 2005	Young men (15–24) rate (%) 2005
Sub-Saharan Africa	4.3	1.5
East Asia	<0.1	0.1
South and Southeast Asia	0.4	0.6
Eastern Europe and Central Asia	0.5	0.9
North Africa and Middle East	0.2	0.1
Caribbean	1.6	0.7
Latin American	0.3	0.5

Source: UNAIDS (2006)

Low levels of knowledge about HIV/AIDS, together with continued higher-risk sexual practices, increase the vulnerability of adolescents to HIV infection. Most young people still lack comprehensive knowledge of HIV/AIDS. According to surveys conducted in 31 countries since 2000, the%age of youth who correctly identify ways of preventing HIV transmission and who reject major misconceptions about HIV transmission ranges between 15 and 54% for males and 9 and 53% for females (Table 24.10). This is far below the target of 90% set by the international community (UNAIDS 2006). Rates of higher-risk sex, as measured by the%age of sexually active young people having sex with non-marital, non-cohabitating partners, are also high. As Table 24.10 shows, in 35 countries with surveys since 2000, the median proportion having high-risk sex is 81% of males and 29% of females. No clear trend has emerged in this indicator (UNAIDS 2006). Moreover, the proportion of young people using a condom during higher-risk sex is still low, although apparently rising in some countries (UNAIDS 2006). Among young males, the proportion ranges from 12% in Madagascar to 86% in Armenia. Among females, the proportion ranges from 5% in Madagascar to 62% in Guyana (Table 24.10). The HIV/AIDS epidemic has also contributed to the growth in the number of adolescent orphans. Of the 130 million orphans worldwide under age 18, about 15 million (11%) have lost one or both parents to HIV/AIDS (UNAIDS 2006). UNAIDS projects this number to grow to 25 million by 2010 (UNAIDS 2007). About half of orphans under 18 are adolescents aged 12–17 (Ruland et al. 2005).

Of the roughly 340 million new cases each year of curable sexually transmitted infections (STIs), between a fifth and half are young people in the age group 10–24 (Bearinger et al. 2007). The disproportionately high burden of STIs among youth reflects the special biological, social, and economic risks they face (WHO 2007b). Many millions more adolescents are infected with incurable viral STIs such as human papilloma virus (HPV), which causes an estimated 500,000 new cases of cervical cancer and 70,000 cases of other types of cancer

Table 24.10 Indicators of HIV/AIDS-related sexual behavior and knowledge, young people aged 15–24, 2000–2006

Country (year of latest survey)	Percent engaging in higher risk sex		Percent using a condom at last higher risk sex		Percent with comprehensive HIV/AIDS knowledge	
	Males	Females	Males	Females	Males	Females
Europe and Central Asia						
Armenia (2005)	78	0	86	–	15	23
Moldova (2005)	84	36	63	44	54	42
Turkmenistan (2000)	–	2	–	–	–	–
Uzbekistan (2002)	45	1	50	–	–	–
Latin American and the Caribbean						
Bolivia (2003)	70	32	37	20	18	15
Colombia (2005)	–	53	–	–	–	–
Dominican Republic (2002)	83	29	52	29	–	–
Guyana (2005)	81	40	68	62	47	53
Haiti (2005)	95	55	43	29	40	32
Honduras (2005)	–	16	–	24	–	30
Nicaragua (2001)	–	14	–	–	–	–
Peru (2000)		29	–	–	–	–
South and Southeast Asia						
Cambodia (2005)	36	1	84	–	45	50
Nepal (2006)	20	–	78	–	44	28
Philippines (2003)	49	6	25	11	18	12
Vietnam (2005)	21	1	68	–	50	42
Sub-Saharan Africa						
Benin (2001)	90	36	34	19	–	–
Burkina Faso (2003)	78	23	67	54	23	15
Cameroon (2004)	91	44	57	46	34	27
Chad (2004)	76	7	25	17	25	17
Congo Brazzaville (2005)	94	60	38	20	22	10
Cote d'Ivoire (2005)	89	54	53	39	28	18
Ethiopia (2005)	37	6	50	28	33	21
Ghana (2003)	83	50	52	33	–	–
Guinea (2005)	95	36	37	26	23	17
Kenya (2003)	84	30	47	25	–	–
Lesotho (2004)	89	42	48	50	18	26
Madagascar (2003/04)	72	31	12	5	16	19
Malawi (2004)	62	14	47	35	36	24
Mali (2001)	85	18	30	14	15	9
Mozambique (2003)	84	37	33	29	33	20
Namibia (2000)	85	80	69	48	41	31
Niger (2006)	38	1	37	18	16	13
Nigeria (2003)	78	29	46	24	21	18
Rwanda (2005)	48	15	40	26	54	51
Senegal (2005)	91	11	52	36	26	20
Tanzania (2004)	83	29	46	39	40	45
Uganda (2006)	65	27	55	38	38	32
Zambia (2001/02)	86	30	42	33	33	31
Zimbabwe (2005/06)	78	16	68	42	46	44

Source: Demographic and Health Surveys (2008)
– = not available

annually (WHO 2007b). Cervical cancer is now the most common type of cancer in women in developing countries (Parkin et al. 2005). The peak years for incidence of HPV infection are between 16 and 20 (WHO and UNFPA 2006b), when most adolescents become sexually active.

Gender-Based Violence

Gender-based violence (GBV) encompasses a range of physical, sexual, and psychological violence directed mainly at women and girls (IGWG 2006). Among the most serious and common forms of these behaviors occur when an intimate male partner abuses his female partner and when a man coerces a woman or girl to have sex. Gender-based violence also encompasses harmful traditional practices such as female genital mutilation (Chapter 10) and human rights violations such as trafficking in girls and women. Gender-based violence is prevalent among young people. A recent WHO study carried out in both developed and less developed countries found that in 11 of the 15 settings worldwide, rates of reported sexual abuse among girls before age 18 were between 7 and 12% (WHO 2005a). Other studies have shown similar results in a wide range of settings (IGWG 2006). Many young women's first sex is coerced. In 10 of the 15 settings studied in the WHO study, over 5% of women reported that their first sexual experience was forced, with more than 14% reporting forced first sex in Bangladesh, Ethiopia, Peru, and the United Republic of Tanzania (WHO 2005a).

Rates of physical violence by intimate male partners against younger women are also high. In 10 of the 15 study sites participating in the recent WHO study, between 20 and 36% of young women aged 15–19 report being subject to at least one act of physical violence in the past year (WHO 2005a). Moreover, in two-thirds of the study sites, rates of current physical violence are highest in the 15–19 age group compared to older women (WHO 2005a). Gender-based violence often has lasting physical, social, emotional, psychological, and economic consequences (Patel et al. 2007) and is linked to many subsequent reproductive health problems (IGWG 2006).

Evidence on Effective Programs to Improve Adolescent Health

The wide range of adolescent health problems and risk behaviors complicates the task of improving adolescent health. Moreover, the enormous number of risks and protective factors potentially influencing adolescent health present daunting challenges for public health programs. To address these complexities, an international consensus has formed around a basic set of principles or framework for approaching adolescent health interventions (WHO 1999). This model promotes a holistic, multi-intervention approach to adolescent health problems centered on providing adolescents with

- Information and skills to make the right decisions about behaviors that affect their health, such as whether and when to have sex and whether to use tobacco
- Access to a broad range of health services that give them the means to act on their knowledge
- A social, legal, and regulatory environment that supports healthy behaviors and protects them from harm

Most adolescent health programs incorporate these goals. Experience to date suggests that effective, youth-focused efforts share a set of common programming principles (Box 24.1).

However, few if any countries have taken an integrated, holistic approach. In practice, to the extent that countries have addressed adolescent health problems at all, it has been piecemeal, by disease or condition. It is worth noting that, in general, the evidence base for effective interventions to improve adolescent health, although expanding, remains weak. However, many youth health interventions are relatively new and not yet well evaluated. Health interventions for youth share this shortcoming with interventions in other areas of youth development (2006b). The following discussion summarizes knowledge of intervention effectiveness and important policy and program gaps, organized by major adolescent health problems.

Interventions to Address Mental Disorders

Patel et al. (2007) note a gradual improvement in treatment of mental health problems in adolescents in recent decades, although evidence for intervention effectiveness and cost remains limited. Mental

---

Box 24.1 General Principles of Health Programming for Adolescents

- *Recognize the diversity of the youth age group*: A sexually inexperienced 11-year-old has vastly different needs than a married 20-year-old. Programs should apply different strategies to reach youth, who vary by age, sex, employment, schooling, and marital status.
- *Involve young people*: Policies and programs are more effective when young people are involved in all aspects of their design, implementation, and evaluation. Involvement must go beyond tokenism and be genuine, meaningful, and sustained.
- *Make health services appealing to youth*: A key to rapidly expanding young people's access to health services is to make them more youth friendly by using specially trained health workers and by bolstering the privacy, confidentiality, and accessibility of care.
- *Address gender inequality*: Gender inequalities expose young girls to coerced sex, HIV infection, unwanted pregnancy, and poor nutrition. Efforts should focus on changing the factors that perpetuate gender inequalities.
- *Address the needs of boys*: Adolescence presents a unique opportunity to help boys form positive notions of gender relations and to raise their awareness of health issues. At the same time, boys seem to be disproportionately exposed to a number of adolescent health risks, including accidents and injuries, suicide, tobacco use, substance abuse, and violence. Program design should take into account the specific needs of boys and young men as well as of girls and young women.
- *Design comprehensive programs*: Comprehensive programs that provide information and services while addressing the social and political context are more effective than narrowly focused interventions.
- *Consider all important benefits*: Many adolescent health interventions focus on only one benefit. For example, a school-based sex education program may focus exclusively on HIV prevention and may neglect other possible benefits from the intervention, such as increased education, averted teen pregnancy and abortions, and other averted STIs.
- *Address the many non-health factors that influence adolescent health*: Linking school and livelihood opportunities to adolescent health programs, at either the policy or the program level, is key to helping young people avoid risky behaviors.
- *Address underlying risk and protective factors*. Factors such as feelings of self-efficacy, attitudes and behaviors of friends, connectedness with parents and other influential adults, and involvement in the community can either increase (risk factor) or decrease (protective factor) the chances that a young person will engage in unhealthy behaviors.

Source: Lule et al. (2006)

---

and behavioral disorders have been responsive to psychotherapy with a behavioral or cognitive-behavioral orientation. Early intervention for psychotic disorders in adolescents has also shown promise. However, there is insufficient evidence for the effectiveness of treatment for depression in adolescents. Large-scale suicide prevention efforts show some promise, and drops in suicide rates among young people have occurred in countries with national programs (Patel et al. 2007). However, very few suicide prevention efforts have proven conclusively effective, particularly over the long term (WHO 2002). Despite mental disorders being the single largest cause of burden of disease in adolescents, countries have done relatively little to address this problem. Few countries have adolescent-specific mental health policies, and services for adolescents in developing countries are almost non-existent. Wealthier countries offer better mental health services, but care tailored to adolescents is not always available (Patel et al. 2007).

Interventions to Prevent Intentional Injury

Table 24.11 shows strategies that proved effective in reducing youth violence or risk factors for youth violence. At the individual level, social development programs to reduce antisocial and aggressive behavior have been found to be effective, beginning in early childhood through adolescence. Such programs that emphasize social and competency skills have been shown to be the most effective and are more effective the earlier they begin (that is, the younger the age group) (WHO 2002).

Another set of interventions try to work on improving relationships young people have with parents, siblings, and peers. Home visitation by a health-care professional and parenting training has been shown to be effective in preventing later youth violence if done when children are still small. Programs that pair adolescents with adult mentors who provide positive role models have been shown to be effective. Family therapy programs that aim to improve parent–child communication and address problems of violence are also effective (WHO 2002). Several types of interventions to reduce youth violence have been tried and proven ineffective, including individual counseling, probation, or parole programs that include meetings with prison inmates describing the brutality of prison life, programs modeled on basic military training, peer mediation or peer counseling, and gang prevention programs. Many other approaches are underway, but still lack evidence of effectiveness (WHO 2002).

Most programs to address youth violence, in both developed and developing nations, are targeted toward managing the consequences of violence and supporting the victims. Countries have neglected prevention efforts, in part because the public and policy makers have not seen violence as something preventable (Dahlberg and Krug 2006). Moreover, much of the effort in youth violence prevention has gone toward untested programs lacking a sound theoretical basis (WHO 2002).

Interventions to Prevent Road Traffic Injuries

Several interventions have proven effective in reducing adolescent deaths and injuries from road crashes (WHO 2007d). Interventions that have reduced speeding (which is a greater factor in crashes involving young drivers) include setting and enforcing speed limits, traffic calming measures such as speed humps, and restrictions on alcohol consumption by youth behind the wheel and on nighttime driving. Mandatory helmet laws, free distribution of helmets, setting quality standards for helmets, and public awareness campaigns to encourage helmet use have increased helmet use for young motorcycle and bicycle

Table 24.11 Effective* youth violence prevention strategies by developmental stage and ecological context

| Ecological context | Developmental stage | | | |
	Infancy (ages 0–3)	Early childhood (ages 3–5)	Middle childhood (ages 6–11)	Adolescence (ages 12–19)
Individual		Social development programs	Social development programs	Social development programs
		Preschool enrichment programs		Providing incentives for youths at high risk for violence to complete secondary schooling
Relationship (e.g., family, peers)	Home visitation			Mentoring programs
	Training in parenting	Training in parenting		Family therapy

*Demonstrated to be effective in reducing youth violence or risk factors for youth violence.
Source: WHO (2002)

riders, who are least likely to wear a helmet. Wearing a motorcycle helmet correctly can cut the risk of death by almost 40% and the risk of severe injury by 72%. Alcohol is a factor in a high proportion of road accidents involving adolescents. Effective measures to reduce drinking and driving among adolescents include restriction of alcohol use by adolescents and enforcement of stricter drinking and driving regulations. Graduated driver licensing systems phase in young beginners to full driving privileges have been shown to improve safety. Young drivers and passengers are less likely to wear seat belts. Effective strategies to encourage seat belt use include seat belt enforcement, ensuring that vehicles are fitted with appropriate seat belts, public awareness campaigns, and community projects involving parents and peers. Several high-income countries have invested in successful, comprehensive, and systematic programs to lower the burden from road traffic injuries (Peden 2004). In developing countries, however, such systematic efforts are almost universally absent, and investments in reducing road traffic injuries among the general population, including those that target adolescents, are extremely low (Norton et al. 2006).

Interventions to Improve Nutrition, Diet, and Physical Activity

To address anemia, a major problem among adolescent girls in developing countries, daily iron supplementation for adolescent girls has been found to effectively reduce anemia and iron deficiency (Elder 2002). Many high-income countries have successfully reduced diet and lifestyle-related chronic diseases rooted in adolescent behaviors and habits. Programs in developing countries are relatively new and have yet to show changes in levels of chronic disease (Willett et al. 2006). Obesity prevention programs, many of them school-based and targeting the adolescent population, have shown mixed results (World Bank 2006a). The key elements of the successful interventions include having an environmental and multidisciplinary approach; generating local adaptations of programs; exploring

cultural norms and fitting the program within those constructs; adhering to a social–ecological model of behavior change; and taking a multifaceted approach to include multiple stakeholders, including health professionals, educators, and policy makers (World Bank 2006a). Studies show that efforts to prevent obesity are more likely to succeed among adolescents than among adults (Delisle et al. 2001). Programs to encourage physical activity among schoolchildren are widespread and an important source of physical activity for adolescents. There is some evidence that such programs have helped keep obesity rates low in countries where such programs are widespread, such as China (Willet et al. 2006).

Nutritional interventions in both developed and developing countries have traditionally neglected adolescents relative to other age groups. The rising importance of diet-related chronic disease has begun to raise the profile of adolescent malnutrition problems, but they still do not receive high priority. In developing countries, lack of financial and institutional capacity coupled with lack of appreciation of the importance of nutrition have hampered the ability to address adolescent nutrition problems (WHO 2005b; World Bank 2006a).

Interventions to Address Tobacco, Alcohol, and Drug Use

Price increases through taxation are a well-established, effective tool for reducing or deterring tobacco use by adolescents. Studies in the United States have shown that price increases have a greater effect on tobacco use by young people than on use by older age groups (Jha et al. 2006). Other interventions such as comprehensive bans on all advertising, including bans on the promotion of tobacco products and trademarks, have also reduced tobacco use among young people (Jha et al. 2006). Another intervention that is effective in reducing youth smoking is comprehensive restrictions on smoking in public spaces and private workplaces (Jha et al. 2006). Programs that give young people the skills to resist peer pressure and other social pressures to smoke have demonstrated consistent and significant reductions or delays in adolescent smoking. School-based programs are also more effective when combined with community-wide supportive efforts. Information campaigns that help young people see how the tobacco industry tries to manipulate their behavior through advertising have been highly effective in changing behavior and attitudes toward smoking among young people in the United States (American Legacy Foundation 2002). With regard to use of alcohol and other drugs, legal and regulatory restrictions on minimum age, quantity, price, place, and time of sale have been shown to be effective in reducing alcohol use. Some prevention programs that aim to reduce the risk factors leading to substance abuse have been shown to be effective, not, however, as short-term, stand-alone interventions. There is also some evidence that early screening for drug problems followed by brief interventions is effective. Harm reduction efforts, such as needle exchange programs for intravenous drug users, have been found to be effective in reducing some of the negative outcomes associated with substance abuse, without affecting use one way or the other (Toumbourou and Stockwell 2007).

Despite the evidence supporting taxation to reduce tobacco use, relatively few countries have deployed such price increases. Only a few developed countries have implemented comprehensive programs that combine taxation with information dissemination and comprehensive bans on advertising. Political constraints and lack of awareness of intervention effectiveness have limited implementation of programs in developing countries (Jha et al. 2006).

Interventions to Address Sexual and Reproductive Health, Including HIV/AIDS

The most recent major review of program effectiveness in this area is the 2006 report by the UNAIDS Inter-agency Task Team on Young People, Preventing HIV/AIDS in Young People: A Systematic Review of the Evidence from Developing Countries (UNAIDS 2006). The report, based on a review of 85 relatively rigorous evaluation studies, divides 23 identified types of interventions into the following four groups according to the strength of evidence of effectiveness, as summarized in Table 24.12:

- Interventions recommended for widespread implementation on a large scale (Go)
- Interventions to be implemented more cautiously along with careful evaluation of their impact on key health outcomes (Ready)
- Interventions requiring further development and demonstration of effectiveness before they can be recommended for widespread implementation (Steady)
- And interventions that should not be implemented because there is sufficient evidence of their lack of effectiveness (Do not go)

Programs with particularly strong evidence for effectiveness include curriculum-based sexuality and reproductive health education programs in schools; clinic-based programs linked with community interventions; and mass media efforts with messages delivered through radio, television, and print media. Several other types of programs delivered promising results but still lack convincing evidence on their effectiveness. Although the focus of the UNAIDS review was on HIV prevention, many of the behavioral outcomes studied are equally applicable to prevention of unwanted pregnancy and other key reproductive health outcomes. These include initiation of sex, number of sexual partners, use of condoms and other contraceptives, and use of other reproductive health services. The findings of the UNAIDS (2006) review are similar to those of the earlier FOCUS on Young Adults (2001) review. Evidence from 70 rigorously evaluated programs in Canada and the United States found evidence that a range of programs are effective in reducing sexual risk-taking, pregnancy, and childbearing among teens (Kirby 2001). Synthesis of developed and developing country studies (Kirby et al. 2006) found that programs are particularly effective for adolescents who are at especially high risk of negative sexual and reproductive behaviors. Of all the programs that have been rigorously evaluated, none has reported a decrease in the age of sexual

Table 24.12 Recommendations on effectiveness of HIV prevention programs for young people

Setting	Type of program
Go – Evidence threshold met	
Schools	Curriculum-based interventions with characteristics that have been found to be effective in developed countries and are led by adults
Health services	Interventions with service providers that include making changes to either the structure or the functioning of the facilities themselves and are linked to interventions in the community to promote the health services for young people
Mass media	Interventions with messages delivered through the radio and other media (for example, print media), except television
	Interventions with messages delivered through the radio and television and other media (for example, print media)
Ready – Evidence threshold partially met	
Health services	Interventions with service providers and in health facilities and in the community that involve other sectors
Geographically defined communities	Interventions targeting youths using existing youth service organizations
Young people most at risk	Facility-based programs that also have outreach and provide information and services
Steady – Evidence threshold not met	
Schools	Schools curriculum based with characteristics found to be effective in developed countries and that are led by peers
	Curriculum based without the characteristics found to be effective in developed countries and that are led by adults
	Curriculum based without the characteristics found to be effective in developed countries and led by peers
	Non-curriculum based without characteristics found to be effective in developed countries and led by adults
	Non-curriculum based without characteristics found to be effective in developed countries and led by peers
Health services	Interventions with service providers and in the community
	Interventions with service providers and involving other sectors
	Interventions with service providers and in facilities and involving other sectors
	Interventions with service providers and in the community and involving other sectors
Mass media	Radio only
Geographically defined communities	Interventions targeting youths through new structures
	Interventions targeting the entire community through traditional networks
	Interventions targeting the entire community through community events
Young people most at risk	Outreach only interventions providing information and services

Source: UNAIDS IATT (2006)

debut or an increase in sexual activity among young people. This finding counters the criticism that opponents of adolescent sexual and reproductive health programs often make, namely that programs hasten or increase sexual activity.

New research has shown the safety and effectiveness of a vaccine to prevent human papillomavirus (HPV), the major cause of cervical cancer. Public health officials are currently recommending that all girls get the vaccine before they become sexually active, between 11 and 12 years old, but as early as age 9. As yet, no country has carried out widespread vaccination programs. Introduction of HPV vaccine in developing countries faces a range of policy challenges, including how to reach the target population of adolescents (WHO 2007c).

Another promising intervention is male circumcision for HIV prevention, which has been shown to cut risk of HIV transmission by more than half in males (Newell and Bärnighausen 2007). Based on these and other studies, experts convened by WHO and UNAIDS in March 2007 recommended including male circumcision as an additional HIV prevention intervention, one for which adolescents and young men are likely to be prime candidates (WHO and UNAIDS 2007). Sexual and reproductive health interventions for adolescents are among the most widespread of adolescent health programs. However, few of these interventions have been large scale, most being small, short-term programs carried out by nongovernmental organizations (Lule et al. 2006). Despite the disparities in health outcomes for the youngest pregnant mothers, maternal and newborn health programs have done relatively little to focus their efforts on pregnant women in the 10–19 age group (WHO and UNFPA 2006a). HIV prevention programs for adolescents increased greatly in scope over the past decade, but they still reach only a small group of adolescents (UNAIDS 2006). Levels of HIV/AIDS education in schools have increased, but still less than half of school children receive such education, and quality is low in many schools (UNAIDS 2006). Even though about half of orphans under 18 are adolescents aged 12–17, programs (including reproductive health-care programs) typically do not focus on the needs of this older age group (Ruland et al. 2005). Countries are increasingly enacting specific national adolescent health policies or addressing adolescent health concerns within national policies on key health issues but many countries have yet to sufficiently carry out such policies.

Cost, Cost-Effectiveness, and Cost–Benefit of Interventions

Good cost studies of adolescent health programs are rare, even in developed countries. The reported cost of such programs varies greatly depending on the country, type of intervention, target group, and so on. For example, such programs cost between US \$0.03 per adolescent reached in a family life education radio program in Kenya and US \$71.00 per year per adolescent reached in a school-based HIV prevention program in Zimbabwe. Only a few programs have documented their cost-effectiveness in terms of DALYs. Cost–benefit analysis, which allows comparison across a range of interventions inside and outside the health sector, has been done for a few interventions (Table 24.13). These studies show that health interventions aimed at adolescents have the potential to be good public investments (Lule et al. 2006; Knowles and Behrman 2003).

Table 24.13 Estimated benefit–cost ratios, selected investments in youth

Investment	Estimated benefit–cost ratio (assuming 3% annual discount rate)	Plausible range of estimated benefit–cost ratio
Scholarship program (Colombia)	4.4	2.8–25.6
Adult basic education and literacy program (Colombia)	27.6	8.1–1,764.0
School-based reproductive health program to prevent HIV/AIDS (Honduras)	0.5	0.1–4.6
Iron supplementation administered to secondary schoolchildren (hypothetical low-income country)	45.2	25.8–45.2
Tobacco tax (hypothetical middle-income country)	20.2	7.0–38.6

Source: Lule et al. (2006)

Conclusions

Adolescence has its own unique health problems, with a disease profile that is different from small children and older adults. Although, relatively speaking, 10–19 years is the healthiest time of life, the adolescent years are still a time of significant disease burden. Moreover, a large portion of the disease burden in adulthood has its roots in adolescent behaviors or conditions. The health problems of adolescence are inter-related, sharing many of the risk and protective factors that influence adolescent behavior and health conditions. These linkages provide opportunities for programs to have multiple positive impacts but also complicate the design of interventions to improve adolescent health. Countries have tried a variety of approaches to improve adolescent health, some of which have proved effective, although generally only modestly (National Research Council and Institute of Medicine 2005). The evidence base for what works is growing but still insufficient. Partly from lack of information about effective interventions and partly because of the perception that many of the health problems of adolescents are "normal" and thus not preventable, countries have been slow to recognize the importance of the burden of disease in adolescence. As a result, almost everywhere, the health system response to adolescent health problems has been inadequate. This is particularly so in developing countries.

Policy and Programmatic Needs

A key message that emerges from the evidence on risk and protective factors and on program effectiveness is the need to move toward a more integrated approach to addressing adolescent health problems. Within each disease area, no single strategy is effective by itself. Comprehensive approaches to road safety, sexual and reproductive health, and violence prevention that use multiple, concurrent strategies are likely to be most effective in addressing adolescent health problems. Moreover, adolescent health programming needs to reach across disease areas to take advantage of the natural synergies and shared risks and protective factors, while also taking advantage of the existing infrastructure and health systems. Nowhere is this more apparent than in the potential synergies between HIV/AIDS and reproductive health programming and in the need to improve effectiveness. For example, in low-HIV prevalence countries, reproductive health programs could be the entry point to increase HIV prevention and in high-prevalence countries, HIV programs could be the entry point to address reproductive health concerns. There is simply not enough human resource capacity (particularly in developing countries) to address each adolescent health problem with separate, vertical programs. In addition, adolescent health programs need to be better integrated with approaches outside the health sector, such as education, which also affect health outcomes.

As is the case with other age groups, poor and disadvantaged adolescents suffer disproportionately from health problems (Lule et al. 2006). Reaching these poor and hard to reach adolescents is another key programmatic need, one in which coordinated action is needed to keep adolescents in school, give them the skills they need to compete in the workforce, and encourage them to become active citizens (World Bank 2006b). Programs also need to do a better job of involving influential gatekeepers such as parents, teachers, employers, administrators, and community leaders, who have significant sway over adolescent behavior and over the programs to be implemented.

To achieve improvements in sexual and reproductive health and HIV prevention, more attention is needed to support marriage delays, address gender inequalities, serve married adolescents, and scale up efforts to serve adolescent males. Finally, it is important for policy makers to recognize that each adolescent experiences the transition to adulthood differently. Policies and programs should focus less on age and more on recognizing the specific health and developmental needs of people as they navigate the passage from childhood to adulthood.

Monitoring and Research Needs

Better monitoring and research on adolescent health problems and interventions is urgently needed to inform policy makers, including the following:

Collecting basic data on adolescent health: Our knowledge is still sparse on many basic facts about adolescent health, including about the cause of death and burden of disease in the adolescent age group. Although information sources are improving, especially in the area of sexual and reproductive health including HIV/AIDS, many gaps remain, particularly around some of the most important health problems of adolescence such as mental illness, road injuries, and violence. Many countries have incomplete or non-existent data on adolescent health problems. Improved methods for collecting and analyzing data are needed.

Documenting the effectiveness of approaches: There are still more questions than answers about the effectiveness of the various adolescent health interventions. Along with better process evaluation to understand the functioning of successful programs, program evaluation necessitates more rigorous research designs including random assignment of treatment so that the effectiveness of programs can be better documented, both in terms of health outcomes and in terms of disease burden. Research could also help better document the non-health effects of adolescent health interventions.

Testing new interventions: A high priority is more research on multi-component programs and on new types of interventions. One promising area of research is the impact of targeted subsidies to keep adolescents in school and in using such subsidies to improve adolescent health behaviors (World Bank 2006b). In relation to sexual and reproductive health, new interventions include approaches such as providing antiretroviral therapy to HIV-infected youth and voluntary counseling and testing for HIV, encouraging adolescents to have fewer sexual partners, reducing the trafficking of young people, preventing and addressing the health consequences of early marriage, and reaching young married women with information and services. Research must better inform interventions so that they reach groups at particularly high risk of poor health outcomes, such as child prostitutes, child

workers, refugees, AIDS orphans, and street children. More research is also needed on a broad range of other adolescent health interventions, especially for those health problems that are among the biggest killers and disablers of young people: HIV/AIDS and mental illnesses for both males and females, maternal conditions for females, and road traffic injuries for males. In addition, research is needed on programs that attempt to influence gender roles and social norms and investments designed to avert drug and alcohol abuse and to improve mental health. Program implementation studies are urgently needed to examine the best way to roll out promising new prevention strategies including male circumcision for HIV prevention and the HPV vaccine. More study is also needed to examine how to integrate prevention and treatment of gender-based violence into adolescent health programming.

Enhancing understanding of the risk and protective factors influencing adolescent behavior: Even though our understanding of the major influences on youth behaviors has come far, more refinement of such understanding is needed, along with a better understanding of how to incorporate such knowledge into the design of programs and policies.

Improving cost, cost-effectiveness, and cost–benefit analysis: Particularly as programs move from small pilot projects to large-scale interventions, more needs to be done to more fully estimate their cost-effectiveness and cost–benefit.

The Way Forward

Global commitment to meeting adolescent health needs has never been higher. The 1994 International Conference on Population and Development (United Nations 1994) and the 2001 UN Special Session on AIDS (United Nations 2001) affirmed the rights of young people to high-quality sexual and reproductive health information and services. Similarly, the *Framework Convention on Tobacco Control*

(WHO 2003) prioritizes the youth dimension of the smoking epidemic. Now, countries need to translate this commitment into national policies and programs. Doing so requires building on and expanding the evidence base on effective and cost-effective interventions. The more countries know about what works, the better the choices adolescents will make – or that will be made for them. These are the choices that will ultimately shape their lives, the welfare of their families, and the future of their communities.

Key Terms

Adolescence	Homicide	School factors
Adolescent behaviors	Human papilloma virus (HPV)	Self-control
Adolescent childbearing	Intentional injuries	Self-efficacy
Adolescent health	Iron deficiency anemia	Self-inflicted injuries
Adolescent orphans	Male circumcision	Sexual abuse
Alcohol use disorder	Malnutrition	Social development programs
Bipolar disorder	Mandatory helmet laws	Substance abuse
Community factors	Overweight	Suicide
Condom	Parental expectations	Teen pregnancy
Demographic transition	Parenting training	Tobacco use
Depression	Peer pressure	Unintentional injuries
Family factors	Psychological factors	Unsafe abortion
Family life education	Reproductive health	Unsafe sex
Gender-based violence (GBV)	Road traffic injuries	
HIV prevention programs	Schizophrenia	

Questions for Discussion

1. Define the term adolescence. Why should national governments and international health agencies be concerned about adolescent health issues?
2. In a narrative of about 1,000 words, describe factors that increase (risk factors) or decrease (protective factors) an adolescent's chance of involvement in unhealthy behaviors. Present your description from the perspectives of the individual, family, institutional, and community.
3. List the major causes of morbidity and mortality among adolescents. How does the prevalence of these causes differ between high- and low-income countries?
4. Outline the nine general principles of health programming for adolescents.
5. Discuss the current state of evidence regarding the effectiveness of interventions to address the following health issues of adolescents:

a. Malnutrition
b. Mental disorders
c. Road traffic accidents
d. Substance abuse
e. Sexual and reproductive health problems (including HIV/AIDS/STIs)

6. What measures would you recommend as priorities for improving the health of adolescents in developing countries?

References

Adeyi O, Smith O, Robles S (2007) Public Policy and the Challenge of Chronic Non-Communicable Diseases. Washington, DC: World Bank Publications

Ahlström SK, Österberg E, Toumbourou J et al. (2004) International perspectives on adolescent and young adult drinking. Alcohol Research and Health, 28(4), 258–268

American Legacy Foundation (2002) New American legacy foundation study shows truth® campaign helping to drive down youth smoking rates. In: American Legacy Foundation. http://www.americanlegacy.org/, cited 8 August 2008

Bearinger L, Sieving R, Ferguson J et al. (2007) Global perspectives on the sexual and reproductive health of adolescents: patterns, prevention, and potential. Lancet, 369, 1220–1231

Behrman JR, Hoddinott J, Maluccio J et al. (2004) The impact of experimental nutritional interventions on education into adulthood in rural Guatemala: preliminary longitudinal analysis. In: The 2004 Population Association of America Annual Meeting. http://repository. upenn.edu/cgi/viewcontent.cgi?article = 1002&context = psc_working_papers, cited 8 August 2008

Birdsall N, Kelley AC, Sinding S.W (Eds.) (2001) Population Matters: Demographic Change, Economic Growth, and Poverty in the Developing World. New York: Oxford University Press

Blum RW, Mmari NK (2005) Risk and Protective Factors Affecting Adolescent Reproductive Health in Developing Countries. Geneva: World Health Organization. http:// www.who.int/child-adolescent-health/New_Publications/ADH/ISBN_92_4_159365_2.pdf, cited 8 August 2008

Dahlberg L, Krug E (2006) Violence as a global public health problem. Ciência and Saúde Coletiva, 11(2), 277–292

Delisle H, Chandra-Mouli V, de Benoist B (2001) Should Adolescents be Specifically Targeted for Nutrition in Developing Countries? To address which problems, and how? Geneva: World Health Organization. www.who. int/child-adolescent-health/New_Publications/NUTRITION/Adolescent_nutrition_paper.pdf, cited 15 Jan 2008

Demographic and Health Surveys (2008) Statcompiler: Measure DHS. http://www.measuredhs.com/accesssurveys/, cited 15 Jan 2008

Elder L (2002) Adolescent Nutrition: Issues and Interventions. Background paper prepared for the World Bank Learning Exchange on Exploring Strategies for Reaching and Working with Adolescents, Washington, DC, June 5

FOCUS on Young Adults (2001) Advancing young adult reproductive health: actions for the next decade. In FOCUS on Young Adults. http://www.fhi.org/en/Youth/YouthNet/Publications/FOCUS/InFOCUS/YouthLivelihoods.htm, cited 15 Jan 2008

Interagency Gender Working Group of USAID (2006) Addressing Gender-Based Violence Through USAID's Health Programs: A Guide for Health Sector Program Officers. http://www.prb.org/pdf05/GBVReportfinal. pdf, cited 15 Jan 2008

Jha P, Chaloupka F, Moore J et al. (2006) Tobacco addiction. In Jamison, D et al. (2nd eds.), Disease Control Priorities in Developing Countries. New York: Oxford University Press

Joint United Nations Programme on HIV/AIDS (UNAIDS) (2006) Report on the Global AIDS Epidemic, 2006. http://data.unaids.org/pub/GlobalReport/2006/2006_GR-ExecutiveSummary_en.pdf, cited 8 August 2008

Kirby D (2001) Emerging Answers: Research Findings on Programs to Reduce Teen Pregnancy. Washington, DC: National Campaign to Prevent Teen Pregnancy. http://www.teenpregnancy.org/resources/data/report_summaries/emerging_answers/, cited 15 Jan 2008

Kirby D, Lepore G, Ryan J (2005) Sexual risk and protective factors: factors affecting teen sexual behavior, pregnancy, childbearing and sexually transmitted disease: which are important? Which can you change? National Campaign to Prevent Teen Pregnancy. http://www.teenpregnancy. org/works/risk_protective_kirby/Kirby_Riskandprotectivefactor_paper.pdf, cited 15 Jan 2008

Kirby D, Laris B, Rolleri L (2006) Impact of sex and HIV education programs on sexual behaviors of youth in developing and developed countries. In: Family Health International Youth Research Working Papers. Global Health Council. http://www.fhi.org/en/Youth/YouthNet/Publications/YouthResearchWorkingPapers, cited 15 Jan 2008

Knowles JC, Behrman JR (2003) Assessing the Economic Benefits of Investing in Youth in Developing Countries. Health, Nutrition, and Population Discussion Paper. http://siteresources.worldbank.org/HEALTHNUTRITIONANDPOPULATION/Resources/281627-1095698140167/Knowles-AssessingTheEconomic-whole.pdf, cited 15 Jan 2008

Lule E, Rosen J, Singh S et al. (2006) Adolescent health programs. In: Jamison D (ed.), Disease Control Priorities in Developing Countries, 2nd ed., 1109–1126. New York: Oxford University Press

MacKay J, Mensah GA (2004) The Atlas of Heart Disease and Stroke. Geneva: World Health Organization

Magnani R, Karim A, Weiss L et al. (2002) Reproductive health risk and protective factors among youth in Lusaka, Zambia. Journal of Adolescent Health, 30, 76–86

Marston C, King E (2006) Factors that shape young people's sexual behaviour: a systematic review. Lancet, 368, 1581–1586

Mathers C (2009) Global burden of disease for women, children and adolescents. In: Ehiri JE, Meremikwu MM (eds.), Global Perspectives on Maternal and Child Health. New York: Springer Publishers.

Mathers C, Loncar D (2006) Projections of global mortality and burden of disease from 2002 to 2030. PLoS Medicine, 3(11), 2011–2030

Mensch BS, Singh S, Casterline J (2003) Trends in the Timing of First Marriage Among Men and Women in the Developing World. Paper Presented at the Annual Meeting of the Population Association of America, Minneapolis, May 1–3

Mochizuki-Kobayashi Y, Fishburn B, Baptiste J et al. (2006) Use of cigarettes and other tobacco products among students aged 13–15 years – worldwide, 1999–2005. Morbidity and Mortality Weekly Report, 55(20), 553–556

National Research Council and Institute of Medicine (2005) Growing Up Global: The Changing Transitions to Adulthood in Developing Countries. Panel on Transitions to Adulthood in Developing Countries. Washington, DC: The National Research Council and Institute of Medicine

Newell ML, Bärnighausen T (2007) Male circumcision to cut HIV risk in the general population. Lancet, 369, 617–619

Norton R, Hyder A, Bishai D et al. (2006) Unintentional injuries. In: Jamison D (ed.), Disease Control Priorities in Developing Countries, 2nd ed. New York: Oxford University Press. http://www.dcp2.org/pubs/DCP/39/Full-Text, cited 15 Jan 2008

Parkin DM, Bray F, Ferlay J et al. (2005) Global cancer statistics, 2002. CA: A Cancer Journal for Clinicians, 55(2), 74–108

Patel V, Flisher A, Hetrick S et al. (2007) Mental health of young people: a global public-health challenge. Lancet, 369, 1302–1313

Peden M (2004) World Report on Road Traffic Injury Prevention. Geneva, Switzerland: World Health Organization. http://www.who.int/violence_injury_prevention/publications/road_traffic/world_report/summary_en_rev.pdf, cited 8 August 2008

Rehm J, Chisholm D, Room R et al. (2006) Alcohol. In Jamison D et al. (eds.), Disease Control Priorities in Developing Countries, 2nd ed., 887–906. New York: Oxford University Press

Rosen J (2004) Adolescent Health and Development: A Resource Guide for World Bank Staff and Government Counterparts. New York: World Bank http://siteresources.worldbank.org/HEALTHNUTRITIONAND-POPULATION/Resources/281627-1095698140167/Rosen-AHDFinal.pdf, cited 8 August 2008

Ruland CD, Finger W, Williamson N, Tahir S et al. (2005) Adolescents: Orphaned and Vulnerable in the Time of HIV/AIDS. [Youth Issues Paper, no. 6] Research Triangle Park, NC: Family Health International. http://www.fhi.org/NR/rdonlyres/ewps7bhbybdcrne4m3sfxvwrj5715nflni2W2jfysko3pkgisuksmumfee3rsngidgn5vuoh6hsl3d/Y16.pdf, cited August 5 2009

Sedgh G, Hussain R, Bankole A et al. (2007) Women with an Unmet Need for Contraception in Developing Countries: Levels and Reasons for Not Using a Method. http://www.guttmacher.org/pubs/2007/07/09/or37.pdf, cited 8 August 2008

Shah I, Ahman E (Eds.) (2004) Unsafe Abortion: Global and Regional Estimates of the Incidence of Unsafe Abortion and Associated Mortality in 2000, 4th ed. http://www.who.int/reproductive-health/publications/unsafeabortion_2000/estimates.pdf, cited 8 August 2008

Toumbourou JW, Stockwell T (2007) Interventions to reduce harm associated with adolescent substance use. Lancet, 369(9570), 1391–1401

UNAIDS Inter-agency Task Team on Young People (UNAIDS IATT) (2006) Preventing HIV/AIDS in Young People. A systematic review of the evidence from developing countries. Geneva: World Health Organization

United Nations (1994) United Nations International Conference on Population and Development (ICPD). http://www.iisd.ca/Cairo.html, cited 8 August 2008

United Nations (2001) General Assembly Special Session on HIV/AIDS. http://www.un.org/ga/aids/coverage/, cited 8 August 2008

United Nations Fund for Population Activities (UNFPA) (2003) The State of World Population, 2003: Making 1 Billion Count – Investing in Adolescents' Health and Rights. New York: United Nations Fund for Population Activities (UNFPA). http://www.unfpa.org/upload/lib_pub_file/221_filename_swp2003_eng.pdf, cited 27 August 2008

United Nations (2006a) World Population Prospects: The 2006 Revision and World Urbanization Prospects. New York: United Nations, Population Division of the Department of Economic and Social Affairs of the United Nations Secretariat. http://esa.un.org/unpp/, cited 8 August 2008

United Nations (2006b) In-Depth Study on All Forms of Violence Against Women. Report of the Secretary-General. United Nations Document A/61/122/Add.1/Corr.1. Division of Advancement of Women. http://daccessdds.un.org/doc/UNDOC/GEN/N06/623/30/PDF/N0662330.pdf?OpenElement, cited 8 August 2008

Willett W, Koplan, Nugent R et al. (2006) Prevention of chronic disease by means of diet and lifestyle changes. In: Jamison D et al. (eds.), Disease Control Priorities in Developing Countries, 2nd ed. New York: Oxford University Press

World Bank (2003) Adolescent Nutrition at a Glance. http://web.worldbank.org/WBSITE/EXTERNAL/TOPICS/EXTHEALTHNUTRITIONANDPOPULATION/EXTNUTRITION/0,contentMDK:20206757~menuPK:282592~pagePK:210058~piPK:210062~theSitePK:282575,00.html, cited 8 August 2008

World Bank (2006a) Repositioning Nutrition as Central to Development: A Strategy for Large-Scale Action. Washington, DC: World Bank. http://siteresources.worldbank.org/NUTRITION/Resources/281846-1131636806329/NutritionStrategy.pdf, cited 8 August 2008

World Bank (2006b) World Development Report 2007: Development and the Next Generation. Washington, DC: World Bank. http://siteresources.worldbank.org/INTWDR2007/Resources/1489782-1158107976655/overview.pdf, cited 8 August 2008

World Health Organization (WHO) (1980) Regional Working Group on Health Needs of Adolescents: Final Report. WHO Document: ICP/MCH/005. Manila: World Health Organization. Regional Office for the Western Pacific

World Health Organization (WHO) (1999) Programming for Adolescent Health and Development. Report of a WHO/UNFPA/UNICEF Study Group on Programming for Adolescent Health. Technical Report 886. Geneva: World Health Organization

World Health Organization (WHO) (2001a) Global Status Report: Alcohol and Young People. Geneva: World Health Organization. WHO Document WHO/MSD/MSB/01.1 http://whqlibdoc.who.int/hq/2001/WHO_MSD_MSB_01.1.pdf, cited 8 August 2008

World Health Organization (WHO) (2001b) The Second Decade: Improving Adolescent Health and Development. Geneva: World Health Organization. WHO Document WHO/FRH/ADH/98.18. http://www.who.int/child-adolescent-health/New_Publications/ADH/WHO_FRH_ADH_98.18.pdf, cited 8 August 2008

World Health Organization (WHO) (2002) World Report on Violence and Health. Geneva: World Health Organization. http://www.who.int/violence_injury_prevention/violence/world_report/en/full_en.pdf, cited 8 August 2008

World Health Organization (WHO) (2003) WHO Framework Convention on Tobacco Control. Geneva: World

Health Organization. http://www.who.int/tobacco/framework/WHO_FCTC_english.pdf, cited 8 August 2008

World Health Organization (WHO) (2004) Global School-Based Student Health Survey (GSHS). Geneva: World Health Organization. http://www.who.int/school_youth_health/assessment/gshs/en/, cited 8 August 2008

World Health Organization (WHO) (2004) Global Status Report on Alcohol 2004. Geneva: World Health Organization. http://www.who.int/substance_abuse/publications/alcohol/en/index.html, cited 8 August 2008

World Health Organization (WHO) (2005a) WHO Multi-Country Study on Women's Health and Domestic Violence Against Women. Geneva: World Health Organization. http://www.who.int/gender/violence/who_multicountry_-study/en/index.html, cited 8 August 2008

World Health Organization (WHO) (2005b) Nutrition in Adolescence – Issues and Challenges for the Health Sector: Issues in Adolescent Health and Development. WHO discussion papers on adolescence, 1–32. Geneva: World Health Organization. http://www.who.int/gender/violence/who_multicountry_study/en/index.html, cited 8 August 2008

World Health Organization (WHO) (2007a) Global Burden of Disease Database. Geneva: World Health Organization. http://www.who.int/whosis/data/Search.jsp?indicators = [Indicator].[MBD].Members, cited 8 August 2008

World Health Organization (WHO) (2007b) Global Strategy for the Prevention and Control of Sexually Transmitted Infections: 2006–2015. Geneva: World Health Organization. http://who.int/reproductive-health/publications/stisstrategy/stis_strategy.pdf, cited 8 August 2008

World Health Organization (WHO) (2007c) Human Papillomavirus and HPV Vaccines. Technical Information for Policy Makers and Health Professionals. Geneva: World Health Organization. http://www.who.int/vaccines-documents/DocsPDF07/866.pdf, cited 8 August 2008

World Health Organization (2007d) Youth and Road Safety. Geneva: World Health Organization. http://whqlibdoc.who.int/publications/2007/9241595116_eng.pdf, cited 8 August 2008

World Health Organization and Joint United Nations Programme on HIV/AIDS (UNAIDS) (2007) New data on male circumcision and HIV prevention: policy and programme implications. In: WHO/UNAIDS Technical Consultation Male Circumcision and HIV Prevention: Research Implications for Policy and Programming. http://data.unaids.org/pub/Report/2007/mc_recommendations_en.pdf, cited 8 August 2008

World Health Organization and United Nations Fund for Population Activities (UNFPA) (2006a) Pregnant Adolescents: Delivery on Global Promises of Hope. Geneva: World Health Organization. http://www.who.int/child-adolescent-health/New_Publications/ADH/ISBN_92_4_159378_4.pdf, cited 8 August 2008

World Health Organization and United Nations Fund for Population Activities (UNFPA) (2006b) Preparing for the Introduction of HPV Vaccines: Policy and Programme Guidance for Countries. Geneva: World Health Organization. http://www.who.int/reproductive-health/publications/hpvvaccines/text.pdf, cited 8 August 2008

World Health Organization (WHO)/United Nations Fund for Population Activities (UNFPA) (2006) Pregnant adolescent: delivering on global promises of hope. Geneva:/New York: WHO/UNFPA. http://whqlibdoc.who.int/publications/2006/9241593784_eng.pdf, cited 27 August 2008

Chapter 25
The Global Burden of Child Maltreatment

Andrea Gottsegen Asnes and John M. Leventhal

Learning Objectives After reading this chapter and answering the discussion questions that follow, you should be able to

- Identify types of child maltreatment and discuss the scope of the problem from a global perspective.
- Discuss the challenges of establishing a universally acceptable operational definition of child maltreatment.
- Analyze risk factors for child maltreatment, including those that relate to the child, parents, family, and society.
- Evaluate measures for prevention of child maltreatment at the individual child level, parent–child relationship level, community and societal levels.

Introduction

Physical and emotional maltreatment, sexual abuse, neglect and negligent treatment of children, as well as their commercial and other exploitation constitute a health challenge that is prevalent in all parts of the world. While deaths associated with child maltreatment represent only the tip of iceberg, millions of children are victims of non-fatal abuse and neglect. Ill-health associated with child abuse contributes significantly to the global burden of diseases among children and increases their predisposition to serious illnesses in adulthood. This chapter

presents an overview of the global problem of child maltreatment. The chapter begins with an examination of the challenges in building a consensus on a universal operational definition of child maltreatment. Types of childhood maltreatment and the scope of the problem are analyzed from a global perspective. The health and economic consequences of the problem are reviewed as are the concomitant risk factors, including child factors, parental factors, family factors, and societal factors. The chapter concludes with an appraisal of strategies for prevention, highlighting action at (i) the societal and community level (e.g., promotion of social, economic, and cultural rights; reducing income and gender inequalities; and eradicating cultural acceptance of violent or exploitative behavior toward children); (ii) the relationship level (e.g., early and frequent home visiting by trained providers who are able to establish a relationship with the parent(s) and teach effective parenting, and (iii) the individual level (e.g., education of children about how to avoid unsafe situations and protect themselves when confronted with threatening situations. This strategy may be most useful in the prevention of child sexual abuse).

Child maltreatment, including physical, sexual, and emotional abuse, neglect, and exploitation, occurs every day and in every corner of the world. Although repeatedly documented in various forms throughout history, child abuse was not recognized as a distinct public health problem until the early 1960s. In 1962, a landmark article entitled "The Battered Child Syndrome" was published in the United States (Kempe et al. 1962). Although previously published scholarly works had addressed inflicted injuries in children, this article (Kempe et al. 1962) was the first to estimate the

A.G. Asnes (✉)
Yale University School of Medicine, New Haven, Connecticut, USA

J.E. Ehiri (ed.), *Maternal and Child Health*, DOI 10.1007/b106524_25,
© Springer Science+Business Media, LLC 2009

incidence of child abuse and to identify the key characteristics of children who were physically abused. Notably, this publication led to public policy in the form of the adoption of a set of laws that mandate the report of child abuse in the United States. In addition, this milestone ignited international interest in child maltreatment that recently culminated in the publication of both *the United Nations Secretary-General's Study on Violence Against Children* (United Nations 2005) and a guide to the prevention of child maltreatment jointly published by the World Health Organization (WHO 2006b) and the International Society for Prevention of Child Abuse and Neglect (ISPCAN).

Defining child maltreatment in an international framework presents challenges not least because of the difficulties in distinguishing between what constitutes discipline or punishment (Box 25.1) across cultures, and even among individual families in the same culture.

Box 25.1 Discipline or Punishment?

Discipline involves training and developing a child's judgment, boundaries, self-control, social conduct, and self-sufficiency. This can be confused with punishment. Corporal punishment is often inappropriately used in an attempt to correct and change a child's behavior. The differences between discipline and punishment are numerous. A child's individual worth should be recognized in positive strategies of discipline. These strategies aim to "strengthen children's belief in themselves and their ability to behave appropriately and to build positive relationships" and should be thought out and intended to encourage a child to understand the expectations of their behavior. However, in punishment a caregiver's anger and desperation is often reflected in the physical and/or emotional punishment of a child. This punishment uses external controls, involves power and dominance, and is frequently not tailored to the child's age and/or developmental level.

Source: World Health Organization (1999)

In 1999, the World Health Organization convened a group of experts on child maltreatment that arrived at the following definition: "Child abuse or maltreatment constitutes all forms of physical and/or emotional ill-treatment, sexual abuse, neglect or negligent treatment or commercial or other exploitation, resulting in actual or potential harm to the child's health, survival, development, or dignity in the context of a relationship of responsibility, trust or power" (WHO 1999). Awareness of differences between developed and developing nations, as well as circumstances present in conflict-ridden nations, is reflected in the fact that the WHO preceded this definition with the following "preamble": "Background or baseline conditions beyond the control of families or caretakers, such as poverty, inaccessible healthcare, inadequate nutrition, unavailability of education can be contributing factors to child abuse. Social upheaval and instability, conflict and war may also contribute to increases in child abuse and neglect" (WHO 1999)

It is notable that prominent recent efforts to address child maltreatment on an international level have focused on defining child maltreatment itself as a primary goal. A unified definition of child maltreatment is widely believed to be crucial to international attempts to address and eradicate child abuse. It is thought that until such a definition can be identified, participation in eradication efforts by countries in which some abusive behaviors toward children are thought to be appropriate will be sorely limited. Cultural and regional variations in the definition of child abuse and neglect are reflected in the responses to a questionnaire developed by ISPCAN. The questionnaire addressed major behaviors included in a country's perception of child maltreatment, the extent of professional response to maltreatment, the scope and availability of interventions to address maltreatment, the public's awareness of the child abuse problem, major barriers to improving the response to maltreatment, and strengths and strategies in preventing maltreatment. Active ISPCAN members with access to national perspectives and data were invited to respond to the survey. Although every country that responded to the questionnaire in 2006 ($N = 72$) agreed that physical and sexual abuse by a parent or caretaker should be considered child abuse, significant variation was noted with respect to specific behaviors, such as the failure to secure medical treatment based on religious beliefs, corporal punishment, or female circumcision (Daroh 2006).

Practices and beliefs regarding corporal punishment provide a good example of the importance of defining what constitutes abusive behavior as opposed to acceptable parenting practice and why a clear definition of child maltreatment is important. Corporal punishment is common and socially acceptable in many societies throughout the world. *The United Nations Secretary-General's Study on Violence Against Children* estimates that between 80 and 98% of children worldwide suffer corporal punishment in their homes and that a third or more of these children are severely punished using implements (United Nations 2005). In the past, an unwill-

value presents enormous difficulty. Of the 72 countries that responded to the questionnaire developed by ISPCAN, only 48.6% of all respondents reported that corporal punishment is considered abusive in their country (WHO 1999). That over one-half of those countries who participated in the survey consider corporal punishment in the home to be an acceptable child-rearing practice highlights the degree to which such a behavior can be ingrained in the culture of a society. The World Health Organization's definition of child maltreatment includes five basic categories of child abuse: physical abuse, sexual abuse, emotional abuse, neglect, and exploitation. Each category requires further definition and will be considered separately. Fig. 25.1 depicts the typology of violence. Although this typology reflects all kinds of interpersonal vio-

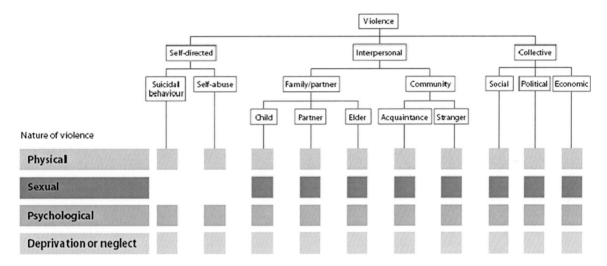

Fig. 25.1 A typology of violence. Source: WHO (2006)

ingness to overstep cultural boundaries in defining such practice as abusive has limited the evolution of a global definition of physical abuse. The United Nations Secretary-General's Study addresses and attempts to dismiss the possibility of an accepted tradition of violence toward children by stating, "the study should mark a turning point – an end to adult justification of violence against children, whether accepted as 'tradition' or disguised as 'discipline'" (United Nations 2005). While the advancement of a universal definition of child abuse is valuable, changing behavior in communities where this practice is a deeply felt cultural

lence, this chapter focuses on one aspect of this typology – that related to child abuse.

Physical Abuse

Box 25.2 presents an overview of some of the common manifestations of child abuse and neglect. A physically abused child can broadly be defined as "any child who receives a non-accidental physical injury as a result of acts . . . on the part of his parents or guardians" (Kempe and Helfer 1972). Some

Box 25.2 Common Manifestations of Child Abuse and Neglect

Manifestations of child abuse and neglect: Injuries inflicted by a caregiver on a child can take many forms. Serious damage or death in abused children is most often the consequence of a head injury or injury to the internal organs. Head trauma as a result of abuse is the most common cause of death in young children, with children in the first 2 years of life being the most vulnerable. Because force applied to the body passes through the skin, patterns of injury to the skin can provide clear signs of abuse. The skeletal manifestations of abuse include multiple fractures at different stages of healing, fractures of bones that are very rarely broken under normal circumstances, and characteristic fractures of the ribs and long bones.

   The shaken infant: Shaking is a prevalent form of abuse seen in very young children. The majority of shaken children are less than 9 months old. Most perpetrators of such abuse are male, though this may be more a reflection of the fact that men, being on average stronger than women, tend to apply greater force, rather than that they are more prone than women to shake children. Intracranial hemorrhages, retinal hemorrhages, and small "chip" fractures at the major joints of the child's extremities can result from very rapid shaking of an infant. They can also follow from a combination of shaking and the head hitting a surface. There is evidence that about one-third of severely shaken infants die and that the majority of the survivors suffer long-term consequences such as mental retardation, cerebral palsy, or blindness.

   The battered child: One of the syndromes of child abuse is the "battered child." This term is generally applied to children showing repeated and devastating injury to the skin, skeletal system, or nervous system. It includes children with multiple fractures of different ages, head trauma, and severe visceral trauma, with evidence of repeated infliction. Fortunately, though the cases are tragic, this pattern is rare.

Sexual abuse

   Children may be brought to professional attention because of physical or behavioral concerns that, on further investigation, turn out to result from sexual abuse. It is not uncommon for children who have been sexually abused to exhibit symptoms of infection, genital injury, abdominal pain, constipation, chronic or recurrent urinary tract infections, or behavioral problems. To be able to detect child sexual abuse requires a high index of suspicion and familiarity with the verbal, behavioral, and physical indicators of abuse. Many children will disclose abuse to caregivers or others spontaneously, though there may also be indirect physical or behavioral signs.

   Neglect: There exist many manifestations of child neglect, including non-compliance with healthcare recommendations, failure to seek appropriate health care, deprivation of food resulting in hunger, and the failure of a child physically to thrive. Other causes for concern include the exposure of children to drugs and inadequate protection from environmental dangers. In addition, abandonment, inadequate supervision, poor hygiene, and being deprived of an education have all been considered as evidence of neglect.

Source: Krug et al. (2002)

define physical abuse as "physical injury (ranging from minor bruises to severe fractures or death) as a result of punching, beating, kicking, biting, shaking, throwing, stabbing, choking, hitting (with a hand, stick, strap, or other object), burning, or otherwise harming a child. Such injury is considered abuse regardless of whether the caretaker intended to hurt the child" (Child Welfare Information Gateway 2006).

   Another definition suggests that a child need not sustain an actual injury to be seen as physically abused. The World Health Organization contends that physical abuse is defined as "the intentional use of physical force against a child that results in – or has a high likelihood of resulting in – harm for the child's health, survival, development or dignity" (WHO 2006).

Sexual Abuse

At its broadest level, sexual abuse can be defined as "the involvement of dependent, developmentally immature children and adolescents in sexual activities that they do not fully comprehend, to which they are unable to give informed consent, or that violate the social taboos of family roles" (Kempe 1978). More simply, sexual abuse can be understood as any sexual contact between an adult and a minor or between two minors when one uses power over the other. Sexual abuse can take many forms. These can include rape, fondling, exhibition, voyeurism, exposure to pornography, and communicating in a sexual manner either directly or by mail, phone, or Internet.

Emotional Abuse

Emotional abuse can be defined as "a pattern of behavior that impairs a child's emotional development or sense of self-worth. This may include constant criticism, threats, or rejection" (Child Welfare Information Gateway 2006). Emotional abuse, or psychological maltreatment, can be seen as distinct from emotional neglect, as in the withholding of love, support, or guidance from a child. Emotional abuse has been defined as a repeated pattern of damaging interaction between parent(s) and child that becomes typical of a relationship. This form of interaction conveys to a child that he or she is "worthless, flawed, unloved, unwanted, endangered, or only of value in meeting another's needs" (Kairys and Johnson 2002). Behaviors that transmit these messages include spurning, terrorizing, ignoring, rejecting, and isolating children, as well as providing inconsistent parenting or exposing children to intimate partner violence. Emotional abuse is a critical component of all other forms of child abuse, and the emotional impact of physical violence or

sexual abuse toward a child may be more severe than the physical aspect and, certainly, more long lasting. By itself, emotional abuse leaves no physical evidence and can be difficult for a child to disclose to others. When emotionally abusive behavior is normalized within a family, an understanding that the behavior is not appropriate may elude a child. Unlike children who are physically abused and may have physical evidence of abuse, emotionally abused children may offer few clues that they are ill-treated at home. For this reason it is thought that emotional abuse may be the most underreported form of child maltreatment.

Neglect

Child neglect is best defined in terms of the basic needs of children. Some needs are material and include adequate food, shelter, and clothing. Also vital are children's needs for education and medical care. Less tangible are children's needs for love, nurturance, guidance, supervision, and protection. If one imagines the provision of each of these needs along a spectrum, it is easy to imagine the absolute absence and absolute presence of each. Difficulties arise toward the middle, where deciding what constitutes actual neglect becomes debatable. The term neglect implies a failure on the part of caretakers to provide adequately for their children. Clearly, poverty and/or lack of education can result in neglectful conditions for a child. Well-meaning and loving parents who are significantly impoverished may be unable to provide for even the most basic of their children's needs. Societal and environmental factors must be taken into account when assessing individual cases of neglect.

Exploitation

The exploitation of a child refers to the use of the child in work or other activities for the benefit of others. Examples of the exploitation of children are child labor and commercial sexual exploitation of children, as well as child trafficking. Child labor is more challenging to define because children may be employed in safe and age-appropriate positions that do not by definition infringe on their other basic needs. Exploitative child labor has been defined by UNICEF as "children...doing things that are harmful to their healthy development [such as] laboring long hours, sacrificing time and energy that they might have spent at school or at home, enjoying the free and formative experience of childhood" (UNICEF 2006). Commercial sexual exploitation of children can be defined as "children engaging in sexual activities for money, profit, or any other consideration due to coercion or influence by any adult, syndicate or group" (UNICEF 2006). Children may be directly forced to labor or engage in sexual activities by adults in order to earn money. They may also be indirectly driven to such activities to survive if they have left otherwise abusive or neglectful conditions at home and are living on the streets.

The Worldwide Scope of Child Abuse and Neglect

Reliable, international statistics for child abuse and neglect are not available. Definitional variations in child maltreatment contribute to the difficulty of accumulating reliable data, as does the variation in the record keeping policies and practices between different nations. Recent attempts to focus worldwide attention on the problem of child maltreatment share a primary goal of more systematic collection of data on child abuse throughout the world. Data on child maltreatment can be collected in several ways, each with advantages and disadvantages. One strategy to collect information is to examine official reports from child protective services, if they exist, or from law enforcement agencies who investigate crimes against children. These data, while important, are likely to underestimate actual numbers of maltreated children because they represent only cases that have been reported or otherwise come to attention of local officials. Furthermore, in countries where physical punishment is not considered to be child abuse, cases of children physically harmed by parents in the name of discipline are not likely to be tabulated. Another

approach is to review child fatality records, but the reported numbers of fatally abused children in a given time period is likely to be small, and numbers are likely to underestimate the phenomenon of child homicides.

Another strategy used to collect data on child maltreatment is the use of interviews of parents about how they care for their own children. For example, in a cross-national collaborative study, investigators in Chile, Egypt, India, and the Philippines queried mothers between 1997 and 2003 about discipline practices. During the 6 months prior to being asked, mothers reported that they hit a child with an object not on the buttocks at incidence rates between 4 and 36%. In Egypt, beating a child within the last 6 months reportedly occurred at a rate of 25%, while in rural India, 10% of mothers reported kicking a child (Krug et al. 2002). Adults also may be interviewed about how they were cared for when they were children. This approach can provide an estimate of the prevalence of the problem. In a random survey of 2,869 young adults conducted in the United Kingdom in 1998 and 1999, 16% of the respondents reported that they had experienced some form of child maltreatment. Serious maltreatment was experienced by 7% of respondents for physical abuse, 6% for emotional abuse, 6% for absence of care, 5% for absence of supervision, and 11% of respondents reported sexual abuse involving contact (May-Chahal and Cawson 2005). Studies of this kind may both underestimate and overestimate the true prevalence levels of child abuse and neglect. Maltreatment occurring during childhood has been found to be underreported in some studies, and adults may not clearly remember events that took place when they were 5 years old or younger (Fergusson et al. 2000). Given that most serious physical abuse occurs in children 3 years old and younger, adults recalling their own childhoods may be likely to underestimate their abuse histories. On the other hand, reporting adults may exaggerate what happened to them as children, and no objective data are available to verify an individual's report.

The United Nations Secretary-General's Study on Violence against Children highlights some early efforts to quantify the problem of child abuse and neglect throughout the world. The study notes that the World Health Organization has used only those data collected by countries themselves to estimate that approximately 53,000 children died worldwide as a result of homicide in 2002 (United Nations 2005). Younger children are killed at significantly higher rates throughout the world than are older children. WHO estimates that children younger than 5 years old are killed at twice the rate of children 5–14 years old. Rates of child fatalities from abuse also vary according to the economic status of the country or region analyzed. The lowest rates are found in high-income countries, and the highest rates are found in the poorest regions. In the WHO Africa Region, 17.9/100,000 boys under the age of 5 years and 12.7/100,000 girls under the age of 5 years were killed (Krug et al. 2002). In contrast, in the United States, child homicides occurred at a rate of 2.04/100,000 children in 2006. Based on data from 39 states, more than three-quarters (78.0%) of children who were killed were younger than 4 years of age. Infant boys (younger than 1 year) had a fatality rate of 18.5 deaths per 100,000 boys of the same age, and infant girls had a fatality rate of 14.7 per 100,000 girls of the same age (U.S. Department of Health and Human Services 2007).

However, the number of fatally abused children in a given time period is likely to be underestimated. Variation in the degree to which child deaths are investigated or even reported contributes significantly to this problem. Undercounting is a significant problem in developed countries as well. For example, a study done in the United States retrospectively analyzed medical examiner data from one state over a 10-year period and found that the state's vital records system underrecorded the coding of child deaths due to battering or abuse by 58.7% (Herman-Giddens et al. 1999). Documenting the numbers of nonfatally abused children throughout the world is significantly more difficult than that of fatally abused children. In the United States in 2006, an estimated 905,000 children were found to be victims of maltreatment in the 52 states (Administration for Children and Families 2008). Not only are these data not routinely collected throughout the world, but what is documented

as maltreatment is likely to consistently undercount the extent of the phenomenon. Physical abuse, for example, in most countries in the world, exists at one end of a spectrum with physical punishment at the other end. As noted by the UN secretary general, when societies condone any form of violence against children, drawing a line between acceptable violence and abusive violence presents a sometimes insurmountable challenge. The subject may fall irretrievably under the category of "private" behavior and, therefore, be unavailable for public scrutiny. If, for example, corporal punishment is seen as acceptable within a culture, setting a standard for what constitutes excessive physical punishment may not be possible. A behavior similar to corporal punishment, in that it is seen as an acceptable practice in some countries and cultures, is that of female "circumcision." UNICEF estimates that in sub-Saharan Africa, Egypt, and the Sudan, 3 million girls and women are subjected to genital cutting/mutilation every year (Ezzati et al. 2004).

The WHO estimates that 150 million girls and 73 million boys under the age of 18 years experienced forced sexual intercourse or other forms of sexual violence during 2002 (UNICEF 2005). Given that sexual abuse of children is often intra-familial and carries social stigma worldwide, it is likely that any approximation of its incidence is a significant underestimate. A different approach to understanding the extent of the problem is to study its prevalence by asking adults about their childhood experiences of sexual abuse. Such studies have been conducted in a variety of countries and cultures, and similar prevalence rates have been determined (Vogeltanz et al. 1999). A review of 19 studies of adults completed in the United States or Canada found that the rates of sexual abuse reported by men were 3–16% and by women 3–62%. The review determined that a summary statistic for women of 20% would be reasonable (Finkelhor 1994). A project in Turkey (Alikasifoglu et al. 2006) used a cross-sectional design in a random sample of high school girls to determine that 13.4% of the girls in the sample reported some form of sexual abuse in childhood, and a study of adult women interviewed in El Salvador found that 17% reported a childhood experience of sexual abuse (Barthauer and Leventhal 1999).

The International Labor Organization estimated in 2002 that 218 million children worldwide could be classified as "child laborers" (International Labor Organization 2002b). Child laborers are a subgroup of those children engaged in "economic activity." Child laborers exclude those children at least 12 years old who work for a few hours a week in light work activities and those children at least 15 years old whose work is not classified as "hazardous." "Hazardous work" is defined as any activity or occupation that "has or leads to adverse effects on the child's safety, health (physical or mental) and moral development." In 2004, the International Labor Organization estimated that 126 million children were engaged in hazardous work (Child Labor Coalition). A sub-classification of hazardous work has been designated by the International Labor Organization as "unconditional worst forms of child labor." These include

a) "all forms of slavery or practices similar to slavery, such as the sale or trafficking of children, debt bondage and serfdom and forced or compulsory labor, including forced or compulsory recruitment of children for use in armed combat;
b) the use, procuring or offering a child for prostitution, for the production of pornography, or for pornographic performances;
c) the use, procuring or offering a child for illicit activities, in particular for the production or trafficking of drugs as defined in the relative international treaties..." (International Labor Organization 2006a).

The International Labor Organization estimated that in 2000, 5.7 million children were in forced or bonded labor, 1.8 million children were engaged in prostitution or pornography, and 1.2 million children were victims of trafficking (International Labor Organization 2002). As striking as these statistics are, they are likely to under-represent the full extent of the global burden of child maltreatment. Infrastructures for tracking child abuse vary enormously; even in developed countries with sophisticated data collection systems, many cases of child maltreatment go unreported, and in countries where no such infrastructure exists, the quantification of child abuse becomes extremely difficult.

Consequences of Child Abuse and Neglect

Health Consequences and Mortality

The immediate health consequences of child abuse are multiple. Table 25.1 presents an overview of the consequences of child abuse and neglect. Infants who survive abusive head trauma have extremely high rates of brain damage and subsequent neurological disability, including blindness, seizure disorders, mental retardation, and paralysis. Even infants who have survived abusive head trauma without major neurological

Table 25.1 Consequences of child abuse and neglect

Physical
　　Abdominal/thoracic injuries
　　Brain injuries
　　Bruises and welts
　　Burns and scalds
　　Central nervous system injuries
　　Disability
　　Fractures
　　Lacerations and abrasions
　　Ocular damage
Sexual and reproductive
　　Reproductive health problems
　　Sexual dysfunction
　　Sexually transmitted diseases, including HIV/AIDS
　　Unwanted pregnancy
Psychological and behavioral
　　Alcohol and drug abuse
　　Cognitive impairment
　　Delinquent, violent, and other risk-taking behaviors
　　Depression and anxiety
　　Developmental delays
　　Eating and sleep disorders
　　Feelings of shame and guilt
　　Hyperactivity
　　Poor relationships
　　Poor school performance
　　Poor self-esteem
　　Post-traumatic stress disorder
　　Psychosomatic disorders
　　Suicidal behavior and self-harm
Other longer-term health consequences
　　Cancer
　　Chronic lung disease
　　Fibromyalgia
　　Irritable bowel syndrome
　　Ischemic heart disease
　　Liver disease
　　Reproductive health problems such as infertility

Source: Krug et al. (2002)

deficit may go on to manifest high rates of cognitive and behavioral dysfunction as they age. Inflicted burns can result in disfiguring scars and restriction of mobility if the skin over moving joints is involved. Long bone fractures that are not properly cared for may result in permanent physical disability. Children who are sexually abused can contract sexually transmitted infections that may impair future fertility or be in and of themselves life threatening, as in the case of HIV/AIDS. Sexually abused girls may become pregnant and incur the health risks associated with pregnancy, a significant burden particularly in developing countries.

Striking long-term consequences of childhood maltreatment that have been repeatedly documented in the literature are adult ill-health (including both physical and mental health problems) and adult engagement in high-risk health behaviors. Adult survivors of childhood abuse suffer at significantly higher rates than others from depression, anxiety disorders, eating disorders, posttraumatic stress disorder, chronic pain syndromes, fibromyalgia, chronic fatigue syndrome, and irritable bowel syndrome. Adults who were abused as children report lower health status and higher use of health services than non-abused adults. The actual worldwide burden of child maltreatment is difficult to estimate. Recently, the World Health Organization analyzed the global and regional burden of diseases attributable to selected risk factors. Among these risk factors was child sexual abuse. Across the world, child sexual abuse is estimated to have contributed to between 4 and 5% of the burden of disease in males and 7 and 8% of the burden of disease in females for depression, alcohol abuse, and drug abuse (Ezzati et al. 2004). These estimations are derived from analyses of available literature describing the relationship between child sexual abuse and adult manifestations of depression and substance abuse.

Furthermore, adults maltreated as children are more likely to be obese or physically inactive, to engage in smoking, substance use, and unsafe sex, to attempt suicide, and to have an unintended pregnancy than non-abused adults (Springer et al. 2003). Possibly because of the link between childhood trauma and high-risk health behaviors, it has been shown that the more adverse experiences an adult had as a child, the more likely that adult is to have heart disease, cancer, stroke, diabetes, skeletal fractures, liver disease, and generally poor health (Felitti et al. 1998). The evidence concerning the links between child maltreatment, high-risk behaviors, poor mental health, and poor physical health suggests a complex interplay between each of these factors.

Financial Costs

The costs associated with child maltreatment are difficult to assess. There are direct costs associated with the immediate medical needs of children who have been physically harmed. There is the tremendous cost of ongoing health care for children with major disability, both physical and mental, that is the direct result of child maltreatment. There are costs associated with the lost yield of children who die prematurely or become physically or mentally disabled as a consequence of child maltreatment. The World Health Organization has summarized the sources of costs incurred by systems responsible for interacting with maltreated children and their families including

- "expenditures related to apprehending and prosecuting offenders,
- the costs to social welfare organizations of investigating reports of maltreatment and protecting children from abuse,
- costs associated with foster care,
- costs to the education system, and
- costs to the employment sector arising from absenteeism and low production" (Krug et al. 2002).

A recent effort to tally the annual direct and indirect costs of child abuse in the United States found that the yearly financial burden in the United States due to child maltreatment was US $103.8 billion. This included $6.6 billion for hospitalizations, $1.1 billion for mental health costs, $25.4 billion for child welfare costs, and $33 million in law enforcement costs. The cost of adult criminality related to child abuse was estimated to be $30 billion (Wang and Holton 2007). Add to these costs those of caring for adults with heart disease, cancer, and diabetes stemming for child abuse, whether directly or as a result of high-risk health behaviors known to be associated with childhood abuse, and these costs become staggering.

Risk Factors for Child Abuse and Neglect

Child maltreatment is a multi-factorial problem, and thus, no single factor can be identified as certain to lead to child maltreatment. Rather, multiple factors at both the individual and the societal level interact to produce this outcome. A helpful ecological model for the etiology of child maltreatment comes from Belsky (1993) who wrote that "there is no one pathway to disturbances in parenting; rather, maltreatment seems to arise when stressors outweigh supports and risks are greater than protective factors" (Belsky 1993). The stressors that can lead to child maltreatment can be broken down into child, parental, family, and societal factors.

Child Factors

The primary characteristic about an individual child most closely correlated with likelihood of maltreatment is the age of the child. Younger children, especially those under 3 years old, are significantly more likely to die from physical abuse throughout the world. Rates of nonfatal physical abuse vary from country to county, perhaps reflecting variation in cultural practices of corporal punishment. Younger children are most dependent on caretakers for meeting basic human needs and are thus most vulnerable to neglect. Peak rates of sexual abuse are thought to rise after the onset of puberty, but younger children are certainly victims of sexual abuse as well (Krug et al. 2002). Children born of unwanted pregnancies, multiple births (twins), and premature infants are at increased risk of child maltreatment. Children who are physically and/or mentally disabled, children who are chronically ill, as well as children who by means of temperament are seen as "needy" are also at increased risk (WHO 2006).

Parent Factors

It is widely believed that parents who were abused as children themselves are more likely than others to abuse their own children. A recent systematic review of the literature has raised concerns about the limited research data to support this claim (Ertem et al. 2000). It is likely that a personal history of maltreatment in childhood is but one of many factors that leads a parent to maltreat his or her own child. Abusive and neglecting parents are more likely to be young, poor, undereducated, and unemployed. They are also more likely to suffer from serious mental illness or retardation. Addiction and substance use by parents are known risk factors for child maltreatment. Substance use has been linked to higher rates of physical and sexual abuse, perhaps by lowering inhibitions and impairing judgment, as well as to higher rates of neglect. Parents who have unrealistic developmental expectations of their children and a poor capacity for empathy with children are more likely to abuse them.

Family Factors

Overcrowded households and especially households containing many small children can contribute to child maltreatment. Violent relationships between adults in a home are associated with violence toward children in the home. Families who are socially isolated and lack external supports are at risk, as are those households whose composition changes frequently. Parents who are prevented from establishing a good relationship with children for any reason, whether by virtue of a personal inability or an inability imposed by outside circumstances, are at increased risk of maltreating their children.

Societal Factors

Poverty is strongly correlated with child maltreatment, especially neglect. Parents living in poverty live with considerable stress that can have an impact on their ability to parent effectively in multiple ways. Poverty and unemployment are related to higher rates of substance use and abuse, as well as mental and physical illness in adults. Poor communities that lack resources and adequate infrastructure offer little or no support to parents with impaired ability to care for children. Desperately poor parents may send children to work in unsafe conditions or even indenture children as workers for others in order to survive. Cultural acceptance of violence contributes to higher rates of child maltreatment, as in the case of corporal punishment. The degree to which a culture values, or devalues, children also is an important societal level risk factor for maltreatment.

Prevention of Child Abuse and Neglect

Child maltreatment is not a new problem. Yet, only very recently has the prevention of child abuse and neglect come to international attention. On October 16, 2006, the World Health Organization issued a news release titled "World Health Organization says violence against children can and must be prevented" (WHO 2006). Efforts to address the issue by entities such as the World Health Organization, the United Nations, and UNICEF can certainly help to illuminate the scope of the problem and are an important first step. They can set an agenda for addressing the problem, as does the recently available guide to prevention of child abuse published jointly by the World Health Organization and the International Society for Prevention of Child Abuse and Neglect. The guide recommends that countries identify a lead agency whose primary purpose is the prevention of child maltreatment. The lead agency would then work to involve other agencies who work with families and children, such as child care services, neighborhood community centers, and religious institution, as well as the media. The lead agency would also take responsibility for preparing a national report on child maltreatment and efforts to prevent it (WHO 2006).

Specific prevention strategies proposed by the guide are stratified into three levels: societal and community, relationship, and individual prevention strategies. On a societal and community level, strategies include promoting social, economic, and

cultural rights, reducing income and gender inequalities, and eradicating cultural acceptance of violent or exploitative behavior toward children (WHO 2006). A sound argument can be made that while it would not rid the world of all child maltreatment, the establishment of worldwide social and economic equality would significantly decrease the amount of child maltreatment throughout the world. While it is beyond the scope of this chapter to offer strategies to combat poverty and social injustice, the degree to which these global problems contribute to child maltreatment must be highlighted. Another societal and community level strategy to prevent child maltreatment is the provision of both early childhood care and education as well as the provision of universal education through the secondary level. Finally, prevention of child maltreatment can be pursued by attempting to change cultural and social norms that support violence against children and adults. Cultural acceptance of certain forms of child maltreatment, such as severe physical punishment and female genital mutilation, can perhaps be addressed by public media and educational campaigns. The degree to which such campaigns are or can be successful is unknown. An example of a governmental effort to change parents' behavior comes from Sweden. In 1979, Sweden passed legislation that effectively abolished corporal punishment as a legitimate child-rearing practice. Recent research has shown that the 1979 legal reform in Sweden did not reduce the level of public support for parental use of corporal punishment as a means of disciplining children (Durrant 1999).

On a relationship level, failures in attachment between parents and children as well as inappropriate developmental expectations contribute significantly to child maltreatment. Single parents and parents who lack social support are more likely to abuse or neglect their children. It is perhaps not surprising, then, that among prevention programs that have been evaluated, home visiting programs are most successful. In order to be successful, however, home visiting must be initiated early, occur frequently, and be carried out by a person able both to establish a relationship with the parent(s) and to teach effective parenting. Such programs are expensive (Leventhal 1996), and in communities where basic social needs are unmet, such as in refugee communities or nations at war, a lofty goal indeed. Another relationship level strategy is the use of training programs in parenting for parents-to-be and new parents.

Children born of unwanted pregnancies, premature, and otherwise disabled children are at higher risk of maltreatment than others. Thus, individual level prevention strategies include the prevention of unwanted pregnancy and improved access to pre- and post-natal care. An additional individual level strategy for prevention is the direct education of children about how to avoid unsafe situations and protect themselves when confronted with a threatening situation (WHO 2006). This strategy may be most useful in the prevention of child sexual abuse. The prevention of child maltreatment is a relatively new and developing field. Child maltreatment was itself once an unrecognized problem. Strategies and programs to prevent child maltreatment are not fully tested in terms of measurable outcomes of success or failure. The identification of appropriate outcome measures is in itself a challenge. It has been proposed that in addition to obvious outcomes for child maltreatment prevention programs such as decreasing child deaths or rates of inflicted injury, protective factors be tracked, such as educational achievement or improved parental expectations of the developmental abilities of children (WHO 2006). The ability to identify and measure meaningful outcomes for child maltreatment prevention programs is crucial to the successful adoption and implementation of such programs. It is likely that only through documented changes in valued outcomes will governments dedicate the financial resources necessary to institutionalize worthwhile prevention efforts (Leventhal 2005).

Conclusions

Improved recognition and tracking of all forms of child maltreatment throughout the world have been identified as important steps in prevention. Epidemiologically sound data on the prevalence of child maltreatment and its consequences, once in hand,

can be used to assess the soundness of prevention programs as they are implemented. Given the huge global burden of child maltreatment, it is apparent that many teachers, heath professionals, social workers, and other professionals interact regularly with victims of child maltreatment, unaware of their plight, and therefore unable to help them. There is an urgent need for all sectors involved in child health promotion to build consensus on common conceptual and operational definitions of child maltreatment in order to facilitate better case detection and reporting. As with other public health problems, early detection and prompt intervention is necessary to prevent long-term health and social consequences of child maltreatment. As the WHO (2006) guide to action and evidence on child maltreatment asserts, professionals who interact on a regular basis with children need training that provides knowledge of

- Myths about child maltreatment
- Physical and behavioral signs of possible and definitive maltreatment – as well as signs that are indicative of maltreatment
- How to respond when possible maltreatment is indicated – including the use of protocols for involving supervisors, reporting cases, and making referrals
- Options for medical and psychosocial treatment of victims

It is germane to note that a number of indicators, algorithms, flowcharts, and checklists (e.g., Fig. 25.2) are currently available to facilitate early detection of child maltreatment. These indicators provide valuable resource for training of primary health-care workers, pediatricians, Emergency Department doctors and nurses. It is important that these tools are evaluated and assessed for their adaptation in various cultures and health-care settings, globally. Health policy makers in all countries must recognize and accord child maltreatment the importance that it deserves given its consequences over the life span. Frontline health and other professionals who are in regular contact with children also need to be assisted not only in identifying and reporting the problem but also in providing appropriate and timely treatment, prevention, and support services to victims.

Fig. 25.2 Simple intervention to improve detection of child abuse in emergency departments. Source: Benger and Pearce (2002)

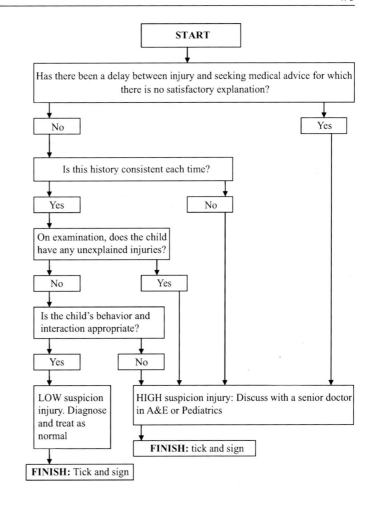

Key Terms

Battered child	Depression	Interpersonal violence
Behavioral dysfunction	Discipline	Long bone fractures
Blindness	Effective parenting	Mental retardation
Brain damage	Emotional abuse	Neglect
Child abuse	Emotional ill-treatment	Negligent treatment
Child factors	Emotional maltreatment	Non-fatally abused children
Child fatality records	Exploitation	Paralysis
Child labor	Exploitative behavior	Parental factors
Child laborers	Family factors	Permanent physical disability
Child maltreatment	Fatally abused children	Physical abuse
Child protective services	Female circumcision	Physical maltreatment
Childhood trauma	Female genital mutilation	Pornography
Cognitive dysfunction	Fondling	Prostitution
Commercial exploitation	Gender inequalities	Punishment
Corporal punishment	Hazardous work	Rape

Seizure	Spurning	Unintended pregnancy
Sexual abuse	Substance abuse	Unsafe sex
Shaken infant	Suicide	Voyeurism
Societal factors	Trafficking	

Questions for Discussion

1. What is child maltreatment? Distinguish between child discipline and corporal punishment.
2. Why is it important to establish a universally acceptable operational definition of child maltreatment? What are the barriers in achieving this?
3. Define the following and provide specific examples of each

   a. Physical abuse
   b. Sexual abuse
   c. Emotional abuse
   d. Neglect
   e. Exploitation

4. Outline the health consequences of child abuse and neglect.
5. List individual, family, community, and societal level strategies for preventing child abuse and neglect.

References

Administration for Children and Families (2008) Child maltreatment 2006. http://www.acf.hhs.gov/programs/cb/pubs/cm06/index.htm, cited 8 August 2008

Alikasifoglu M, Erginoz E, Ercan O et al. (2006) Sexual abuse among female high school students in Istanbul, Turkey. Child Abuse Negl, 30: 247–255

Barthauer LM, Leventhal JM (1999) Prevalence and effects of child sexual abuse in a poor, rural community in El Salvador: a retrospective study of women after 12 years of civil war. Child Abuse Negl, 23: 1117–1126

Belsky J (1993) Etiology of child maltreatment: a developmental-ecological analysis. Psychological Bulletin, 114: 413–434

Benger JR, Pearce V (2002) Simple intervention to improve detection of child abuse in emergency departments. British Medical J 324: 780

Child Labor Coalition (2008) Child labor around the world. Washington, DC: Child Labor Coalition. http://www.stopchildlabor.org/internationalchildlabor/claroundworld.htm, cited 8 August 2008

Child Welfare Information Gateway (2006) Child abuse and neglect. http://www.childwelfare.gov/can Cited 8 August 2008

Daroh D (ed.) (2006) World perspectives on child abuse. West Chicago, IL: The International Society for Prevention of Child Abuse and Neglect

Durrant JE (1999) Evaluating the success of Sweden's corporal punishment ban. Child Abuse Negl, 23: 435–448

Ertem IO, Leventhal JM, Dobbs S (2000) Intergenerational continuity of child physical abuse: how good is the evidence? Lancet, 356: 814–819

Ezzati M, Lopez AD, Rodgers A et al. (eds.) (2004) Comparative quantification of health risks; global and regional burden of disease attributable to selected major risk factors. Geneva: World Health Organization

Felitti,VJ, Anda, RF, Nordenberg D et al. (1998) Relationship of childhood abuse and household dysfunction to many of the leading causes of death in adults: the Adverse Childhood Experience (ACE) Study. Am J Prev Med, 14: 245–258

Fergusson DM, Horwood LJ, Woodward LJ (2000) The stability of child abuse reports: a longitudinal study of the reporting behaviour of young adults. Psychological Medicine, 30: 529–544

Finkelhor D (1994) Current information on the scope and nature of child sexual abuse. Future Child, 4: 31

Herman-Giddens ME, Brown G, Verbiest S et al. (1999) Under-ascertainment of child abuse mortality in the United States. Journal of the American Medical Association, 282: 463–467

International Labour Organization (2002a) A future without child labour, global report under the follow-up to the ILO declaration on fundamental principles and rights at work. International Labour Conference, 90th session, Report 1B. Geneva: ILO. www.ilo.org/dyn/declaris/DECLARATIONWEB.DOWNLOAD_BLOB?Var_DocumentID=1567, cited 8 August 2008

International Labour Organization (ILO) (2002b) Every child counts: new global estimates on child labour. Geneva: ILO, p. 25

International Labour Organization (2006a). The end of child labour: within reach: global report under the follow-up to the ILO declaration on fundamental principles and rights at work. International Labour Conference, 95th session, Report 1B: Geneva: ILO

International Labour Organization (ILO) (2006b) Global child labour trends 2000–2004. International Programme on the Elimination of Child Labor (IPEC) and Statistical information and Monitoring Programme on Child Labor (SIMPOC), International Labour Organization (ILO). Geneva: ILO. http://www.ilo.org/dyn/declaris/DECLARATIONWEB.DOWNLOAD_BLOB?Var_DocumentID=6233, cited 8 August 2008

Kairys SW, Johnson CF and the Committee on Child Abuse and Neglect (2002) The psychological maltreatment of children -technical report. Pediatrics, 109: e68

Kempe CH (1978) Sexual abuse, another hidden pediatric problem. Pediatrics, 62: 382–389

Kempe CH, Helfer RE (1972) Helping the battered child and his family. Philadelphia: JB Lippincott

Kempe CH, Silverman FN, Steele BF et al. (1962) The battered child syndrome. Journal of the American Medical Association, 18: 17–24

Krug EG, Dahlberg LL, Mercy JA (eds.) (2002) World report on violence and health. Geneva: World Health Organization

Leventhal JM (1996) Twenty years later: we do know how to prevent child abuse and neglect. Child Abuse Negl, 20: 647–653

Leventhal JM (2005) Getting prevention right: maintaining the status quo is not an option. Child Abuse Negl, 29: 209–231

May-Chahal C, Cawson P (2005) Measuring child maltreatment in the United Kingdom: a study of the prevalence of child abuse and neglect. Child Abuse Negl, 29: 969–984

Springer KW, Sheridan J, Kuo D et al. (2003) The long-term health outcomes of childhood abuse: an overview and a call to action. J Gen Intern Med, 18: 864–870

United Nations Children's Fund (UNICEF) (2005) Changing a harmful social convention: female genital mutilation/cutting. Innocenti Digest no. 12, Florence, UNICEF Innocenti Research Center

United Nations Children's Fund (UNICEF) (2006) UK's campaign to end child exploitation. http://www.unicef.org.uk/campaigns, cited 8 August 2008

United Nations (2005) The United Nations Secretary-General's study on violence against children. http://www.violencestudy.org/r25, cited 8 August 2008

U.S. Department of Health and Human Services (2007) Child maltreatment 2005. Washington DC: U.S. Department of Health and Human Services Administration on Children, Youth and Families. http://www.acf.hhs.gov/programs/cb/pubs/cm05/cm05.pdf, cited 8 August 2008

Vogeltanz ND, Wilsnack SC, Harris TR et al. (1999) Prevalence and risk factors for childhood sexual abuse in women; national survey findings. Child Abuse Negl, 23: 579–591

Wang CTT, Holton J (2007) Total estimated cost of child abuse and neglect in the United States. Prevent Child Abuse America. http://www.preventchildabuse.org/about_us/media_releases/pcaa_pew_economic_impact_study_final.pdf, cited 8 August 2008

World Health Organization (WHO) (1999) Report of the consultation on child abuse prevention, March 29–31. Geneva, World Health Organization

World Health Organization (WHO) (2006a) Global estimates of health consequences due to violence against children. Background paper for the United Nations study on violence against children. Geneva: World Health Organization

World Health Organization (WHO) (2006b) Preventing child maltreatment: a guide to taking action and generating evidence. Geneva, World Health Organization

World Health Organization (WHO) (2006c) World Health Organization says violence against children can and must be prevented. http://www.who.int/mediacentre/news/releases/2006/pr57/en/index.html, cited 8 August 2008

Chapter 26
Children in Difficult Circumstances

Nancy Mock and Elke de Buhr

Learning Objectives After reading this chapter and answering the discussion questions that follow, you should be able to

- Discuss the challenges in identifying and enumerating children in difficult circumstances.
- Analyze trends in the evolution of the problem of children in difficult circumstances and discuss its public health impact.
- Appraise the status of policies and programs to protect and promote the health of children in difficult circumstances.

Introduction

Children in difficult circumstances represent a large and diverse group. Some form of social disruption is common to all their lives. All of these children have special needs, especially the need for psychosocial support. Their other individual needs vary greatly as the children's specific circumstances are different and ever changing. The public health and medical management of children in difficult circumstances requires intersectoral coordination and a holistic approach to prevention and treatment. This chapter presents a review of definitional and methodological difficulties associated with identifying and enumerating children in difficult circumstances. It examines trends in the evolution of the problem and its public health impact and analyzes the status of policies and strategies to protect and promote the

N. Mock (✉)
International Health and International Development, Tulane University, New Orleans, LA, USA

health of children in difficult circumstances. Since the 1980 s, the public health community has increasingly recognized the needs of children and youth who face particularly difficult circumstances. These children are sometimes referred to as "Children in Especially Difficult Circumstances" (CEDC). These children work in exploitive situations, do not live with their biological or adopted families, and/or are involved in or affected by armed conflict. Categories of children include "street children," Orphans and Vulnerable Children (OVC), and children who are sexually exploited, trafficked, or forced to work at the cost of their education and health (UNICEF/UNAIDS/USAID 2004). While enumeration of children suffering the effects of difficult circumstances is fraught with definitional and methodological problems (Skinner et al. 2006), the global magnitude of children in difficult circumstances is large and is growing because of HIV/AIDS, armed conflict, urbanization, and other developments. For example, the estimated number of orphaned children in 2004 was 85.5 million in Asia and 43.4 million children in Latin America. As a result of HIV/AIDS, this number is expected to grow at least through the next decade (UNICEF 2006).

Although the incidence of violent conflict has been slowing recently, conflict continues to displace children from their families. Conflict may involve the use of child soldiers, increase a child's likelihood of orphanhood and migration as an unaccompanied minor, and/or increase the chance that he/she will be injured and disabled by land mines and other war-associated trauma (see Chapter 7 for discussion of conflict and maternal and child health). No statistical data documenting these affects are sufficiently reliable to report. However, millions of

J.E. Ehiri (ed.), *Maternal and Child Health*, DOI 10.1007/b106524_26,
© Springer Science+Business Media, LLC 2009

children are affected by conflict in the Middle East, Africa, Asia, and Latin America. It has been estimated that 300,000 children under 18 years of age are currently being exploited as child soldiers in armed conflicts worldwide (UNICEF 2006). The numbers of children living on the streets in cities are also not known (Volpe 2002). However, with urbanization, this number of street children is growing in most regions of the world. An increase in numbers of street children has been observed in many African cities (UNICEF 2003).

Child trafficking, sexual exploitation, and unacceptable circumstances of child labor affect millions of children worldwide. More than 317 million of the world's children between 5 and 17 years of age were estimated to be working in 2004. Of these, an estimated 217 million were involved in child labor, and 126 million were estimated to be engaged in hazardous work (Hagemann et al. 2006). In 2002, an estimated 5.7 million children were working as forced or bonded laborers, an estimated 1.2 million children per year are trafficked, and another 1.8 million per year are forced into commercial sexual exploitation (UNICEF 2006).

Definitions and Methodological Issues

The study of children in difficult circumstances is confounded by the breadth of the concept and inconsistent use of the terminology. Box 26.1 presents some common definitions and their sources. Difficult circumstances cover a broad range of problems that are often, but not always, caused by poverty. Frequently, but not always, they are associated with social dislocation from family and community. Many of the categories used to describe certain subpopulations of children in difficult circumstances are used differently by different organizations within the public health community. For example, the term "Orphans and Vulnerable Children" is frequently associated with HIV/AIDS among organizations working in the HIV/AIDS community. However, the term is more broadly applied to orphans and vulnerable children from all causes by other agencies. There is no widely accepted standard definition of the term "orphans and vulnerable children" (OVC). Definitions of

"orphan" tend to distinguish between paternal, maternal, and double orphans. The understanding of "vulnerable children" tends to be broad and poorly defined and may include a variety of different groups of children. The term "street children" also has various meanings and uses and is considered by many social scientists not to be helpful in describing a category of children (Ennew 2003). Children may literally live in the streets, work on the streets, or both. The terms "child work," "child labor," and "worst forms of child labor" are defined in detail by the International Labor Organization (ILO) but often confused in use. An additional problem is in defining the age range of childhood. Again, agencies and countries define eligibility differently, leading to non-comparable research and statistical data.

The concept of "vulnerable children" is used frequently in the context of children affected by AIDS, though the term vulnerability is widely used in the public health literature to identify children who are affected by poverty and other social risks/threats. AIDS orphans are often more vulnerable than other children as they are impacted by AIDS in a much broader sense. This impact often begins long before the death of one or both of their parents. However, vulnerability clearly is not limited to HIV/AIDS. A study by Skinner et al. (2006) suggests a range of factors that may play an important role in causing vulnerability, such as "severe chronic illness of a parent or caregiver, poverty, hunger, lack of access to services, inadequate clothing or shelter, overcrowding, deficient caretakers, and factors specific to the child, including disability, direct experience of physical or sexual violence, or severe chronic illness" (Skinner et al. 2006). More recently, the "vulnerable" group within the OVC rubric is being operationalized. For example, some of the more recent Demographic and Health Surveys (DHS) attempt to measure the category of "vulnerable children" in addition to the general orphan statistics. The Rwanda 2005 DHS (Institut National de la Statistique du Rwanda and ORC Macro 2006), for example, operationalized "vulnerable children" as (a) children "with a very ill parent" either living in the same household with the parent or not, (b) children "living in a household with a very ill adult," and (c) children living in a household with "an adult who died in the last 12 months" (Institut National de la

> ## Box 26.1 Definition of Terms
>
> **Orphan** – Orphan is typically defined as "a child under the age of 18 who has had at least one parent die. A child whose mother has died is known as a maternal orphan; a child whose father has died is a paternal orphan. A child who has lost both parents is a double orphan" (UNAIDS 2004).
>
> **Orphans Due to AIDS** – AIDS orphans are a subgroup within the general orphan population. According to UNAIDS, "a consensus was reached on the definition of an AIDS orphan as 'a child who has at least one parent dead from AIDS', and a dual (or double) AIDS orphan as 'a child whose mother and father have both died, at least one due to AIDS'" (UNAIDS Reference Group 2002).
>
> **Other Vulnerable Children** – According to UNICEF, the term "other vulnerable children" includes "those who are living with HIV/AIDS, those whose parents are sick with HIV/AIDS, and, more generally, children who are especially vulnerable because of poverty, discrimination or exclusion, whether as a consequence of HIV/AIDS or not" (UNICEF 2003).
>
> **Children Living on the Streets** – Street children have been defined by the United Nations as "boys and girls for whom 'the street' (including unoccupied dwellings, wasteland, etc.) has become their home and/or source of livelihood, and who are inadequately protected and supervised by responsible adults" (Wittig et al. 1997).
>
> **Working Children** – According to ILO (ILO 1999), child work is "defined in terms of economic activity. Economic activity covers all market production (paid work) and certain types of non-market production (unpaid work), including production of goods for own use" (Hagemann et al. 2006).
>
> **Child Labor** – ILO (ILO 2006) distinguishes child labor from child work. Child labor "comprises all children under 15 years of age who are economically active, excluding (i) those under 5 years of age and (ii) those aged 12–14 years who spend fewer than 14 hours a week on their jobs, unless their activities or occupations are hazardous by nature or circumstance. Added to this are children aged 15–17 years, who are involved in hazardous work" (Hagemann et al. 2006).
>
> **Worst Forms of Child Labor (WFCL)** – WFCL includes "all forms of slavery or practices similar to slavery" and "work which, by its nature or the circumstances in which it is carried out, is likely to harm the health, safety or morals of children" (International Labor Organization 1999).
>
> **Trafficked Children** – "The recruitment, transportation, transfer, harboring or receipt of a child for the purpose of exploitation is considered 'trafficking in persons'" (United Nations 2000b).
>
> **Forced and Bonded Labor** – "Any institution or practice whereby a child or young person under the age of 18 years, is delivered by either or both of his natural parents or by his guardian to another person, whether for reward or not, with a view to the exploitation of the child or young person or of his labor" (UN Supplemental Convention on the Abolition of Slavery (United Nations 1956)).

Statistique du Rwanda and ORC Macro 2006). For Rwanda, this resulted in a population of "orphans and vulnerable children" (OVC) of 25.6% among children younger than 15 years (17.5% orphans + 8.1% vulnerable children) and 28.6% among all children younger than 18 years (20.5% orphans + 8.1% vulnerable children) (Institut National de la Statistique du Rwanda and ORC Macro 2006).

Trends in the Magnitude of the Problem

Of all groups of children living in difficult circumstances, OVCs and working children, child labor, trafficked children, and sexually exploited children have been the most closely monitored over time. This resulted because of the major international programs aimed at supporting these children. Trends in OVC numbers and characteristics are directly influenced by key demographic indicators such as population growth. The general trend has been a decline in the absolute numbers of orphans in Asia and the Latin American and Caribbean regions. However, the number of orphans in Africa has been increasing and is projected to continue to grow (Fig. 26.1).

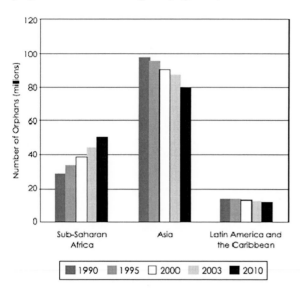

Fig. 26.1 Global trends in orphan numbers. Source: UNICEF/UNAIDS/USAID (2004)

Overall, 28% of these orphaned children are believed to be AIDS orphans. Regional differences within sub-Saharan Africa are considerable, with just 1% of AIDS orphans among all orphaned children in Mauritania and 78% AIDS orphans in Zimbabwe (Fig. 26.2). It has been estimated that 16% of all households in sub-Saharan Africa were caring for orphans between 1997 and 2002 (UNICEF 2003). Again, regional differences are significant. In southern Africa where HIV infection rates are the highest, 20% of all households were estimated to be involved in the care of orphaned children. Other parts of the continent reported this rate to be closer to 15% (UNICEF 2003). In all parts of Africa, the number of orphans per household is expected to continue to grow because of the impact of HIV/AIDS. With orphan numbers growing in HIV/AIDS-affected populations, the HIV/AIDS epidemic is responsible for reversing the global trend of stagnant or decreasing numbers of orphan populations. In sub-Saharan Africa the

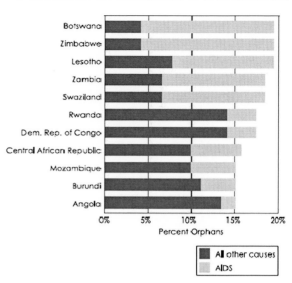

Fig. 26.2 Percent of children orphaned by AIDS versus all other causes in countries with more than 15% orphans. Source: UNICEF/UNAIDS/USAID (2004)

number of orphans is expected to grow by 20 million between 1990 and 2010, while a drop of almost 20 million is expected in Asia during the same period of time. The total number of orphans in Latin America and the Caribbean is expected to remain relatively stable (UNICEF/UNAIDS/USAID 2004).

Methods for Estimating Categories of Children in Difficult Circumstances

It is often a challenge to enumerate children in difficult circumstances while using traditional methods that are used in demographic and health assessments such as the Demographic and Health Surveys (DHS) and the UNICEF Multiple Indicator Cluster Surveys (MICS). These children may not live in households, which are the unit for many enumeration techniques. Instead, the children may live in institutions, on the streets, or they are otherwise on the move. They may be living in communities, but they may still not be included in sampling frames such as child-headed households. They also may be invisible, such as trafficked children or those who are sexually exploited. Therefore, in addition to traditional techniques of census and probability sampling, household surveys that seek to enumerate children in difficult circumstances often require statistical modeling and the application of more recent sampling strategies such as space–time sampling and respondent-driven sampling. The following section provides an overview of the various methods available for estimating the number of children in difficult circumstances.

Population Census

Data derived from a well-executed population census, designed to include all individuals in a population, will present the most accurate picture of the total number of orphans and their population characteristics. A complete census is the preferred method for generating an estimate of the total number of orphans in the population. However, population censuses are high cost, logistically challenging, and usually conducted infrequently. Furthermore, census data tend to undercount some population sub-groups. These are often the smaller but most vulnerable groups like the homeless, migrants, and other mobile or minority populations. For example, while household-based orphans are likely to be covered by a population census, children in orphanages and in particular orphans living on the streets tend to be un- or undercounted. Adjustments for this undercounting can be made, but may be statistically challenging and are often controversial (Rossi et al. 1999).

Population-Based Household Surveys

Sample surveys are another important method for generating estimates of orphan numbers. Household surveys are frequently used to generate estimates of the percentage of orphans in a population. Like a population census, a household survey requires considerable amounts of skill and resources. While the survey sample size is much smaller than a complete population enumeration, thousands of subjects still need to be interviewed to create valid estimates of sub-groups. In addition, sampling on a national level is complex and susceptible to the introduction of a wide range of potential biases.

There are currently two large-scale household survey programs of children that have been implemented in several countries: the USAID Demographic and Health Surveys (DHS) and the UNICEF Multiple Indicators Cluster Surveys (MICS). The DHS and the MICS collect data from stratified and nationally representative population samples on a variety of demographic and health indicators and include some orphan characteristics. Both the DHS and the MICS define an orphan as a child under 15 years of age that has lost one or both of his or her parents; older children are not considered. The sampling frames for these surveys may exclude a significant component of orphaned children. For example, children living in child-headed households, children not living in households, such as children in orphanages and other institutions, and children living on the streets are often excluded. Other children that may not be included in these survey frames include "those in residential transition and those employed as live-in domestic servants" as well as children that are misclassified as non-orphan, having been claimed by adults in the household as their own (the adoption effect) (Bicego et al. 2003).

Model-Based Estimates

As the impact of HIV/AIDS on children became evident, accurate estimates of the number of AIDS orphans were needed to guide public policy and interventions. While orphan estimates can be derived from census or population-based surveys, difficulties in assessing mortality from AIDS makes these methods less feasible for the generation of reliable estimates of this particular subgroup of orphaned children. Model-based orphan estimates that are derived from adult mortality and fertility and child survival statistics promise to overcome some of these obstacles. Efforts to standardize orphan estimation based on models have been led by the UNAIDS Reference Group on Estimates, Modeling, and Projections, with UNICEF, USAID, and the US Census Bureau as participating partners. Building on earlier work by Grassly

Table 26.1 Health risks for different groups of vulnerable children

	Orphans and vulnerable children	Street children	Working children	Children exposed to conflict or disaster
Nutrition	– Several studies have found higher incidence of malnutrition among OVCs than non-OVCs of similar socio-economic backgrounds – Watts et al. (2007) – Miller et al. (2007) – Jayasekera (2006) – A study of Kampala youth found no statistical difference in anthropometric parameters of OVCs and non-OVCs – Sarker et al. (2005) – Maternal orphans had 11% lower height compared to non-orphans – Beegle et al. (2005) – Weight/age Z-scores were not different between orphans and non-orphans; weight/height Z-scores for orphans were 0.3 standard deviations lower than those for non-orphans – Lindblade et al. (2003) – Under-nutrition and stunting are more prevalent among young orphanage children than young non-orphans or village orphans; there is no statistical difference between nutritional status of village orphans and non-orphans – Panpanich et al. (1999)	– There are no significant differences in anthropometric parameters, incidence of stunting, or underweight between street and non-street slum children – Greksa et al. (2007) – There is a high incidence of stunting (52%); street children weighed more and were taller than their socio-economic peers – Gross et al. (1996) – Street children's nutrition is no worse than that of children living at home with similar economic backgrounds – Scanlon et al. (1998)	– There is no association between malnutrition and work (study of boys only) – Duyar and Ozener (2005)	– Nutrition measures are worse for children exposed to disaster (drought/tsunami) – Singh et al. (2006) – Jayatissa et al. (2006) – There is a high prevalence of acute malnutrition among internally displaced and refugee children – Toole and Waldman (1993)
Diseases	– OVCs <5 years are more likely than non-OVCs to suffer from diarrheal illness even after adjusting for extreme poverty – Watts et al. (2007) – There is no difference between orphans and non-orphans in prevalence of fever and malaria parasitemia or history of illness – Lindblade et al. (2003) – Incidence of diarrhea w/in last month among non-orphans is higher than village orphans or orphanage children (30% for	– Prevalence of disease is slightly higher among street children, but most differences are not statistically significant – Greksa et al. (2007) – There is a high prevalence of disease found among the studied street children population – Ayaya and Esamai (2001) – Diseases are common among street children – Anarfi (1997)		– There is a higher incidence of disease among drought-affected children – Singh et al. (2006) – 85% of children <5 years had diarrhea in tsunami-affected Aceh community – Brennan and Rimba (2005)

Table 26.1 (continued)

	Orphans and vulnerable children	Street children	Working children	Children exposed to conflict or disaster
	non-orphans, 10.8% for village orphans, and 6.6% for orphanage children) – Panpanich et al. (1999)	– Many street children suffer from chronic diseases (typhoid, tuberculosis, jaundice, liver, and kidney disorders) – West (2003) – Trauma and certain infections are more common among street-based children than children living with families – Scanlon et al. (1998)		
Sexually transmitted diseases	– There is greater sexual risk behavior (engaging in sexual intercourse, younger age of sexual intercourse) among OVCs than non-OVCs – Thurman et al. (2006) – There is a higher prevalence among female OVCs than non-OVCs, but no difference for male OVCs – Gregson et al. (2005) – HIV-1 seroprevalence rates are higher among orphans than non-orphans; much higher among 0–4 years – Kamali et al. (1996)	– Sexually transmitted infections are not prevalent – Ayaya and Esamai (2001) – There are higher rates of hepatitis B markers found in street-based youth than children living with families – Porto et al. (1994) – There are higher rates of STDs found in street-based youth than children living with families – Pinto et al. (1994) – Sexually transmitted diseases are prevalent among older street children – West (2003) – An increasing number of street children are living with HIV/AIDS – West (2003) – Study of 143 street children (age 7–18) found 112 had genital herpes, 71 had gonorrhea, 39 had HPV, 19 had vaginal trichomoniasis, 24 had chancroids, and 6 had vaginal candidiasis, early latent syphilis, and pubic pediculosis	– Gonorrhea, herpes simplex, and syphilis are common among child prostitutes – United Nations 2000	

Table 26.1 (continued)

	Orphans and vulnerable children	Street children	Working children	Children exposed to conflict or disaster
Injuries		– Traffic-related injuries are one of the main causes of street child morbidity – Solorzano et al. (1992) – Senanayake et al. (1998)	– There is a higher incidence of musculoskeletal disorders – Fassa et al. (2005) – Injuries and illness result from work – Mull and Kirkhorn (2005) – Various health problems/injuries found in sample of working children – Esin et al. (2005) – Gharaibeh and Hoeman (2003) – Manual labor exposes children to injury – Woolf (2002)	– There is a high rate of injury during armed conflict – Pearn (2003) – Majority of those wounded and permanently disabled are women and children – Sapir (1993)
Mental health	– Several studies found higher incidence of mental health problems among OVCs than non-OVCs – Ahmad et al. (2007) – Cluver and Gardner (2006) – Atwine et al. (2005) – A high incidence of PTSD in Rwandan orphans has been reported, but this has not been compared to PTSD incidence among non-orphan population – Schaal and Elbert (2006)		– Emotional/behavioral disorders are more common among working children – Fekadu et al. (2006)	– There was a very high PTSD prevalence after tsunami – John et al. (2007) – There was a high PTSD prevalence (even higher among children in more severely affected areas) following super-cyclone – Kar et al. (2007) – Armed conflict causes psychological trauma in children – Padmanabhan (1992)
Drug abuse	– Alcohol abuse is more prevalent among orphans than non-orphans – Mabiala-Babela et al. (2005)	– Drug abuse is common among street children – Anarfi (1997) – There is a high prevalence – Ayaya and Esamai (2001) – Alcohol and tobacco use are much higher among children living on the street – Forster et al. (1996)		

Table 26.1 (continued)

	Orphans and vulnerable children	Street children	Working children	Children exposed to conflict or disaster

		– 66% of sampled street children reported using drugs
		  – Abt Enterprises (2001)
		– 67.1% of street children sampled reported using drugs the previous month
		  Sherman et al. (2005)		

Violence	– Orphans, especially girls, reported sexual abuse in new households
	  – Salaam (2005)
		– There are high rates of physical and sexual abuse
		  – Lalor (1999)
		– There are higher rates of sexual abuse reported by street-based youth
		  – Pinto et al. (1994)
		– 16% are sexually abused
		  – Senanayake et al. (1998)
		– 80% of street children sampled were exposed to a "real or constant threat of violence"
		  – Abt Enterprises (2001)
			– Physical, verbal, and sexual abuse are common among child workers
			  – Gharaibeh and Hoeman (2003)
			– 8 out of 10 young domestic workers (Fiji) reported being sexually abused by employer
			  – Salaam (2005)
			– Girl soldiers are frequently subjected to rape and other forms of sexual violence
			  – Coalition to Stop the Use of Child Soldiers (2004)
			– In DRC, almost all girls and some boys reported being raped or sexually abused by commanders or other soldiers
			  – Coalition to Stop the Use of Child Soldiers (2004)
			– 38.5% of child prostitutes sampled (Cambodia) reported being beaten or tortured by brothel owner
			  – United Nations (2000)
				– They bear disproportionate consequences of armed conflict
				  – Pearn (2003)
				– Subject to abuse and kidnapping from soldiers
				  – El-nagar (1992)

Source: UNAIDS/UNICEF/USAID (2004)

and Timæus (UNAIDS/UNICEF/USAID 2004) (Table 26.1), the UNAIDS Reference Group proposed a number of models to estimate the number of maternal, paternal, and double orphans; the number of AIDS orphans alone; and the total number of orphans in a population.

The mortality, fertility, and survival data that feed into model-based population estimates are not collected by the UNAIDS Reference Group. They have to be derived from census data, household surveys, demographic projections, and/or other sources. If statistics are not available or if they are of poor quality, model-based orphan estimates either cannot be calculated or they may be inaccurate. Model-based estimates thus rely on the quality of the available data. This quality is likely to differ for each indicator and between countries. In addition, the models depend heavily on the accuracy of their underlying assumptions.

Minorities and High-Risk Populations

Some of the most vulnerable groups of OVC – such as children in orphanages and children living on the streets – are not adequately covered by any of the methods of generating orphan estimates that have been previously described. Not living in a household and often without contact with family, both groups of children are unlikely to be included in population-based surveys that are often focused on surveying heads of households. A population census may include orphanages, but orphans living on the streets will still be overlooked. The model-based estimates are calculated from population data derived from census and household surveys and are thus as likely as the previous methods to exclude orphans in a non-household setting. While this is not a major problem for the population estimates since the numbers of orphaned children in orphanages and on the streets are very small compared to the total number of orphans, it means that separate studies are needed to describe these special populations and serve the information needs of programs serving orphaned, abandoned, and runaway children. These studies may involve sample

surveys, analysis of program records, key informant interviews, focus group discussions, and related methods.

Health Consequences of Living in Difficult Circumstances

The health consequences of being in difficult circumstances are not well documented in the literature. However, violence and psychosocial trauma and social/behavioral problems are most consistently documented across almost all categories of children in difficult circumstances. Other types of health effects are less consistent across the categories of children living in difficult circumstances (Table 26.1).

Street Children

Street children, for example, are not consistently found to have poorer health outcomes than other children in their settings. However, it is consistently reported that drug abuse rates among street children are high, sometimes higher than those of their non-street socio-economic peers (Ayaya and Esamai 2001). The literature also generally agrees that street children suffer from high rates of physical and sexual abuse (Lalor 1999). Some studies have found higher rates of sexually transmitted diseases (STDs) among street-based youth than their non-street-based peers (Pinto et al. 1994).

Working Children

Child workers are not always found to be at greater health risk, except for occupational risk, which may be particularly marked in some industries (Mull and Kirkhorn 2005). Sexually transmitted diseases are common among child prostitutes and injuries frequently result from various types of labor (United Nations 2000a). Working children are often the victims of physical and sexual abuse at the hands of their employers (Salaam 2005). Child soldiers are especially vulnerable to violence and abuse (Coalition to Stop the Use of Child Soldiers 2004).

Orphans and Vulnerable Children

Several studies report higher incidence of malnutrition among OVCs than non-OVCs of similar socioeconomic backgrounds (Watts et al. 2007; Miller et al. 2007; Jayasekera 2006). Higher HIV-1 seroprevalence rates have also been found among orphan populations with rates being particularly high for orphans 0–4 years of age (Kamali et al. 1996). A greater incidence of mental health problems among OVCs has been indicated by many studies (Ahmad et al. 2007; Cluver and Gardner 2006; Atwine et al. 2005).

Children Exposed to Conflict or Disaster

The literature consistently finds that children exposed to conflict, or disaster, are at high risk for various health consequences (Singh et al. 2006). High incidences of post-traumatic stress disorder (PTSD) have been found among children exposed to natural disasters, and armed conflict is associated with psychological trauma in children (John et al. 2007; Kar et al. 2007; Padmanabhan 1992). Armed conflict disproportionately affects children, with abuse, kidnapping, and injury being common consequences. Higher rates of malnutrition and disease have also been reported among populations of children exposed to conflict or disaster (Singh et al. 2006; Toole and Waldman 1993). Studies indicate that children exposed to complex emergencies and disasters are especially vulnerable, even compared to children in orphanages and other centers for unaccompanied children that have not been impacted by conflict. For example, a study by Dowell et al. (1995) found that "the extremely high mortality rates among unaccompanied refugee children during the first 6 weeks after the arrival of Rwandan refugees in Goma, Zaire, illustrates that unaccompanied children in refugee settings are at particular risk for disease and death even after they are placed

in centers specifically created for their care" (Dowell et al. 1995).

A study by Oleke et al. (2006) observed major changes in fosterage patterns under the impact of conflict and HIV/AIDS among the Langi in Uganda, resulting in an unclear and evolving situation. According to the authors "we are witnessing a cultural transition of considerable dimensions: the earlier situation dominated by the voluntary exchange of children for the prime benefit of building closer ties between relatives is today substituted by an *atin kic* scenario, i.e., an orphan scenario in which the customary fostering pattern has almost ceased to exist. The number of orphans is so overwhelming and the burden of taking care of them so immense that there is often little or no room left for considerations of either lending out or taking in children when there is not an acute need to do so" (Oleke et al. 2006). This development is explained by the authors as the likely "transition from 'purposeful' to 'crisis' fostering. Such a transition is characterized by a situation where relatives increasingly have to take on the duty of caring for children due to conditions of death and dying as opposed to a situation where child fostering occurred purposefully for the strengthening of kin relations, for the exchange of labor resources, or for the learning of skills, etc" (Oleke et al. 2006).

Policies and Strategies for Addressing the Problem of Children in Difficult Circumstances

Policies and strategies to address the problem of children in difficult circumstances deal with both causes and consequences of difficult circumstances. A number of policy initiatives attempt to target the factors that can disrupt childhood in the first place. Among these are the Convention on the Rights of the Child and the ILO Convention 182 on Worst Forms of Child Labor, and other global initiatives that aim to combat certain forms of child labor, trafficking, and/or sexual exploitation. These are primary preventive measures that attempt to address the root causes of difficult circumstances. Other types of interventions focus on mitigating the harmful effects of the particular circumstance on children who for any number of reasons are in difficult circumstances. These interventions are discussed below according to the type of circumstance, as programs are usually more specific to the causes of vulnerability. Any interventions in support of children in difficult circumstances must account for the differences in the needs of the various groups of vulnerable children. While the spectrum of interventions that are carried out is wide, best practices are only beginning to emerge.

Street Children

The World Bank has developed a useful categorization of at-risk youth (Box 26.2) that categorizes street children according to their level of social isolation. By category, intervention strategies for each of these three levels are recommended (Volpe 2002). The strategies include primary prevention (poverty alleviation/poverty elimination), secondary prevention (family-targeted support), and tertiary prevention ("treatment" of dislocated children). This framework acknowledges the need for systemic approaches to the problem of street children.

Working Children

In their recent report "The end of child labor: Within reach," the ILO concluded that "child labor elimination and poverty reduction through economic development go hand in hand. The relationship is not automatic, however. Policy choices matter and they must be coherent. The pace of child labor elimination accelerates when strategies open up 'gateways of opportunity' for poor people" (ILO 2006). According to the ILO, Asia's example particularly shows that poverty reduction and access to education are prerequisites for progress in the elimination of child labor. Box 26.3 summarizes the case study of child labor in China.

Orphans and Vulnerable Children

The UK Consortium on AIDS and International Development (2004) suggests a number of core strategies should be used to achieve best practices in OVC programming:

Box 26. 2 Categories of Risk and Intervention Strategies

Youth in *primary risk* are still attached to the family and society. However, because of poverty or other factors of their situation, they could be compromised in the future. Programs at this level are of a preventive nature and typically include universal family and child benefit services, along with programs targeted to poor communities such as school support, health promotion, recreation, and social integration, vocational training, and support to family livelihood.

Youth in *secondary risk* have weaker social ties and are already exposed to some form of specific risk (such as school dropout, abuse, child labor). Programs at this level have a preventive nature but are focused on a specific target group and include specialized family support, protection and organization of working children, abuse prevention, dropout prevention, and other such services. One of the differences between primary and secondary prevention programs is that secondary prevention requires creative and costly assessment and detection of needs to determine which families and youth are at specific risk.

Youth in *tertiary risk* are those for who one or more of the previously mentioned risks are concrete realities. Their ties with society and family are seriously weakened or severed. This group includes children in the street and of the street. This is the place for rehabilitative programs such as group homes, drop-in centers, targeted health and education services, psychological and legal support, job training, children organization, and family and school integration. Interventions can be center based or take place in the street.

Source: Volpe (2002)

Box 26. 3 Addressing Child Labor in China

China ratified ILO Convention No. 138 in 1999 and ILO Convention No. 182 in 2002. Convention No. 138 determined regulations for workers' minimum age requirements by region. New regulations and convention ratifications took effect on December 1, 2002, to ban the employment of any children under the age of 16 years. The new regulations impose fines for violations and require employers to check workers' identification cards.

There are other indications that China is increasingly willing to address the issue of child labor. During the consideration by the United Nations Committee on the Rights of the Child of China's second report in September 2005, there was official recognition that there were children in need of special protection measures, including street children, children of migrants, and those vulnerable to trafficking.

China still faces multiple challenges in child protection owing to visible disparities between urban and rural areas and a traditional culture favoring boys over girls.

Since the proportion of children working is low, the challenge is to reach out and identify the isolated pockets of child labor. One group that is receiving greater attention is the children of migrant workers who are left behind with family members or those who are living with their parents in cities, but without access to education. Moreover, the problem of child labor may spread with the rapid growth of labor-intensive industries.

IPEC has been working in Yunnan Province since 2000 as part of the Mekong sub regional project to combat trafficking in children and women. In 2004, IPEC launched a new project to prevent trafficking in girls and young women for labor exploitation within China. China was also represented at the first regional capacity-building training course on child labor data collection organized by the ILO, together with the inter-agency research project Understanding Children's Work (UCW), held in Bangkok in November 2004. This reflects a growing willingness by China to learn from the experiences of other countries.

Source: IL0 (2006)

- *Strategy 1:* Strengthen capacity of families to protect and care for orphans and vulnerable children by prolonging the lives of parents and providing economic, psychosocial, and other support.
- *Strategy 2:* Mobilize and support community-based responses.
- *Strategy 3:* Ensure access for OVC to essential services, including education, health care, birth registration, and others.
- *Strategy 4:* Ensure that governments protect the most vulnerable children through improved policy and legislation and by channeling resources to communities.
- *Strategy 5:* Raise awareness at all levels through advocacy and social mobilization to create a supportive environment for children and families affected by HIV/AIDS.

The World Vision research reviewed in Box 26.4 further confirms the success of these best practices,

with Strategy 2, "Mobilize and support community-based responses," as its central tenet.

Children Exposed to Conflict or Disaster

Much of the research of OVC in disasters and complex emergencies focuses on care for children that have been orphaned or separated from their parents. This involves questions of physical and emotional well-being as well as long-term options and opportunities. Overall, institutional care is widely discouraged and foster care is often regarded as the preferred option. A study by Duerr et al. (2003) found strong "empirical support for the United Nations recommendation that during acute emergency situations, children should be fostered with other families whenever possible, not isolated from their communities

Box 26. 4 Promising Practices in OVC Responses

World Vision conducted qualitative research exploring and documenting communities' experiences and reflections of OVC programming in six countries – Kenya, Malawi, Rwanda, Swaziland, Uganda, and Zambia, particularly looking at the role of Community Care Coalitions.

Community Care Coalitions with a broad spectrum of stakeholders were viewed very positively in OVC programming. The central role of coalitions is to mobilize and coordinate OVC care activities. Typical members of the coalitions include churches and faith-based organizations (FBOs), teachers, community leaders such as chiefs, people living with HIV/AIDS (PLWHA), traditional birth attendants, home-based care providers, health-care providers, OVC care providers, women's groups, and development committee members. In one case the coalition had a subcommittee consisting of orphans and vulnerable children, and their inclusion was seen as a positive innovation.

Coalitions are a powerful conduit for advocacy, particularly regarding OVC access to education, and child abuse including child labor. Coalitions provide a means for greater accountability in the use of resources. Faith-based organizations in particular are central to the OVC response and provide a range of services individually, as well as core members of community care coalitions. Strengths of FBOs are their wide reach, volunteerism, and mobilization of existing resources.

In terms of mobilizing resources for community responses, the primary source of resources was from within the community itself. Although resources within the community are inadequate, care needs to be taken that the provision of external resources is done in a manner that does not undermine, but rather supplements and enhances, traditional coping mechanisms. Community care coalitions can provide a structure and means of channeling external resources into communities. The coalition members can develop community plans with specific resource requirements and evaluation, ensuring transparency to the wider community. Where there is a need for further training, NGOs are natural allies and can provide both capacity building and resources to coalitions.

There are many unmet training needs, and when training such as proposal writing, home-based care, and counseling was offered, it enhanced coalitions. Educating the community on the roles and objectives of the coalition was essential to avoid unrealistic expectations from the community.

Child participation enhanced the planning, implementation, and monitoring of OVC activities and should become the norm for all coalitions. Child/youth clubs and church activities lend themselves to greater child participation and this opportunity should be utilized. Such clubs are enhanced by endorsement and appropriate support from adult patrons. Child-to-child approaches to care need to be identified and enhanced with appropriate support.

Finally, community-to-community learning demonstrates potential to contribute to the scaling up of OVC response. The methodology should be documented in a user-friendly toolkit and trainings, including documentation of best practice, and monitoring and evaluation.

Source: UK Consortium on AIDS and International Development (2004)

in institutions (Duerr et al. 2003). A study of different groups of orphans impacted by conflict in Eritrea (Wolff and Fesseha 2005) indicates variation in adaptive skills and emotional distress between institutional orphans, group-home orphans, and orphans reunited with their family: "Orphans reunified with extended families had greater adaptive skills than institutional orphans

but as many signs and symptoms of emotional distress as orphanage children. Group-home orphans had fewer signs and symptoms of emotional distress and greater adaptive skills than either reunified or institutional orphans, and they had fewer symptoms of emotional distress than home-reared children. However, placing orphans in small group homes was far more expensive than reunifying them with extended families" (Wolff and Fesseha 2005).

Conclusions

Children are increasingly exposed to an array of difficult circumstances that may jeopardize their growth and development. These circumstances often result in orphanhood, dislocation from families, and social systems of support. Ultimately, these circumstances may lead to adverse emotional and physical health. Unfortunately, the evidence-base available for guiding programs and policies to address this issue is highly limited due to the highly contextual nature of difficult circumstances, the problems of definition and enumeration, and the paucity of epidemiologic research on most categories of children in difficult circumstances.

Key Terms

Child soldiers	Migration	Psychosocial trauma
Child trafficking	Occupational risk	Secondary risk
Community care coalitions	Orphan	Social dislocation
Community responses	Orphanages	Street children
Drug abuse	Orphans and vulnerable	Tertiary risk
Family-targeted support	children (OVC)	Trafficked children
Forced and bonded labor	Population census	Urbanization
Foster care	Post-traumatic stress disorder	Violence
Group-home orphans	(PTSD)	Working children
Household surveys	Poverty alleviation	Worst Forms of Child Labor
Malnutrition	Primary risk	(WFCL)

Questions for Discussion

1. Define and provide examples of the following:

   a. Orphans
   b. Vulnerable children
   c. Street children
   d. Child labor

2. List the factors that contribute to the increasing global trend in the magnitude of the problem of children in difficult circumstances.
3. Outline and critique the methods for estimating categories of children in difficult circumstances.
4. Discuss the health consequences of living in difficult circumstances for the following categories of children:

   a. Street children
   b. Working children
   c. Orphans and vulnerable children
   d. Children exposed to conflict and disaster

5. In an essay of about 1,000 words, present a critique of existing strategies and policies for addressing the problem of children in difficult circumstances.

References

Abt Enterprises (2001) Rapid Situation Assessment Report on The situation of street children in Cairo and Alexandria, including the children's drug abuse and health/nutritional status. http://www.unicef.org/evaldatabase/files/EGY_2001_005.pdf, cited August 8, 2009

Ahmad A, Abdul-Majeed AM, Siddiq AA et al. (2007) Reporting questionnaire for children as a screening instrument for child mental health problems in Iraqi Kurdistan. Transcultural Psychiatry, 44(1), 5–26

Anarfi JK (1997) Vulnerability to sexually transmitted disease: street children in Accra. Health Transit Review, 7, 281–306

Atwine B, Cantor-Graae E, Bajunirwe F (2005) Psychological distress among AIDS orphans in rural Uganda. Social Science and Medicine, 61(3), 555–564

Ayaya SO, Esamai FO (2001) Health problems of street children in Eldoret, Kenya. East African Medical Journal, 78(12), 624–629

Beegle K, De Weerdt J, Dercon S (2005) Orphanhood and the long-run impact on children. World Bank, DANIDA, Economic Research Council (UK). http://www.sarpn.org.za/documents/d0001651/index.php, cited 8 August 2008

Bicego G, Rutstein S, Johnson K (2003) Dimensions of the emerging orphan crisis in sub-Saharan Africa. Social Science and Medicine, 56(6), 1235–1247

Brennan RJ, Rimba K (2005) Rapid health assessment in Aceh Jaya District, Indonesia, following the December 26 tsunami. Emergency Medicine Australasia: EMA, 17(4), 341–350

Cluver L, Gardner F (2006) The psychological well-being of children orphaned by AIDS in Cape Town, South Africa. Annals of General Psychiatry, 19(5), 8

Coalition to Stop the Use of Child Soldiers (2004) Child Soldiers: Global Report 2004. www.child-soldiers.org Cited 8 August 2008

Dowell SF, Toko A, Sita C et al. (1995) Health and nutrition in centers for unaccompanied refugee children: Experience from the 1994 Rwandan refugee crisis. Journal of America Medical Association, 273(22), 1802–1806

Duerr A, Posner SF, Gilbert M (2003) Evidence in support of foster care during acute refugee crisis. American Journal of Public Health, 93(11), 1904–1909

Duyar I, Ozener B (2005) Growth and nutritional status of male adolescent laborers in Ankara, Turkey. American Journal of Physical Anthropology, 128(3), 693–698

El-nagar SE (1992) The impact of war on women and children: case study of Sudan. Women 2000, 5, 9–11

Ennew J (2003) Difficult circumstances: some reflections on "Street Children" in Africa. Children, Youth and Environments, 13, 1

Esin MN, Bulduk S, Ince H (2005) Work related risks and health problems of working children in urban Istanbul, Turkey. Journal of Occupational Health, 47(5), 431–436

Fassa AG, Facchini LA, Dall'Agnol MM et al. (2005) Child labor and musculoskeletal disorders: the Pelotas (Brazil) epidemiological survey. Public Health Reports, 120(6), 665–673

Fekadu D, Alem A, Hagglof B (2006) The prevalence of mental health problems in Ethiopian child laborers. Journal of Child Psychology and Psychiatry, 47(9), 954–959

Forster LM, Tannhauser M, Barros HM (1996) Drug use among street children in southern Brazil. Drug and Alcohol Dependency, 43, 57–62

Gharaibeh M, Hoeman S (2003) Health hazards and risks for abuse among child labor in Jordan. Journal of Pediatric Nursing, 18(2), 140–147

Grassly NC, Phil D, Timæus IM (2005) Methods to estimate the number of orphans as a result of AIDS and other causes in sub-Saharan Africa. Journal of Acquired Immune Deficiency Syndromes, 39, 365–375

Gregson S, Nyamukapa CA, Garnett GP et al. (2005) HIV infection and reproductive health in teenage women orphaned and made vulnerable by AIDS in Zimbabwe. AIDS Care, 17(7), 785–794

Greksa LP, Rie N, Islam AB et al. (2007) Growth and health status of street children in Dhaka, Bangladesh. American Journal of Human Biology, 19(1), 51–60

Gross R, Landfried B, Herman S (1996) Height and weight as a reflection of the nutritional situation of school-aged children working and living in the streets of Jakarta. Social Science Medicine, 43(4), 453–458

Hagemann F, Diallo Y, Etienne A et al. (2006) Global child labor trends 2000 to 2004. Geneva: International Labor Organization (ILO), Statistical Information and Monitoring Programme on Child Labor (SIMPOC)

International Labor Organization (ILO) (1999) ILO Convention No. 182: Convention concerning the prohibition and immediate action for the elimination of the worst forms of child labor. http://www.un.org/children/conflict/keydocuments/english/iloconvention1828.html Cited 8 August 2008

International Labor Organization (ILO) (2006) The end of child labor: Within reach. Global Report under the follow-up to the ILO Declaration on Fundamental Principles and Rights at Work. Geneva: ILO. http://www.ilo.org/public/english/standards/relm/ilc/ilc95/pdf/rep-i-b.pdf Cited 8 August 2008

Institut National de la Statistique du Rwanda and ORC Macro (2006) Enquête Démographique et de Santé, Rwanda 2005 (Rwanda Demographic and Health Survey 2005). Calverton, MD, USA: ORC Macro

Jayasekera CR (2006) Nutritional status of children under five in three state foster care institutions in Sri Lanka. Ceylon Medical Journal, 51(2), 63–65

Jayatissa R, Bekele A, Piyasena CL et al. (2006) Assessment of nutritional status of children under five years of age, pregnant women, and lactating women living in relief camps after the tsunami in Sri Lanka. Food and Nutrition Bulletin, 27(2), 144–152

John PB, Russell S, Russell PS (2007) The prevalence of posttraumatic stress disorder among children and adolescents affected by tsunami disaster in Tamil Nadu. Disaster Management and Response, 5(1), 3–7

Joint United Nations Programme on HIV/AIDS (UNAIDS) Reference Group on Estimates, Modeling and Projections (2002) Improved methods and assumptions for estimation of the HIV/AIDS epidemic and its impact: Recommendations of the UNAIDS Reference Group on Estimates, Modeling and Projections. AIDS, 16, W1–W14

Joint United Nations Programme on HIV/AIDS (UNAIDS) (2004) 2004 report on the global AIDS epidemic. Geneva: Joint United Nations Program on HIV/AIDS. http://www.unaids.org/bangkok2004/GAR2004_html/GAR 2004_00_en.htm Cited 8 August 2008

Kamali A, Seeley JA, Nunn AJ et al. (1996) The orphan problem: experience of a sub-Saharan Africa rural population in the AIDS epidemic. AIDS Care, 8(5), 509–515

Kar N, Mohapatra PK, Nayak KC et al. (2007) Post-traumatic stress disorder in children and adolescents one year after a super- cyclone in Orissa, India: exploring cross-cultural validity and vulnerability factors. BMC Psychiatry, 14, 7–8

Lalor KJ (1999) Street children: a comparative perspective. Child Abuse and Neglect, 23(8): 759–770

Lindblade KA, Odhiambo F, Rosen DH et al. (2003) Health and nutritional status of orphans <6 years old cared for by relatives in western Kenya. Tropical Medicine and International Health, 8(1), 67–72

Mabiala-Babela JR, Mahoungou-Guimbi KC, Massamba A et al. (2005) Alcohol consumption among teenagers in Brazzaville (Congo) Sante, 15(3), 153–160

Miller CM, Gruskin S, Subramanian SV et al. (2007) Emerging health disparities in Botswana: examining the situation of orphans during the AIDS epidemic. Social Science and Medicine, 64(12), 2476–2486

Mull LD, Kirkhorn SR (2005) Child labor in Ghana cocoa production: focus upon agricultural tasks, ergonomic exposures, and associated injuries and illnesses. Public Health Reports, 120(6), 649–655

Oleke C, Blystad A, Moland K et al. (2006) The varying vulnerability of African orphans: the case of the Langi, northern Uganda. Childhood: A Global Journal of Child Research, 13(2), 267–284

Padmanabhan BS (1992) Conflicts and child survival. ICCW News Bulletin, 40(3–4), 66–67

Panpanich R, Brabin B, Gonani A et al. (1999) Are orphans at increased risk of malnutrition in Malawi? Annals of Tropical Pediatrics, 19(3), 279–285

Pearn J (2003) Children and war. Journal of Pediatrics and child health, 39(3), 166–172

Pinto JA, Ruff AJ, Paiva JV et al. (1994) HIV risk behavior and medical status of underprivileged youths in Belo Horizonte, Brazil. The Journal of Adolescent Health, 15(2), 179–185

Porto SO, Cardoso DD, Queiroz DA et al. (1994) Prevalence and risk factors for HBV infection among street youth in central Brazil. The Journal of Adolescent Health, 15(7), 577–581

Rossi PH, Freeman HE, Lipsey MW (1999) Evaluation: a systematic approach. Thousand Oaks: Sage

Salaam T (2005) AIDS orphans and Vulnerable Children (OVC): Problems, Reponses, and Issues for Congress, Congressional Research Service. http://www.sarpn.org.za/documents/d0001829/index.php, cited 8 August 2008

Sapir DG (1993) Natural and man-made disasters: the vulnerability of women-headed households and children without families. World Health Statistics Quarterly, 46(4), 227–233

Sarker M, Neckermann C, Muller O (2005) Assessing the health status of young AIDS and other orphans in Kampala, Uganda. Tropical Medicine and International Health, 10(3), 210–215

Scanlon TJ, Tomkins A, Lynch MA et al. (1998) Street children in Latin America. British Medical Journal, 316(7144), 1596–1600

Schaal S, Elbert T (2006) Ten years after the genocide: trauma confrontation and posttraumatic stress in Rwandan adolescents. Journal of Traumatic Stress, 19(1), 95–105

Senanayake MP, Ranasinghe A, Balasuriya C (1998) Street children – a preliminary study. Ceylon Medical Journal, 43(4), 191–193

Sherman SS, Plitt S, ul Hassan S et al. (2005) Drug use, street survival, and risk behaviours among street children in Lahore, Pakistan. Journal of Urban Health, 82(3), iv113–iv124

Singh MB, Lakshminarayana J, Fotedar R et al. (2006) Childhood illnesses and malnutrition in under five children in drought affected desert area of western Rajasthan, India. Journal of Communicable Diseases, 38(1), 88–96

Skinner D, Tsheko N, Mtero-Munyati S et al. (2006) Towards a definition of orphaned and vulnerable children. AIDS and Behavior, 10(6), 619–626(8)

Solorzano E, Arroyo G, Santizo R et al. (1992) Sexually transmitted diseases in Guatemala City street children. Revista del Colegio de Médicos y Cirujanos de Guatemala, 2, 48–51

Thurman TR, Brown L, Richter L et al. (2006) Sexual risk behavior among South African adolescents: Is orphan status a factor? AIDS and Behavior, 10(6), 627–635

Toole MJ, Waldman RJ (1993) Refugees and displaced persons. War, hunger, and public health. Journal of the American Medical Association, 270(5), 600–605

UK Consortium on AIDS and International Development (2004) Symposium on Sharing of Best Practice in OVC Programming. Workshop report. http://www.aidsconsortium.org.uk/OVCWorkingGroup/OVC%20PDFs%20&%20other%20docs/SymposiumReport04.pdf, cited 8 August 2008

United Nations Children's Fund (UNICEF) (2003) Africa's orphaned generations. New York: United Nations Children's Fund

United Nations Children's Fund (UNICEF), Joint United Nations Programme on HIV/AIDS (UNAIDS), United States Agency for International Development (USAID) (2004) Children on the brink 2004. A Joint Report of New Orphan Estimates and a Framework for Action. New York: United Nations Children's Fund (UNICEF)/Joint United Nations Programme on HIV/AIDS (UNAIDS), US Agency for International Development (USAID).

United Nations Children's Fund (UNICEF) (2006) Fact sheet: child labour. http://www.unicef.org/protection/files/child_labour.pdf, cited August 8 2008

United Nations (1956) Supplementary Convention on the Abolition of Slavery, the Slave Trade, and Institutions and Practices Similar to Slavery Adopted by a Conference of Plenipotentiaries convened by Economic and Social Council resolution 608(XXI) of 30 April 1956 and done at Geneva on 7 September 1956 entry into force 30 April 1957, in accordance with article 13. New York: United Nations. http://www.unhchr.ch/html/menu3/b/30.htm, cited 29 August 2008

United Nations (2000a) Sexually abused and sexually exploited children and youth in Cambodia: a qualitative assessment of their health needs and available services in selected provinces. New York: United Nations.

United Nations (2000b) Protocol to prevent, suppress and punish trafficking in persons, especially women and children, supplementing the United Nations convention against transnational organized crime. http://www.uncjin.org/Documents/Conventions/dcatoc/final_documents_2/convention_%20traff_eng.pdf, cited 8 August 2008

Volpe E (2002) Street children: promising practices and approaches. Washington DC: World Bank Institute. http://www.colorado.edu/journals/cye/13_1/Vol13ArticleReprints/PromisingPractices.pdf, cited 8 August 2008

Watts H, Gregson S, Saito S et al. (2007) Poorer health and nutritional outcomes in orphans and vulnerable young children not explained by greater exposure to extreme poverty in Zimbabwe. Tropical Medicine and International Health, 12(5), 584–593

West A (2003) At the margins: street children in Asia and the Pacific. Asian Development Bank. Regional and Sustainable Development Department. Poverty and Development Papers, 8

Wittig M, Wright JD, Kaminsky DC (1997) Substance use among street children in Honduras. Substance Use and Misuse, 32, 805–827

Wolff PH, Fesseha G (2005) The orphans of Eritrea: what are the choices? American Journal of Orthopsychiatry, 75(4), 475–484

Woolf AD (2002) Health hazards for children at work. Journal of Toxicology Clinical Toxicology, 40(4), 477–482

Chapter 27
Integrated Management of Childhood Illness

Martin Meremikwu and John E. Ehiri

Learning Objectives After reading this chapter and answering the discussion questions that follow, you should be able to

- Discuss milestones in the emergence of IMCI as a strategy for child health promotion in developing countries.
- Discuss the key objectives of the IMCI program.
- Describe the core technical components of IMCI with emphasis on the evidence base of the associated interventions.
- Analyze limitations and challenges of the IMCI initiative.
- Appraise the current status of IMCI and the prospects for scaling it up to improve child health globally.

Introduction

The causes of morbidity and mortality among children in less developed countries are often multiple and inter-related. For this reason, effective and efficient treatment of these conditions requires a comprehensive case management approach that recognizes the complexity of childhood problems in resource-limited settings. The integrated management of childhood illnesses (IMCI) initiative was introduced by the World Health Organization (WHO) and the United Nations Children's Fund (UNICEF) in the 1990s in response to the limitations of the child survival revolution of the 1980s that was based on disparate vertical programs. Its objectives

are to (i) improve the case management skills of health professionals through the provision of locally adapted guidelines and the development of activities to promote the use of such guidelines; (ii) improve health systems needed to allow effective management of childhood illnesses; and (iii) improve family and community practices relevant to child health promotion. This chapter presents a historical perspective on the emergence of IMCI as a strategy for child health promotion in middle- and low-income countries and describes the core technical components of IMCI with emphasis on their evidence base. Case studies of field implementation are described. The chapter concludes with an appraisal of the current status of IMCI and of the prospects for scaling it up to improve child health globally.

Worldwide, children from low- and middle-income countries are 10 times more likely to die before their fifth birthday than their counterparts in industrialized, high-income countries (Global Action for Children 2008). As shown in Fig. 27.1, about 70% of an estimated 10 million deaths among children under 5 years of age in these countries are due to preventable and curable diseases such as malaria, diarrhea, measles, HIV/AIDS, and acute respiratory infections (ARI) (Global Action for Children 2008). Malnutrition, an underlying cause of mortality, contributes to 53% of these deaths (WHO 2003). Several internationally supported public health initiatives often referred to as child survival interventions have, to varying degrees of success, attempted to reduce the high rates of childhood death. Most of these initiatives were coordinated and implemented by UNICEF and the World Health Organization. Notable among these were the control of diarrheal diseases program, including the use of oral rehydration therapy, control of acute

M. Meremikwu (✉)
University of Calabar Teaching Hospital (UCTH), Calabar, Cross River State, Nigeria

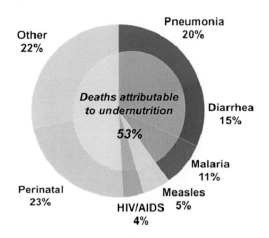

Fig. 27.1 Distribution of 11.6 million deaths among children less than 5 years old in all developing countries, 1995. Source: World Health Report (2003); Caulfield et al. (2004)

Table 27.1 Complexity of childhood illnesses

Presenting complaint	Possible cause or associated condition
Cough and/or fast breathing	Pneumonia
	Severe anemia
	Plasmodium falciparum malaria
Lethargy or unconsciousness	Cerebral malaria
	Meningitis
	Severe dehydration
	Very severe pneumonia
Measles rash	Pneumonia
	Diarrhea
	Ear Infection
"Very sick" young infant	Pneumonia
	Meningitis
	Sepsis

Source: WHO (1999)

respiratory infections program, infant nutrition programs including the promotion of breastfeeding, and the Expanded Program on Immunization (Ehiri and Prowse 1999; Pelletier et al. 1995).

The verticality and multiplicity of these programs pose significant service delivery and administrative problems, especially at health facility levels owing to their limited integrated approach and lack of emphasis on health systems development. In spite of the limitations of these vertical programs, global health policy makers and funding agencies continue to support them. For example, current global initiatives for control and prevention of HIV/AIDS, tuberculosis, and malaria have been mostly vertical or semi-integrated at best. There is comparatively little emphasis on strengthening health systems that lack the capacity to support the large investments in these initiatives. Vertical programs are more likely to achieve rapid short-term results than comprehensive, community-driven approaches advocated in Alma-Ata Declaration of Primary Healthcare (WHO/UNICEF 1978), but they have a tendency to divert resources from programs that offer longer term, sustainable outcomes and opportunities for health system development.

Lessons learned from experimentation with various disease-specific child health initiatives of the 1980s and 1990s in less developed countries (Campbell and Gove 1996) showed that children with severe illnesses often present with overlapping signs and symptoms (Table 27.1).

This means that a single diagnosis may not be possible or appropriate, and treatment may be complicated by the need to combine therapy for several conditions (WHO 1999). Responding to this challenge in the late 1980s and early 1990s, various health programs, professionals, and international development agencies began to experiment with integrated case management strategies (Ehiri and Prowse 1999). Programs that previously targeted individual diseases began to tackle disease complexes. For example, the Technology for Primary Healthcare (PRITECH) program of the United States Agency for International Development (USAID) which initially concentrated on case management of diarrhea began to incorporate malnutrition, aspects of ARI control activities, and hygiene promotion (Ehiri and Prowse 1999). Integrated Management of Childhood Illnesses (IMCI) was subsequently launched by WHO and UNICEF in 1992 and received endorsement by the World Bank in their 1993 report (World Bank 1993). IMCI combines improved management of childhood illness with aspects of nutrition, immunization, and other important factors that influence child health, including maternal health (Fig. 27.2). Its overall goals were to reduce death, the frequency and severity of illness and disability, and to contribute to improved growth and development (WHO 1999). It was perceived that these goals would be achieved by (i) improving the case management skills of health professionals through the provision of locally adapted guidelines and the development

Fig. 27.2 Scope of integrated management of childhood illness. Source: WHO (1999)

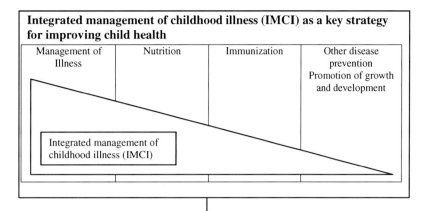

Integrated management of childhood illness (IMCI) as a key strategy for improving child health

Management of Illness	Nutrition	Immunization	Other disease prevention Promotion of growth and development

Integrated management of childhood illness (IMCI)

Interventions currently included in the IMCI strategy

	Promotion of growth Prevention of disease	Response to sickness ("curative care")
Home	-Community/home-based interventions to improve nutrition -Insecticide-impregnated bednets	-Early case management -Appropriate care-seeking -Compliance with treatment
Health Services	-Vaccination -Complementary feeding and breastfeeding counseling -Micronutrient supplementation	-Case management of: ARI, diarrhea, measles, malaria, malnutrition, other serious infection -Complementary feeding and breastfeeding -Iron treatment -Antihelminthic treatment

Interventions included in the IMCI guidelines for first-level health workers

	Conditions covered by case management	Preventive interventions

Generic version	Acute Respiratory infections
	Diarrhea
	  Dehydration
	  Persistent diarrhea
	  Dysentery
	Meningitis, sepsis
	Malaria
	Measles
	Anemia
	Ear infection
		Immunization
		Nutrition counseling
		Breastfeeding support
		Vitamin A supplementation

Using the IMCI Adaptation Guide	HIV/AIDS Dengue hemorrhagic fever Wheeze Sore throat	Periodic de-worming

of activities to promote the use of such guidelines; (ii) improving health systems needed to allow effective management of childhood illnesses; and (iii) improving family and community practices relevant to child health promotion. The core intervention is integrated case management of the five most important causes of childhood deaths – ARI, diarrhea, measles, malaria, and malnutrition (Fig. 27.2).

It also incorporates a range of other preventive and curative interventions that aim to improve practices both in health facilities and at home.

There is an understanding that the combination of interventions that make up IMCI may be modified to include conditions that are important in individual countries and for which there are effective preventive measures and/or treatment. The following section provides further description of the three technical components of IMCI, i.e., (i) improving the case management skills of health professionals through the provision of locally adapted guidelines and the development of activities to promote the use of such guidelines; (ii) improving health systems needed to allow effective management of childhood illnesses; and (iii) improving family and community practices relevant to child health promotion.

Improving the Skills of Health Workers

At the inception of IMCI in the early 1990s, emphasis was placed on training health-care workers to improve the quality of health care at first-level health facilities. Training in approaches for optimum integration of case management is the principal activity of this component. The principles of integration of care are outlined in Box 27.1. They provide the core values for IMCI implementation. Training provided under this component equips health workers with the requisite skills to assess, classify, treat, or make appropriate referral for sick children attending first-level health facilities using a syndromic approach.

As noted in Fig. 27.3, the IMCI approach has identified non-specific signs of serious illness that should be routinely assessed for every sick child. These signs (referred to as "general danger signs") include *convulsions*, *lethargy or unconsciousness*, *vomiting*, and *inability to drink or breastfeed*. A child with one or more of these general danger signs is classified as having severe disease which requires immediate referral to a higher level of care following a pre-referral treatment, where appropriate. The IMCI case management training course involves practical demonstrations and exercises in clinical settings that are aimed at exposing the trainee to the wide spectrum of case scenarios related to integrated case management of the sick child. The WHO first developed a standard and elaborate curriculum, in addition to learning and evaluation tools. The training was originally designed as an 11-day in-service course, but has been modified to a shorter option and a pre-service version for health workers (nurses and community health workers) in

Box 27.1 Principles of Integrated Care

- All sick children must be examined for "general danger signs" which indicate the need for immediate referral or admission to a hospital.
- All sick children must be routinely assessed for major symptoms (for children age 2 months up to 5 years: cough or difficult breathing, diarrhea, fever, ear problems; for young infants age 1 week up to 2 months: bacterial infection and diarrhea). They must also be routinely assessed for nutritional and immunization status, feeding problems, and other potential problems.
- Only a limited number of carefully selected clinical signs are used, based on evidence of their sensitivity and specificity to detect disease. These signs were selected considering the conditions and realities of first-level health facilities.
- A combination of individual signs leads to a child's classification(s) rather than a diagnosis. Classification(s) indicate the severity of condition(s). They call for specific actions based on whether the child (a) should be urgently referred to another level of care, (b) requires specific treatments (such as antibiotics or anti-malarial treatment), or (c) may be safely managed at home. The classifications are color coded: "pink" suggests hospital referral or admission, "yellow" indicates initiation of treatment, and "green" calls for home treatment.
- The IMCI guidelines address most, but not all, of the major reasons a sick child is brought to a clinic. A child returning with chronic problems or less common illnesses may require special care. The guidelines do not describe the management of trauma or other acute emergencies due to accidents or injuries.
- IMCI management procedures use a limited number of essential drugs and encourage active participation of caretakers in the treatment of children.
- An essential component of the IMCI guidelines is the counseling of caretakers about home care, including counseling about feeding fluids and when to return to a health facility.

Source: WHO (2001a)

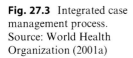

Fig. 27.3 Integrated case management process. Source: World Health Organization (2001a)

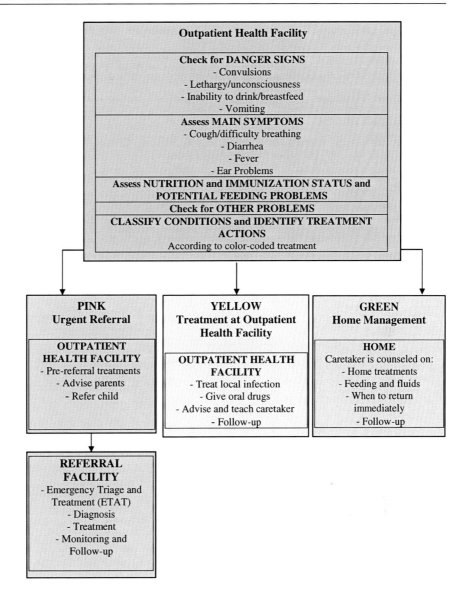

training (WHO 2001a). The course also teaches participants useful skills in communication and client counseling.

Several evaluations of the IMCI approach have highlighted the positive impact of the enhanced counseling and communication skills of the IMCI-trained health workers (WHO 2004). The primary criticism of the first component of IMCI is the slow pace of its implementation (WHO 2004). Several reasons have been given for this slow progress, including the length of training, the challenge of locating suitable training sites

and trainers, and, most prominently, the high cost of project implementation (WHO 2004). Evaluation reports have shown that IMCI is cost-effective in the long term (Bryce et al. 2004). However, the provision of adequate funding for cost-intensive training and early implementation activities remains a challenge. While a few countries have made visible progress in IMCI training of their health workers with donor support, a majority of others have yet to achieve a quarter of their coverage targets for IMCI training (WHO/UNICEF 1999).

Improving the Health-Care System

Improvement of health systems in the context of the IMCI approach includes the following (WHO/UNICEF 1999):

- Improvement in the availability of drugs and supplies at first-level health facilities
- Improvement of service quality and organization of health facilities
- Improvement of referral pathways and care
- Identification of methods for sustainable finance
- Ensuring equity of access
- Linkage of IMCI and health information systems
- Contribution to health sector reform

Efforts to improve health systems through the IMCI approach have received limited implementation support and are the least evaluated of the three components. In reality, initiatives to strengthen the health system cut across all levels, sectors, and programs within the health-care delivery system. It is not feasible to domicile the task of improving the health system within any single health-care initiative. It would also not be appropriate to attribute any improvement in the system to a single program or intervention.

Health system strengthening needs to be reinforced and aggressively supported as a component of the IMCI strategy, since IMCI can only succeed within a strong health system. It is important that the opportunity provided by IMCI implementation is used to leverage resources for health system support. Several cross-cutting issues that address improvement of health-care systems are discussed in Chapter 5 on Health Systems and Maternal and Child Health. Readers are advised to refer to this chapter for more information on health system strengthening.

Community IMCI: Improving Family and Community Practices

This component of IMCI adopts a multi-sectoral approach in order to improve selected behaviors and practices at household and community levels. This component is referred to as Community IMCI or C-IMCI. It focuses on strengthening communities and supporting families in order to adopt health-promoting attitudes and to take action necessary to improve child survival, growth, and development. Based on evidence from research and successful health-care intervention initiatives, community IMCI recommends that families and communities be encouraged and supported to take beneficial actions in order to improve child survival, growth, and development (UNICEF 2001). These practices are grouped into four broad areas that promote (i) the child's physical and mental growth; (ii) disease prevention; (iii) appropriate home care; and (iv) care seeking and compliance. The recommendations for these four areas are outlined hereunder (UNICEF 2001):

Physical and Mental Growth

1. Breastfeed infants exclusively for at least 6 months. Mothers found to be HIV positive require counseling about possible alternatives to breastfeeding.
2. Starting at approximately 6 months of age, children should be fed freshly prepared energy- and nutrient-rich complementary foods, while continuing to breastfeed them for up to 2 + years.
3. Ensure that children receive adequate amounts of micronutrients (vitamin A and iron in particular), either in their diet or through supplementation.
4. Promote mental and social development by responding to a child's needs for care, and through talking, playing, and providing a stimulating environment.

Disease Prevention

5. Take children as scheduled to complete a full course of immunizations (BCG, DPT, OPV, and measles) before their first birthday.
6. Dispose of feces, including children's feces, safely; and wash hands after defecation, before preparing meals, and before feeding children.
7. Protect children in malaria-endemic areas, by ensuring that they sleep under insecticide-treated bed nets.

8. Adopt and sustain appropriate behavior regarding prevention and care for HIV/AIDS-affected people, including orphans.

Appropriate Home Care

9. Continue to feed and offer increased fluids to sick children.
10. Give sick children appropriate home treatment for infections such as diarrhea and malaria.
11. Take appropriate actions to prevent and manage child injuries and accidents.
12. Prevent child abuse and neglect and take appropriate action when it has occurred.
13. Ensure that men actively participate in provision of childcare and are involved in reproductive health initiatives.

Care Seeking and Compliance

14. Recognize when sick children need treatment outside the home and seek care from appropriate providers.
15. Ensure that every pregnant woman has adequate antenatal care. This includes having at least four antenatal visits with an appropriate health-care provider and receiving the recommended doses of the tetanus toxoid vaccination. The mother also needs support from her family and community in seeking care at the time of delivery and during the postpartum and lactation period.
16. Follow the health worker's advice about treatment, follow-up, and referral.

General Principles, Programmatic Elements, and Frameworks for C-IMCI

The Child Survival Collaborations and Resources (CORE) Group, a member of the inter-agency working group on community IMCI, has played a key role in developing the guiding principles for this component of IMCI (CORE Group 2007). The Inter-agency working group for community IMCI includes WHO, UNICEF, and others (notably the CORE Group) and has identified seven general principles to guide the development, implementation, and evaluation of C-IMCI at all levels (Box 27.2).

Box 27.2 General Principles of C-IMCI

1. C-IMCI is implemented at district and community levels, but should be linked to a national strategic plan that provides policy direction and an enabling environment. Links should be established between community and district-level planning and implementation as well as between district, regional, and national levels
2. C-IMCI should identify and build on existing programs and community structures, rather than create new ones
3. Participatory approaches to planning and implementing activities should be utilized to ensure ownership and sustainability
4. Successful implementation of C-IMCI requires effective partnerships at all levels. Clear definitions of roles and responsibilities of all stakeholders are essential
5. C-IMCI recognizes the importance of curative and preventive interventions in the community for reducing child mortality and morbidity and for promoting child growth and development
6. Implementation of C-IMCI requires the other two IMCI technical components to be in place to provide support for families and communities. In some situations, however, where the other two components are not in place, it may be appropriate to implement C-IMCI interventions. In such cases, efforts should be made to ensure that the other two components are introduced
7. Phased introduction of promotion of key family practices is acceptable. Families and communities must not be overwhelmed by the introduction of too much at once, but a good C-IMCI plan should include the eventual phasing in of all the appropriate practices

Source: WHO (2004)

These principles emphasize core values and elements of the Alma-Ata concept of comprehensive primary health care, such as community participation, integration with existing health programs, and inter-sectoral collaboration. This affirms the belief that Alma-Ata remains the ideal and a reference point for initiatives that seek to achieve holistic health care at the community level. It is important to note that these guidelines notwithstanding, the key determinants of outcome are context, culture, and commitment to values and objectives. Results of the multi-country evaluation of IMCI (Bryce et al. 2004) and country-specific experiences (Schellenberg et al. 2004) lend support to proof of effects of the basic principles of the integrated approach. However, coverage or impact remains sparse due to the impact of adverse socio-economic contexts, cultural preferences or limitations, and poor political commitment. The sixth principle (Box 27.2) highlights the critical importance of concurrent implementation of the three components of IMCI but admits that compromise and tendency toward discordant implementation is common. This tends to dilute expected impacts of the strategy.

To give further impetus to the implementation of C-IMCI, two implementation frameworks have been proposed: one by the Child Survival Collaborations and Resources (CORE) Group and USAID's Basic Support for Institutionalizing Child Survival (BASICS II) and the other by WHO Western Pacific Region. The CORE Group/BASICS II proposed three programmatic elements (Table 27.2) that constitute the operational framework for C-IMCI (Winch et al. 2001). This framework shows how the points of intervention could interplay with various inputs to achieve the implementation goals of C-IMCI. The framework highlights the centrality of partnership, community involvement, and integration in the design and implementation of C-IMCI, using experiences and examples of community-based programming.

The C-IMCI framework developed by the WHO Western Pacific Region (WPR) shows the processes by which the three components of IMCI (i.e., improved health provider skills, strengthened health system, and improved family practices) work to improve child health and development. Critical issues in planning C-IMCI services are shown in Fig. 27.4. C-IMCI framework works to improve child health and development through the coordinated effect of four complementary processes (WHO 2004) (Fig. 27.5):

Table 27.2 Three programmatic elements of the C-IMCI

Elements	Examples of corresponding objectives
Element 1 Improving partnership between health facilities and services and the communities they serve	Increase utilization of health facilities and services. Establish mechanisms for community feedback on and/or management of health facilities and services
Element 2 Increasing appropriate, accessible care and information from ommunity-based providers	Increase quality of care from community-based providers. Increase promotion of preventive practices by community-based providers. Decrease harmful practices of community-based providers
Element 3 Integrated promotion of key family practices critical for child health and nutrition	Increased adoption of key family practices for health, nutrition, and development. Engage communities in selecting behaviors to be promoted and identifying actions to be taken

Source: Winch et al. (2001)

1) Partnership and linkages – The implementation of C-IMCI offers a distinct opportunity for health and development programs in private and public sectors to work together in simple collaboration, such as information sharing, or coordination of shared resources. Partnerships in C-IMCI link health facilities, the community, the government (health and other sectors), public and private health providers, different health organizations, and community-based organizations (CBOs) implementing C-IMCI. Effective collaboration leads to coordinated efforts and subsequent improvement of mobilization and utilization of resources. This increases the utilization of health facilities and services at the community level due to increased coordination of communication through direct partnership linkages.

2) Community mobilization and motivation – Promotion of community mobilization and motivation increases the quality of care from

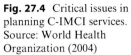

Fig. 27.4 Critical issues in planning C-IMCI services. Source: World Health Organization (2004)

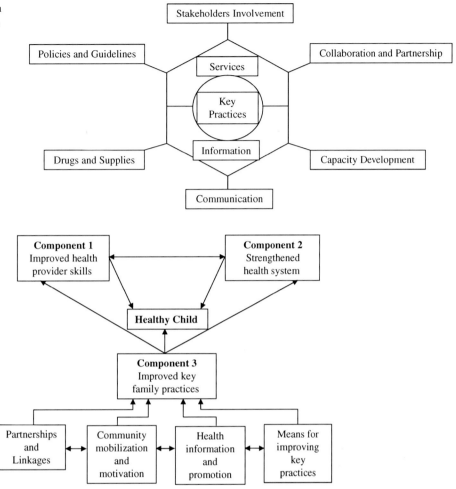

Fig. 27.5 Operational framework for community IMCI (C-IMCI). Source: World Health Organization (2004)

community-based providers by establishing mechanisms for community feedback on and/or management of health facilities and services. It increases appropriate, accessible care and information in addition to promoting preventive practices from community-based providers. Increasing mobilization leads to increased access for families to health providers or facilities that treat sick children and communicate effectively. This increases the prevalence of adequate home care and promotes a home environment that decreases harmful practices of community-based providers and supports children's healthy growth and development.

3) Health information and promotion – Effective, efficient communication is a central strategy for planning and implementing interventions in order to improve key practices. It is a process in which families, community members, and decision makers are engaged in discussions. These discussions enable collaboration and informed decision making for positive behavior change. Promotion activities should enhance the communities' vision for their future and should be complemented by other interventions that focus on community mobilization, training, service-delivery improvement, new or improved technologies, and/or policy change.

4) Means for improving key practices – An increase in the adoption of key family practices for health, nutrition, and development

needs to be targeted in C-IMCI interventions. Improvement of key practices is vital to the enhancement of child health. Communities should engage in selecting key practices that enhance and identify the integrated promotion of key family practices that are critical for the improvement of child health and nutrition.

Evidence Base for IMCI Approach and Implementation Experiences

Most of the disease-based interventions which have been "integrated" within IMCI (viz., treatment of malaria, pneumonia, control of diarrheal and major vaccine preventable diseases) have their basis in sound research evidence. However, the integration approach does not appear to have been supported by direct evidence from well-designed research prior to its implementation. A Cochrane systematic review on health-care integration programs (including the IMCI) found insufficient studies to show whether or not strategies that integrate health-care interventions at the point of delivery are effective (Briggs and Garner 2007). In essence, the IMCI approach could be described as a large implementation research program. The series of multi-country evaluation studies set up by the WHO and its technical partners (Bryce et al. 2004; Tanzania IMCI Multi-Country Evaluation Health Facility Survey Study Group 2004) has been a good attempt at evaluating IMCI as a global health-care initiative and as an implementation research program. There remains a need for more controlled studies that are adequately designed and powered to answer pertinent questions. These questions pertain to the effectiveness of the integration approaches and whether or not it would increase efficiency, improve quality of care, and positively impact childhood morbidity and mortality. Table 27.3 shows the indicators that were used in the WHO multi-country evaluation studies. Box 27.3 presents a summary of interpretation of the findings of the WHO multi-country evaluation of IMCI.

Table 27.3 Indicators of health worker skills, health systems support, assessment, and referral of very sick children

Category	Indicators
Health workers skills	
Assessment of sick children	• Checked for presence of cough, diarrhea, and fever • Weight checked against growth chart • Vaccination status checked • Assessed for feeding practices if under 2 years • Checked for other problems
Correct classification	Correctly classified Correctly classified omitting coughs, colds, no dehydration
Correct treatment	• Pneumonia correctly treated • Malaria correctly treated • Anemia correctly treated • Child needing oral antibiotic and/or oral anti-malarial prescribed drug correctly • Child not needing antibiotic leaves the facility without antibiotic • Child needing vaccinations leaves the facility with all needed vaccinations • First dose of treatment given at facility
Counseling and communication	• Caretaker advised to give extra fluids and continue feeding • Caretaker of child prescribed ORS, oral antibiotic, and/or oral anti-malarial knows how to give the treatment • Caretaker of child prescribed oral medication advised on how to administer treatment • Caretaker advised when to return immediately • Caretaker given or shown a mother's nutrition and counseling card
Health systems support	
Availability of drugs	• Index of availability of essential oral treatments (mean)
Availability of vaccines	• Health facility has equipment and supplies to support vaccination services • Index of availability of four vaccines (mean)
Availability of supplies	• Health facility has essential equipment and materials (includes accessible, working weighing scales for adults and children, timing device, child health cards, source of clean water, spoons, and cups and jugs to mix and administer ORS)

Table 27.3 (continued)

Category	Indicators
Supervision visits	• Health facility has IMCI chart booklet and mother's nutrition and counseling card • Health facility received at least one supervisory visit that included observation of case management during the previous 6 months
Very sick children	
Assessment	• Child checked for three danger signs: – Able to drink or breastfeed – Vomits everything – History of convulsions • Child not visibly awake checked for lethargy
Referral	• Child needing referral is referred • Index of availability of injectable drugs for pre-referral treatment (mean)

Source: Tanzania IMCI Multi-Country Evaluation Health Facility Survey Study Group (2004)

Box 27.3 Summary of Interpretation of Findings of the WHO Multi-country Studies on Evaluation of the Effectiveness of IMCI

- Child survival efforts must begin with local epidemiology, targeting the major causes of death within each region, country, and even district.
- IMCI guidelines for the case management of ill children in health facilities, supported by high-quality training and supportive supervision, are the gold standard and should continue to be implemented widely. New multi-country study findings that IMCI is efficient and costs less than routine care in some settings are encouraging.
- To be successful in reducing child mortality, programs must move beyond health facilities and develop new and more effective ways of reaching children with proven interventions to prevent mortality. In most high-mortality settings, this means providing case management services at community level, as well as focusing on prevention and on reducing rates of under-nutrition.

- Coverage should be the driving force behind district, national, regional, and global child survival programs. Only by paying close attention to whether mothers and children receive interventions can we decipher whether the delivery methods are effective and equitable and whether mortality reductions are likely to occur. Public accountability at all levels can bring delivery bottlenecks to the attention of all and encourage rapid action to address them.
- Countries and districts should be encouraged to prioritize, and to implement first, those interventions known to be cost-effective in reducing under-5 mortality. Better tools to support policy and decision makers in estimating the costs and impact of their choices are needed urgently.
- Ensuring that resources are available, not only for time-limited projects but also in the longer term, is essential to allow sufficient time for planning and implementation to mature and yield impact.
- Much more policy-relevant research is needed and should be conducted at the country level, especially studies that focus on the effectiveness of policies and strategies implemented by Ministries of Health and their partners.

Source: Tanzania IMCI Multi-Country Evaluation Health Facility Survey Study Group (2004)

Implementation Experiences – Successes and Challenges

The implementation of IMCI involves three phases: introduction, early implementation, and expansion. The goal of preliminary visits and activities in the introductory phase is to create a good understanding of IMCI strategy among health professionals and decision makers in the health sector. This will enable them to make informed decisions on whether to adopt the strategy, to encourage their full participation in the planning process, to agree on the management structure for early implementation, and to win the commitment of the national government through the Ministry of Health. While most of these visits succeed in convincing national governments of the majority of countries in developing countries to adopt the IMCI approach, the extent to which these efforts have won adequate political commitment remains unclear.

Given the generally low priority accorded to IMCI in most of the participating countries, it appears that these processes were either not effective to win sufficient political support or failed to offer adequate information to policy makers in regard to cost-implications and benefits. The other potential reason is that the

introductory and early implementation phases were largely donor-supported which gave policy makers the erroneous impression that the approach would always be donor-supported. The result has been that most countries barely go beyond the early implementation phase, since the expansion phase involves relatively high budgets which local authorities do not envisage in the short or medium term and therefore are not prepared to invest in. The continuing effort to summarize the available research reports on the implementation process and effectiveness of IMCI beyond the scope of the WHO multi-country studies is presented in Table 27.4. These studies have addressed diverse outcome variables

Table 27.4 Summary of studies that evaluated different aspects of IMCI implementation

Source/year/location	Study design	Objective	Findings
Victoria et al. (2006) (Brazil, Peru, Tanzania)	Observational study	To describe geographical patterns of implementation of the Integrated Management of Childhood Illness (IMCI) strategy in three countries, Brazil, Peru, and Tanzania, and to assess whether the strategy was implemented in areas with the most pressing child health needs	–Study found that areas of greatest need (district and communities with poor development and health indices) were not prioritized. IMCI implementation strategy lacks guidelines to promote equity –Authors propose "equity analyses" to ensure that geographical deployment of new programs and strategies reach those who need them most
El Arifeen et al. (2004) (Bangladesh (Matlab sub-district)	Cluster-randomized: 20 first-level outpatient facilities in the Matlab sub-district and their catchment areas were randomized to either IMCI or standard care	To determine the effectiveness and efficiency of IMCI implementation in Bangladesh which includes health worker training, health systems support, and community level activities guided by formative research	–Health systems supports were generally available, but implementation of the community activities was slow – Mean index of correct treatment for sick children was 54 in IMCI facilities compared with 9 in comparison facilities (range 0–100) –Use of the IMCI facilities increased from 0.6 visits per child per year at baseline to 1.9 visits per child per year about 21 months after IMCI introduction –19% of sick children in the IMCI area were taken to a health worker compared with 9% in the non-IMCI area

Table 27.4 (continued)

Source/year/location	Study design	Objective	Findings
Ali et al. (2005) (Ethiopia)	Quasi-experimental study	To assess the effect on survival of community-based health promotion activities (community IMCI) in Ethiopia	–Mortality rate was comparable at baseline but significantly lower in the intervention area compared to the control area post-intervention (adjusted hazard ratio = 0.66; 95% confidence interval: 0.46–0.95) –Significant survival advantages for females, children of younger fathers, married parents, living in larger households, and those living near a health center
Bryce et al. (2005) (Tanzania)	Non-randomized controlled trial in two intervention districts (>90% of health-care workers trained in IMCI) and two control districts	To assess the effect of IMCI relative to routine care on the quality and efficiency of providing care for sick children in first-level health facilities in rural Tanzania and to disseminate the results for use in health sector decision making	IMCI training is associated with significantly better child health care in facilities at no additional cost to districts The cost per child visit managed correctly was lower in IMCI than in routine care settings: $4.02 versus $25.70, respectively
Kelly et al. (2007) (Ethiopia)	Randomized controlled trial	To assess caretakers' comprehension and recall of IMCI counseling messages when given under ideal messages	The mean percentage of messages recalled following IMCI counseling was 89.7% immediately after the consultation and 81.9% 1 day later (N = 55 caretakers)
Mohan et al. (2004) (India)	Pair matched, community randomized trial in 12 primary health centers	To assess whether training doctors in counseling improves care-seeking behavior in families with sick children using the IMCI approach	Mothers' appreciation of the need to seek prompt and appropriate care for severe episodes of childhood illness increased, but their care-seeking behavior did not improve significantly
Gilroy et al. (2004) (Mali)	Randomized study in 10 health centers that were either randomized to training or comparison arms	To evaluate the impact of IMCI training on quality of counseling provided to caregivers about administration of anti-malarials to their children	IMCI training showed a non-significant trend overall in improving drug counseling provided to caregivers, with significant improvements in bilingual consultations

using various research methods. Generalizing the results may be misleading. The results are presented here as general information on the scope of research on the subject. As shown, the results highlight varying degrees of effectiveness in different country contexts and underscore the need for further research to fully ascertain the impact of IMCI globally.

The Future of IMCI and Prospects for Scale-Up

Policy environment for scale-up of IMCI: The African Regional Office of the WHO has defined scaling up of IMCI as "the acceleration and expansion of implementation of all components of IMCI in all districts of the country to obtain maximum impact on the reduction of morbidity and mortality due to malaria, pneumonia, diarrhea, measles, malnutrition and HIV/AIDS in children under five years of age" (WHO 2001a). Recent evidence from the multi-country evaluation of IMCI suggests that gains of IMCI in a given country or area of a country would only be significantly attained in the context of at least 80% coverage of the communities and health facilities (Tanzania IMCI Multi-Country Evaluation Health Facility Survey Study Group 2004). The global consensus is that the implementation and scale-up of IMCI has moved at such a snail-speed in most countries that it would take several decades to attain the level of scale-up that would significantly reduce morbidity and mortality in under-5 children. Several reasons have been suggested for this situation, ranging from lack of donor and indigenous resources to insufficient technical and operational experience to serve as lessons to countries that face various forms of bottlenecks. The most critical reason appears to be the lack of political will at local and international levels. This leads to low prioritization of IMCI in the funding program and agenda of national governments and major international donors. The poor policy context of IMCI internationally and within implementing countries has been the key determinant of progress. Table 27.5 provides the results of a qualitative assessment of the IMCI environment using information derived from WHO sources (WHO 2001a). As shown, the results highlight among other notable factors limitations related to political support and commitment and the existence of IMCI implementation framework that is in discord with national strategic objectives and divergent preferences in implementation mechanisms.

Options for private sector participation in IMCI: Involvement of the private sector in IMCI holds enormous opportunities for scale-up and sustainability. Two pathways of private sectors participation options are apparent: (i) IMCI has been promoted as a pro-poor, not-for-profit option. This scenario favors a private–public option in which the government courts private sector participation

Table 27.5 Qualitative appraisal of IMCI policy environment

Desirable determinants of policy environment	Observations on prevailing IMCI policy contexts
• Political support and commitment at all levels, including supportive national policies, laws, and plans	Political support for IMCI has been far from adequate at international and national levels. This is probably the key reason for the slow pace of implementation, limited global experience, and impact of the strategy
• Policies that meet country's expressed needs	The low political commitment and low level of investment in IMCI suggest that the policy framework for IMCI may be discordant with national strategic objectives and preferences in delivery mechanisms. Countries should be encouraged to adopt the IMCI strategy only after careful appraisal shows that IMCI aligns with the strategic direction of health-care programming within that country
• Operational policies that promote access, demand, and quality	All three components of IMCI seek to promote access, demand, and quality of care
• Adequate financial and human resources	International and national funding for IMCI is currently so low that it would be impossible to demonstrate any impact of its contribution to attainment of the health MDGs. Evaluation studies have demonstrated effectiveness of the strategy and potential for impact but adequate financial investment is required to take the implementation to scale and to demonstrate impact
• Active private sector participation	Available reports on implementation experiences lack information on the participation of the private sector in IMCI. Efforts to scale up implementation of IMCI should give careful consideration to mechanisms to involve the private sector
• Implementation of programs according to policies (with efficient processes of evaluation and research)	There is a need to provide adequate resources and structure for efficient monitoring and evaluation of IMCI at international, national, and sub-national levels

through endowments, discounts, and various forms of solicitation for financial support. The private sector comes to this pro-poor option as an altruistic corporate citizen, but would find opportunities to "sell" its image and ultimately its goods. This option raises issues about conflict of interest and ethics on the side of government and the private sector contributors. (ii) The second option which is tagged "pro-quality" marketing option woos the private sector to invest in the IMCI approach as a business venture under well-controlled regulatory conditions. Quality improvement is a central theme of IMCI and is capable of engaging the interest of the private sector. Private sector involvement boosts global resources available for IMCI implementation and leads to a sustainable scale-up. In most developing countries, the non-formal health sector dominates as a leading provider of private health-care services. The bulk of their clientele is the urban and rural poor and middle class (where it still exists). Encouraging the private sector to participate in service provision at the level of primary health care and to adopt IMCI as a key care approach expands the proportion of quality-assured care at that level. It will competitively lead to the contraction of the market share of unorthodox practices.

Implication for Global Health System Reform

IMCI, as a broad-based intervention strategy, is potentially capable of effectively contributing to current global aspirations to reform the health systems of the poorest economies of the world and scale up health-care intervention efforts in order to achieve impact in the short and medium term. Many health systems in developing countries are currently undergoing some type of reform. This is often spurred by a de-centralization of management (WHO 1999). Improvements in equity, efficiency, quality of care, effectiveness, and sustainability are often the stated objectives of global health system reform.

In order for IMCI to be effective within a country, different levels of action are required for health services in the home and community. Coordination and quality of services should be improved to increase the health-care effectiveness and to reduce costs. By providing inclusive standards and valid

training that is country specific, IMCI contributes to improving global quality of care. The IMCI model, when implemented correctly, will improve service delivery. This model could then be applied to other aspects of health care. Table 27.6 shows the areas in which the strengths of IMCI could potentially contribute to the achievement of health system goals, especially as it affects child health, and therefore it should be taken into account early in the reform process.

Table 27.6 Potential IMCI contribution to health system reforms

Common reform aims (World Bank)	Potential IMCI contribution to health reforms
• Increase technical efficiency • Improve allocative efficiency • Improve effectiveness and quality • Prioritize inputs and deliver essential package of cost-effective services • Integrate vertical programs • Decentralize authorities, responsibilities, and accountabilities • Collaborate with private sector • Coordinate donor resources • Improve client responsiveness	• Integration of vertical programs (acute respiratory infection, control of diarrheal disease, expanded program on immunization, malaria control, nutrition) • Increasing technical efficiency • Improving effectiveness (and quality) of diagnosis and treatment • Improving provider motivation • mproving client/patient compliance and motivation • Rationalization of drug use

Conclusions

The technical strengths of IMCI are integration and the expected improvement in technical efficiency and quality of care. The multi-country evaluation has lent reasonable support to the claim that IMCI is a cost-effective approach to improving the quality of health care for children in low-resource settings. While there is need for more evidence from controlled trials to further support or disprove this claim, implementation experiences are relatively sparse. However, they have provided evidence on the relative effectiveness of IMCI compared to routine practice. While these implementation experiences lack statistical power of proof, they show robustness in their contextual link with real national and district health policies and programs. Why then do donor communities ignore an initiative that promises to save cost and deliver on quality? Why are politicians not interested in supporting IMCI? These are pertinent questions for the next round of the IMCI research project.

There are issues about equity in the IMCI. One of the key findings of the multi-country evaluation is that IMCI in its present form has not adopted measures that assure equity in implementation. The result is that those who need health care the most, due to deplorable health and development indices, are the least covered by IMCI in some countries. This presents issues about the next phase of the IMCI scale-up. There should be a strategic decision to target those with the poorest health outcomes and development indices also endeavoring to avoid creation of new levels of inequity by completely ignoring those that currently have relatively better development and health indices within countries.

IMCI has been one of the least supported international public health initiatives. This is despite the fact that it has the potential to provide an efficient pathway for delivery of interventions to control malaria and HIV/AIDS. Effective control of these is crucial to achieving the health-related MDGs. The general principles of IMCI, in addition to the programmatic elements of the C-IMCI framework, are based on the assumption that integration of these major disease interventions would occur at all levels and lead to joint planning, budgeting, implementation, monitoring, and evaluation. The prevailing situation is that these heavily supported programs tend to be implemented disparately, with little or no commitment in human and financial resources. This does not conform to the basic principles of IMCI and detracts from the original goal of primary health care as a holistic approach to the delivery of child health services in low-income countries. Those that fund malaria and HIV/AIDS treatment programs can encourage this integration process by requiring integrated case management as one of the key criteria to fund and appraise program grants. Examples of these programs are the Global Fund to fight against AIDS, TB, and malaria, the US Presidential initiatives for HIV/AIDS and Malaria, respectively, and other equivalent grants made by the Bill and Melinda Gates Foundation.

Key Terms

Acute respiratory infections (ARI)	Expansion phase	Malaria
Case management	Health systems	Malnutrition
Child survival revolution	Health systems development	Measles
Community IMCI	Hygiene promotion	Nutrition
Community mobilization	Immunization	Oral rehydration therapy
Community-based organizations (CBOs)	In-service course	Primary health care
Convulsions	Integrated care	Quality improvement
Diarrhea	Integrated management of childhood illnesses (IMCI)	Quality of care
Early implementation phase	Lethargy	Service delivery
		Vertical programs

Questions for Discussion

1. What is the rationale for adoption of IMCI as a strategy for promoting child health in developing countries?

2. Outline and discuss the three technical components of IMCI.

3. What are the principles of integrated care as defined and used in IMCI?

4. What are the seven principles of community-integrated management of childhood illnesses (C-IMCI)?

5. In an essay of about 300 words, describe the evidence base of the disease-focused interventions that are "integrated" within IMCI (i.e., treatment for malaria, pneumonia, control of diarrhea, and major vaccine preventable diseases).

6. In what ways can IMCI be scaled up to enhance child health improvement in developing countries? What are the barriers?

References

Ali M, Asefaw T, Byass P et al. (2005) Helping northern Ethiopian communities reduce childhood mortality: population-based intervention trial. Bulletin of the World Health Organization, 83: 27–33

Briggs CJ, Garner P (2007) Strategies for integrating primary health services in middle and low income countries at the point of delivery. Cochrane Database of Systematic Reviews, 1

Bryce, J, Victora CG, Habicht J et al. (2004) The multi-country evaluation of the integrated management of childhood illness strategy: lessons for the evaluation of public health interventions. American Journal of Public Health, 94(3): 406–415

Bryce J, Gouws E, Adam T et al. (2005) Improving quality and efficiency of facility based child healthcare through integrated management of childhood illness in Tanzania. Health Policy and Planning, 20(1): i69–i76

Campbell H, Gove S (1996) Integrated management of childhood infections and malnutrition: a global initiative. Archives of Disease in Childhood, 75(6): 468–470

Caulfield LE, de Onis M, Blössner M et al. (2004) Undernutrition as an underlying cause of child deaths associated with diarrhea, pneumonia, malaria, and measles. American Journal of Clinical Nutrition, 80: 193–198

CORE Group (2007) CORE. http://www.coregroup.org/ imci/, cited 21 Feb 2008

Ehiri JE, Prowse JM (1999) Child health promotion in developing countries: the case for integration of environmental and social interventions? Health Policy and Planning, 14(1): 1–10

El Arifeen S, Blum LS, Hoque DM (2004) Integrated management of childhood illness (IMCI) in Bangladesh: early findings from a cluster-randomized study. Lancet, 364: 1595–1602

Gilroy K, Winch PJ, Diawara A et al. (2004) Impact of IMCI training and language used by provider on quality of counseling provided to parents of sick children in Bougouni District, Mali. Patient Education and Counseling, 54(1): 35–44

Global Action for Children (2008) Global action for children: the facts. http://www.globalactionforchildren.org/ static/the_facts/, cited 20 Feb 2008

Kelly JM, Rowe AK, Onikpo F et al. (2007) Care takers' recall of integrated management of childhood illness

counseling messages in Benin. Tropical Doctor, 37(2): 75–79

Mohan P, Iyengar SD, Martines J et al. (2004) Impact of counseling on care seeking behavior in families with sick children: cluster randomized trial in rural India. BMJ, 31, 329: 266

Pelletier DL, Frongillo EA Jr, Schroeder DG et al. (1995) The effects of malnutrition on child mortality in developing countries. Bulletin of the World Health Organization, 73(4): 443–448

Schellenberg A, Adam JR, Mshinda T et al. (2004) Effectiveness and cost of facility-based integrated management of childhood illness (IMCI) in Tanzania. Lancet, 364(9445): 1583–1594

Tanzania IMCI Multi-Country Evaluation Health Facility Survey Study Group (2004) The effect of integrated management of childhood illness on observed quality of care of under fives in rural Tanzania. Health Policy and Planning, 19(1): 1–10

United Nations Children's Fund (UNICEF) (2001) Community IMCI: A Strategy for Accelerating Child Survival and Developmental Interventions. New York: United Nations Children's Fund (UNICEF) Discussion Paper

Victora CG, Huicho L, Amaral JJ et al. (2006) Are health interventions implemented where they are most needed? District uptake of the integrated management of childhood illness strategy in Brazil, Peru and the United Republic of Tanzania. Bulletin of the World Health Organization, 84: 792–801

Winch P, Leban K, Kusha B (2001) Reaching Communities for Child Health and Nutrition: A Framework for Household and Community IMCI. http://www.popline.org/ docs/1580/172408.html, cited 21 Feb 2008

World Bank (1993) World Development Report, 1993: Investing in Health. Washington, DC: World Bank

World Health Organization/United Nations Children's Fund (1978) Declaration of Alma Alta. Report on the International Conference on Primary Healthcare. Alma Alta, USSR. September 6th–12th

World Health Organization/United Nations Children's Fund (1999) Integrated Management of Childhood Illnesses (IMCI) Planning guide, gaining experience with the IMCI strategy in a country. WHO/UNICEF Document: WHO/CHS/CAH/99.1. Geneva/New York: World Health Organization/UNICEF http://whqlibdoc. who.int/hq/1999/WHO_CHS_CAH_99.1_eng.pdf, cited 24 July 2008

World Health Organization (1999) Integrated Management of Childhood Illness and health sector reform. WHO DocumentWHO/CHS/CAH/98.1L. REV.1 1999 http:// libdoc.who.int/hq/1998/WHO_CHS_CAH_98.1L_eng.pdf, cited 10 May 2008

World Health Organization (2001a) Integrated Management of Childhood Illnesses: Planning, Implementing and Evaluating Pre-service Training. Geneva: World Health Organization, Department of Child and Adolescent Health and Development (CAH), Family and Community Health (FCH). http://www.who.int/child_ adolescent_health/documents/pdfs/planning_implementing_ evaluating.pdf, cited July 24, 2008

World Health Organization (2001b) WHO Regional Office for Africa's Annual IMCI Report 2001. Brazzaville, Congo: WHO Regional Office for Africa.http://www.afro.who.int/imci/reports/imci_annual_report.pdf, cited 21 Feb 2008

World Health Organization (2003) World Health Report – Shaping the Future. Geneva: World Health Organization: http://www.usaid.gov/our_work/global_health/nut/techareas/malnutrition_chart.html, cited 20 Feb 2008

World Health Organization (2004) Child Health in the Community: Community IMCI: Briefing Package for Facilitators. Geneva: World Health Organization.http://whqlibdoc.who.int/publications/2004/9241591951_V1.pdf, cited 21 Feb 2008

Chapter 28
Planning, Development, and Maintenance of the MCH Workforce

Jeffrey M. Smith and Anne Hyre

Learning Objectives After reading this chapter and answering the discussion questions that follow, you should be able to

- Discuss the relationship between health worker density and maternal and child health indicators.
- Critically analyze the challenges in health sector human resource planning, development, and maintenance in developing countries.
- Identify and discuss elements of successful training programs with respect to deployment, integration, supervision, support, and retention of MCH workers.
- Evaluate factors that influence the performance MCH workers and discuss gender issues related to MCH workforce in developing countries.

Introduction

As the World health Organization observed in the 2000 World Health Report entitled, "Health Systems – Improving Performance" (WHO 2000), human resources, the different kinds of clinical and non-clinical staff who provide services to individuals and families, are the most important of the health system's inputs. The performance of health-care systems depends ultimately on the knowledge, skills, and motivation of the people responsible for delivering services. The provision of maternal and child health (MCH) services at service delivery sites requires three basic elements: skilled personnel who provide the services; an enabling environment for services (including infrastructure, supplies, and drugs), and organizational processes and policy framework that define the package of services and how they are to be provided. Thus, the process of preparing, enabling, and supporting health workers is central to the mission of providing high-quality MCH services. Given that two-thirds of the health budget in any given country is typically devoted to the salary support for health workers (Vujicic 2005), maximizing the efficiency and effectiveness of that workforce should be a priority in the health sector. Also, in developing countries, MCH services represent a large proportion of the health services consumed by the public. In some populations, the combination of children under 5 years of age and women of reproductive age can reach 40% of the total. Yet, the ability to provide these services is continually challenged by lack of human resources, maldistribution of the limited available health workers, verticalization of health services, issues of competency, and retention of health staff. This chapter explores the nature of the MCH workforce, those factors necessary to develop and support these workers and help them to perform, and the unique elements that influence their ability to effectively provide MCH services. To provide a common understanding, some of the terminologies used in this chapter are defined in Box 28.1.

J.M. Smith (✉)
JHPIEGO Corporation/Johns Hopkins University
Bloomberg School of Public Health, Baltimore,
Maryland, USA

J.E. Ehiri (ed.), *Maternal and Child Health*, DOI 10.1007/b106524_28,
© Springer Science+Business Media, LLC 2009

Box 28.1 Key Definitions

Pre-service Education: The process by which students enrolled in a recognized educational institution are given the knowledge, skills, and professional foundation to enter the health workforce upon completion of their course of study. Graduates are awarded a diploma or degree upon successfully completing all of the requirements of the curriculum and then must obtain a license to practice from an appropriate regulatory agency or professional body (Schaefer 2002).

In-service Training: Continuing study by a health-care provider in order to gain new knowledge and/or skills or refresh and strengthen the knowledge and skills used in his/her current practice. The provider retains his/her original qualification and professional designation at the end of the course (Sullivan 1995).

Competency-Based Training: The training process for developing the specific knowledge, attitudes, and skills needed to provide a particular service or activity. It is skill focused and requires that the participant demonstrate that he or she can perform the skill or activity by the end of the training (Sullivan 1995).

Skilled Birth Attendant: The term "skilled attendant" refers exclusively to people with midwifery skills (for example, midwives, doctors, and nurses) who have been trained to proficiency in the skills necessary to manage normal deliveries and diagnose, manage, or refer obstetric complications. At minimum, the person must be competent to manage normal childbirth and be able to provide emergency (first-line) obstetric care. Not all skilled attendants can provide comprehensive emergency obstetric care although they should have the skills to diagnose when such interventions are needed and should have the capacity to refer women to a higher level of care (WHO 2004).

Midwife: A midwife is a person who, having been regularly admitted to a midwifery educational program, duly recognized in the country in which it is located, has successfully completed the prescribed course of studies in midwifery and has acquired the requisite qualifications to be registered and/or legally licensed to practice midwifery (International Confederation of Midwives 2005).

The Crisis in Human Resources for Health in Resource-Poor Settings

In many countries in all regions of the world, the absolute number of health workers is not adequate to provide the necessary services. This results in rationing of services, concentration of services in the urban areas, and reduction in the quality of services due to the overburdening of health-care workers. Table 28.1 presents data on health worker density, life expectancy, and infant and adult mortality rates for selected countries.

While there is no absolute recommendation for the number of health workers per population, some data suggest that a certain density of health workers is necessary to achieve certain health goals, including two indicators related to the Millennium Development Goals (MDGs) – measles immunization and skilled attendance at birth (Fig. 28.1). Analysis of the health worker density necessary to achieve these outputs suggests that a density of about 1.5 health workers per 1,000 population is associated with 80% coverage of measles immunization and that 2.5 skilled birth attendants per 1,000 population is necessary to provide 80% of women with a skilled attendant at birth (Joint Learning Initiative 2004). Studies have also examined the effect of reductions in health sector human resources on maternal and child health outcomes within countries. Beginning in 1992 in Indonesia health centers began reducing their staffing levels in response to budget cuts imposed by the government in its bid to reduce its fiscal deficit. The large reduction in staffing (1.8 to 1.2 physicians per health centre) led to a 39% increase in the child

Table 28.1 Ratios of health workers to populations and selected health indicators, selected countries, 2000–2005

	Country				
	Afghanistan	Zambia	Ethiopia	Bolivia	Sweden
Population 2004 (000)	28,574	11,479	75,600	9,009	9,008
Health Worker Density					
(per 1,000 population)					
Physicians	0.19	0.12	0.03	1.22	3.28
Midwives	0.01	0.27	0.01	0.01	0.70
Nurses	0.22	1.74	0.23	3.19	10.24
Life expectancy at birth (years) – males	42	40	49	63	78
Life expectancy at birth (years) – females	42	40	51	66	83
Adult mortality rate – males aged 15–60	509	683	451	248	82
Adult mortality rate – females aged 15–60	448	656	389	184	51
Infant mortality rate	257	182	166	69	4

Sources: Management Sciences for Health and Health and Development Service (2003); WHO (2006a)

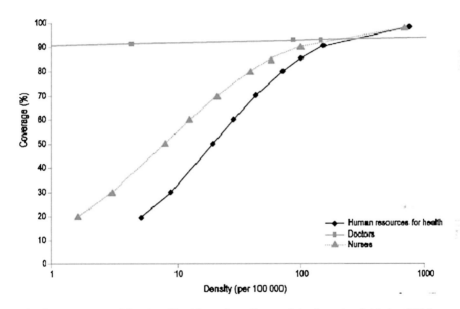

Fig. 28.1 Immunization coverage and density of health workers. Source: Joint Learning Initiative (2004)

stunting rate (Barber and Gertler 2005). In the United States and Canada there is evidence to suggest that reductions in nurse staffing levels in hospitals led to a decrease in quality of care and to an increase in mortality and complications for certain procedures (Aiken et al. 2002).

Similarly, the availability of health workers has a direct and positive effect on the morbidity and mortality of mothers, infants, and children. When income, education, and poverty levels are controlled for, a 10% increase in the number of health workers per 1,000 population leads to a 2–5% decrease in child mortality rates (Fig. 28.2). The benefit to

maternal mortality is even higher, given that the presence of a health worker will more directly affect the types of morbidities that lead to maternal death than those that lead to infant or under-5 deaths (Joint Learning Initiative 2004).

Currently, there is a substantial shortage globally in the number of health workers able to provide MCH services. This shortage is especially acute in Africa (Fig. 28.3). It is estimated that in the next 10 years, an additional 334,000 midwives (above current development plans) will be needed globally. Furthermore, knowledge and skill updates will be required for another 27,000 doctors and technicians

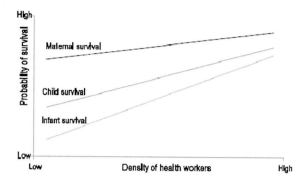

Fig. 28.2 Health worker density and child mortality. Source: WHO (2006a)

to enable them to provide appropriate consultation to these midwives. In the next 10 years, the expansion, updating, and upgrading of the health workforce for MCH will require an additional investment of US $25 billion (WHO 2005).

This crisis in health workforce capacity and capability puts at risk other investments and initiatives to address health challenges. Limitations in human resources may impede current investments in health care, including those that address MCH. For example, although more resources are available from such groups as the GAVI Alliance and the Global Fund to Fight AIDS, Tuberculosis and Malaria, limitations in the health workforce reduce the capacity of countries to benefit optimally from these resources (Dussault

and Dubois 2003). Simply put, in some countries, there are not enough health workers to do the job, regardless of the available funding to fight disease.

There are numerous factors contributing to the health workforce crisis. The economic migration and brain drain of health workers deepen the health crisis in the countries they leave. In a recent article, Stilwell et al. (2004) analyzed the extent of the problem of health worker migration, examining the determinants, effects on health systems, and strategic approaches to its management. As they noted, the trend in health personnel migration is neither different from the overall trend in international migration nor a new phenomenon. However, globalization and global acute shortage of skilled health personnel in both rich and poor countries mean that these personnel are highly sought after globally. With aging populations in many high-income countries and the growing shortage of health workers (especially nurses), countries such as the United Kingdom and the United States have programs that specifically recruit health workers from developing countries to fill their vacancies (Stilwell et al. 2004). Factors that encourage migration of health personnel from poor to rich countries (Fig. 28.4) have been shown to include low wages, household poverty (the money sent back to their home countries by migrants is the most stable source of external finance in some countries; the figures for the 1990s exceeded the

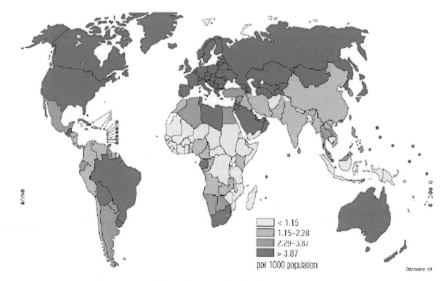

This map is an approximation of actual country borders.

Fig. 28.3 Density of health-care providers (doctors, nurses, and midwives). Source: WHO (2006a)

Reasons for leaving

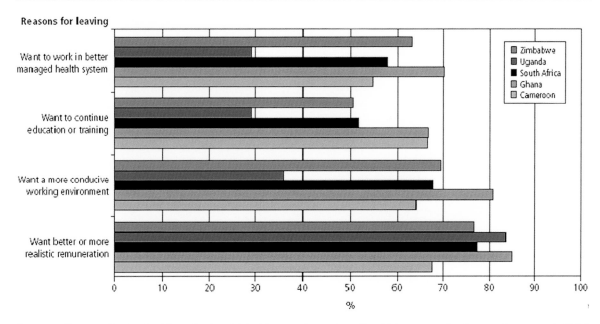

Fig. 28.4 Factors affecting health professionals' decision to migrate from five African countries. Source: Awases et al. (2003)

amount of official development aid flowing into source countries (Connell 2002)), poor working conditions, lack of opportunities for promotion, desire to gain experience, changes in labor and visa regulations, and active recruitment drives from poor countries by rich nations (Awases et al. 2003).

Within countries, there is a concentration of health workers in urban areas, as a result of challenging working conditions, poor work environments, quality-of-life issues, and low salaries. Health workers are either leaving the public sector in favor of the private sector or engaging in dual practice scenarios, due to salary pressure, unclear career advancement, or restrictions on practice patterns. The economic migration and maldistribution are compounded in some areas by loss of health workers due to HIV/AIDS. This constellation of factors leads to lack of motivation, decreased performance, and a downward spiral of greater migration from the health workforce.

Who Provides Health Care to Mothers, Newborns, and Children?

As the components of MCH vary from country to country, so does the constellation of workers who provide the services. Within a health-care system,

MCH services are provided by a team of professionals (Table 28.2) that depend on the scope of services provided. Often, the midwife is the central worker since her skill set most closely matches the needs of the MCH population and because women often state a preference for a female health worker for these services due to cultural norms and customs.

A strategy for training and deploying a midwife to a health center, and supporting her to deliver basic emergency obstetric care, is considered a central strategy for reducing maternal and newborn mortality (Campbell and Graham 2006). This "health center intrapartum care strategy" advocates that women deliver in a health center under the care of a midwife who is supported by a team of other health-care providers. As opposed to a strategy that promotes home-based care by a skilled attendant, this strategy enables women to receive care from a provider who can address the majority of complications, in a location that allows timely intervention and easy transport to other facilities if referral is deemed necessary. This strategy also facilitates support and supervision of midwives and provides midwives with sufficient caseload to maintain their clinical skills. The success of this strategy, however, is contingent upon improving the quality of care offered at health centers and modifying health

Table 28.2 Typology of health workers

Category	Worker type	Education	Skills/tasks
Informal workers	• Volunteers • Family and home carers	Variable, none specific to caring role	• Practical care • Supervising medication • Transporting individuals
Traditional healers	• Curanderas • Shamans	Variable	• Healing • Counseling • Use of traditional and natural medicines
Community workers	• Village health workers • Community health workers	Primary-secondary school with brief pre-service and on-the-job training	• Ambulatory home and community-based care (immunization, oral rehydration, nutrition, etc.) • Prevention, promotion, and management of basic health problems • Public health outreach • Referral function
Vocational workers	• Medical assistants • Nursing and dental aides • Laboratory technicians	Secondary school, college	• Assisting health professionals • Technical support • Home-based care
Health professionals	• Doctors • Nurses • Dentists • Pharmacists • Midwives • Psychologists • Physician's assistants • Public health officers	Tertiary – professional college, university	• Diagnosing and treating acute and chronic illnesses • Hospital and community care • Health promotion and education • Palliative care • Record-keeping of past medical histories • Referral function
Teachers and researchers	• Faculty lecturers • Laboratory researchers • Epidemiologists • Pharmaceutical developers	Post-basic university (e.g., Master's, PhD)	• Developing new knowledge • Preparing health professionals for entry to the workforce • Working with policy makers to implement new knowledge into policy and practice
Non-medical workers	• Managers • Accountants • Drivers • Policy makers	All kinds	• Various support functions to health systems and health workers

Source: Joint Learning Initiative (2004)

center birthing environments to address cultural and personal concerns of women and their families.

Given the nature of MCH, facility-based services and personnel should be complemented by community-based services and a variety of community health workers. Community health workers or health volunteers provide a spectrum of MCH services that vary widely from country to country, but typically include preventative health activities, counseling and information sharing, and services such as family planning (WHO 1995), treatment of newborn infections (Bang et al. 2005), and prevention of postpartum hemorrhage (JHPIEGO/MNH Program 2004). Specifically, community-based health workers include village health volunteers, community health extension workers, traditional birth attendants (TBAs), health promoters, and other workers. In some countries, skilled care has been taken to the community level where community midwives reside in the villages they serve and provide services from their own homes or in the homes of their clients.

Planning for the MCH Workforce

Health workforce planning requires the articulation of clear government policies that define the package of health-care services to be provided, the types of personnel who are needed to provide these services, and the job descriptions of those personnel. Thus, health workforce planning is a process of estimating the number and types of health personnel needed to achieve predetermined health targets. The process of planning has to answer the question "How many of each type of health worker does the health system need?" for example, how many midwives are needed to provide essential obstetric care to the current and future population of women of reproductive age? It must also address "Where and when these human resources are needed to accomplish the goals of the health sector" and thus requires a level of microplanning that uses good data about the resources for, and distribution of, health services (Joint Learning Initiative 2004).

Human resource planning requires highly specialized technical skills because multiple and complex variables intervene in determining human resources needs. There are different methodologies, based on different underlying assumptions, for developing plans for the health-care workforce. Planning can

- Determine the health-care personnel needed in ratio to the population distribution (population-based methodology)
- Assume that the populations will be served in the future in the way they are currently being served (utilization-based methodology)
- Estimate the requirements to meet all or part of the expected health-care needs in response to the types of diseases in the populations (needs-based methodology)
- Establish the requirements to satisfy the expected development of health-care services and the

preferences of the population (effective demand-based methodology)

The planning methodology chosen by a particular country depends on the specific characteristics of the country's health system and, frequently, on the availability and quality of data necessary for planning and decision making. A single planning methodology may not fit the requirements of every situation. Many countries have expressed a commitment to reduce maternal mortality by increasing the number of births attended by a skilled birth attendant (SBA) (Sachs and McArthur 2005). These efforts provide an excellent illustration of the application of health workforce planning concepts. To increase the number of births attended by a skilled birth attendant, there must be a policy in place that describes what a skilled birth attendant is, what the skill set is for that attendant and, specifically, which cadres of health workers are or will be considered as skilled birth attendants.

Once the cadres for skilled attendants are clarified in a country, the job description must be updated to reflect the new or amended responsibilities of these personnel. In-service training courses (or pre-service education curricula) must be designed or redesigned, based on national clinical service delivery guidelines, so that providers are trained in a manner consistent with the country's service delivery processes. The training materials and the training process must be competency based, so that health workers acquire the skills in processes that most efficiently and effectively use the limited time, resources, and effort available.

Developing the MCH Workforce

Health workforce development is the process by which the supply of skilled health workers is made available. Development of the MCH workforce in most countries includes the process of pre-service education – the production of new health workers, as well as in-service training to maintain the skills of those workers. While certain elements are recognized as critical to the success of both pre-service education and in-service training, health worker development must consider elements of human capacity development in order to increase the impact of training on health services. These are discussed below.

Elements of Successful Training Programs

Training programs must be designed to effectively transfer and assess the knowledge, skills, and attitudes of MCH workers. Often, training programs focus on acquisition of knowledge (technical updates or classroom-based courses) and the observation or discussion of clinical procedures, rather than on the acquisition of competency in these skills. If managed in a systematic and results-oriented manner, training has a positive impact on knowledge and skills (Fogarty et al. 2004). Competency-based training courses, which enable providers to individually develop clinical skills or modify attitudes, are typically more time-consuming, resource-intensive, and challenging to implement. While challenging, this approach is a far more effective mechanism for transferring critical clinical skills (Limpaphayom et al. 1997).

Decisions to conduct training interventions should be made following an assessment of the performance of health workers and the ability of the health system to meet predetermined targets or objectives. If that assessment suggests that limitations in MCH services are due to a gap in the knowledge and skills of providers, a training intervention should be considered. Further assessments, often called training needs assessments, must be done to identify whether an in-service training program or a pre-service program is necessary. Training needs assessments also look at the current training and education system, the policy environment in which health workers learn and work, the learning materials and methodologies used, and the capacity and capability of the training institutions and trainers/teachers.

To improve clinical care, training institutions and programs must ensure structured opportunities for participants to develop necessary clinical skills. To achieve these improvements, participants require adequate time to review the clinical procedure with experienced trainers, practice the skill in a simulated setting (such as a skill learning lab) in which they can master the steps of target psychomotor skills, and then apply the skill in a clinical setting under supervision. Through this process, they are more likely to achieve clinical competence and thus improve clinical care. Whether the training program is a pre-service education program (e.g., in a medical or midwifery school) or an in-service training program, there are several elements that increase the quality of training and thus the likelihood that it will result in competent providers.

Policy, Curricula, Service Delivery Guidelines, and Learning Materials

Evidence-based training materials that are supported by clear reference documents should be developed for both trainers and learners. Learners' materials should include the information to be learned, and the tools necessary for learning this information (e.g., case studies for learning clinical decision making, role plays for building communication and counseling skills), and detailed and explicit skill learning guides for developing clinical skills. These should be complemented by materials for teachers and trainers, such as knowledge assessment questionnaires, answer keys for case studies, and skill checklists for assessing the development of clinical skills. All of these materials should be based on national service delivery guidelines and policies that facilitate student learning and appropriate practice following the completion of learning. If students are taught to provide care that is not supported by national clinical norms and guidelines, or vice versa, they will be unprepared for the clinical workplace, leading to the need for retraining and waste of resources.

High-Quality Clinical Practice Sites

The development of clinical competency requires that learners be given an opportunity to practice the desired clinical skills in actual clinical facilities. During clinical practice they will use the knowledge, skills, and attitudes being learned in the classrooms. The standard of clinical care in these facilities should be consistent with service delivery guidelines and the theory described in the curriculum. There is an

Box 28.2 Indonesia Case Study: Promoting High-Quality Training – The Indonesian National Clinical Training Network

Since 1991, reducing maternal mortality has been a priority for Indonesia's Ministry of Health. Early efforts to tackle the problem focused on rapidly educating large numbers of midwives who would be distributed widely across the country, and within a few years a remarkable 57,000 *bidan de desa* (village midwives) were produced. Over time, however, concern was raised about the midwives' skills, and it seemed that the desire for quantity had overtaken a focus on quality. Many midwives lacked the essential skills to deliver effective services, and the impact of the program was questioned. In 1997, a major initiative was launched to upgrade the skills of these midwives using standardized, competency-based training as the centerpiece of the strategy.

The Indonesian Association of Obstetricians and Gynecologists and the Indonesian Midwives Association, together with partners and stakeholders, formed the National Clinical Training Network (NCTN). The NCTN established standards for high-quality training, including standards for training centers, training materials, and trainers. They realized the importance of high-quality clinical experience and paid particular attention to the environments in which participants learned and practiced their clinical skills. The quality of care at the clinical training sites was upgraded, the clinical preceptors were given coaching skills, and training and assessment materials were revised. Additional clinical practice sites were developed and students were taught in smaller batches. All of these efforts were made to ensure that trainees were achieving competency.

The systematic process of training had an impact. The trainers and the government saw the difference made by a high-quality training process that focused on skill development. The midwives were providing more services and increasing their coverage in the communities. In 1999, the Ministry of Health endorsed a policy that identified the NCTN as the sole provider of clinical training in reproductive health in Indonesia. The principles of sound training demonstrated by the NCTN became the standard throughout the country.

As a result of these efforts, the NCTN currently has the capacity to offer high-quality training in maternal and newborn health. Since 2001, approximately 14,000 midwives have undergone training through the NCTN. Quality has won out over quantity, and the country is on the path to achieving its goal of reduced maternal mortality.

expected and desired process of professional socialization that begins in training and extends to the workplace. Students or workers who have learned new skills will adopt the clinical behaviors that are prevalent in the facilities where they learn and practice. Therefore, the clinical practices of clinical staff and clinical preceptors may need to be standardized so that they are modeling the specific clinical behaviors that are being taught. Often, initial work is necessary to upgrade and standardize the practices in these clinical learning sites, in an effort to reduce the gap between classroom theory and clinical practice. Although this is a challenging component of any initiative to improve clinical training, if it is not done, the other efforts are not likely to succeed. The

National Clinical Training Network in Indonesia (Box 28.2) provides a good example of in-service training that incorporates the elements of a successful training system, from the use of standardized curricula to the development of high-quality classroom and clinical training environments.

Qualified Teachers and Trainers

Effective teaching requires that trainers and faculty have the appropriate skills to enable them to correctly and efficiently transfer the course content. Teachers need up-to-date clinical skills so that they are proficient in the knowledge and skills they are teaching. In addition, they need strong training skills to allow them to correctly use modern pedagogic approaches such as competency-based training. These skills include mastery of adult learning theories and principles (Brookfield 1986), the use of effective presentation techniques, management of small-group activities, clinical coaching to support learners as they develop clinical skills, and the ability to coordinate and manage the development of clinical skills in both simulated and real health facility environments.

Well-Equipped Teaching Environments

Competency-based education and training require that learning environments be appropriately equipped to facilitate knowledge and skill transfer and assessment. Classrooms must have necessary audiovisual equipment such as overhead projectors or video players. Clinical skill development laboratories must be adequately equipped with anatomic models and instruments to allow all students to have adequate opportunity for supervised practice before providing services and performing procedures on real patients. In addition, clinical practice sites must be relevant to the reality of where learners will practice after their training is completed. Use of clinical practice sites should be managed to ensure that students are supervised and allowed to practice the skills in the curriculum. If a midwifery curriculum includes the care of patients in both inpatient and outpatient environments, suitable practice sites for both of these areas must be employed. The number of students going to an individual site must be limited to allow for both the development of student competencies and the maintenance of clients' rights and privacy.

Evaluation of Training Interventions

The systematic evaluation of training is essential for ensuring that training interventions achieve the objectives of improved performance and greater availability of services. Evaluation approaches are typically conducted at five levels as follows:

- *Level 1 – Participant reaction*: How participants liked the course and perceived its value. The responses should be used by trainers to improve their training skills.
- *Level 2 – Participant learning*: Whether participants learned the required knowledge and skills. These are assessments of knowledge and skills gained in the course. This information is used as a basis for determining whether participants can receive a certificate of competency and thus guides post-training follow-up. It is also used for assessing the design of the training and its ability to achieve the stated objectives of the training.
- *Level 3 – On-the-job performance*: How and whether participants applied the newly acquired knowledge, skills, and attitudes on the job. It is measured through changes in on-the-job performance, and the results are used to reassess the quality of training courses and the extent to which trainees were able to transfer new skills to the workplace.
- *Level 4 – Effect of training*: The extent to which the quality or availability of services changed as a result of the training intervention. It uses service delivery statistics and quality indicators and helps determine the appropriateness of using training as the intervention to address service provision gaps.
- *Level 4 – Impact of training*: This is a measure of the long-term contribution of training to improvements in population health outcomes – reduction in diarrheal diseases among infants and children, reductions in infant and maternal mortality, etc. Training impact is more difficult to measure since improvements in population health outcomes cannot result from training alone, but from a range of medical and nonmedical programs and policies.

Deployment of Health-Care Workers

After health-care providers are prepared, they must be deployed to health-care facilities where they can apply their knowledge and skills to address the needs of the community they are meant to serve. Deployment may be through voluntary choices of the graduates/trainees; through enticements such as salary differentials, priority for professional advancement, etc.; or mandatory, based on compulsory service programs or service requirements. Planning for successful deployment requires substantial coordination and collaboration between the producers of human resources (typically the Ministry of Education and private schools) and the consumers of human resources (typically the Ministry of Health). The goal of deployment is to successfully link a newly trained and skilled health worker with a facility or community prepared to employ and utilize the worker. A key factor in effective deployment is successful recruitment and selection of students prior to enrollment. If students are selected from the major urban centers in a country, it is challenging and often unlikely that these students will be successfully deployed to rural health centers upon graduation. To achieve a higher level of deployment, especially of midwives and female nurses, a strategy of targeted recruitment from locations near the sites of deployment may have a better result. Factors such as origin, ethnicity, marital status, and gender may need to be considered when deployment of graduates is planned (Fritzen 2007).

Depending on the nature of the health system and its relation to the education system in the country, graduates either enter the marketplace upon graduation, where they are expected to find their own employment, or enter government service and are employed, either partly or entirely, by the government. To ensure public welfare, health systems must be highly regulated if graduates are expected to identify their own work opportunities. More commonly in developing countries, graduates from medical, nursing, and midwifery colleges enter government service and are meant to be deployed to government facilities. Deployment of graduates into government service is facilitated by careful recruitment of students from priority areas where health workers are needed. Selection of students who are from areas that have a demonstrated need increases the likelihood that these students will return to their home districts upon graduation. The alternative is that students enter the program without discrimination on the basis of geographic origin and then are asked to accept posts. A robust strategy for deployment (including to underserved areas) is needed to ensure that the financial, material, and technical resources invested in the production of human resources for health are not wasted by large losses due to attrition (WHO 2007).

Integration, Supervision, and Support of MCH Workers

Successful deployment of new graduates must go beyond the identification of appropriate posts for these health workers to fill. Especially, in the case of nurses and midwives who are trained in an expanded set of skills or who learn new skills through in-service training programs, efforts to support the integration of those health workers into, or back into, their health facilities must be undertaken. In a study of quality of child health services in primary health-care facilities in southeastern Nigeria, Ehiri et al. (2005) reported that much of the supervisory activities of primary health-care coordinators and national immunization program managers were in the form of "surprise visits," usually for punitive reasons (e.g., to identify those who had not reported to work on time). Supervision of health workers must reflect not simply administrative supervision, whereby workers' attendance and adherence to stated policies are monitored. Supportive clinical supervision should focus on the care provided, the quality of that care, and the ability of the provider to perform the job according to standards. Supervisory processes and checklists should reflect the clinical elements of the job, and the supervisor must make every effort to assess the provider in the actual performance of clinical duties. To conduct this type of supervision, clear performance standards must be available and must be known and understood by both the supervision team and the health worker.

In the case of MCH, this supervision can be difficult, since provision of services, such as care during labor and birth, cannot be scheduled, and therefore frequently cannot be assessed in real time. It also requires that the supervisor understand and possess the same clinical skills as the person being supervised. When actual clinical care is to be observed but actual clients are not available, external supervisors should have the capacity to devise simulated scenarios in which the health-care worker can demonstrate how he or she would typically perform. This approach gives a much more realistic assessment of quality of care and offers the supervisor the chance to make specific recommendations and give constructive feedback (Garrison et al. 2004). In their study of quality of child health services in primary health-care centers in southeastern Nigeria, Ehiri et al. (2005) concluded that inadequacy in the quality of child health services in the facilities was a product of failures in a range of quality measures – structural (lack of equipment and essential drugs), process failings (non-use of the national case management algorithm and lack of a protocol of systematic supervision of health workers). Thus, supervision of health workers is one element that ultimately supports performance. Other elements include the physical and material resources available to ensure the provision of care, as well as the attitude and approach of co-workers. Workers who struggle to provide care according to standards should be asked what they need in order to solve the problem. When health workers participate in devising the solutions to their own problems, they are more likely to follow through with the interventions and be motivated to solve other problems in the future.

Factors That Influence the Performance of Health Workers

Six general factors are thought to have a central impact on performance (Stolovitch and Keeps 1999):

- *Job Expectations*: Health workers need clear job descriptions that outline what is expected of them, what is allowed, and what skills they require to do their jobs. These may be national documents that can be adapted in the workplace.
- *Performance Feedback*: Regular systems of feedback should be established to allow health workers to know how they are performing. This feedback should come from managers, peers, and clients to capture the opinion of all those who are affected by the workers' performance.
- *Tools/Environment*: The health workers' physical, professional, and psychological environment has a profound impact on performance. The availability of equipment, supplies, and drugs, as well as the physical infrastructure, including power, water, and security, will either impede or enhance performance of health workers.

- *Incentives*: Incentives for performance need not be only financial incentives. Motivation can be related to social and moral imperatives; pride and recognition by peers, supervisors, and clients; and social and professional advancement. Certainly, there is a financial threshold below which health workers are demotivated; however, increases in salary do not necessarily lead to improved job performance.
- *Skills/Knowledge*: Workers need the appropriate knowledge and skills to do their jobs well. Training can be an important intervention to improve performance. However, training in a vacuum without accounting for other factors that influence performance will rarely result in improved performance.
- *Organizational Support*: The managerial, strategic, and operational mechanisms of the organization must be aligned with those of the workers. If the organization asks the workers to achieve one objective, yet it is focused on the achievement of another competing objective, the workers will ultimately become frustrated and face limitations in their ability to perform.

These factors can be grouped into three categories: the capability to perform one's job, the opportunity to do one's job, and the motivation to do one's job (Necochea and Bossemeyer 2005) (Fig. 28.5). Performance is at the center of these three areas, and interventions to improve performance must address all of these areas.

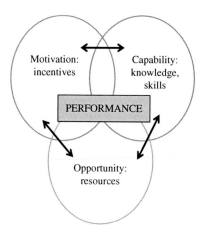

Fig. 28.5 Influences on performance: a holistic and systemic approach

Retention of MCH Workers

Retaining health workers in their jobs is an ongoing and challenging problem that threatens the advances made in health services and health system development. The migration of health workers to more urban areas within a country and to international posts outside their home country is at the center of the issue. One study estimated that in a 10-year period from 1986 to 1995, 61% of doctors who qualified from one medical school in Ghana left the country (Dovlo and Nyonator 1999). The extent of loss of capacity is greatest in Africa, but examples can be cited from every region of the world.

Loss of health workers represents a substantial loss of time, financial resources, and energy consumed to educate and develop them. Furthermore, faculty and educational institutions begin to see as futile their efforts to educate new workers if the wastage from the health system is substantial. The health workers and educators who remain are burdened with additional workload and greater responsibility. In addition, the lack of expertise in workforce management in many countries results in further inefficient use of health workers, inappropriate skill mix to address health priorities, and reduced performance, quality, and morale, in an already underperforming and demoralized system.

Efforts to resolve the problem must look beyond simply enhancing remuneration. Solutions must look comprehensively at the multiple factors that lead to health workers' decisions to migrate away from their posts. Numerous solutions have been proposed, including policies for the active recruitment of students from rural backgrounds, development of more positive rural rotations during preservice education, and efforts to address quality-of-life concerns (Kotzee and Couper 2006). In addition to efforts to address the movement of current workers, attention must be given to identifying ways to prepare the next generation of health-care workers, with an eye toward presenting rural or simply domestic health service in a more positive light. There have been efforts to revise medical education to make the curriculum more geared to the preparation of community-focused physicians (Bor 2002). There must be further research on mechanisms to foster rural service and on creative approaches for deployment of health workers to rural and underserved areas.

While approaches are being implemented to address the loss of workers from the health system, efforts to increase the skill mix of health-care teams should also be considered. The training or retraining of selected workers to take on new and expanded scopes of practice may represent a temporary solution. The evidence comes from both the developed world and several African countries. While nomenclature varies, the principles of enhancement (increasing the scope of practice of a health worker), delegation (shifting tasks from one worker to another, typically a more junior cadre), and innovation (creating a new cadre that assumes some of the responsibilities of the other cadre) are prevalent in all efforts (Dovlo and Nyonator 1999).

Gender in Relation to MCH Workforce Development

Health workers involved in the care of women, newborns, and children are more likely to be female than male. This is especially true in cultures in which women express a preference for a female provider for both their own and their children's health care. This gender differential has an impact on the health workforce, especially as it relates to MCH services and providers. Although careers and employment patterns of female health workers in developing countries have not been studied extensively, it is likely that the greater challenges and outside responsibilities that women face would affect their availability to provide services. Female health professionals typically shoulder a greater proportion of the family responsibilities in the home and work a greater number of hours caring for children and maintaining the home. A study of Canadian physicians with children found that male physicians spent an average of 11.4 hours per week on child care, whereas female physicians spent an average of 39.7 hours per week on child care (Woodward et al. 1996). The figures for less developed countries would undoubtedly reflect similar, if not much wider, disparity.

In addition, there is a tendency to promote a "fast-track" approach to the education and development of cadres of workers exclusively dedicated to the care of women. Some countries have advocated the shortening of midwifery education, thus risking the quality of professional development in favor of quantity and speed of production. Often the extent to which the courses are shortened, or requested to be shortened, for example, from a 2- or 3-year course of study to a 6- to 12-month program of preparation, is below the threshold necessary for student midwives to achieve competency in the various skills necessary for them to be called skilled attendants. This could be due to an unspoken, and probably unintended, sense that the competencies necessary for the care of pregnancy and childbirth are somehow less complex or more easily learned. Calls for shortening midwifery education in countries are not typically accompanied by similar calls for shortening the education of nurses or physicians, potentially suggesting that the education of those cadres involved in the care of men is somehow of greater value. Fortunately, recent clarifications of the definition and scope of practice of a skilled attendant are beginning to result in a more uniform approach to the preparation of midwives and other cadres with responsibility for maternal and childbirth care.

MCH at the Community Level

The provision of some MCH services at the community level is thought to be effective and feasible, and community-based services play an important role in MCH services. Programs have demonstrated that trained community-level health workers can effectively provide certain forms of family planning (Douthwaite and Ward 2002), treat newborn infections, provide immunizations, prevent postpartum hemorrhage (Derman et al. 2006), and educate and mobilize the community toward better health services. The prevailing global opinion at present is that efforts should be made to ensure that all women have access to a skilled provider to assist them during birth. A meta-analysis of 63 traditional birth attendant (TBA) training programs showed that while training has a positive effect on TBAs' knowledge, attitude, behavior, and advice, this training actually had a negative effect on maternal mortality and a limited effect on perinatal/neonatal mortality (Sibley and Sipe 2002). Furthermore, a study of

TBA training in Ghana showed that while TBA training resulted in a significant decrease in intrapartum fever and retained placenta, this finding was counterbalanced by an increase in the rate of women with prolonged labor >18 hours. The authors conclude that "the evidence for beneficial impact of TBA training on the health of mothers and newborns is not compelling" (Smith et al. 2000). A study comparing the practices of trained and untrained TBAs in Bangladesh showed that although trained TBAs were more likely to practice clean delivery, the infection rates among patients of trained and untrained TBAs were no different (Goodburn et al. 2000).

The WHO, in collaboration with United Nations Fund for Population Activities (UNFPA), the United Nations Children's Fund (UNICEF), and the World Bank, makes the following statement regarding the skilled attendant (WHO 2004):

> The term "skilled attendant" refers exclusively to people with midwifery skills (for example midwives, doctors and nurses) who have been trained to proficiency in the skills necessary to manage normal deliveries and diagnose, manage or refer obstetric complications. At minimum the person must be competent to manage normal childbirth and be able to provide emergency (first-line) obstetric care. Not all skilled attendants can provide comprehensive emergency obstetric care although they should have the skills to diagnose when such interventions are needed and the capacity to refer women to a higher level of care. Traditional birth attendants, either trained or not, are excluded from the category of skilled attendant at delivery.

TBAs and other types of community health workers can and do serve a vital role in the lives and experiences of pregnant women. The efforts of community health workers can be focused along the lines of provision of selected, evidence-based interventions, including

- Acting as community educators for accurate maternal and neonatal health messages (e.g., nutrition, tetanus toxoid vaccination, etc.)
- Identifying pregnant women in the community and linking them with appropriate maternal health services
- Partnering with skilled providers (especially midwives and community midwives)
- Promoting birth preparedness and complication readiness
- Providing directed, limited antenatal care, including the distribution of iron and folate, tetanus immunization, etc.

- Identifying, treating, and referring sick newborns
- Understanding and accessing referral systems more readily and ensuring the continuum of care during the referral process
- Providing selected family planning methods

The participation of TBAs in assisting births will continue for many years; it is neither practical nor realistic to expect their activities to cease. Countries should seek an evolution of the role of the TBA into one in which she advocates for women and skilled birthing care, and countries should engage TBAs in a partnership to achieve this goal. The substantial reductions in maternal mortality in countries such as Malaysia, Sri Lanka, China, Egypt, and Honduras have all included a policy of enhancing skilled attendance and partnering with TBAs, while reducing their utilization as isolated caregivers at birth. At present, the evidence does not suggest that scarce resources should be devoted to training, supervising, or equipping TBAs as birth attendants. In summary, partnerships should be advocated, but material or strategic support will likely have limited impact.

Conclusion

Improving MCH will be accomplished only by strengthening the delivery of health services by health workers. As stated by Chen et al. (2004) in their work on human resources for health, "The only route to reaching the health MDGs is through the health worker; there are no shortcuts." Specific strategies have been suggested for analyzing the root causes of gaps in education, deployment, and retention and for addressing the problems that have resulted from the chronic underinvestment and lack of attention to human resources. The increased profile of the problem and the launch of several global initiatives to address the problem are promising. The capacity of countries to plan, develop, and maintain human resources for MCH must be strengthened. Governments, donors, and implementing partners must come together under a common framework to implement creative interventions that have the

potential for lasting results. Departments of ministries responsible for human resources for MCH must be strengthened and must achieve greater coordination and specialists in health workforce planning and management must be developed and utilized. Inter-ministerial collaboration mechanisms must bring together those responsible for the production and the consumption of human resources for health.

The issue of migration of health workers must be addressed in line with the strategic approaches suggested by Stilwell et al. (2004). This calls for development of mechanism to regulate the flow of health workers between countries. It is suggested that each country has to develop its own strategy to influence the retention, recruitment, deployment, and development of health workers. Mechanisms for collection of data on migration of health workers must be developed and strengthened as a tool for good workforce planning. Establishing and maintaining appropriate information systems on human resources, including a database on migration, is a vital first step. Triangulation of data from different sources (e.g., destination countries and countries of origin) to provide the most comprehensive overall picture has also been recommended (Diallo 2004).

There is evidence (Korte et al. 2003) that non-financial incentives (e.g., training, study leave, the opportunity to work in a team, support and feedback from supervisors, and for those working in rural areas provision of housing and transport, agreement on the number of years that will be spent in a rural location (rather than expecting a worker to remain there indefinitely), offering further training, and offering financial incentives) may be important in motivating heath-care workers and improving retention.

Finally, the knowledge base regarding planning and development of the MCH workforce must be expanded. Additional effort must be given to developing systems for counting health workers, analyzing their work as well as their needs, and supporting their performance. The education of health workers should be revitalized to decrease inefficiencies and outdated practices, increase connectedness to workplace expectations, and develop a sense of critical and evidence-based self-appraisal.

Key Terms

Brain drain	Health worker density	Skilled attendance at birth
Community health extension workers	Health worker development	Skilled birth attendant
Community health workers	Health worker life expectancy	Staffing levels
Competency-based training	Health workforce planning	Traditional birth attendants (TBAs)
Delegation	Human resource planning	Training needs assessments
Economic migration	Incentives	Village health volunteers
Emergency obstetric care	Innovation	Measles immunization
Enhancement	In-service training	Midwife
Globalization	Job Expectations	Organizational support
Health-care worker deployment	MCH human resource development	Performance feedback
Health promoters	MCH worker retention	Pre-service education
Health volunteers	MCH workforce	

Questions for Discussion

1. In an essay of about 1,000 words, discuss the relationship between health worker density and the following health indices:

   a. Life expectancy
   b. Child mortality rates
   c. Maternal mortality rates

2. Briefly discuss the factors that influence health worker migration. What are the effects of such migration on health systems?

3. You have been posted as the MCH Advisor for a country in sub-Saharan Africa. The country's federal ministry of health is planning a comprehensive training program for all the nation's primary health-care workers. What advise would you give the ministry to ensure the success of the training program?

4. You are the director of MCH services in a developing country. There is concern that your MCH workers are emigrating from the country in large numbers and that the few remaining personnel are not performing at optimum levels. What recommendations would you present to the government for increasing retention and improving the performance of the workers?

References

Aiken LH, Clarke SP, Sloane DM et al. (2002) Hospital nurse staffing and patient mortality, nurse burnout, and job dissatisfaction. *Journal of the American Medical Association*, 288(16): 1987–1993

Awases M, Gbary A, Nyoni J, Chatora R (2003) Migration of Health Professionals in Six Countries: A Synthesis Report. Brazzaville: WHO Regional Office for Africa. http://www.afdb.org/pls/portal/docs/PAGE/JAI/RESOURCE_MATERIALS/COURSE_MATERIALS/HEALTH%20SECTOR%20REFORM%20FOR%20PORTUGESE%20COUNTRIES/MIGRATION%20STUDY%20AFRO.PDF Cited 2 August 2008

Bang AT, Deshmukh MD, Baitule SB, Bang RA (2005) Neonatal and infant mortality in the ten years (1993 to 2003) of the Gadchiroli field trial: effect of home-based neonatal care. *Journal of Perinatology*, 25(1): S92–S107

Barber S, Gertler P (2005) Child Health and the Quality of Medical Care in Indonesia. Berkeley: University of California. http://faculty.haas.berkeley.edu/gertler/working_papers/02.28.02_childheight.pdf Cited 2 August 2008

Bor D (2002) Community-Based Education for Health Professionals. The Network for Unity Towards Health. http://www.the-networktufh.org/publications_resources/positioncontent.asp?id=2&t=Position+Papers Cited 2 August 2008

Brookfield SD (1986) Understanding and Facilitating Adult Learning. San Francisco: Jossey-Bass Publishers.

Campbell OMR, Graham WJ (2006) Strategies for reducing maternal mortality: getting on with what works. *Lancet*, 368(9543): 1284–1299

Chen L, Evans T, Anand S et al. (2004) Human resources for health: overcoming the crisis. *Lancet* 364: 1984–1990

Connell J (2002) The Migration of Skilled Health Personnel in the Pacific Region: 2002 Report of Study Commissioned by WHO Western Pacific Regional Office. Manila: Western Pacific Regional Office, WHO

Derman RJ, Kodkany BS, Goudar SS et al. (2006) Oral misoprostol in preventing postpartum haemorrhage in resource-poor communities: a randomized controlled trial. *Lancet*, 368(9543): 1248–1253

Douthwaite M, Ward P (2002) Increasing contraceptive use in rural Pakistan: an evaluation of the Lady Health Worker Programme. *Health Policy and Planning*, 20(2): 117–123

Diallo K (2004) Data on the migration of health-care workers: sources, uses, and challenges. *Bulletin of the World Health Organization*, 82: 601–617

Dovlo D, Nyonator F (1999) Migration of graduates of the University of Ghana Medical School: a preliminary rapid appraisal. *Human Resources for Health Development Journal*, 3: 45

Dussault G, Dubois CA (2003) Human resources for health policies: a critical component in health policies. *Human Resources for Health*, 1: 1

Ehiri JE, Oyo-Ita AE, Anyanwu EC et al. (2005) Quality of child health services in primary health care facilities in Calabar, Southeastern Nigeria. *Child Care: Health and Development*, 31(2): 181–191

Fogarty LA et al. (2004) Performance Evaluation of Recent Graduates of a Strengthened Registered Midwifery Training Program in Zambia. Baltimore, MD: JHPIEGO

Fritzen SA (2007) Strategic management of the health workforce in developing countries: what have we learned? *Human Resources for Health*, 5: 4

Garrison K, Caiola N, Sullivan R, Lynam P (2004) Supervising Healthcare Services: Improving the Performance of People. Baltimore, MD: JHPIEGO

Goodburn EA, Chowdhury M, Gazi R et al. (2000) Training traditional birth attendants in clean delivery does not prevent postpartum infection. *Health Policy and Planning*, 15(4): 394–399

International Confederation of Midwives (2005) Definition of a Midwife. http://www.medicalknowledgeinstitute. com/files/ICM%20Definition%20of%20the%20Midwife%202005.pdf, cited 2 August 2008

JHPIEGO/Maternal and Neonatal Health Program (2004) Prevention of Postpartum Hemorrhage Study: West Java, Indonesia. Baltimore, MD: JHPIEGO. http://www. jhpiego.org/resources/pubs/mnh/pphjavastudy.pdf, cited 2 August 2008

Joint Learning Initiative (2004) Human Resources for Health: Overcoming the Crisis. Cambridge, MA: Harvard University. http://www.hup.harvard.edu/catalog/ JOIHUM.html, cited 2 August 2008

Korte R et al. (2003) Proceedings of the Migration and Development Conference: Using Opportunities Together. Berlin, Germany, October 20–21

Kotzee T, Couper ID (2006) What interventions do South African qualified doctors think will retain them in rural hospitals of the Limpopo province of South Africa? *Rural and Remote Health*, 6: 581. http://www.rrh.org.au/ publishedarticles/article_print_581.pdf, cited 2 August 2008

Limpaphayom K, Ajello C, Reinprayoon D et al. (1997) The effectiveness of model-based training in accelerating IUD skill acquisition. *British Journal of Family Planning*, 23(2): 58–61

Necochea E, Bossemeyer D (2005) Standards-Based Management and Recognition: A Field Guide. Baltimore, MD: JHPIEGO

Sachs JD, McArthur JW (2005) The Millennium project: a plan for meeting the Millennium Development Goals. *Lancet*, 365: 347–353

Schaefer L (2002) Pre-service Implementation Guide: A Process for Strengthening Pre-service Education. Baltimore, MD: JHPIEGO. http://www.jhpiego.org/resources/pubs/ psguide/psimpgden.pdf, cited 2 August 2008

Sibley LM, Sipe T (2002) Traditional Birth Attendant Training Effectiveness: A Meta-Analysis. Washington, DC: Academy for Educational Development. http://www.sciencedirect. com/science?_ob=ArticleURL&_udi=B6T7M-490 H3T8-2&_user=10&_rdoc=1&_fmt=&_orig=search &_sort=d&view=c&_acct=C000050221&_version= 1&_urlVersion=0&_userid=10&md5=bc9cdeb336d3945 f0a170143e871c662, cited 2 August 2008

Smith JB, Coleman NA, Fortney JA et al. (2000) The impact of traditional birth attendant training on delivery complications in Ghana. *Health Policy and Planning*, 15(3): 326–331

Stilwell B, Diallo K, Zurn P et al. (2004) Migration of health-care workers from developing countries: strategic approaches to its management. *Bulletin of the World Health Organization*, 82(8): 595–600

Stolovitch HD, Keeps EJ (1999) Handbook of Human Performance Technology: Improving Individual and Organizational Performance Worldwide. Silver Spring, MD: International Society for Performance Improvement

Sullivan R (1995) The Competency-Based Approach to Training. Baltimore, MD: JHPIEGO. http://www.reproline.jhu.edu/english/6read/6training/cbt/cbt.htm, cited 2 August 2008

Vujicic M (2005) Macroeconomic and Fiscal Issues in Scaling Up Human Resources for Health in Low-Income Countries. Washington, DC: Human Development Network, The World Bank. http://www.who.int/hrh/documents/ macroeconomic_fiscal_issues.pdf, cited 2 August 2008

Woodward CA, Williams AP, Ferrier B, Cohen M (1996) Time spent on professional activities and unwaged domestic work: is it different for male and female primary care physicians who have children at home? *Canadian Family Physician*, 42: 1935–1938

World Health Organization (1995) Community-Based Distribution of Contraceptives: A Guide for Programme Managers. Geneva: WHO

World Health Organization (WHO) (2000) The World Health Report 2000: Health Systems – Improving Performance. Geneva: WHO. http://www.who.int/whr/2000/ en/, cited 2 August 2008

World Health Organization (WHO) (2004) Skilled Attendant at Birth: Definitions. http://www.who.int/reproductivehealth/global_monitoring/skilled_attendance.html, cited 2 August 2008

World Health Organization (WHO) (2005) The World Health Report 2005: Make Every Mother and Child

Count. Geneva: WHO. http://www.who.int/whr/2005/en/index.html, cited 2 August 2008

World Health Organization (WHO) (2006) The World Health Report 2006: Working Together for Health. Geneva: WHO. http://www.who.int/whr/2006/en/, cited 2 August 2008

World Health Organization (WHO) (2007) Scaling up Health Workforce Production: A Concept Paper towards the Implementation of World Health Assembly Resolution WHA59.23. Geneva: WHO http://www.who.int/hrh/documents/scalingup_concept_paper.pdf, cited 2 August 2008

Chapter 29
An Agenda for Child Health Policy in Developing Countries

John E. Ehiri

Learning Objectives After reading this chapter and answering the discussion questions that follow, you should be able to

- Identify and discuss the environmental, social, and political factors that influence child health in less-developed countries.
- Discuss the limitations of global child health policies and programs that are based mostly on vertical, disease-focused programs.
- Analyze the background to, and rationale for, the Alma Ata Declaration of Primary Health Care.
- Present a coherent case for the adoption of a global child health policy that is based on the tenets of the Alma Declaration of Primary Health Care.

Introduction

There is considerable information on the effectiveness of several simple interventions to promote child health in less-developed countries. The knowledge and technology to implement these interventions also exist. Nevertheless, each year, millions of infants and children suffer and die from conditions that can be easily prevented at minimal cost. Much progress has been made with regard to improvement of child health over the past six decades. Yet, there seems to be comparatively very little to show for the huge resources and efforts that governments, bilateral agencies, foundations, and other global health agencies invest annually in child health promotion in less-developed countries. This is mostly because the resources and efforts are often expended on specific disease conditions, with little attention to the environmental, socioeconomic, and health system factors that underlie the diseases. Disease-focused child health interventions may reduce mortality, but because they are usually not designed to modify the "environmental" conditions that make children sick, their effectiveness in reducing the burden of childhood disease is usually very limited. As a typical example, childhood diarrheal disease control efforts of the 1980s targeted the reduction of mortality from dehydration by promoting the use of oral rehydration solution (ORS) during diarrheal episodes. Increased intake of fluids supplemented by ORS together with continued feeding has proven to be a powerful intervention for the prevention of childhood deaths from diarrhea (Victora et al. 2000). Estimates have shown a steady decline ever since: 3.3 million deaths in the 1990s (Bern et al. 1992) and 2.5 million in the year 2000 (Kosek et al. 2003). In spite of this decline, diarrhea is still the second leading cause of under-5 mortality globally. This chapter presents a critical review of current strategies for child health promotion in less-developed countries and discusses the limitations of disease-focused approaches that do not address environmental and socioeconomic factors that underlie morbidity and mortality among children in poor countries. It is noted that after several years of investment in disparate vertical interventions, preventable diseases still remain a major challenge for child health in less-developed countries. The chapter concludes with a call for a return to the tenets of the Alma Ata Declaration of Primary Health Care which emphasize action on social determinants of health, a focus on health systems development and access to basic services.

J.E. Ehiri (✉)
Division of Health Promotion Sciences, Mel & Enid
Zuckerman College of Public Health, University of Arizona,
Tucson, AZ 85724, USA

The Role of Medicine in Child Health

There is a perception that much of the improvement in population health recorded in many countries over the past century has resulted from advances in medical technology, pharmaceutical discoveries, and therapeutic innovations. Today, health-care systems of many high-income countries have a range of innovative technologies and procedures for diagnosing and treating disease conditions for which medicine had no cure six decades ago, including cancers and cardiovascular diseases. Within the global health sphere, the successful eradication of smallpox and typhus, significant declines in maternal and child mortality, and increases in life expectancy have helped to shape the view that medicine and therapeutic interventions were the major contributors to the overall improvement in global health over the years. Informed by this view, global health agencies and national governments of less-developed countries continue to lay emphasis on therapeutic interventions to the neglect of investment in health systems development, infrastructure strengthening, and environmental and economic empowerment programs. Moreover, health-care systems in many of these countries have emerged from colonial medical services that focused to a huge extent on large hospitals in urban centers, even in situations where a majority of the population live in remote rural areas with limited physical and financial access to the most basic health services. Thus, during the 1950s and 1960s, when many less-developed countries gained their independence, they essentially inherited health-care systems that were based on high-technology, urban-based curative care. Because many of these countries have not invested efforts in purposefully creating and maintaining health systems that reflected their population's dynamics and level of socioeconomic development, they have perpetually continued to suffer from the effects of inadequate or non-existent health systems and infrastructures with grave impacts on the health of women and children.

Over the years, each childhood disease eradication program of major players in global health (bilateral agencies and non-governmental organizations) has operated autonomously, each disease program with its own administration and budget and with very little integration into the recipient nations' health systems. These disparate programs have been credited with some successes, including the eradication of smallpox and a decrease in tuberculosis prior to the HIV/AIDS pandemic. However, their impact on overall burden of disease among populations in less-developed countries has been minimal, and sustainability has been an abiding problem. It has been argued (Ehiri and Prowse 1999; Magnussen et al. 2004) that this limitation in overall impact is inevitable, given that these disparate disease-focused interventions do not address the social determinants of disease in these settings. Although one disease might be controlled or eliminated by an intervention, recipients of that intervention might die of other diseases or their complications if the factors that underlie the proliferation of disease in the environment are not addressed. For example, when smallpox vaccination became available in the early 19th century, smallpox deaths, which occurred mostly among children, fell precipitously, but the overall mortality remained relatively unaffected as deaths from diarrhea and related conditions subsequently increased (Ehiri and Prowse 1999; McKeown 1979). As Sagan (1989) observed, "one cause of mortality simply replaced another." This problem is a major weakness in current strategies adopted to reduce childhood diseases by donor agencies and governments in less-developed countries.

Child Health Problems Have Multifactorial Causes and Consequences

Evidence shows that in many less-developed countries, a significant proportion of the problems of ill-health and disease among infants and children are closely linked to both environmental conditions and poverty. The problem confronting Tanzania, for example, is similar to that in many other less-developed countries – high incidence of infectious and parasitic diseases, low nutritional levels, and problems relating to pregnancy and childbirth (Sunguya et al. 2006; Mhalu 2005). There is general acceptance (WHO 1995) that the primary cause of these problems is poverty, which operates through inadequate food intake, low educational levels, lack of safe drinking water, poor environmental conditions, and lack of access to basic care. The brunt of the problem is borne by infants and children under the age of 5, who although constitute about 18% of the population account for 63% of all deaths (Armstrong Schellenberg et al. 2008). It was not surprising that the 10th Edition of the International Classification of Diseases (ICD-10) (WHO 1992) includes a code for extreme poverty, *Z59.5*. As the World Health Organization noted in its 1995 World Health Report (WHO 1995), "poverty is the main reason why babies are not vaccinated, clean water and sanitation are not provided, and curative drugs and other treatments are unavailable, and why mothers die in childbirth. Poverty is the main cause of reduced life expectancy, of handicap and disability, and of starvation" (WHO 1995). Tackling child health problems too narrowly in less-developed countries and paying minimal attention to primary prevention through action on household and community social and environmental health factors are expensive and unsustainable.

Research conducted on the impact of disease-specific interventions in less-developed countries shows that children with severe illness often present with multiple problems that call for a comprehensive approach that recognizes the complexity of the problem (Campbell and Gove 1996). Responding to the challenge posed by this predicament, international health agencies led by the World Health Organization (WHO) and the United Nations Children's Fund (UNICEF) introduced the Integrated Management of Childhood Illnesses (IMCI) in the 1990s (WHO 1999). Details of this strategy, including its objectives and country implementation experiences, are discussed in Chapter 27. The objectives of IMCI include improvement in health systems and family and community practices. However, its actual implementation remains largely focused on case management. As Rowe et al. (1999) noted, the focus of IMCI on case management does not significantly distinguish it from other disease-focused policy initiatives of the past that have been criticized for their lack of attention to social determinants of health and disease in less-developed countries. The primary aim of the IMCI strategy is to prevent deaths and disabilities by improving the case management of sick children in outpatient health facilities. Its guidelines have therefore been focused on the treatment of individual children (Rowe et al. 1999).

Factors That Contributed to Population Health Improvements in High-Income Countries

In considering the best options for child health promotion in less-developed countries, it is important to analyze and draw parallels with factors that contributed to population health improvements in high-income countries over the past century. This parallel is not unreasonable given that many less-developed countries are more or less currently at the level of health and social economic development that many high-income countries were several decades ago. In his analysis of factors that contributed to improvements in health and growth of the population of England and Wales, McKeown (1979) showed that the high death rates of the past were largely attributable to a combination of infectious diseases, nutritional, and environmental factors. He estimated that from the beginning of the 18th century to the mid-1970s, 80–90% of the total reduction in death rate in England and Wales was as a result of the decline in deaths caused by infections and water- and food-borne diarrheal diseases. He noted that with the exception of vaccination against smallpox (associated with less than 2% of the decline in death rate from 1848 to 1871), it was unlikely that immunization or therapy had any significant effect on infectious diseases before the 20th century given that much of the reduction in mortality from tuberculosis, respiratory, water- and food-borne diseases had already occurred before effective immunization or treatment was available. In conclusion, he asserted that these improvements in health had resulted more from "environmental public health," political, economic, and social measures than from specific medical or therapeutic interventions.

Several other analyses (Lucas 2003; United Nations 1973) have yielded similar conclusions. Box 29.1 presents a summary of the factors that contributed to early reductions in mortality in Europe and North America. While it is important to question the validity of these retrospective reviews, it is interesting to note the consensus among many authors regarding the importance of social and environmental factors. Beaver (1973) noted that in the second half of the 18th century, infant mortality

Box 29.1 Causes of Mortality Decline in the 18th and 19th Centuries in Europe, North America, Australia, and New Zealand

Improved agriculture: Increased food production and better nutrition (e.g., the Agricultural Revolution in England included better fertilizers, crop rotation, and winter crops).

Industrialization: The development of the factory system led to wider availability of manufactured goods. Factory production of machinery (e.g., iron plough, team engine) also contributed to improved agriculture.

Improved transport: Facilitated the distribution of food and other goods (e.g., in Europe, railways enabled food supplies to be sent rapidly from rural to urban areas).

Social reforms: Various health and social welfare schemes and regulations, including the regulation of child labor in factories.

Greater control of temperature and humidity: Regulation of temperature and humidity in homes and at work may have contributed to the decline of some diseases.

Public sanitation: Including improved sewage disposal, water supplies, and water purification (e.g., filters that eliminated cholera and typhoid from the water).

Improved personal hygiene: The availability of cheap and easy-to-wash cotton clothing, potable water supplies, and soap facilitated improved personal hygiene.

Asepsis and antisepsis: The exclusion and killing of disease-causing organisms was developed by Joseph Lister in the late 19th century (e.g., the sterilization of surgical instruments).

Immunology: For example, Edward Jenner's inoculation against smallpox and discoveries by Koch and Pasteur that inoculation with a mild form of the disease will prevent a serious case.

Biological factors: Increased resistance to some diseases and some diseases becoming more benign (e.g., scarlet fever).

Source: Thomlinson (1976)

fell in England and Wales when supplies of cheap cow's milk became generally available throughout the year. With regard to smallpox, for example, Razzell (1974) noted the role of immunization, but stressed the huge influence of improved hygiene, including the use of soap and washable cotton clothes in the first 40 years of the 19th century. In France, Preston and van de Walle (1978) found that mortality was relatively high in three urban areas, but after 1850, mortality in these settings declined dramatically as a result of improvements in water supply and sewerage. As they noted, medical improvements did not become important until diphtheria immunizations in the 1890s.

In considering the foregoing evidence, it is reasonable to argue that the key to sustainable improvement in child health in less-developed countries may lie in the development of infrastructures to improve environmental public health, efforts to alleviate poverty, and enhancement of people's overall living standards.

Recommendations for a New Strategy

Given the limitations of the current disease-specific approach to child health promotion in less-developed countries, a rethink of global child health policy is needed. A historical analysis of specific country experiences shows that comprehensive approaches to child health promotion are effective and sustainable. These include, for example, the creation of the Bhore Commission in India (Government of India 1946) which demonstrated significant improvements in child and population health through the establishment of rural health centers, staffed by community health workers; the implementation of "community-based health programs" in Nicaragua, Costa Rica, Guatemala, Honduras, Mexico, Bangladesh, and the Philippines; and the barefoot doctor program in China which deployed trained community health workers to rural areas as the gatekeepers of the nation's health who provided basic preventive and curative services to people in their environments (Magnussen et al. 2004). As part of the overall efforts to improve population health, these countries brought a new theme to global health discourse: a commitment to social justice and equity in health services. Contrary to the top-down, high-technology approach that continues to drive international cooperation in child health, the foundation of these country experiences is essentially a bottom-up approach that emphasized prevention and managed health problems in their social contexts. These countries' experiences also embodied the tenets of the Alma Ata's Declaration of Primary Health Care by the WHO and the UNICEF in 1978, which made it the responsibility of governments and agencies to promote equity and ensure that segments of the population were not unduly suffering for the benefits received by others. The Declaration defined primary health care as "essential care based on practical, scientifically sound and socially acceptable methods, made technologically and universally available to individuals and families in the communities through their full participation, and at a cost the community and country can afford to maintain at every stage of their development, in the spirit of self-determination and self-reliance" (WHO/ UNICEF 1978). WHO/UNICEF asserts that primary health care forms an integral part of a country's development and health system. It is the first level of contact for the individual, family, and community with the health system, bringing health care as close as possible to where people live and work, and constitutes the first element of a continuing health-care process (WHO/UNICEF 1978). Primary health care was intended to cover the following key areas:

- Health education
- Food supply and nutrition
- Water and sanitation
- Maternal and child health
- Immunization
- Prevention and control of locally endemic diseases
- Treatment of common diseases and injuries
- Provision of essential drugs

The selective approach to primary health care which used results of cost-effective studies (Walsh and Warren 1979) to determine a package of disease-focused interventions to be funded and implemented in less-developed countries has been tested and the results show that its inability to tackle broader environmental and social

determinants of health is a major limitation (WHO 2008; Magnussen et al. 2004; Ehiri and Prowse 1999). Thus, the intent of this chapter is not to revisit the protracted debate regarding the merits of selective versus comprehensive approaches to primary health care but rather to propose that the comprehensive approach envisioned in the Alma Ata Declaration (WHO/UNI-CEF 1978) be given a chance as a key element of an evolving policy for child health promotion in less-developed countries. Three decades after the Alma Ata Declaration, and on account of the apparent limitations of the selective approach to primary health care, the 2008 report of the World Health Organization (WHO 2008) has chosen as its title "Primary Health Care: Now More Than Ever," thus revisiting the ambitious vision of primary health care as a set of values and principles for guiding the development of health systems. As the director general of the World Health Organization, Dr. Margaret Chan observes the report represents an important opportunity to draw on the lessons of the past, consider the challenges that lie ahead, and identify major avenues for health systems to narrow the intolerable gaps between aspiration and implementation (WHO 2008). In embarking on this important policy shift, the focus should not be on generalities but on a number-specific action steps, some of which are discussed below.

Development and Maintenance of Infrastructures to Support Integrated Systems of Care

Many less-developed countries continue to rely on vertical programs, with less emphasis on people's involvement and development of systems and infrastructures to sustain those programs. Whilst not undermining the contributions of medicine to public health, medical care should underpin the health of a population or a group only when prevention fails (Ashton and Seymour 1993). Reliance on case management of specific diseases as a framework for health improvement in less-developed countries is expensive, unsustainable, and will result in few real health benefits if the underlying environmental and social causes are not addressed. For example, although the current initiative on vaccines and immunization (GAVI Alliance), designed to help countries to incorporate new vaccines into their national health systems, has benefits for addressing specific communicable diseases as discussed in Chapter 23, their full potential will be difficult to achieve in the absence of effective health systems and supporting infrastructures. Limited assessment of this initiative undertaken in Mozambique, Ghana, Lesotho, and Tanzania (Brugha et al. 2002) revealed that the infrastructural foundation needed for successful implementation and sustainability was inadequate. Moreover, maintaining the cost of expensive new vaccines after donor support ceases is financially unsustainable for many less-developed countries. As with most vertical programs, analysts have expressed concern that raising poor countries' awareness of new vaccines and immunization programs without support in implementing such programs could end up creating markets for these vaccines while doing little to tackle major health problems (Fleck 2002). Given that disease-focused models continue to be funded and promoted in less-developed countries, it is apparent that adequate lessons have not been learned from experimentation with selective, vertical approaches; that the notion of self-reliance, community participation, and health systems development proposed at Alma Ata have diminished in importance; and that inadequate consideration is given to the link between health and socioeconomic development. Global health policy for the 21st century should recognize that expensive high-technology models to address diseases of poverty will not be sustainable where the infrastructures needed for operationalization and institutionalization of those technologies do not exist.

Community-Focused Approach to Intervention Development and Implementation

The Alma Ata Declaration requires that interventions come from the needs of the community, expressed and subsequently led by community members. Global health problems cannot be solved by distant policy makers and planners (Bichmann 1988) as involvement of individuals and communities fosters the mobilization of needed local resources (Askew 1991). Implied in the concept of participation is decentralized physical location of hospitals and health centers, which emphasizes that programs need to be founded and researched in the locality in which they will be applied. The Alma Ata Declaration also recognizes that the issue of accessibility to health services and resources has historically been a barrier to effective care and that placing emphasis on curative, tertiary care hospitals located in urban centers often precludes access for a mostly rural population.

Greater Collaboration and Reduction of Overlap and Waste Among the Various Key Players in Global Child Health Practice

Countries need to strengthen their primary health care through the development of intersectoral forums at every level. Human health should be a cross-cutting issue throughout the decision-making process in different sectors and at different levels. Health policy development should involve those sectors, agencies, and social groups that are critical to achieving better health. This can be achieved through advocacy for health objectives as integral to socioeconomic development and through engagement of different sectoral partners and community structures in the consensual process. Because health does not occur in isolation, the various sectors, including those within a national government and among aid agencies, need to work together at every level of practice. The ministry of health is not the sole agency charged with production of health; the departments of agriculture, housing, sanitation, and education, along with food distribution, are all involved in achieving optimal health. Integrated planning, management, and execution of public health policies and practices by these different governmental departments is essential to the promotion of public health in less-developed countries.

Development of Pro-poor Policies

Health policy makers should be aware that macroeconomic, labor, and social policies have the potential to limit or enhance health opportunities for different groups in the population. International aid agencies and governments in less-developed countries should be aware that the pursuit of liberal macroeconomic pro-growth policies has the tendency to provide better opportunities to those with resources and high levels of education, while large segments of the population without these assets are unlikely to benefit and may in fact become casualties of economic transition. Thus, it is the duty of health policy makers to signal when other policies may undermine efforts to promote health equity (McIntyre and Gilson 2000).

Emphasis on Effective Training, Development, and Deployment of Child Health Professionals

As shown in Chapter 28, ensuring the quality of primary health care and reform of the health sector under primary health care should include coherent human resource development plans at the village, district, state/regional, and national levels. Strategies for retention of trained personnel in remote and rural areas are also important. Primary health-care systems in developing countries provide interventions that are already known to be effective. This means that achievement of quality in primary health-care facilities requires the proper performance of these interventions according to prescribed standards. However, the most common challenge is that often, these interventions are not properly executed (Ehiri et al. 2005; Gilson et al. 1995). In a recent study in southeast Nigeria, Ehiri et al. (2005) revealed that inadequacy in the quality of services provided by community-based primary health-care workers is a product of failures in a range of quality measures: structural, process failings, and lack of a protocol for systematic supervision of health workers. Thus, quality improvement in this context is not simply a matter of providing infrastructural resources but one of paying attention to improvement in process, especially through training and supervision.

Political Commitment

Although the challenges of addressing the socioeconomic root causes of disease in less-developed countries may seem insurmountable, analyses of factors that contributed to health improvements in developed countries provide cause for optimism. For example, the appalling health conditions described in the Report of the Sanitary Commission of Massachusetts to the Massachusetts State Legislature in 1850 were similar to those that prevail in many less-developed countries today (Evans et al. 1981). The report embodied the essential elements of comprehensive primary health care – communicable disease control, promotion of child health, housing improvement, sanitation, training of community health workers, public health education, promotion of individual responsibility for one's own health, mobilization of community participation through sanitary associations, and creation of multidisciplinary boards of health to assess needs and plan programs. Recognizing the importance of political commitment, the report called for establishment of a strong public health constituency and addressed inequity by highlighting major differences in life expectancies between US rural and urban areas. Thus, many of the improvements in Americans' health have been attributed to the ensuing political commitment and emphasis on public health and socioeconomic interventions implemented by the various arms of the US government over time. Governments in less-developed countries must commit to funding for sustaining community involvement in health. This can be achieved through, for example, private-sector involvement and through hosting village, district, or regional people's health assemblies so that the voices and opinions of the people can be represented in the design and implementation of health policies.

Conclusion

This chapter posits that global child health policies and programs based on vertical therapeutic interventions will not greatly alleviate the overall burden of childhood disease in less-developed countries unless the socioeconomic, political, and health system factors that underlie child health and disease in these countries are challenged. The chapter further argues that progress lies in a fundamental shift in emphasis from vertical, short-term measures to a revitalization of Alma Ata's primary health care, with emphasis on poverty alleviation, community participation, and the development of health systems and infrastructures to create and sustain health. To engender real change, a rethink of the current disease-focused policy is urgently needed. As evidence has shown, treating children of environmentally induced ailments, whilst at the same time, tackling the causative environmental and social factors, is a most comprehensive and sustainable alternative.

Key Terms

Alma Ata Declaration	Health system	Poverty
Bilateral agencies	Health care system	Smallpox
Bottom-up approach	Integrated Management of	Selective primary health care
Comprehensive primary	Childhood Illnesses (IMCI)	Social determinants
health care	International Classification of	Sustainability
Equity	Diseases (ICD)	Top-down approach
Essential drugs	Macroeconomics	
Disease-focused interventions	Non-governmental	
GAVI Alliance	Organizations (NGOs)	

Questions for Discussion

1. It is said that diseases occurring among infants and children in less-developed countries are closely linked to poor environmental conditions and poverty. Discuss, using specific examples.
2. Starting with poverty on one end and child survival on the other end, use a flow chart to illustrate how poverty affects child health.
3. What is the Alma Ata Declaration of Primary Health Care? Distinguish between comprehensive and selective approaches to primary healthcare implementation.
4. Medical interventions are needed to reduce the burden of mortality among infants and children in less-developed countries. To ensure sustainable reductions in morbidity and overall improvements in quality of life, investments in environmental, social, and economic interventions, and health systems development would be necessary. Discuss this statement, using specific diseases and country examples as appropriate.

References

Armstrong Schellenberg JR, Mrisho M, Manzi F et al. (2008) Health and survival of young children in southern Tanzania. BMC Public Health, 8: 194

Ashton J, Seymour H (1993) The New Public Health: The Liverpool Experience. Open University Press, Milton Keynes, UK

Askew I (1991) Planning and implementing community participation in health programs. In: Healthcare Patterns and Planning in Developing Countries. Akhtar R (Ed.) Contributions in Medical Studies # 29. Greenwood Press, New York

Beaver S (1973) Population, infant mortality and milk. Population Studies, 27(2): 243–254

Bern C, Martines J, de Zoysa I, Glass RI (1992) The magnitude of the global problem of diarrheal disease: a ten-year update. Bulletin of the World Health Organization, 70: 705–714

Bichmann W (1988) Translation summary from Grodos? and de bethune? les interventions sanitaires selectives. Social Science and Medicine, 26(9): 889

Brugha R, Starling M, Watt G (2002) GAVI, the first steps: lessons for the global fund. Lancet, 359(9304): 435–438

Campbell H, Gove S (1996) Integrated management of childhood infections and malnutrition: a global initiative. Archives of Disease in Childhood, 75(6): 468–470

Ehiri, JE, Oyo-Ita AE, Anyanwu EC et al. (2005) Quality of child health services in primary healthcare facilities in

Calabar, Southeastern Nigeria. Child Care: Health and Development, 31(2): 181–191

Ehiri JE, Prowse JM (1999) Child health promotion in developing countries: the case for integration of environmental and social interventions? Health Policy and Planning, 14(1): 1–10

Evans JR, Hall KL, Warford J (1981) Shattuck lecture – healthcare in the developing world: problems of scarcity and choice. New England Journal of Medicine, 305(19): 1117–1127

Fleck J (2002) Children's charity criticizes global immunization initiative. British Medical Journal, 324(7330): 129

Gilson L, Magomi M, Mkangaa E (1995) The structural quality of Tanzanian primary healthcare facilities. Bulletin of the World Health Organization, 73(1): 105–114

Government of India (1946) Report of the Health Survey and Development Committee (Chairman Sir Joseph Bhore). Government of India, Ministry of Health, New Delhi, pp. 157–167

Kosek M, Bern C, Guerrant R (2003) The global burden of diarrheal disease as estimated from studies published between 1992 and 2000. Bulletin of the World Health Organization, 81: 197–204

Lucas D (2003) World population growth. Beginning Australian Population Studies. The Australian National University, Canberra, Australia. Chapter 3. http://adsri.anu.edu.au/pubs/BAPS/BAPSChap3.pdf Cited 28 September 2008

Magnussen L, Ehiri JE, Jolly P (2004) Comprehensive versus selective primary health-care: lessons for global health policy. Health Affairs, 23(3): 167–176

McIntyre D, Gilson L (2000) Redressing disadvantage: promoting vertical equity within South Africa. Healthcare Analysis, 8(3): 235–258

McKeown T (1979) The Role of Medicine: Dream, Mirage, or Nemesis? Princeton University Press, Princeton, NJ

Mhalu FS (2005) Burden of diseases in poor resource countries: meeting the challenges of combating HIV/AIDS, tuberculosis and malaria. Tanzania Health Research Bulletin, 7(3): 179–184

Preston SH, van de Walle E (1978) Urban French mortality in the nineteenth century. Population Studies, 32(2): 275–297

Razzell R (1974) An interpretation of the modern rise of population in Europe – critique. Population Studies, 28(1): 5–17

Rowe AK, Hirnschall 1G, Lambrechts T et al. (1999) Linking the integrated management of childhood illness (IMCI) and health information system (HIS) classifications: issues and options. Bulletin of the World Health Organization, 77(12): 988–995

Sagan LA (1989) The Health of Nations: True Causes of Sickness and Wellbeing. Basic Books, New York

Sunguya BF, Koola JI, Atkinson S (2006) Infections Associated with Severe Malnutrition Among Hospitalized Children in East Africa. Tanzania Health Research Bulletin, 8(3): 189–192

Thomlinson R (1976) Population Dynamics. Random House, New York

United Nations (1973) The Determinants and Consequences of Population Trends. United Nations, New York

Victora CG, Bryce J, Fontaine O et al. (2000) Reducing deaths from diarrhea through oral rehydration therapy. Bulletin of the World Health Organization, 78: 1246–1255

Walsh J, Warren K (1979) Selective Primary Healthcare: An Interim Strategy for Disease Control in Developing Countries. New England Journal of Medicine, 301(18): 967–974

WHO/UNICEF (1978) Declaration of Alma Ata. Report on the International Conference on Primary Healthcare, Alma Ata, USSR, September, 6–12, 1978

World Health Organization (WHO) (1992) International Statistical Classification of Diseases and Related Health Problems, 10th revision. World Health Organization, Geneva

World Health Organization (WHO) (1995) World Health Report, 1995: Bridging the Gaps. World Health Organization, Geneva

World Health Organization (1999) Integrated Management of Childhood Illness and health sector reform. WHO DocumentWHO/CHS/CAH/98.1L. REV.1 1999 http://libdoc.who.int/hq/1998/WHO_CHS_CAH_98.1L_eng.pdf Cited 28 September, 2008

World Health Organization (WHO) (2008) The World Health Report 2008 – Primary Health Care – Now More Than Ever. World Health Organization, Geneva. http://www.who.int/whr/2008/whr08_en.pdf Cited 28 September 2008

About the Editor

John Ehiri, MSc (Econ.), MPH, PhD, is Professor and Director, Division of Health Promotion Sciences, Mel and Enid Zuckerman College of Public Health (MEZCOPH), the University of Arizona, Tucson, Arizona, USA. His research and teaching focus on social and behavioral aspects of disease prevention, and on global maternal, child and adolescent health – all linked by program intervention design, evaluation methodology and evidence-based policy/practice. He has over 20 years of research, teaching and service experience in global health.

Prior to joining the University of Arizona College of Public Health, Dr. Ehiri was Associate Professor in the Department of Maternal and Child Health at the University of Alabama at Birmingham (UAB) School of Public Health. He was Principal Investigator and Chair, Executive Committee, UAB Framework Program for Global Health, an initiative funded by the Fogarty International Center of the US National Institutes of Health that builds global health education and research capacity in the United States abroad, by supporting the development of innovative, multidisciplinary global health programs. At UAB, Dr. Ehiri taught core courses in the University's Global Health Studies Program and was the recipient of the President's Award for Excellence in Teaching (School of Public Health) in 2006. Prior to joining UAB, he was a Lecturer in International Health, and Director of the Master of Community Health (MCommH) Program at the Liverpool School of Tropical Medicine, England, United Kingdom. Dr. Ehiri has provided technical assistance on various aspects of maternal, child, and adolescent health to United Nations and bilateral agencies, and has supervised students' field projects in over 20 countries.

Dr. Ehiri obtained his PhD and MPH degrees from the University of Glasgow, Scotland, United Kingdom. He also holds an MSc (Econ) in health policy and planning from the University of Wales, Swansea, United Kingdom. He has authored/co-authored over 70 peer-reviewed articles on critical issues in global maternal, child, and adolescent health.

J.E. Ehiri (ed.), *Maternal and Child Health*, DOI 10.1007/b106524,
© Springer Science+Business Media, LLC 2009

About the Contributors

Rebecca Affolder, M.Phil., is head of the Executive Office of the GAVI Alliance. Prior to joining the GAVI Alliance, she was part of the Secretariat to the Commission for Africa, chaired by the UK Prime Minister. She was responsible for the health section of the Commission's Report, as well as for consultation and presentation of the overall human development recommendations following its publication in March 2005. From 2003 to 2004, Rebecca worked with the UK Department for the Environment, Food and Rural Affairs on the Modernizing Rural Delivery Programme. Prior to this, she held posts with the Canadian International Development Agency (CIDA), both in the Policy Branch and the Programme Against Hunger, Malnutrition and Disease. She holds a BA (Hons) in History from the University of Alberta and an M.Phil. from the University of Cambridge, where she studied the political and social history of famine in Africa.

Ebere Anyanwu, B.Sc., MS, Ph.D., FRSH, M.Biol., C.Biol., was a lead researcher at the Medical Center for Immune and Toxic Disorders and adjunct professor of Anatomy and Physiology at the North Harris and Montgomery Colleges in Houston, Texas. He has taught at various institutions of higher education in the United Kingdom and the United States and has published over 84 papers in international peer-reviewed health science journals. In 2004, Ebere Anyanwu was awarded the International Health Professional of the 2004 by the International Biographical Society, Cambridge, United Kingdom. He is a fellow of the Royal Society (1979), a chartered biologist, clinically certified forensic counselor, and diplomate of the American College of Forensic Counselors. He is currently an independent international health research scientist and consultant.

Robert E. Black, MD, MPH, is the Edgar Berman professor, chair of the Department of International Health, and director of the Institute for International Programs at the Johns Hopkins Bloomberg School of Public Health, Baltimore, Maryland. Dr. Black is trained in medicine, infectious diseases, and epidemiology. He has served as a medical epidemiologist at the US Centers for Disease Control and worked at institutions in Bangladesh and Peru on research related to childhood infectious diseases and nutritional problems. His current research includes field trials of vaccines, micronutrients and other nutritional interventions, effectiveness studies of health programs such as the Integrated Management of Childhood Illness approach, and evaluation of preventive and curative health programs in low- and middle-income countries. His other interests are related to the use of evidence in policy and programs, including estimates of burden of disease, the development of research capacity, and the strengthening of public health training in less-developed countries. As a member of the US Institute of Medicine and advisory bodies of the World Health Organization, the International Vaccine Institute, and other international organizations, he assists with the development of policies intended to improve global child health. He currently chairs the Child Health Epidemiology Reference Group (CHERG) established by the WHO in 2001 to provide external technical guidance and global leadership in the development and improvement of epidemiological estimates for children under 5 years of age. He also chairs the Child Health and Nutrition Research Initiative (CHNRI), an international network of interested partners registered as a Swiss Foundation and supported by the Global Forum for Health Research (GFHR) in Geneva, Switzerland. He currently has projects in Bangladesh, Benin, Ghana, India, Mali, Pakistan, Peru, Senegal, Zanzibar, and Zimbabwe. He has more than 450 scientific journal publications and is coeditor of the textbook *International Public Health* (Jones & Bartlett Publishers, Inc., 2006, 3rd Edition).

Cynthia Boschi-Pinto, MD, MPH, Ph.D., is a medical officer in the Department of Child and Adolescent Health and Development at the World Health Organization, Geneva, Switzerland. She is responsible for activities related to child health epidemiology and is the coordinator of WHO's Child Health Epidemiology Reference Group (CHERG). Her previous researches were on spatial distribution of mortality, heterosexual transmission of HIV, and cancer epidemiology. Her current interests are child mortality, burden of childhood disease, and the use of evidence for priority setting and planning. Prior to joining the WHO office in Geneva, Dr. Boschi-Pinto held several research and teaching positions in epidemiology, child, and adolescent health. She was professor at Universidade Federal Fluminense, head of the Department of Epidemiology at the Institute of Public Health, and researcher at Oswaldo Cruz Foundation (FIOCRUZ) in Rio de Janeiro, Brazil. She received her medical degree from Universidade Federal Fluminense, an MPH with specialization in epidemiology from FIOCRUZ, and a Ph.D. from the Harvard School of Public Health.

Elke de Buhr, MS, Ph.D., is assistant professor at the Payson Center for International Development, Tulane University, New Orleans. Her research focuses on the rights and protection of children, and the health and well-being of people of all ages. She currently is the monitoring/data collection specialist on the Tulane University team that oversees the implementation of the Harkin-Engel Protocol and the efforts undertaken by the international cocoa/chocolate industry to eliminate the worst forms of child labor in the cocoa sector in West Africa. This project, which involves repeated representative survey research as well as other research and monitoring tasks, reports yearly to the US Congress on progress made toward the implementation of the Protocol. Her earlier research and projects include the study of orphans and vulnerable children in the Democratic Republic of Congo, research on street children in Eastern Europe and the Middle East, HIV/AIDS monitoring and evaluation in Rwanda, data management and capacity building in the health sector in Ethiopia, and participation in the evaluation of the international response to the 2004 Indian Ocean tsunami in South-East Asia. Elke de Buhr has worked as a consultant on projects financed by CDC, UN-OCHA, UNAIDS, World Vision, among others. She has a Ph.D. from Tulane University, an MS in International Development from Tulane University, and a diploma in Political Science from Free University of Berlin, Germany.

Lisa Byers, MSW, Ph.D., is a member of the Cherokee Nation in Oklahoma and an assistant professor at the University of Oklahoma's School of Social Work, Tulsa Campus. She has dedicated her education and activities to the promotion of tribal well-being. This endeavor has included an acknowledgment of both the disparities that Native people face and the appreciation for the resilience of tribal people, particularly elders. Dr. Byers was a National Institute of Mental Health pre-doctoral fellow and a Council for Social Work Education minority research fellow, which led to her focus on depression, discrimination, trauma, and American Indian ethnic identity. She is codeveloper of a social work course module for Oklahoma Native elders funded by the Council of Social Work Education. In addition, she is working in the area of early childhood intervention research within urban American Indian contexts through the Indigenous Early Intervention Alliance in Phoenix, Arizona.

Andrew L. Cherry, Jr., DSW, ACSW, is endowed professor in Mental Health at the School of Social Work, University of Oklahoma. He has worked in the helping professions since receiving his BS degree from Troy State University, Troy, Alabama, in 1969. While working as a child welfare worker in Alabama, he became interested in the growing phenomena of teenage pregnancy. He received his Master of Social Work from the University of Alabama in 1974 and worked as a psychiatric social worker at Bryce Hospital, Tuscaloosa, Alabama. He received his doctorate from Columbia University School of Social Work in 1986. Over the next few years as the incidence of teenage pregnancy rapidly increased, he conducted several extensive studies of teenage pregnancy that resulted in two books: *Social Bonds and Teen Pregnancy* (1992) and *The Socialization Instinct: Individual, Family and Social Bonds* (1994). More recently he was the series advisor for a set of 18 books entitled *A World View of Social Issues*. He coedited and wrote several chapters in one of the books, *Adolescent and Teen Pregnancy: A Global View* (Greenwood Press, 2001). Dr. Cherry conducts research and evaluations in the areas of co-occurring disorders, homelessness, services to children and families, teenage pregnancy, and the influence of social bonds on human behavior. Professor Cherry has authored four other books and two research textbooks.

Ian G. Child, MSHA, Ph.D. (ABD), is chairman and CEO of IRISS-International, Inc. and an adjunct professor of Global Health at University of Alabama at Birmingham. Early in his career he was a laboratory research biochemist and then director of European product development for a major British pharmaceutical company. Over a period of 30 years, he was president of the UK, Canada, Australia, and New Zealand subsidiaries of the world's largest medical data research company; then joint founder of the leading United States pharmacy computer services company; information systems advisor in six

Far East countries; president of a medical artificial intelligence software company; and advisor to a joint clinical research organization in four US universities. For many years he has had a deep interest in health-care systems and social determinants of health in OECD countries and the complexities of care delivery in developing countries.

Hoosen M. (Jerry) Coovadia, MBBS, M.Sc., MD, D.Sc., is Victor Daitz chair in HIV/AIDS Research and is the director of Biomedical Science at the Centre for HIV/AIDS Networking, Nelson R. Mandela School of Medicine, University of Natal, South Africa. Prior to this, he was professor and head of Pediatrics and Child Health at the same university. His research interest is in pediatric HIV/AIDS, with particular emphasis on mother-to-child transmission. He has published a number of groundbreaking research articles on this subject. He and his team were the first to suggest, contrary to popular opinion, that transmission of HIV from mother-to-child via breastfeeding could be significantly reduced by exclusive breastfeeding. He has authored or coauthored more than 200 articles in peer-reviewed journals and is coeditor of *Paediatrics and Child Health* (Oxford University Press, 2000), a manual that covers all aspects of child care in developed and less-developed countries and is widely used by medical students and junior doctors around the world. Dr. Coovadia has received numerous national and international honors and awards. He was elected a fellow of the University of Natal in 1995 and was awarded an honorary D.Sc. by the University of Durban, Westville, South Africa in 1996. In 1999, President Nelson Mandela honored him with the Star of South Africa for his contribution to democracy and health and he received a silver medal from the Medical Research Council for excellence in research. In 2000, he received the International Association of Physicians in AIDS and Care Award, the Heroes in Medicine Award in Toronto, Canada, the Nelson Mandela Award for Health and Human Rights, and was elected a Foreign Member of the Institute of Medicine of the National Academy of Sciences, USA – an honor that is seldom awarded. He was awarded a second honorary D.Sc. by the University of Witwatersrand, South Africa, in 2007 and received the Science for Society Gold Medal from the Academy of Science of South Africa. He was appointed by the National Department of Health as chairperson of the National Advisory Group on the HIV/AIDS and STD Programme from 1995 to 1997, while his international stature in the area of HIV/AIDS led to his election as chairperson of the XIIIth International Conference on AIDS held in Durban in July 2000. Dr. Coovadia received his medical degree from the University of Bombay, India, an M.Sc. in Immunology from the University of Birmingham, England, and an MD from the University of Natal, South Africa.

Emmanuel d'Harcourt, MD, MPH, is senior technical advisor for Child Survival at the International Rescue Committee. His work focuses on developing community health networks to deliver essential health services in sub-Saharan African countries affected by conflict, including the Democratic Republic of Congo, Rwanda, Sierra Leone, and South Sudan. His interests include the development of alternative models for rebuilding health systems and the use of information technology in infrastructure-poor countries. He is author of the forthcoming *Community Case Management Essentials Manual*. Emmanuel holds degrees from Yale, Johns Hopkins, and Harvard and completed his pediatric residency at the Children's Hospital of Philadelphia. He is a member of the board of the CORE Group.

Mary Dillon, Ed.D., MSW, is an adjunct professor at the University of Oklahoma, School of Social Work, and has been working in the social services field since the late 1980s. Her current research focus is on the effects of protective services on girls and women who present with the co-occurring disorders of mental illness and substance abuse. Her interest in teenage pregnancy and women's issues in general began in the 1980s when she was the program director at a day shelter for homeless women and children. Later, she worked as the executive director of a nonprofit afterschool program for at-risk adolescent girls and their families. Her research and interest in teenage pregnancy and the impact of drug and alcohol abuse led to the publication of two books. She coedited and wrote several chapters in *Adolescent and Teen Pregnancy: A Global View* (Greenwood Press, 2001) and *Abuse of Alcohol and other drugs: A Global View* (Greenwood Press, 2002). Mary received her Master of Social Work degree from Barry University in Miami, Florida, in 1993, and her doctorate in Education and Human Services from Nova Southeastern University in 2007.

Emmanuel Ezedinachi, MD, DTMH, is a professor of Medicine and consultant physician at the University of Calabar Teaching Hospital, Calabar, Nigeria. He is also founder and pioneer director of the Institute of Tropical Diseases Research and Prevention, the University of Calabar Teaching Hospital, Calabar, Nigeria. His research focuses on tropical and emerging diseases, especially malaria, HIV/AIDS, and tuberculosis. He was the national professional officer the World Health Organization's Roll Back Malaria (RBM) program between 2000 and 2007. Dr. Ezedinachi has published many articles and made numerous national and international presentations on malaria and other tropical diseases and continues to provide technical assistance to United Nations agencies. He obtained his medical degree from the University Düsseldorf, Germany, in 1974 and a diploma in Tropical Medicine & Hygiene from the Tropical Medicine Institute, Hamburg, Germany, in 1978.

Nancy Gerein, Ph.D., M.Sc., is a senior lecturer and deputy head, Nuffield Centre for International Health and Development. She has worked extensively in health planning, and health sector reforms in many countries, including India, Cameroon, Indonesia, and Bangladesh. As a health advisor for the Canadian International Development Agency (CIDA), she was responsible for the planning, management, and evaluation of health programs in Africa and Asia. She joined the Nuffield Centre for International Health and Development at the University of Leeds in 1999. Her teaching, research, and consultancy interest is focused in the areas of reproductive health, health systems development, and monitoring and evaluation. Nancy holds a Ph.D. in Healthcare Epidemiology from the London School of Hygiene and Tropical Medicine, England, and an M.Sc. in Health Policy and Planning from the University of British Columbia in Canada.

Robert Gilman, MD, DTMH, is a Professor in the Department of International Health, Bloomberg School of Public Health, Johns Hopkins University, Baltimore, Maryland. He is also a Research Professor at the Universidad

Peruana Cayetano Heredia. His research focuses on tropical diseases including parasitic diseases such as Cysticercosis and Cyclospora cayetanensis. He has also published widely on various aspects of tuberculosis and is best known for his development of the diagnostic technique of Microscopic Observation and Detection and Susceptibility (MODS) for use in tuberculosis. He continues to spend at least six months each year in Peru working on locally endemic diseases, including tuberculosis, Chagas and cysticercosis. Dr. Gilman received his medical degree from Downstate Medical School in 1965 and his Diplomate of Internal Medicine and Fellowship in Infectious Diseases from the Department of Medicine, University of Maryland Hospital in 1973.

Andrea Gottsegen Asnes, MD, MSW, is an assistant professor in the Department of Pediatrics, Yale University School of Medicine. Her area of expertise is medical evaluation of suspected child maltreatment. Her research focuses on the forensic evaluation of children who disclose sexual abuse and the experience of nonoffending parents of sexually abused children. Dr. Asnes also teaches communication skills and professionalism. She obtained her medical degree from the Mount Sinai School of Medicine, her MSW from New York University, and is a graduate of the Robert Wood Johnson Clinical Scholar's Program at the University of Michigan.

Andrew Green, MA, Ph.D., is head of the Nuffield Centre for International Health and Development, a member of the Senior Management Team for the Institute of Health Sciences, and chair of the International Management Committee at the University of Leeds, England, UK. His research interests are in health planning and policy, health sector reform, health economics, and nongovernmental organizations; he has published widely in these areas. His book *An Introduction to Health Planning for Developing Health Systems* (published by Open University Press, 3rd Edition, 2007) is a well-known text on the subject. He has carried out numerous consultancies for various organizations including the Department for International Development (DFID), London, the World Bank, and the World Health Organization. Dr. Green holds a Ph.D. from the University of Leeds, England, and an MA in Development Economics from the University of Sussex, England.

Anne Hyre, CNM, MSN, MPH, is a certified nurse-midwife with experience in strengthening midwifery education and clinical practice in 15 countries. She has more than 15 years of experience in strategic planning, program design, implementation, and program evaluation for maternal and reproductive health in the United States and abroad. She also has a solid record of success in business development with donors, foundations, and corporations. She currently works as the director of Global Outreach for the American College of Nurse-Midwives (ACNM). Prior to joining ACNM, she spent 15 years with Jhpiego, including 8 years based in Jakarta, Indonesia. With Jhpiego, she provided technical leadership and support to programs in preservice education, training systems development, human resource capacity building, and clinical performance improvement.

Monir Islam, MD, MPH, FRCOG, is director of the Department of Making Pregnancy Safer, World Health Organization, Geneva, Switzerland. He graduated with a degree in medicine from Dhaka University, Bangladesh, and received his MPH from the Royal Tropical Institute, University of Amsterdam, the Netherlands. He is a fellow of the Royal College of Obstetricians and Gynaecologists (FRCOG), UK. Prior to joining the Making Pregnancy Safer at WHO, Geneva, he was the director of Family and Community Health at the WHO Regional Office for South-East Asia, New Delhi, India.

Albrecht Jahn, MD, Ph.D., is scientific officer, European Commission Directorate General for Research, Brussels, Belgium. Prior to joining the European Commission, he was a senior lecturer in the Department of Tropical Hygiene and Public Health at the University of Heidelberg, Germany. With specializations in obstetrics and gynecology, public health, and tropical infectious diseases, Dr. Jahn worked for several years in rural hospitals in Kenya and Tanzania focusing on mother and child health, including malnutrition. After establishing an interdisciplinary research group at Heidelberg University, his research collaborations extended to Pakistan, Nepal, Burkina Faso, Cape Verde, and South Africa with a focus on assessing and improving maternity-related health systems and services as well as related procedures and technologies.

Chuks Kamanu, MBBCh, FWACS, FICS, is an honorary consultant and head of the Department of Obstetrics and Gynecology, Abia State University Teaching Hospital, Aba, Nigeria. He is also a senior lecturer in the College of Medicine, Abia State University, Uturu. He is actively involved in medical education at both the undergraduate and postgraduate levels, and is an external examiner for several Medical Schools in Nigeria. His research focuses on to reduce maternal morbidity and mortality. He is involved in grassroots advocacy against harmful traditional practices on women, and is a coveted speaker in academic and religious conferences on this issue. Presently, he is working on a research publication for the Surgery in Africa Review on destructive operations in obstetrics (set of operations carried out in neglected obstructed labor when the fetus is dead). Dr. Kamanu obtained his medical degree from the College of Medicine, University of Calabar, Nigeria, where he also received his specialist training in Obstetrics and Gynecology. He is a fellow of the West African College of Surgeons and a fellow of the International College of Surgeons.

Andrzej Kulczycki, Ph.D., is an associate professor in the Department of Health Care Organization and Policy, University of Alabama at Birmingham (UAB). His research and teaching focus on strengthening reproductive health systems and demography. He has published on various aspects of abortion, including a landmark comparative study of abortion practice and policy centered on the transnational dimensions involved (*The Abortion Debate in the World Arena*; London: Macmillan; New York: Routledge). He obtained his Ph.D. from the University of Michigan and also holds degrees from the Universities of London and Durham, United Kingdom.

Claudio F. Lanata, MD, PPH, is a senior researcher at the Nutritional Research Institute in Lima, Peru, which he joined in 1983, after his postgraduate training in the United States. His research focuses on the relationship between poverty and maternal and child health. He has led in Peru, an extensive research in child health and nutrition focusing on diarrheal and respiratory diseases, micronutrients, and vaccine development. His work has resulted in one book, 23 chapters, and more than 80 journal publications, mostly in major international journals. An active collaborator with World Health Organization and the Pan American Health Organization, he has served as a trustee of the International Center for Diarrhoeal Disease Research, Bangladesh (ICDDR,B) and continues to participate in several expert committees on diarrheal diseases and vaccine development. Dr. Lanata is a member of the Child Health Epidemiology Reference Group (CHERG), the Food-borne Epidemiology Reference Group (FERG) of the World Health Organization, and founder of the Child Health and Nutrition Research Initiative (CHNRI) in Switzerland.

John M. Leventhal, MD, is a professor of Pediatrics at the Child Study Center, Yale University School of Medicine and an attending pediatrician at Yale-New Haven Children's Hospital. At the Children's Hospital, he is medical director of the Child Abuse Prevention Programs. Dr. Leventhal has worked in the field of child maltreatment for over 25 years. From 2001 to 2006, he served as editor-in-chief of *Child Abuse & Neglect, The International Journal*. During his tenure as editor, he developed a "midwife" program to help international authors improve their manuscripts so that they would be suitable for publication. His research has focused on the epidemiology of child maltreatment, risk factors for abuse and neglect, and distinguishing abusive from unintentional injuries. He has published over 125 peer-reviewed articles and chapters.

Julian Lob-Levyt, MBChB, DRCOG joined the GAVI Alliance in January 2005 as the executive secretary of the GAVI Alliance, and CEO and president of the GAVI Fund. Prior to this, he worked with UNAIDS as senior policy advisor to the executive director. His career in global health has included work with both bilateral and multilateral organizations. He was chief health advisor at the UK Department for International Development (DFID) from 2000 to 2004. His other key posts include regional health advisor for the European Commission (EC) in Zimbabwe (1998–1999) and health sector reform coordinator for WHO in Cambodia (1994–1997). Dr. Lob-Levyt represented the United Kingdom as a founding board member of the Global Fund to Fight AIDS, TB and Malaria. He is currently a board member of the International AIDS Vaccine Initiative (IAVI) and the Global Health Workforce Alliance.

Elizabeth Lule, M.Sc., is manager of the AIDS Campaign Team for Africa (ACTafrica), which is responsible for policy direction and coordination of the World Bank's HIV/AIDS work in Africa. She oversees implementation of the Multi-Country HIV/AIDS Program (MAP) for Africa that has committed over US $1.7 billion in more than 30 countries. Prior to 2006, she was the World Bank's advisor for Population and Reproductive and Child Health. Before joining the World Bank, Elizabeth was Africa regional vice president for Pathfinder International. She also worked with USAID in Nigeria as program manager and technical advisor for the health, nutrition, and population program. She taught Statistics and Demography at the University of Swaziland and worked as epidemiologist with the Ministry of Health in Nigeria. Elizabeth has advanced degrees from the London School of Hygiene and Tropical Medicine and the London School of Economics.

Colin Mathers, Ph.D., is the coordinator for Epidemiology and Burden of Disease in the Information, Evidence and Research Cluster at the World Health Organization, Geneva, Switzerland. He manages the WHO's work on global, regional, and country-level estimates of mortality and burden of disease. His principal research interests are in the measurement and reporting of population health and its determinants, the burden of disease methods and applications, the measurement of health-state prevalences, and cross-population comparability. Colin graduated with an honors degree and University Medal in Physics from the University of Sydney in 1975 and received his Ph.D. in Theoretical Physics from the same institution in 1979.

Martin Meremikwu, MBBS, M.Sc., FMCPed, is professor of Child Health & Consultant Pediatrician in the Department of Pediatrics, University of Calabar Teaching Hospital (UCTH), Calabar, Cross River State, Nigeria. He obtained his medical degree from the University of Nigeria, Nsukka, and also holds a Master of Science degree in Mother and Child Health from the Institute of Child Health (ICH), University of London, England. Dr. Meremikwu contributes actively to assessment of the evidence base of maternal and child health interventions and programs in developing countries, working as an editor with the Cochrane Collaboration (Infectious Diseases Group), based at the Liverpool School of Tropical Medicine, England. He has authored several Cochrane systematic reviews of key issues in maternal and child health and has supported the development of several others. He served on the Board of the Cochrane Child Health Field and is head of the Evidence-based Medicine and Clinical Trials Unit at the Institute of Tropical Diseases Research, University of Calabar Teaching Hospital, Nigeria. He serves as a consultant to several national governments, nongovernmental organizations, and international development agencies. In the past 5 years, he has provided technical assistance to WHO's programs on integrated management of childhood illnesses (IMCI), and monitoring and evaluation of malaria control, including management of malaria in pregnancy.

Caroline J. Min, MPH, DrPH, is research associate in the Dean's Office, Mailman School of Public Health, Columbia University. Prior to this, she served as a research scientist at the New York City Department of Health and Mental Hygiene, senior legislative assistant, FH/GPC Healthcare Practice, Washington, DC, and senior program assistant, Management Sciences for Health (MSH), Boston, MA. Caroline has an MPH in Population and Family Health from Columbia University and a DrPH in Population, Family and Reproductive Health from Johns Hopkins University.

Tolib Mirzoev, MD, MA, is a lecturer in International Health Systems at the Nuffield Centre for International Health and Development, University of Leeds, England. Before joining the University of Leeds, Tolib practiced medicine in Russia and worked with the National Ministry of Health on health reform projects where he developed expertise in the areas of health planning, health reforms, human resources, health management information system, and project management in the context of Tajikistan. He also has interest in health sector-wide approaches (SWAps). Dr. Mirzoev received his medical degree from the University of Saint Petersburg (Russia) and also holds a master's degree from the University of Leeds.

Nancy Mock, DrPH, currently serves as the interim executive director of the Newcomb College Center for Research on Women and is an associate professor of International Health and International Development at Tulane University.

Dr. Mock has over 30 years of experience in humanitarian and development work, where she has concentrated on the problems of difficult to reach and especially vulnerable populations. She has worked in more than 30 countries in Africa, Asia, Latin America, and Eastern Europe including Angola, Mozambique, Russia, Rwanda, Guatemala, and Sudan. She is the codeveloper of a partnership between universities and private voluntary organizations to combine efforts to address the problems of children in especially difficult circumstances. She works extensively in Rwanda on the problem of HIV/AIDS and Orphans and Vulnerable Children. She has published more than 30 peer-reviewed articles and more than 50 technical reports. She has organized and co-organized major conferences on Gender, Conflict, and HIV/AIDS; the psychosocial aspects of complex emergencies; and best practices in programming related to Orphans and Vulnerable Children. Dr. Mock has a doctoral degree in Public Health from Tulane University. She received her Bachelor of Science degree from Yale University.

David Moore, MD, is reader in Infectious Disease and Tropical Medicine at Imperial College London, England. He is a Wellcome fellow in Clinical Tropical Medicine. He lives in Peru, where his work is focused on the development, evaluation, and implementation of novel diagnostic tests and testing strategies for tuberculosis and multidrug-resistant tuberculosis (MDRTB). He has published widely in this area, including breakthrough work in the *New England Journal of Medicine* on the MODS assay. David received his medical degree from the University of Birmingham, England. He also has an M.Sc. in Epidemiology from the London School of Hygiene and Tropical Medicine where he holds an honorary lecturer position. He is a principal investigator in the Peruvian nongovernmental organization AB PRISMA and an associate in the Department of International Health at Johns Hopkins Bloomberg School of Public Health. He is currently chair of the subgroup for culture-based diagnostics of the New Diagnostics Working Group of the STOP TB Partnership.

Olaf Müller, MD, Ph.D., is a professor of public health and head of the interdisciplinary working group on *Disease Control in Disadvantaged Populations,* Department of Tropical Hygiene and Public Health, Medical Faculty, Ruprecht-Karls-University of Heidelberg, Germany. He studied biology, medicine, and public health at the Technical University of Hannover and the Free University of Berlin, Germany, and received his Ph.D. in Tropical Medicine in 1990. Before being employed at the Heidelberg University, he was trained in pediatrics and internal medicine at the University Hospital in Berlin/Germany. Afterward, he worked in the field of infectious disease control for several organizations including the International Red Cross in Kampala/Uganda, the German Federal Health Office in Berlin/Germany, the GTZ in Kinshasa/Zaire and Eschborn/Germany, and the British Medical Research Council Laboratories in Farafenni/The Gambia. His research interests are in the areas of tropical infectious disease control, particularly malaria and HIV/AIDS, but also in the area of neglected tropical diseases and malnutrition. He was and is the principal investigator of a number of health facility and community-based clinical trials, mainly in the field of malaria control interventions in Africa.

Marianne Nichol, M.Sc., is an epidemiologist working in the area of chronic disease surveillance at Queens University, Kingston, Canada. Her research focuses on effects of the built environment on physical activity among adolescence. She holds a master's degree in Epidemiology from Queen's University, Kingston, Canada.

Mary Ann Pass, MD, MPH, is a research professor in the Department of Health Care Organization and Policy, University of Alabama at Birmingham (UAB). Her research and teaching focus on infectious diseases, children with special health-care needs, global health, and public health practice. She has served as a local and regional health officer in Alabama and consultant for Alabama state agencies on MCH services. She obtained her medical and public health degrees from the University of Alabama at Birmingham.

Rebecca Pass, MPA, was most recently a fellow with the United Nations World Food Programme in Dakar Senegal. A graduate of Columbia University's School of International and Public Affairs with a degree in Environmental Science and Policy, she has worked as a health-care consultant for hospitals, health systems, and medical schools. Her research interests include the ability of gene–gene interactions to buffer an organism against environmental perturbations. She received an AB from Princeton University in 2002.

Stephen Pearson, Ph.D., is a senior research fellow at the Nuffield Centre for International Health and Development, University of Leeds, England. He is a social scientist and demographer with specialization in qualitative and quantitative research on men's and young people's reproductive health. He has extensive experience as a consultant to several global health and development agencies, including the Population Council, New York, and WHO, Geneva. He received his Ph.D. in Environmental Science from the University of Southampton, England.

William Pickett, BSc, MSc, PhD, is Associate Professor in the Department of Community Health and Epidemiology at Queen's University, Kingston, Ontario, Canada. He teaches epidemiology in both the graduate school and medical school at Queen's. He and his colleagues have an active and international research program that focuses upon children and their health, with a special emphasis on injury, trauma and their prevention. Areas of special focus include adolescent risk-taking and its effects on injury, pediatric trauma on farms, and youth violence. This program of research is funded by the Canadian Institutes of Health Research, the Public Health Agency of Canada, and the National Institutes of Health in the United States.

Susan Purdin, RN, MPH, is Deputy Health Director, International Rescue Committee, New York. She also holds an adjunct faculty position in Columbia University's Forced Migration and Health Program, teaching courses on program planning, reproductive health, and HIV/AIDS prevention in situations of forced migration. In 1999, she received the Global Health Council's award for "Best Practice in the Field of Global

Health" for providing field-based, on-site, technical assistance to reproductive health projects in conflict settings.

Joanna Raven, MCommH, Ph.D., is a research associate in health systems research in the International Health Group at the Liverpool School of Tropical Medicine, England. Her research interests are maternal and reproductive health and vulnerability, quality of care, and health systems. She has extensive experience of working with partners from Europe, China, and Vietnam to design and conduct research projects on maternal health, health insurance, and health systems development. She is a registered midwife and holds a master's degree in Community Health from the Liverpool School of Tropical Medicine, England.

Krishna Reddy, MD, is a resident in internal medicine at the Massachusetts General Hospital in Boston, USA. He was an NIH Fogarty International Clinical Research Scholar in Peru, where he conducted research on novel methods of diagnosing tuberculosis. Krishna obtained his medical degree from Harvard Medical School.

Nigel C. Rollins, MB, BCH, MRCP, MD, is a professor and head of the Department of Maternal and Child Health at the University of KwaZulu-Natal, South Africa. His research focuses on risk of HIV transmission associated with exclusive breastfeeding. He is involved in a multicenter trial of maternal highly active antiretroviral therapy (HAART) and postnatal transmission of HIV. He is also principal investigator of a health systems improvement intervention project that is aimed at improving the quality of prevention of mother-to-child transmission (PMTCT) services at the district level, as well as PMTCT surveillance projects in South Africa. Dr. Rollins is chair of the WHO Technical Advisory Group on HIV and Nutrition and is a member of several national and international professional committees, including the South Africa National PMTCT Steering Committee, Research Ethics Committee of the University of KwaZulu-Natal, and Executive Committee, Commonwealth Association of Paediatric Gastroenterology and Nutrition. He is an honorary senior lecturer at the Institute of Child Health, University College, London (UCL), England. He joined the Department of Child and Adolescent Health of WHO in July 2008 to work on PMTCT, infant feeding, and broader pediatric HIV issues, particularly nutrition. A member of the UK Royal College of Physicians, Dr. Rollins obtained his MB, BCH, and MD degrees from Queen's University, Belfast, in Northern Ireland.

James Rosen, MS, is an independent consultant and economist by training who has worked for over two decades in the field of global health. Jim's most recent work has focused on mainstreaming adolescent pregnancy concerns into safe motherhood strategies, analyzing user-fee systems for sexual and reproductive health care, making sure HIV programs include a proper focus on young people, identifying ways to mainstream youth issues in poverty-reduction strategies, measuring the impacts of health sector reform, and searching for sensible and cost-effective linkages between HIV and other reproductive health programs. Before becoming an independent consultant in 2000, he worked for 5 years as a senior research associate at Population Action International, Washington, DC.

He previously held positions at Development Associates, Inc., Southborough, MA, the Population Council, New York, and the World Bank, Washington, DC. Jim has worked in over 20 less-developed countries, providing technical assistance to health programs and policy makers and carrying out research and program evaluation. He received his master's degree in Economics from the University of Wisconsin.

Allan Rosenfield, MD, was emeritus professor at Columbia University, New York until he passed away in 2008. He was Delamar professor of Public Health Practice and dean of the Mailman School of Public Health at Columbia University for more than 20 years. He wrote extensively (with over 140 published articles) on major domestic and global issues in the field of maternal and child health. World renowned for his work on women's reproductive health and human rights, Dr. Rosenfield was among the first to draw attention to the burden of maternal mortality in less-developed countries. He established the pioneering Averting Maternal Death and Disability program, supporting more than 85 projects to improve obstetric care in 50 countries. His publication *"Maternal Mortality: A Neglected Tragedy: Where is the M in MCH?"* (*Lancet* 1985, 2: 83–85), which questioned the neglect of maternal health in global maternal and child health programs, drew considerable debate and attention to reduction of maternal mortality during the child survival revolution era of the 1980s and 1990s. He was the 2007 recipient of the United Nations (UN) Population Award, an award that recognized his high-level advocacy efforts, having served on the boards of many organizations and advisory groups including those of the UN Millennium Project and the World Health Organization. He was also a recipient of the reproductive health movement's highest award, the Planned Parenthood Federation of America's Margaret Sanger Award. Dr. Rosenfield obtained his medical degree from Columbia University, New York.

Jeffrey M. Smith, MD, Ph.D., is assistant professor in the Department of Gynecology and Obstetrics, Johns Hopkins University School of Medicine. He is also an assistant professor in the Department of Population and Family Health. He currently works as the technical director for Jhpiego based in Bangkok, Thailand. He is one of the key contributors to the manual *"Managing Complications in Pregnancy and Childbirth (MCPC): A Guide for Midwives and Doctors"* published by the WHO in partnership with the World Bank, the United Nations Children's Fund (UNICEF), and the United Nations Fund for Population Activities (UNFPA). He has written numerous national and international strategic policy documents related to reproductive health and human capacity development.

Alan Tita, MD, MPH, Ph.D., is assistant professor in the Divisions of Maternal-Fetal Medicine and International Women's Health in the Department of Obstetrics and Gynecology at the University of Alabama at Birmingham (UAB). He is also an investigator in the Center for Women's Reproductive Health, which houses UAB's site for the NICHD Maternal-Fetal Medicine Units Network. His research activities focus on improving maternal and perinatal health globally, with a focus on preterm birth, obstetric infections, obstetric and medical complications of pregnancy, evidence-based maternal and child health, and epidemiology. He has written several peer-reviewed publications and book chapters in these areas. He previously worked as a medical officer in both the governmental and the NGO sectors in Cameroon, Africa. Dr. Tita holds an MD degree from the University of Yaoundé, Cameroon, an MPH (International Health) from the University of Leeds, UK, and a Ph.D. in Epidemiology from the School of Public Health, University of Texas Health Sciences Center at Houston. He is trained in obstetrics and gynecology (Baylor College of Medicine, Houston) and maternal-fetal medicine (UAB). He is a diplomate of the American Board of Obstetrics and Gynecology.

Sally Theobald, MA, Ph.D., is a senior lecturer in social science and international health in the International Health Research Group, Liverpool School of Tropical Medicine (LSTM), England. She has been at LSTM since 1999, with a 2-year secondment to work as technical advisor to the Research for Equity and Community Health (REACH) Trust in Malawi. Her current research interests are captured under the umbrella of equitable and gender-sensitive health development, especially in relation to TB, HIV, and sexual and reproductive health. She has experience in designing and implementing gender-sensitive qualitative research projects in health and has worked collaboratively on qualitative research projects on HIV, tuberculosis, sexual and reproductive health, maternal and child health, and health systems in Thailand, South Africa, Burkina Faso, Malawi, and Kenya. She holds a BA in Geography from the University of Newcastle Upon Tyne, England, and an MA and PhD in Gender, Health, and Development from the University of East Anglia, England.

Rachel Tolhurst, PhD, is a Lecturer in Social Science and International Health in the International Health Research Group at the Liverpool School of Tropical Medicine. UK. She gained her MA in Gender Analysis in Development at the University of East Anglia and her PhD from the Faculty of Medicine at the University of Liverpool. Her research interests and experience centre on qualitative research on gender and equity issues in relation to health systems development, including health financing, maternal health and communicable disease (with a focus on malaria, tuberculosis and HIV). She has been working on gender and health for 10 years, and has designed, conducted and supported research in China, Ghana, Malawi, and Vietnam. She has also provided technical assistance on mainstreaming gender in Sector Wide Approaches in Ghana and Bangladesh.

L. Lewis Wall, MD, D.Phil., is an obstetrician–gynecologist and medical anthropologist who has been active in the field of obstetric fistula surgery for many years. He studied at the Institute of Social Anthropology in Oxford, England, as a Rhodes Scholar and carried out anthropological field research in northern Nigeria. This work was subsequently published as *Hausa Medicine: Illness and Well-being in a West African Culture*" (Duke University Press, 1988). The author of many peer-reviewed medical articles and book chapters in the field of urogynecology and reconstructive pelvic surgery, he was named national "Continence Care Champion" by the National Association for Continence (NAFC) in 2005. He is president of The Worldwide Fistula Fund (a not-for-profit charity), which is currently building a model fistula surgery and training center in Danja, Niger. Dr. Wall also has a master's degree in Bioethics and writes frequently in medical journals about issues of social and ethical concern.

Sarah Wamala, B.Sc., M.Sc., Ph.D., is the newly appointed director general of the Swedish National Institute of Public Health by the Swedish government. Prior to this, she worked as the head of Department of Health Promotion and Disease Prevention at Stockholm Centre for Public Health. She has also previously worked as research manager and head of Unit of Social Epidemiology at the Swedish National Institute of Public Health. She is associate professor and senior lecturer in Public Health at Karolinska Institute. Dr. Wamala is trained in economics, public health, and epidemiology at various universities including Makerere University (Uganda), Stockholm University (Sweden), Karolinska Institute (Sweden), Tufts University (USA), and Cambridge University School of Public Health (UK). She was the 2000 recipient of the Knut and Alice Wallenberg's Award for promising young scientists. Dr. Wamala (together with Dr. Ichiro Kawachi at Harvard School of Public Health) is among the first to edit a text book on globalization and health (by Oxford University Press, New York), including a critical analysis of the benefits and shortfalls of globalization for health. She is also the principal investigator of one of the first international research projects empirically investigating the effects of globalization on women's health in sub-Saharan Africa.

Amy T. Wilson, Ph.D., is associate professor and director of the International Development Programs at Gallaudet University, Washington, DC. Her research focuses on how Northern governments and global health agencies can best bring development assistance to people living with disability in less-developed countries. Amy has traveled globally to work with and evaluate the work of American federal agencies, American and foreign nongovernmental organizations, faith-based organizations, and foreign development assistance agencies. Dr. Wilson recently completed a 2-year, eight-country evaluation of an American NGO's work with children who have multiple disabilities.

Sarah Windle, MPH, is a specialist in global maternal and child health with an interest in social determinants of health and the development of theory-based interventions for the promotion of sexual and reproductive health among women and adolescents. She recently facilitated the development of sexual health training materials for Réseau Matoutou, a nonprofit health promotion agency in French Guiana, South America. Sarah received a Bachelor of Science degree in Psychology from McGill University, Canada, and an MPH with specialization in international maternal and child health from the University of Alabama at Birmingham, USA.

Victor Y.H. Yu, AM, MBBS, M.Sc. (Oxon.) MD, FRACP, FRCP (Lond.), FRCP (Edin.), FRCP (Glasg.), is professor and clinical director of the Ritchie Centre for Baby Health Research. He is also professor of neonatology at Monash University, Australia, president of the Australian Perinatal Society, president of the Federation of Asia-Oceania Perinatal Societies, and vice president of the World Association of Perinatal Medicine. He has been invited as visiting professor and guest speaker to lecture in 44 countries on over 250 occasions. He is a consultant to the World Health Organization and to the Singapore and Hong Kong Governments on issues related to perinatal health. He has published 10 books, 170 book chapters, 270 papers, and 370 abstracts. He has supervised neonatal training for about 200 pediatricians from 41 countries other than Australia. Victor graduated from Hong Kong University Medical School in 1968. He went to Oxford University in England in 1972 and McMaster University in Canada in 1975 for his postgraduate neonatal training and became the founding director of the Neonatal Intensive Care Unit at Monash Medical Centre in Melbourne, Australia, in 1977.

Michel Zaffran, M.Sc., is the deputy executive secretary and chief technical and policy officer, GAVI Alliance. A French national, Michel received his engineering degree from Ecole Centrale, France, and Technische Hochschule, Darmstadt, Germany, with subsequent training in Tropical Epidemiology at the Heidelberg University. After 2 years in Morocco with the French Government, he joined GRET, a French NGO for which he worked in Burkina Faso and the Democratic Republic of Congo. He then spent 18 years with WHO Vaccines and Immunization Department, in cold chain and logistics, overseeing the work on quality of immunization services and as program manager in charge of the departmental strategic planning. His last assignment with WHO was as coordinator of the Access to Technologies team where he led efforts in Vaccine Quality, Vaccine Management, Vaccine Supply, and Immunization Financing. From 1998 to 2003 he was the WHO representative on the Working Group which helped to design and launch GAVI.

Index

CPI Antony Rowe
Chippenham, UK
2019-01-11 10:48